The Health Professional's Guide to

Popular Dietary Supplements

2nd Edition

The Health Professional's Guide to

Popular Dietary Supplements

2nd Edition

Allison Sarubin Fragakis, MS, RD

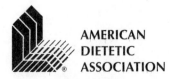

**AMERICAN
DIETETIC
ASSOCIATION**

Diana Faulhaber, Publisher
Laura Brown, Development Editor
Judith Clayton, Managing Editor
Composition by Book Comp, Inc.
Cover Design by Nykiel Design

The views expressed in this publication are those of the authors and do not necessarily reflect policies and/or official positions of the American Dietetic Association. Mention of product names in this publication does not constitute endorsement by the authors or the American Dietetic Association. The American Dietetic Association disclaims responsibility for the application of the information contained herein.

10 9 8 7 6 5 4 3 2 1

Library of Congress Cataloging-in-Publication Data

Sarubin Fragakis, Allison.
   The health professional's guide to popular dietary supplements /Allison Sarubin Fragakis.— 2nd ed.
        p. ; cm.
Includes bibliographical references and index.
   ISBN 0-88091-173-5
   1. Dietary supplements—Handbooks, manuals, etc.
      [DNLM: 1. Dietary Supplements—Handbooks. QU 39 S251h 2002] I. American Dietetic Association. II. Title.

RM258.5 .S27 2002
613.2'8—dc21

                                                    2002013465

To Chris,
my husband and best friend

REVIEWERS

Annette Dickinson, PhD
Vice President, Scientific & Regulatory Affairs
Council for Responsible Nutrition
Washington, D.C.
(Reviewed Appendix A, Government Regulation
of Dietary Supplements)

Norman R. Farnsworth, PhD
Research Professor of Pharmacognosy and
    Distinguished University Professor
College of Pharmacy
University of Illinois at Chicago
Chicago, Illinois
(Reviewed Black Cohosh, Bromelain, Cranberry,
Dong quai, Echinacea, Flaxseed, Gamma
Oryzanol, Garlic, Ginkgo biloba, Ginseng, Gold-
enseal, Hydroxycitric Acid, Kava, Ma Huang,
Noni Juice, St. John's Wort, Valerian, Wheat
Grass and Barley Grass, Saw Palmetto, and
Yohimbine entries)

Tracy A. Fox, MPH, RD
President
Food, Nutrition & Policy Consultants, LLC
Bethesda, Maryland
(Reviewed Appendix A, Government Regulation
of Dietary Supplements)

Kristin A. Franco, Associate
American Dietetic Association
Washington, D.C.
(Reviewed Appendix A, Government Regulation
of Dietary Supplements)

Barbara F. Harland, PhD, RD, FADA
Department of Nutritional Sciences
College of Pharmacy, Nursing, and Allied
    Health Sciences
Howard University
Washington, D.C.

Harold Holler, RD
Director, Governance
American Dietetic Association
Chicago, Illinois
(Reviewed Appendix B, Ethical Issues and
Dietary Supplements)

Amy B. Howell, PhD
Associate Research Scientist
Marucci Center for Blueberry Cranberry
    Research
Rutgers, The State University of New Jersey
Chatsworth, New Jersey
(Reviewed Cranberry Extract entry)

Cathy Kapica, PhD, RD, CFCS
Director, Nutrition Education
The Quaker Oats Company
Barrington, Illinois
(Formerly Assistant Professor, Nutrition and
    Clinical Dietetics, Finch University of
    Health Sciences/The Chicago Medical
    School, Chicago, Illinois)

Sharon L. Miller, PhD
Director Nutrition Research
National Dairy Council
Rosemont, Illinois
(Reviewed Whey Protein entry)

Sylvia Moore, PhD, RD, FADA
Director/Professor, University of Wyoming
Division of Medical Education & Public Health
Assistant Dean for WWAMI in Wyoming
University of Washington School of Medicine
Laramie, Wyoming

Michael W. Pariza, PhD
Wisconsin Distinguished Professor
Director, Food Research Institute
Chair, Department of Food Microbiology and
    Toxicology
University of Wisconsin-Madison
Madison, Wisconsin
(Reviewed Conjugated Linoleic Acid entry)

Carol Seaborn, PhD, RD
Department of Food & Nutrition
College of Human Development
University of Wisconsin-Stout
Menomonie, Wisconsin

Cynthia Thomson, PhD, RD, FADA,
    CNSD
Assistant Professor
Department of Nutritional Sciences
University of Arizona
Tucson, Arizona

John Westerdahl, PhD, MPH, RD
Director, Wellness and Lifestyle Medicine and
    Nutritional Services Departments
Castle Medical Center
Kailua, Hawaii

Pamela Williams, MPH, RD
Nutrilite
Buena Park, California

First Edition Reviewers:
Lisa K. Fieber, MS, RD; Constance J. Geiger, PhD, RD; Sylvia Moore, PhD, RD; Carol Seaborn, PhD, RD; Cynthia Thomson, PhD, RD, FADA, CNSD

Martha A. Belury, PhD; Jeffrey Blumberg, PhD, FACN; Kathryn Carroll, PhD; Ellen Coleman, MA, MPH, RD; John R. Crouse III, MD; Mary A. Carey, PhD, RD; Jane W. Folkman, MS, RD; Bruce D. Rengers, PhD, RD; Norman R. Farnsworth, PhD; John Finley, PhD; Tracy Fox, MPH, RD; William Harris, PhD; Steve Hertzler, PhD, RD; Cathy Kapica, PhD, RD, CFCS; Todd R. Klaenhammer, PhD; Mindy Kurzer, PhD; Alice J. Lenihan, MPH, RD, Joel Mason, MD; Forrest Nielson, PhD; Donna Porter, PhD, RD; Susan M. Potter, PhD; Dennis Savaino, PhD; V. Srini Srinivasan, PhD; Connie M. Weaver, PhD; John Westerdahl, PhD, MPH, RD; Pamela Williams, MPH, RD; Steven Zeisel, MD, PhD

CONTENTS

Preface xi

Acknowledgments xiii

Introduction xv

PART ONE
ALPHABETICAL GUIDE TO DIETARY SUPPLEMENTS

Acidophilus/*Lactobacillus Acidophilus* (LA)	2
Alanine	8
Alpha-Lipoic Acid (ALA)	11
Androstenedione and Androstenediol	16
Arginine	20
Aspartic Acid/Asparagine	30
Bee Pollen	33
Black Cohosh (*Cimicifuga racemosa*)	36
Boron	41
Branched Chain Amino Acid (BCAA)	45
Bromelain	51
Calcium	58
Carnitine (L-Carnitine)	68
Chitosan	77
Chondroitin Sulfate	82
Chromium	85
Coenzyme Q$_{10}$	94
Colostrum/Bovine Colostrum	102
Conjugated Linoleic Acid	108
Cranberry Extract	115
Creatine	119
Dehydroepiandosterone (DHEA)	129
Dong quai (*Angelica sinensis*)	138
Echinacea	141
Fish Oil	147
Flaxseed	160
Folate/Folic Acid	167
Fructooligosacharides (FOS)	175
Gamma Linolenic Acid (GLA)	180
Gamma Oryzanol (Phytosterols)	191
Garlic	194
Ginkgo biloba	204
Ginseng	211
Glucosamine	221
Glutamine	227
Glycerol	231
Goldenseal (*Hydrastis canadensis*)	236
Green Tea Extract	239
5-Hydroxy-Tryptophan (5-HTP)	246
β-Hydroxy -Methylbutyrate (HMB)	251
Hydroxycitric Acid (*Garcinia cambogia*)	256
Kava (*Piper methysticum*)	259
Lecithin/Choline	264
Lysine	269
Ma Huang (*Ephedra sinica*)	273
Magnesium	280
Melatonin	291
Methylsulfonylmethane (MSM)	300
N-Acetylcysteine (NAC)	302
Noni Juice	308
Pancreatin	310
Pantothenic Acid	313
Phosphatidylserine	317
Potassium	321
Pyruvate	326
Royal Jelly	332
S-adenosylmethionine (SAM-e)	335
St. John's Wort (*Hypericum perforatum*)	344

Saw Palmetto (*Serenoa repens*) 350
Selenium 353
Shark Cartilage 359
Sodium Bicarbonate 363
Soy Protein and Isoflavoness 365
Spirulina/ Blue-Green Algae 377
Valerian (*Valeriana officinalis*) 382
Vanadium 387
Vitamin A/Beta-Carotene 392
Vitamin B$_1$ (Thiamine) 405
Vitamin B$_2$ (Riboflavin) 410

Vitamin B$_3$ (Niacin) 412
Vitamin B$_6$ (Pyridoxine) 418
Vitamin B$_{12}$ (Cobalamin) 426
Vitamin C 433
Vitamin D 445
Vitamin E 451
Wheat Grass and Barley Grass 467
Whey Protein 470
Yohimbine/ Yohimbe 474
Zinc 478

PART TWO
APPENDIXES

Appendix A: Government Regulation of Dietary Supplements 491

Appendix B: Ethical Issues and Dietary Supplements 503

Appendix C: Supplements Sorted by Purported Use 507

Appendix D: Dietary Intake Tables 512

Appendix E: Additional Resources 519

Appendix F: Dietary Supplement Intake Assessment 525

PREFACE

The seed for this book was first planted by SCAN (the Sports, Cardiovascular, and Wellness Nutritionists practice group of the American Dietetic Association). In 1996, the editors at SCAN asked me to summarize research on sports supplements for their annual *Guide*. Realizing there was a need for a large-scale version of SCAN's publication, I began working with the American Dietetic Association on the first edition of *The Health Professional's Guide to Popular Dietary Supplements*. An advisory panel of five dietitians and several experts were signed on to help shape and review the book.

As more and more information became available, it became clear that a second edition was needed. New Dietary Reference Intakes (DRIs) for several vitamins and minerals had been released by the Food and Nutrition Board, new safety data (including drug/supplement interactions) for a variety of supplements had accumulated, and more clinical research results had been published since the first edition was released.

This second edition reflects these changes. In addition to all the new studies and safety information (over 340 new references are included), ten more supplements have been added. New summary tables at the beginning of each supplement entry replace the single, lengthy table of the first edition. The new tables evaluate the scientific validity of media and marketing claims, based on available evidence; summarize any advisories/cautions associated with the supplement; and list potential drug/supplement interactions. The appendix on government regulations (Appendix A) has also been updated to reflect the latest legal developments. The Additional Resources in Appendix E have been revised to provide the most recent Internet links and contact information for a variety of organizations. Finally, complete charts with the new DRIs for vitamins and minerals (including a listing of Tolerable Upper Intake Levels) have been added in Appendix D.

As the public, along with the medical community, are becoming more "supplement-savvy," they are demanding evidence that dietary supplements are safe, effective, and reliable. This book is all evidence-based and aims to provide the reader with straightforward and objective information. Despite this goal, the content of the book seemed controversial at times during the review process. For instance, reviewers often had differing opinions on whether there was enough evidence to rate a supplement as effective or not effective. Some noted that the book seemed biased toward using supplements; others suggested that the book was too conservative; still others felt that more decisive recommendations were needed. For certain, the reader can be assured that the opinions and comments of more than thirty expert reviewers have been incorporated into this edition.

The bottom line is that regardless of whether you work with these products, it is important to be aware of their potential beneficial or harmful effects. No matter what your opinion about supplementation, my aim is that you find this book helpful in making sense of the claims and facts surrounding the numerous dietary supplements on the market.

Allison Sarubin Fragakis, MS, RD

ACKNOWLEDGMENTS

Many thanks go to the numerous people involved in reviewing and fine-tuning both editions of *The Health Professional's Guide to Popular Dietary Supplements*. A number of people were integral to the development of this second edition: Thank you to Laura Brown, ADA development editor, for organizing the revision process with such skill that it appeared easy (even though it was hard work). Also, thank you from the bottom of my heart to the reviewers who spent hours looking over manuscript pages. I would especially like to acknowledge the time and effort spent by Cynthia Thomson, PhD, RD, Cathy Kapica, PhD, RD, and Barbara Harland, PhD, RD. Thank you to Jude Clayton; her attention to detail while overseeing production of both editions was so important to the final product. And, the research assistance from nutrition students Lynn Goldstein and Lindsay de Jongh was a tremendous help.

I am ever-grateful to those who contributed to the first edition: A special thank you to June Zaragoza, MPH, RD, for her incredible dedication, patience, and editorial skills, and for kindly guiding me along the publishing road. This book would not be the same without the expert advice of Kathryn Carroll, ADA's former nutrition scientist, nor ADA intern Beth Birnbaum's researching, fact-checking, food table conversions, and resource compilations. I am especially grateful for the highly qualified panel of dietitians and expert reviewers who critiqued the manuscript during its development and to Lisa Fieber, MS, RD, and Samuel Fieber, JD, for contributing the ethics appendix; to Ruth DeBusk, PhD, and the Nutrition in Complementary Care (NCC) practice group for providing information for the resource appendix; to former ADA librarians Chuck Williams and Cathy Colette for locating hundreds of journal articles; and to Lynn Brown and Daniel Connor, for their fine copyediting at lightning speed.

And, thank you to Chris, my dear husband, for his ongoing support, encouragement, and bright smile. Thank you to my beautiful new baby, Cassidy, my marvelous parents, and my entire family for all of their love. And of course, thanks to my dog, Marley, for letting me know when it was time to take a break.

INTRODUCTION

National surveys show that more than 40 percent of Americans take some form of dietary supplement (1, 2). The US Food and Drug Administration (FDA) estimates that more than 29,000 supplement products are on the market, supplied by approximately 500 to 850 manufacturers. Table 1 illustrates the growth in sales of natural remedies and dietary supplements.

Table 1

US Supplement Industry in Consumer Sales from All Retail Channels, Direct Sales, Multilevel Marketing, Mail Order, and Practitioner Sales
(Figures are in millions of dollars.)

Products	1994	1995	1996	1997	1998	1999	2000
Vitamins	3,870	4,250	4,720	5,220	5,610	5,780	5,850
Botanicals/herbs	2,020	2,470	2,990	3,530	3,960	4,070	4,120
Sports nutrition	900	990	1,070	1,190	1,340	1,450	1,590
Minerals	690	800	890	1,020	1,140	1,290	1,350
Meal supplements	450	560	590	1,720	1,840	1,970	2,140
Specialty/other*	670	750	920	1,210	1,210	1,500	1,680
Total sales	$8,600	$9,820	$11,180	$13,890	$15,100	$16,060	$16,730

Source: *Nutrition Business Journal* (3).

*Because NBJ's estimates constantly evolve as more information is accumulated, the sales numbers reported here have changed slightly from those previously reported in the first edition.

According to *Nutrition Business Journal* (NBJ), supplement sales have been steadily increasing and reached $16.7 billion in 2000 (3). Tables 1 and 2 summarize components of these sales figures. Although total supplement sales have increased over the last seven years, the rate of growth in sales is slowing. NBJ projects that supplement sales will grow 3 percent to 5 percent between 2001 and 2004, compared to 10.5 percent in 1998.

Table 2

The U.S. Supplement Industry, 1998 and 2000. Breakdown of Product Types

Product	Percent of Sales 1998	Percent of Sales 2000
Vitamins	40	35
Botanicals	29	25
Sports nutrition	10	9
Minerals	8	8
Specialty supplements/other*	8	10
Meal supplements	5	13
	100%	100%

Source: *Nutrition Business Journal* (3).

*"Specialty supplements/other" includes supplements such as amino acids, hormones, and fish oil.

Given these statistics, health professionals must fully understand the beneficial and harmful effects of dietary supplements marketed to the public. Most Western-educated health professionals have had little, if any, training in this area. To stay abreast of the latest supplement trends, in order to advise patients or clients appropriately, it is important to research the literature and evaluate studies.

The Health Professional's Guide to Popular Dietary Supplements, Second Edition is designed to inform health professionals about approximately 80 dietary supplements. The science behind dietary supplements is constantly evolving; thus, the information presented in this book is not exhaustive but aims rather to familiarize readers with the scope and types of currently available research. Because in many cases the state of the research is rapidly changing, it is important to also check other resources such as Medline and the new database made available by the National Institutes of Health (NIH) Office of Dietary Supplements (see Appendix E) to keep up to date on new studies and safety issues.

HOW TO USE THIS BOOK

There are many ways to use this book. Practitioners can scan for information to answer a patient's or colleague's question, to prepare for a presentation or television interview, to use as background for writing consumer nutrition articles, or simply to become better educated about today's supplement market.

Supplements are presented alphabetically, with information provided in an easy-to-read bullet format for quick access. In cases where a supplement is known by more than one name, or where two or more supplements are grouped in a single entry, cross-references appear within the text. For example, a reader looking under "Beta-Carotene" is advised to "see Vitamin A/Beta-Carotene." To locate the names of supplements by purported use, see Appendix C.

The content of each entry is organized in the same sequence: a brief overview of the dietary supplement; a table summarizing media and marketing claims, efficacy, cautions, and drug-supplement interactions; key points about the supplement; food sources; dosage information and bioavailability; relevant research; safety considerations; and references.

SUMMARY TABLE

The summary table for each supplement provides a quick reference to media and marketing claims, advisory issues, and drug/supplement interactions.

Media and Marketing Claims

The media and marketing claims listed for each supplement were gathered from Web sites, product literature, magazine articles and advertisements, books and newsletters promoting supplement use, and health food stores. The claims are *not* based on scientific facts. Many of the media and marketing claims listed in this section—for example, "Lowers cholesterol"—would not be considered legal if printed on supplement labels or in promotional materials. However, the claims illustrate how many books, magazine articles, and some practitioners refer to the benefits of the supplement. (Refer to Appendix A, "Government Regulation of Dietary Supplements" for more details about allowable health claims for dietary supplements.)

Efficacy

In the "Efficacy" column of the table, a coding system indicates whether available scientific evidence supports the media and marketing claims.

The following symbols appear in this column:

↑   Evidence from several controlled trials in humans (*in vivo*) supports efficacy claims.

?↑ Preliminary evidence from a few controlled trials in humans support efficacy claims, but more research is needed. (Research that is positive and has only been performed *in vitro* is so designated in the column.)

↔   Evidence from conflicting controlled research in humans is equivocal.

↓   Research in humans does not support efficacy claims.

NR Not enough research in humans is available to evaluate the efficacy of the claims, or the quality of research is poor.

Advisory

The advisory section of the table lists safety issues and concerns for the supplement. In cases where the National Academy of Science Food and Nutrition Board has developed a Tolerable Upper Intake Level (UL), the highest daily intake level that is not likely to pose risk of adverse effects to almost all individuals in the general population, the UL is also included.

Drug/Supplement Interactions

This section provides a list of possible or known interactions between the supplement and any drug or other supplement. This information was derived from a variety of sources including a Medline search and the following resources:

- Ang-Lee MK, Moss J, Yuan CS. Herbal Medicines and Perioperative Care. *JAMA.* 2000;286:208–216.

- Blumenthal M. Interactions between herbs and conventional drugs: introductory considerations. *HerbalGram.* 2000;49:52–63.

- Brinker F. *Herb Contraindications and Drug Interactions,* 2nd edition. Sandy, OR: Eclectic Medical Publications; 1998

- Cupp MJ. Herbal remedies: adverse effects and drug interactions. *Am Fam Phys.* 1999;59:1239–1244.

- Fugh-Berman A. Herb-drug interactions. *Lancet.* 2000;355:134–138.

- Jellin JM, Gregory P, Batz F, et al. *Pharmacist's Letter/Prescriber's Letter Natural Medicines Comprehensive Database,* 3rd edition. Stockton, CA: Therapeutic Research Faculty; 2000.

- Lininger SW, Jr (ed.) *A–Z Guide to Drug-Herb-Vitamin Interactions.* Rocklin, CA: Healthnotes; 1999.

- Miller L. Herbal medicinals: selected clinical considerations focusing on known or potential drug-herb interactions. *Arch Int Med.* 1998;158:2200–2211.

KEY POINTS

This section gives a general summary of the supplement. Each key point specifically addresses whether available scientific evidence supports the media and marketing claims for a particular supplement. The conclusions should be considered a snapshot in time, which can potentially change as science emerges. Refer to the Key Points when time is short and a brief overview is needed.

FOOD SOURCES

This section lists food sources of a particular supplement (if applicable). Because the science and safety of ingesting isolated nutrients in pill form is still relatively understudied and because foods contain a wide array of known and unknown nutrients and health-promoting constituents, food sources are recommended as a first choice whenever possible. Dietary supplements should be viewed as "supplemental" to a healthy diet. Not only may food sources of a particular nutrient or phytochemical contain additional nutrients and health benefits but they are also often less expensive than supplement forms. However, in some instances, one would have to consume an excessive amount of food to get the desired quantity of a certain nutrient, and supplementation is therefore appropriate. Use this section to encourage individuals to make appropriate food selections within the context of a balanced eating plan.

Note: Unless otherwise indicated, the serving sizes noted in Food Sources tables are for cooked foods.

DOSAGE INFORMATION/BIOAVAILABILITY

This section reports the range of doses suggested on supplement labels and the doses used in clinical trials. It indicates whether supplements are available in tablet, capsule, tincture, or powder form and whether products are voluntarily standardized. (See following definitions.) The Dosage Information/Bioavailability section also notes the various chemical compounds found in different products (e.g., chromium is available in the form of chromium picolinate or chromium chloride supplements). If there are data on bioavailability and absorption, they are also included under this heading.

Definitions for Dosage and Bioavailability Items (4–6)

Extract: A concentrated preparation of liquid or dry consistency made from dried plant materials.

Liquid Extract: A preparation created by dissolving dried extract in alcohol or water or by soaking or percolating dried plant material with solvent and evaporating it to produce a specified ratio of dry matter to solvent. Usually the solvent is evaporated to produce a ratio of 1:1 of dry plant material to solvent.

Dried Extract: A preparation created by evaporating all of the liquid solvent from the liquid extract. The powdered material can then be processed into tablets, capsules, or lozenges.

Standardized Extract: A preparation created by adjusting extract to a consistent strength. Standardization may be done by dilution with inert materials or by mixing several different strengths to achieve desired levels.

Tincture: A preparation created by steeping dried or fresh plant material with a mixture of water and alcohol to extract the plant material at room temperature. (If glycerol is used as the solvent, the preparation is referred to as a glycerite.) Tinctures are often made into strengths with ratios of 1:5 or 1:10 of plant to solvent and are not as concentrated as liquid extracts. Tinctures frequently contain alcohol.

Infusion/"Tea": A preparation created by pouring boiling water over chopped plant material and straining after steeping.

Decoction: A preparation created by adding cold water to chopped plant material, bringing it to a boil, then simmering before cooling and straining.

Strength: The ratio of plant material to solvent.

When reviewing information in this section, it is important to keep in mind certain issues facing consumers and the supplement industry (see also Appendix A, "Government Regulation of Dietary Supplements"). For example:

- The FDA does not have the resources, nor is it the agency's duty, to monitor and ensure the reliability and safety of every supplement on the market.

- The activity and content of herbs vary depending on manufacturer, harvest time, climate, soil, portion of plant used (root or leaves), method of extraction, formulation, and storage.

- Even when an herbal product states that it is standardized to contain a certain amount of an "active" ingredient, the constituents that are biologically active may not be known. In many cases, there may be several compounds that are potentially bioactive. Therefore, standardizing a product to one ingredient does not always ensure a superior product. This is an area of research that is sure to remain controversial and inconclusive for some time.

- Studies have documented inaccuracies in dietary supplement labels. It is not uncommon for the level of ingredients analyzed from individual pills or capsules to differ from the amount stated on the label (even though such deviations are not legally permissible).

RELEVANT RESEARCH

The Relevant Research discussion is generally the largest part of each supplement's entry. Studies and review articles from peer-reviewed journals are briefly summarized and listed by relevant category (e.g., diabetes, cardiovascular disease, weight loss, exercise performance, etc.). The entries are brief overviews and are not intended to be in-depth analyses of the literature. When a study is reported as having a "significant" result, this is stated as a statistical significance at a p-value of 0.05 or less. In general, only journal articles in English are included. This book does not cover research about supplement use during pregnancy, lactation, infancy, or childhood. More information on a particular study can be found in its references at the end of the dietary supplement entry.

Some of the studies listed under this heading have serious limitations, and these are generally identified for the reader. Both well-designed and flawed studies are included because some supplement manufacturers cite small or uncontrolled studies to promote their products. Thus, the descriptions help to point out the scientific nature of the supporting research. In a few cases, published abstracts are described and noted as such. These abstracts were only included if they are frequently cited in promotional literature.

No study is perfect. It is imperative to critically review research designs. Because research on dietary supplements is emerging so rapidly, readers are encouraged to be proactive in developing critical appraisals of the validity and significance of study results. Even though a trial may report a *statistically* significant result, it does not necessarily equate with *biological* significance. Nor does it follow that the research was methodologically sound. Because scientific discovery emerges through often-contradictory findings, it is important to consider the totality of evidence rather than the results of one study. When reviewing research articles, readers should consider the following questions:

- Was the study double-blinded and placebo-controlled?

- Were the subjects randomly assigned to treatment and control groups?

- What was the sample size? (Results from trials with less than 80 subjects should be viewed as preliminary.)

- What is the population being studied? To whom do the results apply?

- Do the subjects represent the population to whom the supplements are marketed?

- How long did the study last? Was there ample time to assess biological effects?

- Were important variables controlled (age, weight, diet, fitness level, medication)?

- What endpoint biomarker was used? A subjective measure, such as perceived pain, or a biological marker of health status, such as serum cholesterol level?

- Could there have been a publication bias (i.e., were only positive papers printed)?

- Is the journal peer-reviewed? (Check *Ulrich International Periodicals Directory* or contact the journal's publisher directly.)

Definitions for Research (7,8)

Case-Control Study: A retrospective observational study in which the subjects are selected based on whether they have a disease or condition. Subjects with the disease are the "cases" and subjects without are the "controls." Case-control studies explore associations only, not causality (e.g., a study of the history of the use of vitamin C supplements by subjects with breast cancer compared to subjects without breast cancer.)

Cross-Sectional Study: A cross-sectional assessment of exposure to possible risk factors and prevalence of disease or health problems in a population at one point or period of time (e.g., National Food Consumption Surveys). Cross-sectional studies do not provide information on the etiology of the disease or condition being studied.

Prospective Cohort Study: An epidemiological study that follows a group of subjects for a certain period of time to observe the effect of certain variables on outcome variables such as disease incidence or mortality.

Relative Risk: A statistical formula used in a cohort study/cross-sectional epidemiological study. It is calculated by dividing the cumulative incidence of disease among those exposed to the variable by the cumulative incidence of the disease among those not exposed.

Retrospective Cohort Study: An epidemiological study that requires subjects to recall past behaviors or examines previously recorded information to determine the effect of certain variables on disease incidence. This study design is inferior to prospective research because of errors in recall and the likelihood that behaviors change after diagnosis.

Terminology Used in Controlled Clinical Research

Controlled Study: An interventional study where a comparable group of subjects is also examined, but does not receive the treatment. A placebo-controlled study is an interventional study where subjects receive either treatment or a placebo (inert or inactive substance). The gold standard in clinical research is a study that is randomized, double-blinded, and placebo-controlled.

Crossover-Design Study: A controlled study comparing two or more treatments whereby subjects complete one course of treatment and then are switched to the other. Typically, assignment to the first treatment is randomized. Well-designed crossover studies include a wash-out period between treatments to avoid the possibility of run-over effects.

Double-Blind Study: Through the use of a "blinded" or masked coding system, neither the researchers nor the subjects know which subjects are in the treatment and control groups until after the study. This process is only effective when the intervention used is easily masked.

Meta-analysis: A statistical technique in which the results of many studies are pooled to make overall conclusions. Meta-analyses must select studies that are well-designed and have similar protocols. However, if studies chosen for grouped analysis are flawed or if a publication bias exists, meta-analyses will not provide accurate information.

Randomization: The process of assigning subjects randomly to treatment or control group so that each subject has an equal chance of being assigned to either group.

SAFETY

Safety is the most important factor when deciding to use supplements, and yet in many cases this is difficult to assess given the dearth of supporting data. There is often very little human research regarding food-herbal, drug-herbal, or multiple herbal interactions. The Safety subsection lists reported information about toxicity, known drug interactions, or adverse events associated with supplementation. It also discusses whether any long-term studies have been completed. Use this section to help evaluate the pros and cons of a particular supplement.

Note: Pregnant or lactating women should not use any dietary supplement without the advice of their physician. This population should clearly avoid supplements that are associated with serious adverse effects, including those listed in the Safety subsection. However, routine supplementation during pregnancy should include a prenatal multivitamin and mineral supplement with particular attention to the nutrients folic acid, iron, and calcium in healthy populations (9–10).

If an adverse effect occurs in association with a dietary supplement, it should be reported to MedWatch, the FDA's Medical Products Reporting Program. MedWatch is a postmarket surveillance program designed to educate health professionals about the critical importance of being aware of, monitoring, and reporting adverse events and product problems to the FDA and/or manufacturer. Health professionals may report a problem by calling the MedWatch hotline at 800-FDA-1088 (800-332-1088) or by using its Web site (http://www.fda.gov/medwatch/report/hcp.htm). Consumers may also report an adverse effect by calling the hotline or using a separate Web site (http://www.fda.gov/medwatch/report/consumer/consumer.htm).

APPENDIXES

Appendix A: Government Regulation of Dietary Supplements explains how the supplement industry is regulated and discusses the Dietary Supplement Health and Education Act (DSHEA) of 1994, the proper labeling of dietary supplements, quality control, and how to choose quality dietary supplements.

Appendix B: Ethical Issues and Dietary Supplements discusses the ethical and legal considerations that arise with widespread use of dietary supplements. This appendix is contributed by Lisa K. Fieber, MS, RD, and Samuel L. Fieber, JD.

Appendix C: Supplements Sorted by Purported Use lists selected supplements in 45 categories, such as cardiovascular disease and weight management.

Appendix D: Dietary Intake Tables summarizes Dietary Reference Intakes (DRIs), Recommended Dietary Allowances (RDAs), and other information.

Appendix E: Additional Resources provides information about relevant organizations, publications, Web sites, and books.

Appendix F: Dietary Supplement Intake Assment offers a number of questions for practitioners to ask patients and clients in order to assess their use of supplements.

REFERENCES

1. Eisenberg DM, Davis RB, Ettner SL, et al. Trends in alternative medicine use in the United States, 1990–1997: results of a follow-up national survey. *JAMA.* 1998;280:1569–1575.
2. Slesinski MJ, Subar AF, Kahle LL. Trends in use of vitamin and mineral supplements in the United States: The 1987 and 1992 National Health Interview Surveys. *J Am Diet Assoc.* 1995;95:921–923.
3. Nutrition Business Journal. *Industry Overview.* 1999, volume IV, no. 6:1–5.
4. Blumethal M, ed. *The Complete German Commission E Monographs Therapeutic Guide to Herbal Medicines.* Boston, Mass: Integrative Medicine Communications, 1998.
5. Schulz V, Hansel R, Tyler VE. *Rational Phytotherapy: A Physician's Guide to Herbal Medicine.* 3rd ed. Berlin, Germany: Springer-Verlag, 1998.
6. Ody P. *The Complete Medicinal Herbal.* New York, NY: Dorling Kindersley Limited, 1993.
7. Monsen ER, ed. *Research: Successful Approaches.* Chicago, Ill: American Dietetic Association, 1992.
8. Fennick JH. Studies Show: *A Popular Guide to Understanding Scientific Studies.* Amherst, NY: Prometheus Books, 1997.
9. Hunt, JR. Position of the American Dietetic Association: vitamin mineral supplementation. *J Am Diet Assoc.* 1996;96:73–77.
10. American Dietetic Association. Position of the American Dietetic Association: food fortification and dietary supplements. *J Am Diet Assoc.* 2001;101:115–125.

Part One

ALPHABETICAL GUIDE TO DIETARY SUPPLEMENTS

A
B
C
D
E
F
G
H
K
L
M
N
P
R
S
V
W
Y
Z

Acidophilus/*Lactobacillus Acidophilus* (LA)

Lactic acid bacteria are a heterogeneous group of gram-positive rods and cocci that use carbohydrates for energy and produce lactic acid, hydrogen peroxide, enzymes, and B vitamins via fermentation in food and dairy products as well as the gut. *L acidophilus* (LA) is one of many strains of lactic acid bacteria found in the human gastrointestinal tract that appears to play a role in stimulating the immune response and in combating intestinal and food borne pathogens. Within the LA species, there also exist individual strains each with differing actions. After ingestion, LA withstands the stomach pH and travels to the lower intestine. Some portion of a bacterial load may adhere to the epithelium and thus have the potential to help defend the host against harmful bacteria. Antibiotics, oral contraceptives, physical stress, and malnutrition may affect the delicate balance of microflora in the intestine. Some researchers suggest that recolonizing the gut with LA and other *Lactobacillus* bacteria (via food or supplements) will create a healthy microflora and reduce gastrointestinal symptoms and vaginal infections associated with harmful bacteria overgrowth (1–3).

Media and Marketing Claims	Efficacy
Improves digestion of dairy products and reduces diarrhea	↔
Prevents antibiotic-associated and traveler's diarrhea	↔
Prevents vaginal yeast infections	↔
Lowers cholesterol	↔
May protect against cancer	NR
Clears skin problems	NR

Advisory

No reported serious adverse effects

Drug/Supplement Interactions

May have a positive effect on gut flora when administered with antibiotics

KEY POINTS

- There is evidence that LA cultured dairy products may improve absorption of lactose and reduce associated symptoms such as cramps and diarrhea in individuals with lactose intolerance. Currently, different strains of LA are being tested for their relative effectiveness in this condition.

- There is preliminary evidence that LA cultured yogurt (2 cups/day) may reduce episodes of vaginal infections. More work is needed to determine the efficacy of LA supplements. Women suffering from vaginitis may wish to try LA cultured dairy products, not only for their potential ability to improve the infection, but also because they are good sources of calcium, which is important for women's health in general.

- As discussed in several review articles, LA and other probiotic bacteria administered in dairy products or supplements may reduce diarrhea associated with antibiotic use and *C difficile* and other pathogens. Whether LA can prevent traveler's diarrhea needs further investigation.

- There is preliminary evidence that dairy products fermented with LA may reduce cholesterol levels in hyperlipidemic and normal subjects. Larger controlled trials testing LA foods and supplements are needed to verify this lipid-lowering effect.

- Although there is preliminary evidence from observational data and animal experiments that LA may have anticarcinogenic properties, no clinical studies have specifically tested the influence of LA dairy products or supplements on biomarkers of cancer in humans.

- Studies are needed to determine the role, if any, LA foods or supplements play in acne, dermatitis, and other skin disorders.

- Conflicting data regarding efficacy of LA may be a result of differing experimental designs, differing *Lactobacillus* strains, variations in preparation and storage of LA, and the use of nonviable bacteria in studies (4). According to one review article, "Until strains with specific properties are scientifically selected, characterized and used carefully in commercial preparations … they are unlikely to prevent infection in the intestine. … This may be one explanation for failures with *Lactobacillus* therapy" (4).

FOOD SOURCES

Yogurt containing live LA cultures, kefir, and acidophilus milk

DOSAGE INFORMATION/BIOAVAILABILITY

LA supplements are sold in powders, tablets, or capsules often with other *Lactobacilli* (*L casei, L delbruekii*) or *Bifidobacteria* (*B adolescentis, B bifidum, B longum, B infantis*). Dosages are expressed in millions or billions of viable bacteria. Most manufacturers recommend taking 1 to 10 billion viable LA cells daily. LA supplements must be used by the expiration date and most require refrigeration to maintain viability. Some companies market their products as being heat stable and therefore not requiring refrigeration.

RELEVANT RESEARCH

LA and Lactose Intolerance

- During fermentation of yogurt and acidophilus milk, *Lactobacilli* produce lactase that hydrolyzes milk lactose to glucose and galactose. Thus, up to 50 percent of lactose in acidophilus milk and yogurt is predigested by lactase during the fermentation process, which potentially reduces symptoms associated with lactose ingestion in intolerant individuals (5).

- In a double-blind, controlled trial, 11 clinically confirmed lactose maldigesting subjects were given one of four strains of acidophilus milk (2 percent fat) or a control milk without LA. Lactose malabsorption was assessed by measuring breath H_2 excretion. Consumption of acidophilus milk containing strains B, N1, and E resulted in a significant reduced mean total H_2 production compared with that of the control. Milk containing strain ATCC 4356 did not differ from the control. Strain N1 was the most effective of the acidophilus milks in improving lactose digestion and tolerance (6).

- Review articles have reported several studies demonstrating that fermented dairy products (acidophilus milk, yogurt [not pasteurized or heated]) are absorbed better as measured by breath hydrogen and are associated with fewer intestinal symptoms than nonfermented dairy foods (2, 5).

LA and Intestinal Infections

- Possible mechanisms for the protective role of LA against intestinal and vaginal disorders include: (1) LA forms antimicrobial compounds such as lactic acid; acetic acid; hydrogen peroxide; broad-range, antibiotic-like compounds and bacteriocins that inhibit the growth of pathogenic bacteria; (2) LA by-products such as short chain fatty acids create a lower pH and inhibit pathogenic organisms; and (3) LA competes with pathogenic bacteria for nutrients and adhesion sites (1, 3).

- According to a detailed review published in *JAMA* that evaluated all available placebo-controlled, human studies supplementing biotherapeutic agents (*L acidophilus, Bifidobacterium longum, Lactobacillus casei GG*, and other selected microorganisms) from 1966 to 1995 concluded that these studies "have shown that biotherapeutic agents have been used successfully to prevent antibiotic-associated diarrhea, to prevent acute infantile diarrhea, to treat recurrent *Clostridium difficile* disease, and to treat various other diarrheal illnesses. The authors noted that many of the studies included small numbers of subjects (7).

- In a double-blind, controlled study, 30 healthy subjects were given the antibiotic cefpodoxime proxetil for one week and were randomized to receive one of three treatments for 21 days: (1) fermented milk supplement with *B longum* BB 536 and acidophilus NCFB 1748 and 15 g oligofructose; (2) fermented milk supplement with 15 g oligofructose; or (3) fermented milk supplement (placebo). Treatment started on the same day as antibiotic administration. In all three groups there was an elimination of *Escherichia coli*, followed by an overgrowth of enterococci and loss of bifidobacteria as a result of the antibiotic therapy. Also, gastrointestinal symptoms (flatulence, loose stools, increased defecation) were most pronounced in groups 1 and 2 compared to the placebo group. The authors attributed these side-effects to oligofructose. The number of lactobacilli also decreased but was significantly higher in groups 1 and 2 compared to group 3 at the end of antibiotic treatment. Interestingly, there was a significant increase in yeasts (*Candida albicans*) only in groups 1 and 2, but not in 3 (placebo). Since *C difficile* overgrowth that causes diarrhea and colitis is a common side-effect during antibiotic treatment, the researchers measured fecal *C difficile*. Six of 10 subjects in each of groups 2 and 3 were colonized by strains of *C difficile.*, compared to only one subject in group 1. The two bacterial strains given to group 1 were isolated in fecal samples, and this indicated that they survived intestinal passage. The authors suggested that further studies are needed in patients at risk of developing *C difficile* disease (8).

- In a double-blind, placebo-controlled study, 820 Finnish subjects traveling to southern Turkey to two destinations were randomized to receive 2×10^9 *Lactobacillus GG* powder (a new *Lactobacillus* strain isolated from human intestine) or placebo twice daily before departure and continuing during the trip. A total of 756 subjects completed the study. A physician was available during the trip at both destinations (Marmaris and Alayna) to record the participants' cases of diarrhea, to observe side-effects, and to administer medical treatment if necessary. During the return flight subjects completed questionnaires recording the incidence of diarrhea and related symptoms. The total number of subjects with diarrhea reported during the trip was 331 (43.8 percent), of whom 178 (46.5 percent) were in the placebo group and 153 (41 percent) were in the *Lactobacillus* group; the difference was not significant (p = 0.065). When the two destinations were analyzed separately, there were no significant differences in Marmaris. However, in Alayna, the number of travelers with diarrhea was 30 (39.5 percent) in the placebo group and 17 (23.9 percent) in the *Lactobacillus* group during the first week; the difference was significant. In subjects staying for two weeks, there was an insignificant trend toward less diarrhea in *Lactobacillus* supplemented subjects. Protection rate against diarrhea (calculated as percent diarrhea in placebo group minus percent diarrhea in *Lactobacillus* group divided by percent diarrhea in placebo group) showed *Lactobacillus* resulted in a significant increase in protection against traveler's diarrhea in Alayna, but not Marmaris. There were no reported side-effects associated with treatment (9).

- Twenty-seven patients diagnosed with ear, sinus, or throat infections were randomly assigned to receive amoxicillin/clavulanate only or in combination with LA (1.2×10^8 organisms/4 times/day). Duration of administration was not specified. LA combined with antibiotic therapy resulted in a significant reduction in gastrointestinal discomfort (nausea, cramping, yeast superinfection, and flatulence) compared to antibiotic therapy alone. However, this study was not blinded to patients or clinicians, which may have introduced a reporting bias (10).

LA and Vaginal Yeast Infections

- In a double-blind, controlled, crossover study of 46 women with a history of vaginal infections, participants were assigned in random order to consume LA yogurt (150 mL/day) containing live organisms/active cultures for two months or pasteurized yogurt (150 mL/day) for two months each, with a two-month washout period between treatments. Only 28 of the subjects completed the first four months and only 7 subjects completed the entire study protocol because of "inconvenience to subjects." The authors did not give any additional explanation for the high dropout rate. LA yogurt containing active cultures was associated with a significant increased prevalence of LA colonization in the rectum and vagina and a significant reduction in episodes of bacterial vaginosis. Both yogurts were associated with a decrease in candidal vaginitis, with no statistical difference between treatments (11).

A

LA and Cholesterol

- Several hypotheses have been offered to explain the observed effect of LA in lowering serum cholesterol. For example, LA may (1) inhibit 3-hydroxy-3-methylglutaryl CoA reductase, a rate-limiting enzyme in endogenous cholesterol synthesis; or (2) bind with cholesterol in the intestinal lumen, thus reducing absorption into the blood stream (1, 5).

- According to two review articles of more than 25 animal and *in vitro* studies, isolated LA and lactic acid bacteria found in fermented dairy products were associated with hypocholesterolemic effects (1, 5).

- In a double-blind, placebo-controlled, crossover study, 40 hypercholesterolemic subjects were randomized to receive 200 mL yogurt containing live cultures of LA or placebo daily for four weeks each, with a two-week washout. LA yogurt (strain L1) was associated with a significant 2.9 percent reduction of serum cholesterol. The authors concluded: "Since every 1 percent reduction on serum cholesterol is associated with an estimated 2 to 3 percent reduction in risk for coronary heart disease, regular intake of fermented milk (yogurt) containing an appropriate strain of LA has the potential of reducing risk for coronary heart disease by 6 to 10 percent" (12).

- In a double-blind, placebo-controlled, crossover trial, 30 healthy male subjects with borderline elevated cholesterol levels were randomized to receive 125 mL yogurt fermented with LA with added fructooligosaccharides (2.5 percent) or a traditional yogurt fermented only with yogurt strains. Subjects consumed 3 _ 125 mL yogurt daily for three weeks each with a one-week washout period. Blood samples were taken before the study, and at the end of both treatments. Compared to the control product, LA yogurt resulted in significantly lower values for serum total and LDL cholesterol, and the LDL/HDL ratio by 4.4, 5.4, and 5.3 percent, respectively. Serum HDL cholesterol, triglycerides, and blood glucose levels were unaffected (13).

LA and Cancer

- Several possible mechanisms of the potential anticarcinogenic action of LA have been hypothesized. These hypotheses include the production of compounds that inhibit tumor cell growth, antagonistic action against organisms that convert procarcinogens into carcinogens, and degradation of carcinogens (1).

- Observational studies have suggested that consumption of fermented dairy products is correlated with a lower prevalence of colon cancer (1).

- According to a review article of several animal studies, orally administered LA (fermented dairy products and single preparations) may slow tumor development in animals. However, the researchers stressed that there is currently no proof in humans that *Lactobacilli* or their fermented products can prevent cancer (5).

- A study of mice with induced mammary tumors showed that neither the initiation nor the promotion phase of cancer was affected by supplementation of LA, *bifidobacteria*, or fermented yogurt powder (14).

SAFETY

- There have been no reports of any negative side effects in human studies supplementing LA at dose levels of 10^{10} or 10^{11} colony-forming units/day. In addition, various *Lactobacillus* products (milk, yogurt, sweet acidophilus milk) have been on the market for decades with no reports of bacteremic infections (15).

- One case of liver abscess attributed to LA was reported in a 39-year-old man with chronic pancreatitis and with a choledoco-duodenostomy (16).

REFERENCES

1. Mital BK, Garg SK. Anticarcinogenic, hypocholesterolemic, and antagonistic activities of *Lactobacillus acidophilus*. *Crit Rev Microbiol*. 1995;21:175–214.
2. Canganella F, Paganini S, Ovidi M, et al. A microbiology investigation on probiotic pharmaceutical products used for human health. *Microbiol Res*. 1997;152:171–179.
3. Salminen S, Deighton M. Lactic acid bacteria in the gut in normal and disordered states. *Dig Dis*. 1992;10:227–238.
4. Reid G, Bruce AW, McGroarty JA, et al. Is there a role for lactobacilli in prevention of urogenital and intestinal infections? *Clin Microbiol Rev*. 1990;3:335–344.
5. Gorbach SL. Lactic acid bacteria and human health. *Ann Med*. 1990;22:37–41.
6. Mustapha A, Jiang T, Savaino DA. Improvement of lactose digestion by humans following ingestion of unfermented acidophilus milk: influence of bile sensitivity, lactose transport, and acid tolerance of *Lactobacillus acidophilus*. *J Dairy Sci*. 1997;80:1537–1545.
7. Elmer GW, Surawicz CM, McFarland LV. Biotherapeutic agents. A neglected modality for the treatment and prevention of selected intestinal and vaginal infections. *JAMA*. 1996;275:870–876.
8. Orrhage K, Sjostedt S, Nord CE. Effect of supplements with lactic acid bacteria and oligofructose on the intestinal microflora during administration of cefpodoxime proxetil. *J Antimicrob Chemo*. 2000;46:603–611.
9. Oksanen PJ, Salminen S, Saxelin M, et al. Prevention of traveller's diarrhea by *Lactobacillus* GG. *Ann Med*. 1990;22:53–56.
10. Witsell DL, Garrett CG, Yarbrough WG, et al. Effect of *Lactobacillus acidophilus* on antibiotic-associated gastrointestinal morbidity: a prospective randomized trial. *J Otolaryngol*. 1995;24:230–233.
11. Shalev E, Battino S, Weiner E, et al. Ingestion of yogurt containing *Lactobacillus acidophilus* compared with pasteurized yogurt as prophylaxis for recurrent candidal vaginitis and bacterial vaginosis. *Arch Fam Med*. 1996;5:593–596.
12. Anderson JW, Gilliland SE. Effect of fermented milk (yogurt) containing *Lactobacillus acidophilus* L1 on serum cholesterol in hypercholesterolemic humans. *J Am Coll Nutr*. 1999;18:43–50.
13. Schaafsma G, Meuling WJ, van Dokkum W, et al. Effects of a milk product, fermented by *Lactobacillus acidophilus* and with fructo-oligosaccharides added, on blood lipids in male volunteers. *Eur J Clin Nutr*. 1998;52:436–440.

14. Rice LJ, Chai YJ, Conti CJ, et al. The effects of dietary fermented milk products and lactic acid bacteria on the initiation and promotion stages of mammary carcinogenesis. *Nutr Cancer.* 1995;24:99–109.

15. Slaminen S. Functional dairy foods with *Lactobacillus* strain GG. *Nutr Rev.* 1996;54(11 pt 2):S99—S101.

16. Larvol L, Monier A, Besnier P, et al. Liver abscess caused by *Lactobacillus acidophilus. Gastroenterol Clin Biol.* 1996;20:193–195.

Alanine

L-alanine is a nonessential amino acid involved in glucose metabolism when the exogenous glucose supply is low. In the process known as the alanine cycle, pyruvate from glucose oxidation in skeletal muscle is aminated to form alanine, which is transported to the liver, deaminated, and converted into glucose. Alanine also carries nitrogen from peripheral tissues to the liver for excretion (1).

Media and Marketing Claims	Efficacy
Stabilizes blood sugar in hypoglycemia	↔
Protects the liver	NR
Spares muscle during intense training	NR

Advisory

No reported serious adverse effects

Drug/Supplement Interactions

Potential interaction with diabetic drugs used to lower blood glucose

KEY POINTS

- There is preliminary evidence that high doses of alanine (20 g to 40 g) in solution with 10 g glucose may prevent or treat nocturnal hypoglycemia in type 1 diabetes mellitus patients. Larger, controlled studies are needed to further explore the effects of alanine on hypoglycemia. Until more information is available, self-supplementation with alanine is not recommended in this population without the knowledge of a physician because of possible adverse effects on glycemic control.

- There is preliminary evidence in animal studies that alanine has a protective effect on hepatocyte function and regeneration. However, there are no human studies testing alanine in patients with liver disease. At this time, alanine supplements are not recommended for this population because the safety and efficacy have not been determined in controlled clinical trials.

- Although alanine is a glucogenic amino acid and plasma levels increase during exercise (2), there is currently no evidence that supplemental alanine spares muscle during exercise or enhances exercise performance.

FOOD SOURCES

Protein-rich foods such as egg, dairy, meat, fish, poultry

Food	Alanine (g/Serving)
Beef, lean (3 oz)	1.498
Chicken, skinless, boneless (3 oz)	1.455
Salmon (3 oz)	1.025
Egg (1 large)	0.348
Beans, kidney (½ c)	0.322
Milk (1 c)	0.276

Source: USDA Nutrient Database (www.nal.usda.gov/fnic)

DOSAGE INFORMATION/BIOAVAILABILITY

Alanine is found in single preparations of 450-mg capsules or as a powder. It is also found in supplements with a variety of amino acids and in some sports beverages. There is no dietary requirement for alanine because it is synthesized *in vivo*.

RELEVANT RESEARCH

Alanine and Hypoglycemia

- In a controlled, crossover (not blinded) study, 15 type 1 diabetes mellitus patients were given the same individualized dose of NPH insulin during four occasions separated by two weeks completed in random order at 10 p.m.: (1) NPH with no treatment (control); (2) 200-kcal snack (2 percent milk and toast); (3) 40 g alanine, plus 10 g glucose (200 kcal); and (4) 5 mg terbutaline (stimulates the B_2-adrenergic actions of epinephrine that increase plasma glucose). During the first half of the night, plasma glucose concentrations were significantly higher after the snack, alanine and glucose or terbutaline compared to control. During the second half of the night, mean plasma glucose levels were not different from control after the snack but tended to be higher after alanine (did not reach statistical significance) and were significantly higher after terbutaline. Nocturnal hypoglycemia, ie, plasma glucose levels of 40 mg/dL or less, occurred on 13 occasions in 7 patients in the control arm and 10 occasions in 6 patients in the snack arm (not statistically significant). There was only one occasion in the alanine-plus glucose arm (significant compared to control) and the terbutaline arm. The authors concluded that an evening dose of NPH insulin with a conventional snack exerts an inconsistent glycemic effect during the first half of the night, and bedtime ingestion of

A

alanine prevents nocturnal hypoglycemia more effectively than a snack. The authors point out that alanine must be taken in solution which has an unpleasant taste (3).

- Hypoglycemia was artificially induced by subcutaneous insulin injection in nine patients with type 1 diabetes mellitus and eight normal controls. During hypoglycemia, subjects with diabetes were given in random order: (1) 10 and 20 g glucose, (2) glucagon injection, (3) 40 g alanine, (4) oral terbutaline, (5) terbutaline injection, or (6) a placebo. All diabetic subjects participated in the placebo arm; six participated in the two oral glucose arms and the glucagon arm; and six participated in the oral and subcutaneous terbutaline arms and alanine arm of the study. Nondiabetic subjects only participated in the placebo arm. Oral alanine raised glucose levels within 30 minutes, with a gradual rise over practical hours in subjects with diabetes when compared to placebo ingestion. Oral terbutaline had a similar effect to alanine. Glucose and glucagon initially raised plasma glucose, but the effects were transient. The authors concluded that alanine produced sustained glucose recovery from hypoglycemia in diabetes and is potentially useful for the treatment and prevention of mild or moderate iatrogenic hypoglycemia when food intake is not possible for several hours (4).

- A study by the same researchers with a similar protocol found that alanine supplementation (20 g and 40 g) raised plasma glucagon and insulin, with no significant changes in blood glucose in nondiabetic subjects. In subjects with type 1 diabetes, alanine raised glucagon and plasma glucose but had no effect on insulin levels (5).

Alanine and Liver Function

- Rats with induced acute liver failure from a lethal dose of D-galactosamine were given alanine or a placebo. Liver function parameters improved in alanine-treated rats and the hepatic ATP content was significantly greater than in control rats. The authors concluded, "alanine is effective for the treatment of experimental acute liver failure, probably caused by the promotion of ATP synthesis. Alanine may be a good candidate for clinical application because of its preventative effect on hepatocyte necrosis and its promotive effect on liver regeneration" (6).

- Other animal studies reported a protective effect of alanine on damaged liver cells (7–9).

SAFETY

- In these limited studies with small numbers of subjects, alanine appears to be safe in the doses administered (20 g to 40 g). However, there are no studies testing the long-term safety of high-dose alanine supplementation.

REFERENCES

1. Matthews DE. Proteins and amino acids. In: Shils ME, Olson JA, Shike M, Ross AC, eds. *Modern Nutrition in Health and Disease.* 9th ed. Baltimore, Md: Williams & Wilkins; 1999:11–48.

2. Williams BD, Chinkes DL, Wolfe RR. Alanine and glutamine kinetics at rest and during exercise in humans. *Med Sci Sports Exerc.* 1998;30:1053–1058.

3. Saleh TY, Cryer PE. Alanine and terbutaline in the prevention of nocturnal hypoglycemia in IDDM. *Diabetes Care.* 1997;20:1231–1236.

4. Wiethop BV, Cryer PE. Alanine and terbutaline in treatment of hypoglycemia in IDDM. *Diabetes Care.* 1993;16:1131–1136.

5. Wiethop BV, Cryer PE. Glycemic actions of alanine and terbutaline in IDDM. *Diabetes Care.* 1993;16:1124–1130.

6. Maezono K, Mawatari K, Kjiwara K, et al. Effect of alanine on D-galactosamine-induced acute liver failure in rats. *Hepatology.* 1996;24:1211–1216.

7. Moriyama M, Makiyama I, Shiota M, et al. Decreased ureagenesis from alanine, but not from ammonia and glutamine, in the perfused rat liver after partial hepatectomy. *Hepatology.* 1996;23:1584–1590.

8. Maezono K, Kajiwara K, Mawatari K, et al. Alanine protects liver from injury caused by F-galactosamine and CC14. *Hepatology.* 1996;24:185–191.

9. Tanaka T, Ando M, Yamashita T, et al. Effects of alanine and glutamine administration on the inhibition of liver regeneration by acute ethanol treatment. *Alcohol Suppl.* 1993;1B:41–45.

Alpha-Lipoic Acid (ALA)

Alpha-lipoic (thioctic) acid or ALA is classified as a nonessential "vitamin-like" compound that contains sulfur. Synthesized in the mitochondria, it is involved in intermediary cell metabolism and is believed to possess antioxidant activity. ALA absorbed from the diet crosses the blood-brain barrier where it is taken into the cells and tissues. There ALA acid is reduced to dihydrolipoate that can travel to the extracelluar fluid, thereby providing antioxidant protection in both intra- and extracellular compartments. It functions in the pyruvate dehydrogenase complex, where it assists thiamin to form acetyl CoA. Lipoate and dihydrolipoate are believed to scavenge free radicals and protect membranes by interacting with vitamin C and glutathione, which may recycle vitamin E. Because of its potential antioxidant properties, ALA has been investigated for its protective role in conditions believed to be related to oxidative stress, including diabetes, cataracts, HIV, nerve degeneration, and radiation injury (1, 2).

Media and Marketing Claims	Efficacy
Normalizes blood sugar level	NR
Inhibits HIV	NR
Supports a healthy liver	NR
Improves exercise performance	NR
Slows aging	NR

Advisory

- No reported serious adverse effects
- May lower blood glucose level; should be monitored by physician

Drug/Supplement Interactions

Potential interactions with diabetes medications; may lower blood glucose

KEY POINTS

- Though there is preliminary evidence that intravenous ALA supplementation may improve diabetic neuropathy, two large controlled trials of oral ALA showed no improvement in neuropathic subjects' symptoms. Additionally, though there is evidence from *in vitro* and animal trials that ALA may play a beneficial role in conditions related to diabetes (cataracts, glucose utilization, oxidative stress), controlled clinical trials in humans are needed before recommendations can be made. A long-term study is currently in progress and will add to the body of research.

- There is preliminary evidence that ALA may play a role in slowing HIV replication *in vitro*; however, no human studies have tested whether ALA affects morbidity or prolong the lives of HIV patients. According to one study, ALA did not improve HIV-associated dementia.

- There is also preliminary evidence from *in vitro* and animal studies that ALA may play a role in neurodegenerative diseases. However, to date there is no research testing ALA in human subjects.

- There is no evidence from controlled trials at this time to substantiate claims that ALA has a favorable effect on body mass, enhances exercise, or slows the aging process.

FOOD SOURCES

Yeast and liver (3)

DOSAGE INFORMATION/BIOAVAILABILITY

Manufacturers provide ALA in pills and capsules in doses ranging from 50 mg to 300 mg. Most studies have used 100 mg/day to 800 mg/day doses. Lipoic acid is easily absorbed due to its low molecular weight (1).

RELEVANT RESEARCH

ALA and Diabetes

- In a double-blind, placebo-controlled trial, 73 patients with type 2 diabetes with cardiac autonomic neuropathy (CAN) were randomly assigned to receive 800 mg/day ALA or a placebo for four months. Seventeen patients dropped out of the study for various reasons (noncompliance, relocation, lack of efficacy). Parameters of heart rate variability at rest using an electrocardiogram included: coefficient of variation (CV); root mean square successive difference (RMSSD); and spectral power in the low- and high-frequency (LF and HF). Cardiovascular autonomic symptoms were also assessed. There were no significant differences in symptoms, mean blood pressure and HbA_{1c} levels between groups at baseline and during the study. There was a significant improvement in two out of four parameters of heart rate variability (CV and RMSSD) in the ALA group compared to the placebo. The authors concluded that ALA may slightly improve CAN in NIDDM patients and "Long-term studies of oral treatment with alpha-lipoic acid are now needed to confirm the observed improvement in CAN and to address the following questions: Can it be applied to IDDM patients? Can it be accompanied by effects on clinical endpoints?" (4).

- In a double-blind, placebo-controlled multicenter study, 509 type 2 diabetic patients with polyneuropathy were randomized to receive one of three treatments: (1) 600 mg intravenous (IV) ALA daily for three weeks, followed by 1,800 mg oral ALA/day for 6 months; (2) 600 mg IV alpha-lipoic acid daily for three weeks, followed by oral placebo daily for six months; or 3) placebo IV followed by oral placebo for six months. Outcome measures included the Total Symptom Score (TSS) for neuropathic symptoms (pain, burning, paresthesias, and numbness) in the feet and the Neuropathy Impairment Score (NIS). At the end of the study, ALA had no effect on neuropathic symptoms (TSS) compared to placebo. The authors suggested that this may have been a result of intercenter variability in symptom scoring. Subjects administered IV ALA did have significantly improved NIS scores after three weeks, but not after six months of oral treatment compared to subjects receiving placebos (5).

- In a double-blind, placebo-controlled trial, 328 patients with type 2 diabetes and diabetic neuropathy were randomized to receive treatment with intravenous infusion of ALA (1,200 mg, 600 mg, or 100 mg) daily or a placebo for three weeks. Neuropathic symptoms were scored at the baseline and throughout the study. The Hamburg Pain Adjective List and the Neuropathy Symptom and Disability Scores were assessed at the baseline and at day 19. The total symptom score in the feet was significantly decreased in ALA patients compared to the placebo. There was a significant improvement in the response rates after 19 days (defined as improvement of at least 30 percent in total symptom score) and in the Pain Adjective List with ALA supplementation compared to the placebo (6)

- In a placebo-controlled, pilot study, 74 patients with type 2 diabetes were randomized to receive either placebo or 600 mg, 1,200 mg, or 1,800 mg ALA daily for four weeks. Subjects underwent an isoglycemic glucose-clamp at the beginning and end of the study. When compared to subjects receiving the placebo, ALA-supplemented subjects had an increase in insulin-stimulated glucose disposal at the study's end. There was no difference in effect seen among the three different doses of ALA (7).

- Animal studies have shown that ALA may improve glucose utilization by the heart (8), and may improve nerve blood flow, reduce oxidative stress, and improve distal nerve conduction in experimental diabetic neuropathy (9).

A

- A review article discussed ALA studies demonstrating inhibition of diabetic cataractogenesis in rat lens cell cultures exposed to high concentrations of glucose and in animal models with induced cataracts (2).

- In Germany, ALA is frequently used to treat diabetic polyneuropathy (10). In one small, placebo-controlled, German study, 1,000 mg ALA administered intravenously resulted in increased insulin-stimulated glucose clearance in 13 type 2 diabetic patients (10).

- A long-term, large multicenter trial (NATHAN I) is being conducted in North America and Europe to examine the effect of oral ALA on the progression of diabetic neuropathy.

ALA and HIV

- In a randomized, double-blind, placebo-controlled trial using a parallel group 2 × 2 factorial design, 36 patients with HIV-associated cognitive impairment received deprenyl (a monoamine oxidase B inhibitor and putative antiapoptic agent) or ALA. There was no improvement in cognitive function in patients supplemented with ALA compared to a placebo, whereas deprenyl resulted in significant improvement (11).

- *In vitro* studies have shown that ALA inhibits nuclear factor kappa B (NF-kappa B) which is believed to play an important role in the activation of human immunodeficiency virus (12, 13). One *in vitro* experiment showed that ALA administration raised cellular levels of glutathione and "is therefore a potential therapeutic agent in an array of diseases with glutathione anomalies, including HIV infection" (14).

ALA and Liver Disease

- One review reported that no well-controlled research supports the use of ALA in the treatment of alcoholic liver disease. Most studies showing benefit were flawed and one double-blind, placebo-controlled, long-term study showed no effect (1).

ALA in Other In Vitro Studies

- Review articles have cited other potential uses of ALA supplements including the treatment of radiation damage, heavy metal poisoning, neurodegenerative diseases, and cerebral and myocardial ischemic-reperfusion injury. However, in most of these cases, ALA has only been tested *in vitro* and in animals (1, 2).

SAFETY

- ALA in doses up to 2,000 mg/day have been well-tolerated with few reported adverse effects.

- Reported side-effects include allergic skin reactions and possible hypoglycemia as a consequence of improved glucose utilization (1).

- Because one study showed ALA had lethal effects on rats that were severely thiamin-deficient, researchers recommend that patients who may be thiamin-deficient (eg, alcoholics) should supplement thiamin while taking ALA (2).

- The lethal dose (LD_{50}) of ALA in animals is 400 mg/kg to 500 mg/kg body weight.

- Some *in vitro* data indicates that a metabolic breakdown product of ALA (dihydrolipoate) may exert a prooxidant effect in the presence of iron. The physiological consequences are not known, though researchers do not believe this occurs *in vivo* (2).

REFERENCES

1. Packer L, Tritschler HJ, Wessel K. Neuroprotection by the metabolic antioxidant alpha-lipoic acid. *Free Radic Biol Med.* 1997;22:359–378.
2. Packer L, Witt EH, Tritschler HJ. Alpha-lipoic acid as a biological antioxidant. *Free Radic Biol Med.* 1995;19:227–250.
3. Linder MC. Nutrition and metabolism of vitamins. In: Linder MC, ed. *Nutritional Biochemistry and Metabolism with Clinical Applications.* 2nd ed. Norwalk, Conn: Appleton & Lange; 1991:112–122.
4. Ziegler D, Schatz H, Conrad F, et al. Effects of treatment with the antioxidant alpha-lipoic acid on cardiac autonomic neuropathy in NIDDM patients. A 4-month randomized controlled multicenter trial (DEKAN Study). *Diabetes Care.* 1997;20:369–373.
5. Ziegler D, Hanefeld M, Ruhnau KJ, et al. Treatment of symptomatic diabetic polyneuropathy with the antioxidant alpha-lipoic acid: a seven month multicenter randomized controlled trial (ALADIN III Study). ALADIN III Study Group. Alpha-lipoic Acid in Diabetic Neuropathy. *Diabetes Care.* 1999;22:1296–1301.
6. Ziegler D, Hanefeld M, Ruhnau KJ, et al. Treatment of symptomatic diabetic neuropathy with the anti-oxidant alpha-lipoic acid. *Diabetologia.* 1995;38:1425–1433.
7. Jacob S, Ruus P, Hermann R, et al. Oral administration of RAC-alpha-lipoic acid modulates sensitivity in patients with type-2 diabetes mellitus: a placebo-controlled pilot trial. *Free Radic Biol Med.* 1999;27:309–314.
8. Strodter D, Lehmann E, Lehmann U, et al. The influence of thioctic acid on metabolism and function of the diabetic heart. *Diabetes Res Clin Pract.* 1995;29:19–26.
9. Nagamatsu M, Nickander KK, Schmelzer JD, et al. Lipoic acid improves nerve blood flow, reduces oxidative stress, and improves distal nerve conduction in experimental diabetic neuropathy. *Diabetes Care.* 1995;18:1160–1167.
10. Jacob S, Henriksen EJ, Schiemann AL, et al. Enhancement of glucose disposal in patients with type 2 diabetes by alpha-lipoic acid. *Arzneimittelforschung.* 1995;45:872–874.
11. A randomized, double-blind, placebo-controlled trial of deprenyl and thioctic acid in human immunodeficiency virus-associated cognitive impairment. Dana Consortium of the Therapy of HIV Dementia and Related Cognitive Disorders. *Neurology.* 1998;50:645–651.
12. Packer L, Suzuki YJ. Vitamin E and alpha-lipoate: role in antioxidant recycling and activation of the NF-kappa B transcription factor. *Mol Aspects Med.* 1993;14:229–239.
13. Suzuki YJ, Aggarwal BB, Packer L. Alpha-lipoic acid is a potent inhibitor of NF-kappa B activation in human cells. *Biochem Biophys Res Commun.* 1992;189:1709–1715.

A

14. Han D, Tritschler HJ, Packer L. Alpha-lipoic acid increases intracellular glutathione in a human T-lymphocyte Jurkat cell line. *Biochem Biophys Res Commun.* 1995; 20:258–264.

Androstenedione and Androstenediol

Androstenedione (4-Androstene-3β, 17β-dione) is one of the primary androgens secreted by the human adrenal glands. Androgens are steroid hormones that increase male characteristics. Androstenedione has weak androgenic activity; however, it can be converted into the active steroids testosterone and dihydrotestosterone(1). Androstenediol (4 or 5-Androstene-3β, 17β-diol), a metabolite of dehydroepiandrosterone (DHEA), is also an androgen possessing weak activity. Androgen-based supplements have become popular among professional athletes and weight lifters for their purported anabolic effects on muscle. Although legally available over-the-counter, androstenedione and androstenediol are banned by the U.S. Olympic Committee, the National Collegiate Athletic Association, and the National Football League (2).

Media and Marketing Claims	Efficacy
Increases testosterone production	↔
Increases muscle mass and strength	NR
Enhances recovery from exercise	NR
Improves libido	NR

Advisory

- Causes increased androgen levels that could stimulate breast and prostate cancers
- May promote masculinization hormonal effects in women and feminizing hormonal effects in men
- May increase risk of heart disease by adversely affecting lipid levels

Drug/Nutrient Interactions

- No reported adverse interactions
- Theoretical interaction with androgenic and estrogenic drugs

KEY POINTS

- Most of the research does not suggest that androstenedione/-diol supplements raise testosterone levels in men. However, two studies have reported increases in testosterone levels, but also in those of the hormones estradiol and estrone.
- Androgen supplements do not appear to affect muscle size and strength or body composition of athletically trained or untrained males. No research has been performed in women.

- There is currently no evidence published in peer-reviewed journals to support the claims that androstenedione or androstenediol enhances recovery from exercise or improves libido.

- Because of the potential dangers of self-administration with an adrenal hormone, supplementation is not recommended.

FOOD SOURCES

None

DOSAGE INFORMATION/BIOAVAILABILITY

Androstenedione is sold in capsules with labels suggesting doses of 100 mg to 600 mg daily. Androstenediol is sold in capsules providing 200-mg doses. Androstenedione and androstenediol are also often sold in combination. Some manufacturers recommend taking supplements in one dose prior to physical activity. Of seven brands of over-the-counter androstenedione supplements analyzed, one had no androstenedione, one contained 10 mg testosterone, and four had less than 90 percent of the dose reported on the label (3).

RELEVANT RESEARCH

Effect on Testosterone Levels, Muscle Mass, and Muscle Strength

- In a double-blind, placebo-controlled study, 50 healthy men (aged 35 y to 65 y) with normal testosterone levels were randomized to receive 200 mg of androstenedione, or 200 mg androstenediol, or a placebo daily for 12 weeks. Subjects participated in a high intensity resistance training program during the study. Serum sex hormone profile, body composition, muscular strength, and lipid profiles were analyzed. Throughout the study, both the androstenedione and androstenediol groups had significantly elevated estrone and estradiol levels. Total testosterone levels increased significantly by 16 percent in the androstenedione group after one month, but returned to baseline by 12 weeks. Neither treatment enhanced body composition or muscular strength compared to the placebo. However, both andro treatments were associated with significant reductions in HDL-cholesterol, and had a negative effect on lipid ratios (LDL-cholesterol/HDL-cholesterol/apolipoprotein A/apolipoprotein B). In contrast, the placebo group had significant improvements in HDL and lipid ratios (4).

- In a double-blind, placebo-controlled, crossover design trial, 10 healthy males received in random order 200 mg of androstenedione/day or a placebo for two days. Treatments were separated by a two-week washout period. On day two, subjects performed heavy resistance exercise with blood drawn before, after, and 90 minutes postexercise. Androstenedione treatment resulted in elevated plasma androstenedione and luteinizing hormone, but had no effect on testosterone levels. Androstenedione also significantly elevated plasma estradiol by 83 percent for 90 minutes after exercise. In this

A

small study of short duration, the authors concluded that androstenedione does not appear to provide male athletes with anabolic benefits and may elevate estrogen levels with heavy weight training (5)

- In a double-blind, placebo-controlled study, 40 healthy, trained men (aged 40 y to 60 y) were randomized to receive one of three treatments for 12 weeks: (1) 100 mg androstenedione (divided into two doses); (2) 100 mg DHEA; or (3) a placebo. Blood samples, body composition, and performance were assessed at baseline, 6 weeks, and 12 weeks. Subjects met with a nutritionist and exercise physiologist who instructed them to maintain their normal diet, not to use other supplements, and to keep exercise logs. Compliance was measured by analyzing three-day dietary food records throughout the study. Supplementation with either androstenedione or DHEA had no statistically significant effect on lean body mass, strength, or plasma testosterone or androstenedione levels compared to placebo. Three months of supplementation had no adverse effects on liver function or blood levels of prostate-specific antigen (PSA), insulin, glucose, insulin, LDL cholesterol, or HDL cholesterol (6).

- In a double-blind, placebo-controlled study, 42 healthy male subjects (aged 20 y to 40 y) were randomized to one of three groups for seven days, receiving: (1) 100 mg androstendione/day; (2) 300 mg androstenedione/day; or (3) a placebo. Serum androstenedione, testosterone, estrone, and estradiol were measured at 0, 15, 30, 45, 60, 90, 120, 180, 240, 360, and 480 minutes after administration on days 1 and 7. On days 2 to 6, hormone concentrations were measured just prior to taking supplements. The high-dose androstenedione was associated with a significant increase in serum testosterone compared to the placebo group. In contrast, the 100-mg dose did not raise testosterone levels. Both doses resulted in increases in serum estradiol and estrone, with greater increases observed in the 300-mg dose group. There were no significant changes in liver function tests, serum creatinine, cholesterol, or hematocrit levels in any treatment group. The authors noted that there was considerable variability in changes of circulating sex hormones among the subjects, and that some men may be more prone to develop androgenic or estrogenic responses to androstenedione supplements (7).

- In a double-blind, placebo-controlled study, 20 normotestosterogenic, untrained men (age 19 y to 29 y) performed eight weeks of whole-body resistance training. During weeks 1, 2, 4, 5, 7, and 8, the men were randomized to receive 300 mg androstenedione daily or a placebo. The effect of a single 100-mg androstenedione dose on serum testosterone and estrogen was determined in 10 men. Serum-free and total testosterone concentrations were not changed by short- or long-term androstenedione supplementation. Serum estradiol was significantly higher in the androstenedione group after weeks 2, 5, and 8 compared to baseline values. Serum estrone concentrations were significantly higher after two and five weeks of androstenedione supplementation compared to the baseline. There were no differences between groups in knee extension strength, muscle fiber cross-sectional area, or body composition. Androstenedione subjects had reduced HDL cholesterol levels after two weeks that persisted after five and eight weeks of training and supplementation (8).

■ In a double-blind, placebo-controlled, crossover study, eight male subjects were randomly administered oral supplements in one dose of 200 mg androstenedione (4-androstene-3β, 17β-dione), 200 mg androstenediol (4-androstene-3β, 17β-diol), or a placebo. Treatments were separated by seven days. During each trial, blood collection was taken at 30, 60, 90, and 120 minutes after ingestion. Androstenedione resulted in a significant increase in serum androstenedione levels and a significant rise in both free and total testosterone compared to the placebo. Androstenediol ingestion was associated with an insignificant rise in free and total testosterone. The placebo caused a significant decline in free and total testosterone. The authors concluded that oral adrostenedione is capable of increasing blood testosterone concentrations and may be beneficial in conditions of androgen deficiency (9).

SAFETY

■ No long-term studies have tested the safety of androstenedione or androstenediol supplementation.

■ Some studies have reported adverse effects on HDL cholesterol levels and cholesterol ratios in men taking androstenedione supplements (4, 8).

■ It is not known whether androgen supplements could interfere with natural androgen steroid production.

■ Androgen excess in women could cause deepening of the voice, increased facial hair, decreased breast size, and genital enlargement. One review hypothesized that in young males, supplemental androgen may have fewer adverse effects because of the already high circulating levels of natural testosterone. However, excessive amounts could lead to increased levels of testosterone and estrogen resulting in emotional outbursts, acne, early puberty, growth stunting, hair loss, and possibly stimulation of breast development and reduction in testes size. In older men, increased androgen levels could result in cancerous growth of the prostate, elevation of blood lipids, and acceleration of male pattern baldness (2).

■ Elevated serum androstenediol (5-androstene-3β, 17β-diol) levels have been associated with increased risk of breast cancer in postmenopausal women (10). *In vitro* studies show that androstenediol binds to estrogen receptors and stimulates proliferation of estrogen-sensitive MCF-7 breast cancer cells in estradiol-poor environments (postmenopausal women have reduced estradiol concentrations) (10).

■ Tumor growth was stimulated by high levels of androstenedione in rats transplanted with human prostate tumor (PC-82). The authors hypothesized that an increase in tumor growth was caused by peripheral conversion of androstenedione into testosterone and 5-alpha-dihydrotestosterone (1).

A

REFERENCES

1. van Weerden WM, van Kreuningen A, Elissen NMJ, et al. Effects of adrenal androgens on the transplantable human prostate tumor PC-82. *Endocrinology.* 1992;131:2909–2913.
2. Gwartney DL, Stout JR. Androstenedione: Physical and ethical considerations relative to its use as an ergogenic aid. *Strength Cond.* 1999;21:65–66.
3. Catlin, DH, Leder BZ, Ahrens B, et al. Trace contamination of Over-the-Counter Androstenedione and Positive Urine Test Results for a nandrolone metabolite. *JAMA.* 2000;284:2618–2621.
4. King DS, Sharp RL, Vukovich MD, et al. Effect of oral androstenedione on serum testosterone and adaptations to resistance training in young men: a randomized controlled trial. *JAMA.* 1999;281:2020–2028.
5. Broeder CE, Quindry J, Brittingham K, et al. The Andro Profect: physiological and hormonal influences of androstenedione supplementation in men 35 to 65 years old participating in a high-intensity resistance training program. *Arch Intern Med.* 2000;160:3093–3104.
6. Ballantyne CS, Phillips SM, MacDonald JR, et al. The acute effects of androstenedione supplementation in healthy young males. *Can J Appl Physiol.* 2000;25:68–78.
7. Wallace MB, Lim J, Cutler A, et al. Effects of dehydroepiandrosterone vs androstenedione supplementation in men. *Med Sci Sport Exerc.* 1999;31:1788–1792.
8. Leder BZ, Longcope C, Catlin DH, et al. Oral androstenedione administration and serum testosterone concentrations in young men. *JAMA.* 2000;283:779–782.
9. Earnest CP, Olson MA, Broeder CE, et al. In vivo 4-androstene-3,17-dione and 4-androstene-3,17-diol supplementation in young men. *Eur J Appl Physiol.* 2000; 81:229–232.
10. Dorgan JF, Stanczyk FZ, Longcope C, et al. Relationship of serum dehydroepiandrosterone (DHEA), DHEA sulfate, and 5-androstene-3·,17·-diol to risk of breast cancer in postmenopausal women. *Cancer Epidemiol Biomark Prev.* 1997;6:177–181.

Arginine

Arginine and its precursors, ornithine and citrulline, are nonessential amino acids involved in the synthesis of urea in the liver. Arginine becomes essential during growth and catabolic states because it is thought to stimulate anabolic hormone secretion (human growth hormone [GH] and insulin) (1). Arginine is also precursor to nitric oxide, which has potent vasodilating properties in endothelial cells. There is a large body of literature on the role of nitric oxide in hypertension, myocardial dysfunction, inflammation, cell death, and protection against oxidative damage (2). Some researchers believe that a reduction in nitric oxide synthesis or activity may contribute to the initiation and progression of atherosclerosis (3). Because arginine is a substrate for nitric oxide, the potential role of L-arginine supplements has been examined in cardiovascular disease, cancer, and immune function (2, 4).

Media and Marketing Claims	Efficacy
Builds muscle by increasing growth hormone level	↔
Improves cardiovascular health	?↑
Enhances immune system in cancer patients	?↑
Important for immune function in elderly	↔
Important for wound healing	?↑
Improves immune parametes in HIV+ patients	NR

Advisory

- No reported serious adverse effects
- Long-term effects of high-dose supplementing are not known
- Potentially could aggravate herpes simplex virus

Drug/Nutrient Interactions

Interacts with the amino acid lysine by competing for absorption and reducing serum lysine levels

KEY POINTS

- Research in small numbers of subjects is conflicting on the acute effect of arginine in raising basal growth hormone secretion. The claim that arginine and other amino acids "build muscle" is unsubstantiated at this time.

- As a precursor to nitric oxide, it is possible that arginine may benefit patients with cardiovascular disease. Preliminary studies in small numbers of subjects have suggested that arginine supplements may reduce cell adhesion, improve blood flow, and enhance exercise function. More research is needed to clarify the role of arginine supplements in this population.

- High doses of arginine (30 g) before chemotherapy treatment have been shown in preliminary studies to improve some immune parameters in breast cancer and colon cancer patients. However, until more information is available, cancer patients should not use arginine supplements without their physician's knowledge and approval. Additional controlled research is needed before recommendations can be made.

- Preliminary studies suggest arginine/ornithine supplements may improve nutritional status in the elderly. However, improvements may arise from the additional protein in the diet and not specifically due to ornithine because protein intake was not controlled in these studies. Arginine supplements enhanced wound healing and immune function in one study of elderly patients.

- Preliminary evidence in humans suggests that arginine supplements enhance wound healing and immune response. Studies in animals have also reported improved healing with arginine supplementation.

- In the only study on HIV-positive patients, arginine supplements had no effect on any immune parameters measured.

A

FOOD SOURCES

The average American diet provides about 5.5 g arginine daily mainly from meat and fish (4). Arginine, citrulline, and ornithine are found in protein-rich foods and also in nuts, whole grains, and chocolate.

Food	Arginine (mg)(5)
Beef, ground (3.5 oz)	1,437
Beans, garbanzo (1 c)	1,369
Salmon, Atlantic (3 oz)	1,124
Peanuts, roasted (1 oz)	803
Soy milk (1 c)	514
Rice, brown (1 c)	382
Egg (1)	378
Milk, nonfat (1 c)	301
Cheese, cheddar (1 oz)	267
Baking chocolate (1 oz square)	163
Shredded wheat cereal (1 oz)	160

Source: Data from Pennington (5)

DOSAGE INFORMATION/BIOAVAILABILITY

Arginine, citrulline, and ornithine are found in tablets, capsules, drinks, and protein powders in various dosages (500 mg, 2 g to 3 g, 25 g). They are also commercially available with several other amino acid combinations and in creatine monohydrate supplements.

RELEVANT RESEARCH

Effects of Arginine and Ornithine on Exercise Hormones

- In a double-blind, placebo-controlled, crossover study, 16 male subjects (mean age = 22 y) completed four trials in random order with one-week washout periods: (1) placebo ingestion followed by resistance exercise session; (2) ingestion of 1,500 mg L-arginine and 1,500 mg L-lysine, immediately followed by exercise; (3) ingestion of same amino acids with no exercise; or (4) a placebo ingestion and no exercise. Dietary protein intake was not controlled nor assessed. All subjects were tested to ensure normal growth hormone metabolism. Growth hormone levels were higher during the exercise trials (1 and 2) compared to the resting trials (3 and 4). There was no effect of arginine and lysine on GH during the exercise trials. However, a small but significant rise in GH was seen during resting conditions 60 minutes after amino acid ingestion compared to the placebo trial (6).

- In a randomized, controlled study, seven male body builders (mean age = 22 y) were supplemented after an eight-hour fast on four separate occasions, in random order with: (1) a placebo; (2) 2.4 g arginine/lysine in solution; (3) 1.85 g ornithine/tyrosine in solution; and (4) a commercial drink containing 7.8 g protein (438 mg arginine, 412 mg lysine, 362 mg leucine, 312 mg valine, 238 mg phenyalanine, 200 mg isoleucine). The commercial drink was not blinded, but all other treatments were. Blood samples were drawn every 30 minutes for 180 minutes following ingestion while subjects sat quietly. Subjects were tested to confirm that GH concentrations were normal and all maintained protein intakes of 1.2 to 2.2 g/kg. Serum GH concentrations were not affected by any of the amino acid supplements. The authors concluded: "Ingestion of arginine/lysine supplements, ornithine/tyrosine supplements, or protein drinks, in the quantities recommended by the manufacturers and used by sport participants, does not consistently increase serum GH concentrations. There is no apparent reason why these supplements should be effective as ergogenic aids" (7).

- In a double-blind, placebo-controlled study, 22 untrained male subjects (mean age = 37 y) participating in a five-week progressive strength-training program were randomized to receive 1 g each of L-arginine and L-ornithine or a placebo. At the end of the study, subjects were tested for total strength on a series of weight machines, lean body mass (LBM), and urinary hydroxyproline (a marker of exercise-induced soreness and tissue damage). Dietary protein intake was neither controlled nor assessed. Compared to the placebo group, the arginine-ornithine supplemented subjects scored higher on total strength and LBM measures and lower in hydroxyproline excretion. The results of this study should be viewed with caution because subjects were not matched to controls and not pretested for strength and body mass (8).

Arginine and Cardiovascular Disease

- In a double-blind, placebo-controlled study, 41 subjects with intermittent claudication were randomized to one of three groups for two weeks: (1) two HeartBars™ (6.6 g L-arginine); (2) one HeartBar (3.3 g L-arginine); or one placebo bar; or (3) two placebo bars. Pain-free and total walking distances were measured by treadmill exercise testing, and quality of life was assessed by the Medical Outcome Survey. There were no differences in walking distances at baseline. After two weeks, the pain-free walking distance in the 6.6-g L-arginine group was significantly 66 percent greater and the total walking distance was significantly increased by 23 percent. These effects were not seen in the lower dose arginine or placebo groups. Likewise, there was a significant benefit in perceived general, emotional, and social function in the 6.6 g L-arginine group, but not in the other treatments (9).

- In a double-blind, comparative study, 39 patients with intermittent claudication were randomized to receive one of three treatments for three weeks: (1) 16 g L-arginine/day in two doses, (2) 80 (g prostaglandin E₁ (PGE₁)/day in two doses, or (3) control (no active treatment). The pain-free and absolute walking distances were assessed on a treadmill and nitric oxide mediated, flow-induced vasodilation of the femoral artery was assessed by ultrasonography at baseline, at weeks 1, 2, and 3 of therapy and six weeks after the end of treatment. Urinary nitrate and cyclic guanosine-3', 5'-monophosphate (GMP) were assessed as indices of endogenous nitric oxide production. Arginine treatment, but not PGE₁ treatment, increased urinary nitrate and cyclic GMP excretion rates, indicating normalized endogenous nitric oxide formation. Arginine supplements significantly improved pain-free walking distance by 230 ± 63 per-

A

cent and absolute walking distance by 155 ± 48 percent. PGE_1 also resulted in significant improvements, whereas control patients experienced no significant change. In both the arginine group and the PGE_1 group, there was a significant improvement in subjective assessment of pain on a visual analogue scale (10).

- In a double-blind, placebo-controlled trial, 22 patients with stable angina pectoris and healed myocardial infarction were randomized to receive 6 g L-arginine divided into three doses or placebo for three days. Blood samples were obtained and performance on an exercise test was determined before and after treatment. Blood pressure and an electrocardiogram were recorded during exercise. Arginine improved exercise capacity compared to the placebo (significant increase in maximum workload and mean exercise time to maximal ST-depression on an electrocardiogram). The authors hypothesized that supplements possibly improve an inefficient L-arginine/nitric oxide system that contributes to impaired heart muscle perfusion and/or poor vasodilation during exercise (11).

- In a double-blind, placebo-controlled, crossover design trial, 15 patients with heart failure were given L-arginine chloride (5.6 g arginine/day to 12.6 g/day) for six weeks and six weeks of placebo capsules in random sequence. Dietary intake of L-arginine was not assessed. Forearm blood flow during exercise was significantly increased during arginine supplementation compared to a placebo. Functional status (distance in a six-minute walk test) along with scores on the Living with Heart Failure questionnaire were significantly better during arginine intake. Furthermore, arginine supplements significantly improved arterial compliance and reduced circulating levels of endothelin (a vasoconstrictor) compared to a placebo (12).

- In an *ex vivo* study (20 hypercholesterolemic patients and 12 healthy controls), it was determined that human mononuclear cells (MNC) from subjects with high blood cholesterol levels had increased adhesiveness compared to normal subjects. To determine the effect of arginine on adhesiveness, in a double-blind, placebo-controlled study, 10 subjects with elevated blood cholesterol were randomized to receive arginine hydrochloride (8.4 g arginine/day) or placebo for two weeks. MNC adhesion remained statistically significantly elevated in placebo-treated subjects in contrast to arginine, which normalized adhesiveness. The authors concluded: "It remains to be seen whether supplements of the nitric oxide precursor [arginine] will inhibit atherogenesis in humans" (13).

- In a prospective, double-blind, placebo-controlled, crossover study, 10 men (mean age = 41 y) with angiographically proven coronary atherosclerosis were randomized to receive 21 g L-arginine divided into three doses or placebo for 3 days each, with a 10-day washout period. After arginine treatment, there was a significant increase in plasma arginine levels and a significant improvement in endothelium-dependent dilation of the brachial artery (measured as the change in diameter in response to increased blood flow from external vascular ultrasound). No changes were observed in endothelium-independent dilation of the brachial artery (measured as the change in diameter in response to sublingual nitroglycerine), blood pressure, heart rate, or fasting lipid levels. In an *ex vivo* analysis, monocyte adhesion to endothelial cells was significantly reduced following arginine supplementation compared to a placebo (14).

- In a double-blind, placebo-controlled, crossover study, 27 hypercholesterolemic subjects (19 y to 40 y) with known endothelial dysfunction and average LDL cholesterol levels of 238 mg/dL were assigned in random order to receive 21 g L-arginine (divided into three doses) or placebo for four weeks each, with a four-week washout period. Dietary intake was not controlled. Brachial artery diameter was measured at rest, during increased flow (causing endothelium-dependent dilation [EDD]) and after sublingual glyceryl trinitrate (causing endothelium-independent dilation). After arginine supplementation, there was a statistically significant rise in plasma arginine levels and a significant improvement in brachial artery diameter measured during increased flow (EDD). There were no significant changes in response to glyceryl trinitrate. After placebo, there were no changes in endothelium-dependent or independent vascular responses. Lipid levels were unchanged after arginine and placebo. The authors speculated that arginine improves EDD, and this may slow atherogenic progression (15).

- In a double-blind, placebo-controlled crossover study, 10 healthy postmenopausal women received in random order 9 g L-arginine or a placebo each day for one month (separated by a month washout period). Nitric oxide levels in serum, brachial artery endothelium-dependent dilator (EDD) responses, and cell adhesion molecules (markers of inflammation in blood) were measured at the end of each treatment period. L-arginine levels were increased in all women during L-arginine administration. However, there was no change in serum nitric oxide levels nor an effect on EDD during hyperemia compared to the placebo. There was also no effect of L-arginine on cell adhesion molecules compared to placebo. From this small study, the authors concluded that L-arginine does not appear to augment endothelial nitric oxide synthesis and release in healthy postmenopausal women and thus probably does not have a protective effect against atheroslerosis development (16).

- Acute intravenous infusion of L-arginine significantly improved brachial artery flow-mediated dilation in hypercholesterolemic patients (n = 9) and smokers (n = 9), but had no effect on subjects with type 1 diabetes (n = 9) or healthy controls (n = 9) (17).

Arginine and Cancer

- In a double-blind, placebo-controlled study, 96 breast cancer patients were randomized to receive 30 g L-arginine or a placebo for 3 days prior to each of six chemotherapy treatments during 21 days. There was no difference in the overall response rate between groups. However, in patients with tumors less than 6 cm in initial diameter, histopathological responses were significantly improved in the L-arginine supplemented group (88 percent responded) compared to the placebo group (52 percent responded) (18).

- A smaller study with a similar protocol found 30 g L-arginine administered to 10 breast cancer patients (aged 42 y to 73 y) before chemotherapy delayed the onset and severity of immunosuppression compared to that of patients not taking arginine (n = 6) prior to chemotherapy. Arginine supplementation also stimulated natural killer and lymphokine-activated killer cell activity (19).

- In a randomized, controlled (not blinded) study, 18 colorectal cancer patients received either a standard diet (60 g protein/3.2 g arginine) or the same standard diet supplemented with 30 g of L-arginine for three days before surgery. Tumor biopsies and blood samples were taken during surgery. Arginine supplementation resulted in significant alterations in tumor-infiltrating lymphocytes (believed to be involved in regulating tumor growth). Specifically, there was a significant increase in the number of cells expressing characteristics of natural killer and lymphokine activated killer cells. However, there was no change in the number of T and B cells, T helper and T suppresser cells. The authors concluded: "These findings confirm the potentially powerful therapeutic effects of dietary manipulation and have important implications for the immunotherapeutic treatment of malignant disease in humans" (20).

Arginine and Ornithine for the Elderly

- In a placebo-controlled, double-blind study, 45 healthy elderly subjects were given 17 g free arginine as arginine-aspartate (n = 30) or a placebo (n = 15) for two weeks. Dietary intake was not controlled. Arginine supplementation resulted in a significant increase in serum insulin-like growth factor and improved nitrogen balance compared to the placebo. Arginine supplementation also was associated with reduced total cholesterol without a decrease in high-density lipoprotein cholesterol (21).

- In a double-blind, placebo-controlled trial, 194 elderly patients (mean age = 74 y) recovering from acute illness were randomized to receive 10 g ornithine oxoglutarate (containing 1.3 g nitrogen) or a placebo (isocaloric maltodextrin) for two months. One-hundred-eighty-five patients completed the study (93 in the ornithine group, 92 in the placebo group). After 30 and 60 days of supplementation, the ornithine group had significantly improved appetite, body weight and independence compared to the placebo group. Two months after treatment, there was still an improvement in the quality-of-life index and the medical-cost index (overall cost savings of 37 percent). The authors hypothesized that the benefits may be attributed to the stimulation of insulin and growth hormone (not measured) and by the promotion of anabolism by endogenous production of proteins in the liver and fibroblasts (22).

Arginine and Ornithine for Wound Healing

- In a double-blind, placebo-controlled study, 32 elderly subjects with pressure ulcers were randomized to receive one of three enteral formulas daily for one month: (1) 0 g L-arginine (placebo); (2) 8.5 g L-arginine; or (3) 17 g L-arginine. Subjects were recruited from two nursing homes. Markers of immune function (lymphocyte proliferation to phytohemagglutinin and interleukin 2 production) were measured at baseline and at four weeks. Supplemental arginine significantly increased plasma arginine levels and was easily tolerated by subjects. Markers of immune function were not enhanced by arginine. The authors noted that the elderly can tolerate nitrogen loads from arginine supplements if their baseline renal function is normal and fluid intake is encouraged (23).

- In a double-blind, placebo-controlled study, 60 healthy, male and female elderly subjects (> 65 y) were randomized to receive 30 g arginine-aspartate (17 g free arginine) or placebo for two weeks. Fibroplastic wound responses were assessed by inserting a catheter subcutaneously into the right deltoid region. Epithelialization was examined by creating a 2×2 cm split-thickness wound on the upper thigh. Mitogenic response of peripheral lymphocytes to concanavalin A, phytohemagglutinin, pokeweed mitogen, and allogeneic stimuli was assayed at the beginning and end of supplementation. Arginine supplementation significantly enhanced wound catheter hydroxyproline (index of reparative collagen synthesis) and total protein content. Arginine did not influence the DNA content (index of cellular infiltration) of the catheters or the rate of epithelialization of the skin defect. Responses to mitogenic and allogenic stimulation were significantly greater in the arginine-supplemented group. Serum insulin-like-growth factor-1 levels were also significantly elevated in the arginine group. The authors concluded that the arginine supplementation may improve wound healing and immune responses in the elderly (24).

- In a double-blind, placebo-controlled study (similar protocol as in the study just cited), 36 healthy, nonsmoking subjects were randomized to receive one of three treatments for two weeks: (1) 24.8 g arginine/day, (2) 30 g arginine-aspartate (17 g free arginine)/day, or (3) a placebo. Prior to randomization, subjects underwent local anesthesia while a catheter was inserted subcutaneously into the right deltoid region. Dietary intake was not controlled. Mitogenic responses of peripheral blood lymphocytes were assayed at the start of the study, and at one and two weeks after supplementation. At two weeks, the catheters were removed, and the amount of hydroxyproline was determined as an index of new collagen synthesis and deposition. Arginine supplementation (both doses) significantly enhanced the amount of collagen deposited into a standardized wound as assessed by the amount of hydroxyproline present. Both arginine-supplemented groups also had increased lymphocyte mitogenesis in response to phytohemagglutinin and concanavalin A (25).

- Arginine supplementation increased wound strength and collagen deposition in rats, whereas arginine-deficient diets in rats have the opposite effect (2).

- Plasma fluxes of arginine, citrulline, and ornithine were studied in nine burn patients. Arginine fluxes were higher in burn patients than healthy controls, leading the researchers to hypothesize that higher rates of arginine loss from the body after burn injury would need to be balanced by exogenous intake of preformed arginine to maintain protein homeostasis and promote recovery (26).

Arginine and AIDS

- In a randomized, double-blind, placebo-controlled study, 55 HIV-infected outpatients received a daily nutritional supplement (606 calories) or the nutritional supplement plus 7.4 g arginine and 1.7 g omega-3 fatty acids for six months. The arginine and omega-3 supplement had no effect on body weight or immunologic parameters (CD4 and CD8 lymphocyte counts, tumor necrosis factor soluble receptors, viremia) (27).

SAFETY

- There are no human studies testing the safety of long-term supplementation of arginine, ornithine, or citrulline.

A

- In general, arginine supplements have been well tolerated, although possible detrimental effects of supplements observed include increased sodium and water losses and reduced plasma free lysine concentrations (28)

- High intakes of any one amino acid may interfere with the metabolism of other amino acids. In one study, arginine supplements (561 mg/day) reduced plasma free lysine (28).

- Arginine is required for the herpes simplex virus to replicate, whereas the amino acid lysine has an inhibitory effect on replication. Because arginine and lysine are antagonistic, patients with herpes simplex virus may be adversely affected by taking arginine supplements (29, 30) (*see* Lysine).

- If, in fact, arginine increases growth hormone levels, long-term supplementation could theoretically have a negative effect on normal regulation of pituitary growth hormone secretion.

REFERENCES

1. Cynober L. Can arginine and ornithine support gut functions? *Gut.* 1994;35:S42—S45.
2. Abcouwer SF, Souba WW. Glutamine and arginine. In: Shils ME, Olson JA, Shike M, Ross AC, eds. *Modern Nutrition in Health and Disease.* 9th ed. Baltimore, Md: Williams & Wilkins; 1999:559–569.
3. Cooke JP. Is atherosclerosis an arginine deficiency disease? *J Investig Med.* 1998;46:377–380.
4. Tenenbaum A, Fisman EZ, Motro M. L-arginine: rediscovery in progress. *Cardiology.* 1998;90:153–159.
5. Pennington JAT. *Bowes and Church's Food Values of Portions Commonly Used.* 17th ed. Philadelphia, Pa: Lippincott-Raven Publishers; 1998.
6. Suminski RR, Robertson RJ, Goss FL, et al. Acute effects of amino acid ingestion and resistance exercise on plasma growth hormone concentration in young men. *Int J Sport Nutr.* 1997;7:48–60.
7. Lambert MI, Hefer JA, Millar RP, et al. Failure of commercial amino acid supplements to increase serum growth hormone concentrations in male body-builders. Int J Sport Nutr. 1993;3:298–305.
8. Elam RP, Hardin DH, Sutton RA, et al. Effects of arginine and ornithine on strength, lean body mass, and urinary hydroxyproline in adult males. *J Sports Med.* 1989;29:52–56.
9. Boger RH, Bode-Boger SM, Thiele W, et al. Restoring vascular nitric oxide formation by L-arginine improves the symptoms of intermittent claudication in patients with peripheral arterial occlusive disease. *J Am Coll Cardiol.* 1998;32:1336–1344.
10. Maxwell AJ, Anderson BE, Cooke JP. Nutritional therapy for peripheral arterial disease: a double-blind, placebo-controlled, randomized trial of HeartBar. *Vasc Med.* 2000;5:11–19.

11. Ceremuzynski L, Chamiec T, Herbaczynska-Cedro K. Effect of supplemental oral L-arginine on exercise capacity in patients with stable angina pectoris. *Am J Cardiol.* 1997;80:331–333.

12. Rector TS, Bank AJ, Mullen KA, et al. Randomized, double-blind, placebo-controlled study of supplemental oral L-arginine in patients with heart failure. *Circulation.* 1996;93:2135–2141.

13. Theilmeier G, Chan JR, Zalpour C, et al. Adhesiveness of mononuclear cells in hypercholesterolemic humans is normalized by dietary L-arginine. *Arterioscler Thromb Vasc Biol.* 1997;17:3557–3564.

14. Adams MR, McCredie R, Jessup W, et al. Oral L-arginine improves endothelium-dependent dilatation and reduces monocyte adhesion to endothelial cells in young men with coronary artery disease. *Atherosclerosis.* 1997;129:261–269.

15. Clarkson P, Adams MR, Powe AJ, et al. Oral L-arginine improves endothelium-dependent dilation in hypercholesterolemic young adults. *J Clin Invest.* 1996;97:1989–1994.

16. Blum A, Hathaway L, Mincemoyer R, et al. Effects of oral L-arginine on endothelium-dependent vasodilation and markers of inflammation in healthy post-menopausal women. *J Am Coll Cardiol.* 2001;35:271–276.

17. Thorne S, Mullen MJ, Clarkson P, et al. Early endothelial dysfunction in adults at risk from atherosclerosis: different responses to L-arginine. *J Am Coll Cardiol.* 1998;32:110–116.

18. Heys S, Ogston K, Miller I, et al. Potentiation of the response to chemotherapy in patients with breast cancer by dietary supplementation with L-arginine: results of a randomized controlled trial. *Int J Oncol.* 1998;12:221–225.

19. Brittendon J, Heys SD, Ross J, et al. Natural cytotoxicity in breast cancer patients receiving neoadjuvant chemotherapy: effects of L-arginine supplementation. *Eur J Surg Oncol.* 1994;20:467–472.

20. Heys SD, Segar A, Payne S, et al. Dietary supplementation with L-arginine: modulation of tumor-infiltrating lymphocytes in patients with colorectal cancer. *Br J Surg.* 1997;84:238–241.

21. Hurson M, Regan MC, Kirk SJ, et al. Metabolic effects of arginine in a healthy elderly population. *JPEN.* 1995;19:227–230.

22. Brocker P, Vellas B, Albarede JL, et al. A two-center, randomized, double-blind trial of ornithine oxoglutarate in 194 elderly, ambulatory, convalescent subjects. *Age Ageing.* 1994;23:303–306.

23. Langkamp-Henken B, Herrlinger-Garcia KA, Stechmiller JK, et al. Arginine supplementation is well tolerated but does not enhance mitogen-induced lymphocyte proliferation in elderly nursing home residents with pressure ulcers. *J Parenter Enteral Nutr.* 2000;24:280–287.

24. Kirk SJ, Hurson M, Regan MC, et al. Arginine stimulates wound healing and immune function in elderly human beings. *Surgery.* 1993;114:155–159.

25. Barbul A, Lazarou SA, Efron DT, et al. Arginine enhances wound healing and lymphocyte immune responses in humans. *Surgery.* 1990;108:331–337.

26. Yu YM, Ryan CM, Burke JF, et al. Relations among arginine, citrulline, ornithine, and leucine kinetics in adult burn patients. *Am J Clin Nutr.* 1995;62:960–968.
27. Pichard C, Sudre P, Karsegard V, et al. A randomized double-blind controlled study of 6 months of oral nutritional supplementation with arginine and omega-3 fatty acids in HIV-infected patients. Swiss HIV cohort study. *AIDS.* 1998;12:53–63.
28. Beaumier L, Castillo L, Ajami AM, et al. Urea cycle intermediate kinetics and nitrate excretion at normal and "therapeutic" intakes of arginine in humans. *Am J Physiol.* 1995;269(5 pt 1):E844—E896.
29. Griffith RD, DeLong DC, Nelson JD. Relation of arginine-lysine antagonism to herpes simplex growth in tissue culture. *Chemotherapy.* 1981;27:209–213.
30. Flodin NW. The metabolic roles, pharmacology, and toxicology of lysine. *J Am Coll Nutr.* 1997;16:7–21.

Aspartic Acid/Asparagine

Aspartic acid (aspartate) is a nonessential amino acid involved in urea synthesis and is a glucogenic and pyrimidine precursor. In the TCA (Krebs) cycle, aspartic acid and oxaloacetic acid are interconvertible. Asparagine is also a nonessential amino acid that can be hydrolyzed into aspartic acid. Asparagine acts as a reservoir of amino groups throughout the body. It has been hypothesized that aspartate salts enhance athletic performance. The proposed mechanism of action is that aspartate spares glycogen by increasing the availability of free fatty acids (FFAs) for fuel and potentially reduces exercise fatigue by clearing excess ammonia from the blood through urea synthesis (1).

Media and Marketing Claims	Efficacy
Improves stamina and fights fatigue	NR
Clinically useful in depression	NR

Advisory

No reported serious adverse effects

Drug/Supplement Interactions

No reported negative interactions; however, it is not known whether high doses of aspartic acid or asparagine negatively affect absorption and metabolism of other amino acids

KEY POINTS

- The ergogenic effect of aspartate salts on exercise performance is controversial. None of the studies evaluated serum aspartate levels. In addition, the small number of subjects makes interpretation of the data difficult. Aspartate salts do not appear to reduce accumulation of ammonia in plasma. Most studies do not show a benefit, and until additional controlled trials with larger sample sizes are conducted, supplementation is not warranted.

- Although there has been research (not discussed here) investigating serum amino acid concentrations in relation to depression, there is currently no evidence that aspartate salts or asparagine supplements are effective in treating depression.

FOOD SOURCES

Aspartic acid and asparagine are found in protein-rich animal foods. The sugar-free sweetener aspartame is a combination of aspartic acid and phenylalanine (40 percent aspartic acid).

Food	Aspartic Acid (g/Serving)
Beef, ground (3 oz)	6.683
Chicken breast (½)	2.377
Flour, whole wheat (1 c)	0.844
Egg (1 large)	0.627
Corn (1 ear)	0.194

Source: USDA Nutrient Database (http://www.nal.usda.gov/fnic/

DOSAGE INFORMATION/BIOAVAILABILITY

L-aspartic acid is available in single or mixed amino acid preparations providing 500 mg to 1,200 mg as potassium, calcium, or magnesium aspartate. L-asparagine is usually only found in mixed amino acid supplements in 60-mg doses.

RELEVANT RESEARCH

Aspartic Acid and Asparagine for Exercise

- In a double-blind, comparative crossover trial, 12 male weight trainers were randomly assigned to receive aspartate salts (150 mg/kg) or vitamin C (150 mg/kg) over a two-hour period, five hours before a resistance workout. Trials were separated by one week. Vitamin C was chosen as the placebo because it has no known effects on ammonia production or clearance. Plasma ammonia levels increased between pre- and post-exercise. However, there were no significant differences in plasma ammonia levels or bench-press tests between treatments. The authors concluded: "Acute aspartate supplementation does not reduce ammonia during and after a high intensity resistance training workout in weight-trained subjects" (2).

- In a double-blind, crossover study, seven trained subjects were given 10 g of potassium and magnesium aspartic salts providing 5 g aspartate or a placebo 24 hours prior to an exercise-to-exhaustion on a cycle ergometer, separated by a one-week washout. Fol-

A

lowing aspartate ingestion, there was a significant increase in time to exhaustion and postexercise free fatty acid (FFA) levels. There was a significant decrease in lactate concentrations. Blood ammonia levels were significantly lower throughout exercise in the aspartate trial compared to the placebo. The researchers hypothesized that the ergogenic benefit of aspartates was attributable to improved ammonia clearance (3).

▪ In a double-blind, placebo-controlled, crossover study, eight young male subjects received 6 g aspartic acid salts (as magnesium-potassium aspartate) or a placebo over a 24-hour period before exercising to exhaustion on a cycle ergometer (75 percent maximum oxygen uptake), with a week washout period. There were no differences in blood glucose, lactate, ammonia, or plasma FFA levels between treatment groups during or after exercise. There was also no effect on respiratory exchange ratio. The authors concluded: "These results show no beneficial effect of oral aspartate administration on work capacity in man and also suggest that the metabolic processes that occur during exercise are not influenced by this treatment" (4).

▪ In an animal study, rats' diets were supplemented with 1) aspartic acid and asparagine (45 mg/kg body weight of each) plus carnitine (90 mg/kg) or 2) a placebo. Additionally, they were sedentary, allowed to run in a rotating wheel, or were swimming-trained for five weeks. Supplementation of amino acids enhanced the capacity of the muscle to use FFAs and spare glycogen as indicated by plasma glucose, FFA, lactate concentrations and muscle glycogen content. In addition, time to exhaustion was longer in the swimming-trained rats supplemented with amino acids compared to the placebo group (5).

▪ Intravenous aspartate administration (1 g/kg) to rats before swimming exercise had no effect on swimming time to exhaustion of the test group compared to saline-injected rats. Aspartate resulted in lower plasma FFA concentrations after swimming compared to saline injection, not suggestive of an ergogenic benefit. In addition, aspartate had no effect on liver or muscle glycogen (6).

SAFETY

▪ There are no long-term studies testing the safety of aspartic acid or asparagine. Acute ingestion (5 g to 10 g aspartate) was not associated with any reported adverse effects in the previously described human studies.

▪ Sedentary or swimming-trained rats supplemented with 45 mg aspartate/kg body weight and 90 mg carnitine/kg for one week experienced myofibrillar and mitochondrial disorganization and dissolution along with other dysfunctional changes in the soleus muscle similar to changes observed after prolonged periods of ischemia. The authors hypothesized that amino acids given in excess could impair the process of protein synthesis and lead to muscle damage (7).

▪ It is not known whether high doses of aspartic acid or asparagine negatively affect absorption and metabolism of other amino acids.

REFERENCES

1. Abcouwer SF, Souba WW. Glutamine and arginine. In: Shils ME, Olson JA, Shike M, Ross AC, eds. *Modern Nutrition in Health and Disease.* 9th ed. Baltimore, Md: Williams & Wilkins; 1999:561.
2. Tuttle JL, Potteiger JA, Evans BW, et al. Effect of acute potassium-magnesium aspartate supplementation on ammonia concentrations during and after resistance training. *Int J Sport Nutr.* 1995;5:102–109.
3. Wesson M, McNaughton L, Davies P, et al. Effects of oral administration of aspartic acid salts on the endurance capacity of trained athletes. *Res Q Exerc Sport.* 1988;59:234–239.
4. Maughan RJ, Sadler DJ. The effects of oral administration of salts of aspartic acid on the metabolic response to prolonged exhausting exercise in man. *Int J Sports Med.* 1983;4:119–123.
5. Lancha AH, Recco MB, Abdalla DS, et al. Effect of aspartate, asparagine, and carnitine supplementation in the diet on metabolism of skeletal muscle during moderate exercise. *Physiol Behav.* 1995;57:367–371.
6. Trudeau F, Murphy R. Effects of potassium-aspartate salt administration on glycogen use in the rat during a swimming stress. *Physiol Behav.* 1993;54:7–12.
7. Lancha AH, Santos MF, Palanch AC, et al. Supplementation of aspartate, asparagine, and carnitine in the diet causes marked changes in the ultrastructure of soleus muscle. *J Submicrosc Cytol Pathol.* 1997;29:405–408.

Bee Pollen

Bee pollen is a powder form of non-airborne pollen collected by bees from male seed flowers. The pollen is mixed with secretions from the bee and formed into granules for the bee to carry back to the hive on its hind legs. Bees store pollen in the hive as food for larvae. Bee pollen as a dietary supplement has been used extensively in Europe and Asia because of purported nutritional benefits (1). In one study, the composition of two types of bee pollen from Western Australia were estimated to contain 57 percent carbohydrates, 1 percent fat, and 20 percent to 28 percent protein, with lysine as the limiting amino (2). Considerable variation in the nutritional content of pollen exists (ie, protein content varies from 7 percent to 40 percent) (2). Analysis of the mineral composition of these pollens showed that potassium, phosphorus, calcium, and sodium were present in the highest concentration (no analysis of vitamin content) (2). However, when calculated to determine the amounts found in a typical dose of a commercial bee pollen supplement (7 g), the actual quantities of these nutrients are relatively insignificant (4 mg to 8 mg calcium, 33 mg potassium, 0.31 mg to 0.46 mg zinc, 6 mg magnesium, 1.8 g protein, 4 mg carbohydrates, and < 1 g fat).

B

Media and Marketing Claims	Efficacy
Nature's perfect food—a complete balance of protein, carbohydrate, fat, vitamins, and minerals	↓
Increases vitality, memory and concentration, and well-being	NR
Improves exercise performance	NR
Improves respiratory tract infections, endocrine diseases, colitis, and allergies	NR

Advisory

- Should be avoided by people with asthma or allergies to honey or bee stings
- Can cause anaphylactic reactions in allergic individuals

Drug/Supplement Interactions

No reported adverse interactions

KEY POINTS

- The typical dose of bee pollen (½ teaspoon to 1 teaspoon) provides insignificant quantities of protein, carbohydrate, fat, and most vitamins and minerals.

- Currently, there is no scientific evidence to substantiate the claims regarding bee pollen supplementation. Instead of taking bee pollen as a dietary supplement, a regular multivitamin/mineral supplement may be a less costly, more efficient, and safer alternative given the possibility of an allergic reaction. Although relatively rare, an anaphylactic reaction can occur in some sensitive individuals. Accordingly, bee pollen is contraindicated for people with asthma or allergies to honey or bee stings.

FOOD SOURCES

Small amounts found in honey

DOSAGE INFORMATION/BIOAVAILABILITY

Bee pollen is sold in powder, granules, or capsule forms. Some manufacturers suggest taking ½ to 1 teaspoon (≈ 3 g to 7 g) pure bee pollen powder or 1,000 mg to 1,500 mg in capsule form daily. Bee pollen is also a popular ingredient added to fruit "smoothies" and certain multivitamin/mineral supplements. In one study, the digestibility of the protein in two different bee pollens ranged from 52 to 59 percent compared to 89 percent for casein. The authors of this study noted: "Their relatively low digestibility will be a limiting factor in their usefulness as a food for humans" (2). In addition, the amounts of protein consumed from supplements contribute minimally to overall protein intake.

RELEVANT RESEARCH

- In general, research on bee pollen is scant, though some studies, mostly using experimental animals, have been published in Chinese and Russian journals.

- In 1978, 18 high school cross-country runners participated in a double-blind, placebo-controlled study. Subjects were given bee pollen extract capsules (dose not specified), protein capsules, or a placebo every day for 12 weeks. There were no significant differences among groups for blood levels of potassium, hemoglobin, or hematocrit. There was also no effect of supplements on the mean velocity of a pre- and post-three-mile run (3).

- A double-blind, placebo-controlled, crossover trial of 100 elderly Danish subjects with self-reported memory deterioration tested the effects of a traditional Chinese mixture known as NaO Li Su containing bee pollen and a variety of Chinese herbs. There were no improvements in memory functions between groups as assessed by a battery of psychological and biochemical tests. There was a statistically significant increase in red blood cell count and serum creatinine concentration in supplemented subjects (4). Because bee pollen was not administered singly, the pharmacological effect of bee pollen cannot be determined from this study.

SAFETY

- There have been several reports of anaphylactic reaction resulting from bee pollen in individuals with a sensitivity to bee stings and honey allergies (5, 6). However, not all reactive individuals had a prior allergic reaction to bee stings (1). One 19-year-old asthmatic man had a fatal hypersensitive reaction to bee pollen (5). Another patient experienced hypereosinophilia (indicative of an allergic response), neurological, and gastrointestinal symptoms after six weeks of bee pollen supplementation. An open challenge with the bee pollen later reproduced the presenting symptoms (7). Acute hepatitis occurred after ingestion of pure bee pollen in one case and bee pollen with the herb chaparral in another case were reported (8).

REFERENCES

1. Geyman JP. Anaphylactic reaction after ingestion of bee pollen. *J Am Board Fam Pract.* 1994;7:250–253.
2. Bell RR, Thornber EJ, Seet JL, et al. Composition and protein quality of honeybee-collected pollen of *Eucalyptus marginata* and *Eucalyptus calophylla. J Nutr.* 1983;113:2479–2484.
3. Steben RE, Boudreaux P. The effects of pollen and protein extracts on selected blood factors and performance of athletes. *J Sports Med Phys Fitness.* 1978;18:221–226.
4. Iversen T, Fiigaard KM, Schriver P, et al. The effect of NaO Li Su on memory functions and blood chemistry in elderly people. *J Ethnopharmacol.* 1997;56:109–116.

5. Prichard M, Turner KJ. Acute hypersensitivity to ingested processed pollen. *Aust N Z J Med.* 1985;15:346–347.

6. Greenberger PA, Flais MJ. Bee pollen-induced anaphylactic reaction in an unknowingly sensitized subject. *Ann Allergy Asthma Immunol.* 2001;86:239–242.

7. Lin FL, Vaughan TR, Vandewalker ML, et al. Hypereosinophilia, neurologic, and gastrointestinal symptoms after bee-pollen ingestion. *J Allergy Clin Immunol.* 1989;83:793–796.

8. Shad JA, Chinn CG, Brann OS. Acute hepatitis after ingestion of herbs. *South Med J.* 1999;92:1095–1097.

Beta-Carotene

See Vitamin A.

Black Cohosh (Cimicifuga racemosa)

Black cohosh is a member of the buttercup family. Eighteen species grow in Europe, North America, and Asia. The "black" refers to the dark color of the rhizome. "Cohosh" comes from an Algonquian word meaning rough, referring to the feel of the rhizome. Traditionally the root of the plant was used for treatment of dysmenorrhea, dyspepsia, and rheumatism. In the 1800s, black cohosh was a main ingredient in "Lydia Pinkhams's Vegetable Compound," a popular remedy used for a variety of female complaints. Black cohosh has been investigated and used in Germany since the 1950s and is approved by the German Commission E for premenstrual discomfort, dysmennorrhea, or menopausal ailments. Remifemin, the brand name of the standardized extract, has been used in all the clinical trials and is available in the United States (1–3).

The exact mechanism of action and particular active components of the herb are not fully understood. The biologically active compounds in the herb are credited triterpene glycosides including actein, cimicifugoside, deoxyacetylacteol, and 27-deoxyactein.[1]

Originally, researchers suggested that isoflavones in black cohosh exerted weak estrogenic effects that lessened menopausal symptoms. However, recent studies have not found the herb to be estrogenic, nor does it contain isoflavones. Another theory was that black cohosh suppressed luteinizing hormone (LH), a hormone that typically increases with menopause and is believed to contribute to hot flashes. Although some research has shown that black cohosh lowers LH, other data are conflicting. Although the actions of this herb need further study, more and more women are choosing to use black cohosh as an alternative to hormone replacement therapy (HRT) for the management of menopausal symptoms (1–3).

---

[1] Recent research has shown that this compound was initially and erroneously named as such, but the proper name is 23-epi-26-deoxyactein.

Media and Marketing Claims	Efficacy
Helpful for menopause	↑?
May relieve PMS symptoms	NR

Advisory

- Appears to be safe in studies of up to six months' duration
- Avoid during pregnancy—may stimulate uterine contractions
- More research needed to determine safety in women with breast cancer

Drug/Supplement Interactions

No reported adverse interactions

KEY POINTS

- There is some evidence from a few controlled and several uncontrolled studies that black cohosh relieves menopausal symptoms such as hot flashes, irritability, and anxiety. However, the lack of controls in the majority of the studies makes it difficult to evaluate the efficacy. Standard hormone replacement therapy is associated with beneficial effects on bone density and possibly cardiovascular health. Whether black cohosh has the same positive effects is not known.

- The National Institutes of Health has funded a double-blind, placebo-controlled study to help determine whether black cohosh is beneficial for menopausal women. This study will attempt to make up for the limitations of previous research, and should provide further answers on efficacy, safety, and dosage.

- Although black cohosh has been used for centuries for a variety of female complaints, more research is needed to evaluate the role of the herb on premenstrual syndrome and dysmenorrhea.

FOOD SOURCES

None

DOSAGE INFORMATION/BIOAVAILABILITY

Black cohosh is most commonly sold in capsules, tablets, tinctures, and teas. In the United States, black cohosh is marketed as Remifemin, a standardized black cohosh root and rhizome extract (standardized for triterpene glycosides, calculated as 23-epi-26-deoxyactein). Most studies have used 80 mg to 160 mg daily of Remifemin (a total of 4 mg to 8 mg of 23-epi-26-deoxyactein/day). Because of improved extraction processes, the current recommended dose of Remifemin is 40 mg/day or two tablets (3).

Data on bioavailability has not been studied. The upcoming NIH study will provide pharmacology information.

RELEVANT RESEARCH

Black Cohosh and Menopause

- In a double-blind, placebo-controlled study, 85 patients who were diagnosed with breast cancer who had completed their primary treatment were randomly assigned black cohosh or a placebo, stratified on tamoxifen use. Upon beginning the study, subjects completed a questionnaire about demographic factors and menopausal symptoms. The same questionnaire was given at 30 days and then again at 60 days. In addition, subjects completed a four-day hot flash diary. FSH and LH levels were measured upon the first and final days of the study. Of the 85 patients, 59 were taking tamoxifen and 26 were not. Both treatment and placebo groups reported declines in the number and intensity of hot flashes. There were no significant differences between groups. Both groups also reported improvements in menopausal symptoms. FSH and LH also did not differ between the two groups. The researchers concluded that black cohosh was not better than the placebo in the treatment of menopausal symptoms in this population of women, most of whom were taking tamoxifen (4).

- In a double-blind, placebo-controlled trial, 80 menopausal women received either 0.625 mg of estrogen, 80 mg of a standardized black cohosh extract, or a placebo for 12 weeks. Hot flashes, night sweats, heart palpitations, headaches, nervousness, irritability, insomnia, depressive moods, and changes in vaginal cell proliferation were assessed by the Kupperman Menopausal Index and the Hamilton Anxiety Scale. Altogether 16 women discontinued treatment before the study ended (13 subjects stopped after five to eight weeks because of inefficacy—12 in the estrogen group, one in the placebo group; two placebo subjects stopped treatment due to side effects; one subject with varicosis in the black cohosh group stopped treatment due to thrombophlebitis at week 8). Black cohosh-treated subjects showed significant improvement in both measures. The estrogen proved to be given in too low a dose for reliable comparison (5).

- In a double-blind, placebo-controlled study, 60 women aged < 40 y who had at least one ovary removed and complained of climacteric symptoms were randomly divided into four groups. These four groups of equal number were treated with either 1 mg estriol, 1.25 mg of conjugated estrogens, estrogen-gestagen conbination, or Remifemin (80 mg/day). The Menopausal Index with evaluation of the trophic disturbances of the genitals and FSH and LH serum concentrations were used as the efficacy criteria. In all four groups there was improvement in the profile of complaints of postoperative ovarian functional deficits, a significant decline in the modified Menopausal Index, and a moderate decline in the serum gonadotropin concentrations. There was no significant therapeutic difference among the individual medication groups. Remifemin was shown to be just as effective in improving postoperative ovarian functional deficits after hysterectomy in the women as estriol-gestagen combination (6).

- In a placebo-controlled (not blinded) study, 110 menopausal women received 8 mg of black cohosh or placebo daily for eight weeks. The black cohosh provided was concentrated to contain three types of endocrinologically active fractions of a commercial extract (Remifemin). The isolated fraction of the root reduced LH production compared to placebo. There was no effect on FSH. The findings of this study would have been strengthened if it had been double-blinded (7).

- In a multicenter, open German study, 629 menopausal women received 4 mg of a black cohosh extract twice daily for six to eight weeks. Of the total subjects, 367 women were not previously treated, 204 were treated previously with hormones, 35 were treated with psychopharmaceuticals, 11 were treated with a combination of hormones and psychopharmaceuticals, and 12 were lacking specific treatment data. Forty-nine percent of the participants reported a dramatic reduction in hot flashes, sweating, headaches, vertigo, palpitations, and tinnitus attributed to menopause. More than 39 percent noted a decrease in nervousness, irritability, and depression. Seven percent reported minor gastric discomfort. The results of the study should be viewed with caution because there was no placebo-control, randomization, or blinding (8).

- In an open, controlled comparative study on 60 patients in a gynecologic practice through the course of 12 weeks, Remifemin was compared to estrogen and diazepam on menopausal symptoms. Group one received Remifemin daily, group 2 received conjugated estrogens, 0.625 mg per day and group 3 received diazepam, 2 mg per day. A positive estrogen-like stimulation of the vaginal mucosa occurred with Remifemin and with estrogen therapy with a clear increase in the cytologic indices under the herbal and estrogen therapy within four weeks. No changes in the cytologic parameter were observed with psychopharmaceutical therapy. All three forms of therapy influenced menopausal symptoms as measured by a significant reduction of the SDS Index and a significant reduction in the modified Menopausal Index of symptoms of hot flashes, night sweats, nervousness, headaches, and heart palpitations. The results of the study should be viewed with caution because it was not double-blinded (9).

- The National Institutes of Health, through the National Center for Complementary and Alternative Medicine, is funding Phase I and II studies of black cohosh use by women suffering from premenstrual syndrome. The study is being conducted at the University of Illinois at Chicago, College of Pharmacy and College of Medicine. During the Phase I study, three groups of five women each will receive one dose (escalating) of a biologically and chemically standardized extract of black cohosh to determine a safe dose to be used in the Phase II study. The Phase II study will involve a larger group of women who will receive the extract for one year. Efficacy and metabolism and pharmacokinetic studies will be carried out in a double-blind, placebo-controlled, randomized protocol.

SAFETY

- Black cohosh was not associated with any serious adverse effects in studies lasting up to six months. Because of a lack of long-term trials, the German Commission E Monographs recommends limiting the use of black cohosh to six months (10).

- Mild side-effects may include some gastrointestinal upset (10).

- Experimental studies demonstrate no toxic, mutagenic, or carcinogenic properties with black cohosh (11).

- The question of whether black cohosh can be used safely by women with breast cancer needs further research. If the herb is estrogenic, some postulate that it would exacerbate estrogen-stimulated cancers. On the other hand, some researchers cite evidence that black cohosh is not estrogenic and therefore can be used safely by women with breast cancer.

- There is a possibility that using black cohosh during pregnancy can stimulate uterine contractions.

REFERENCES

1. Foster, S. Black cohosh: *Cimicifuga racemosa* a literature review. *HerbalGram.* 1999;45:34–49.

2. Taylor M. Botanicals: Medicines and menopause. *Clin Obstet Gynecol.* 2001;44:853–863.

3. Pepping J. Black cohosh: *Cimicifuga racemosa. Am J Health-Syst Pharm.* 1999;56:1400–1402.

4. Jacobson JS, Troxel AB, Evans J. Randomized trial of black cohosh for the treatment of hot flashes among women with a history of breast cancer. *Clin Oncol.* 2001; 19:2739–2745.

5. Stoll W. Phytopharmacon influences atrophic vaginal epithelium: Double blind study—cimicifuga vs. estrogenic substances. *Therapeuticum.* 1987;1:23–31.

6. Lehman-Willenbrock, E. Reidel, H. Clinical and endocrinologic examinations concerning therapy of climacteric symptoms following hysterectomy with remaining ovaries. *Zentralbl Gynakol* 1998;110:611–618.

7. Duker EM, Lopanski L, Jarry H, Wuttke W. Effects of extracts from *Cimifuga racemosa* on gonadotropin release in menopausal women and ovariectomized rats. *Planta Med* 1991;57: 420–424.

8. Stolze, H. An alternative to treat menopausal complaints. *Gynecology.* 1982; 3:14–16.

9. Warnecke G. Influencing menopausal symptoms with a phytotherapeutic agent: successful therapy with Cimicifuga mono-extract. *Med Welt.*1985;36:871–874.

10. Blumenthal M, ed. *The Complete German Commission E Monographs Therapeutic Guide to Herbal Medicines.* Austin, Tex: American Botanical Council; 1998.

11. Liske E. Therapeutic efficacy and safety of *Cimicifuga racemosa* for gynecologic disorders. *Adv Ther.* 1998;15:45–54.

Black Currant Oil (Ribes nigrum)

See Gamma-Linolenic Acid.

Borage Oil (Borago officinalis)

See Gamma-Linlenic Acid.

Boron

Originally known as essential in plants, boron, an ultratrace mineral, has recently been recognized as essential for some animals and thus is likely to be essential for humans. Boron is distributed throughout the body with the highest concentrations found in the bone, fingernails, teeth, hair, spleen, and thyroid. Although the functions of boron in the human body are unclear, research during more than 20 years has shown that boron may be involved in bone formation and maintenance (1).

Media and Marketing Claims	Efficacy
Prevents osteoporosis	NR
Prevents and treats osteoarthritis	NR
Increases muscle mass by raising testosterone level	NR
Improves memory	NR
Suppresses hot flashes	NR
Improves sex drive	NR

Advisory

- Tolerable Upper Intake Level for adults = 20 mg/day
- Doses above 50 mg associated with toxicity

Drug/Supplement Interactions

- No reported adverse interactions
- Theoretical interaction with estrogenic drugs

KEY POINTS

- There is evidence that boron deprivation can be detrimental to calcium metabolism, but currently no studies clearly demonstrate that boron supplements can prevent or treat osteoporosis. Boron appears to have raised estrogen levels, which may indirectly impact bone metabolism.

- There is a lack of well-controlled, clinical research supporting the role of boron in osteoarthritis. Large-scale, controlled studies are needed before boron can be recommended to treat this population.

- Despite the marketing of boron supplements as a way to increase testosterone, the limited research does not suggest that boron affects lean body mass, testosterone levels, or strength in body builders.

- There is preliminary evidence that chronically low-boron diets (< 0.25 mg/day for 42 days to 63 days) may have a negative effect on cognitive function. However, doses above the amount found naturally in the diet do not appear to enhance brain function.

- Although one small study reported that boron supplements (3 mg) mimicked some of the effects of estrogen therapy, there is currently no evidence from controlled clinical trials that supplemental boron reduces symptoms of menopause such as hot flashes in women.

- There are currently no trials testing the effect of boron on libido.

- In general, Americans appear to consume diets adequate in boron. Based on the limited evidence available, additional boron supplementation provides little or no further benefit if an individual consumes the recommended five fruit and vegetable servings per day, which supply approximately 1 mg to 10 mg boron. Supplementing with no more than 3 mg to 10 mg boron appears to be relatively safe but is probably not warranted, based on the current scientific evidence.

FOOD SOURCES

Non-citrus fruits and leafy vegetables are the main dietary sources of boron. Other rich sources include nuts, dried fruit, avocado, legumes, wine, cider, and beer. Dairy and meat products are low in boron. Coffee and milk, although low in boron, are the top two contributors of boron in the American diet because they are consumed in high amounts (2).

Food	Boron (µg/Serving) (2)*
Raisins (½ c)	1,760
Peanuts, roasted (⅓ c)	833
Wine (3.5 oz)	628
Applesauce (½ c)	342
Broccoli (½ c)	195
Coffee (1 c)	69
Milk, 2% (1 c)	44

Source: Data from Rainey CJ, Nyquist LA, Christensen RE, et al (2)
*Serving sizes calculated from values in Reference 2.

DOSAGE INFORMATION/BIOAVAILABILITY

There is no RDA or AI set for boron; however, boron researchers suggest daily intakes of approximately 1 mg/day (3, 4). The average American diet provides an estimated 0.96 mg to 1.17 mg boron/day (2, 4). Most boron supplements in the form of sodium borate, boron chelates (citrate, aspartate, glycinate), and sodium tetraborate decahydrate provide 3 mg doses and are often combined with other minerals such as calcium and magnesium. Absorption of dietary boron is inefficient because most of the boron is excreted in the urine after three to seven days (1).

B

RELEVANT RESEARCH

Boron and Bone Health

- In the first nutritional human study of boron, 12 postmenopausal women initially were fed a boron-deficient diet that provided 0.25 mg boron/2,000 calories for 119 days, and then subjects were fed the same diet with a supplement of 3 mg boron (sodium borate)/day for 48 days. Boron supplementation reduced total plasma calcium and altered calcium and magnesium metabolism, and elevated serum levels of 17β-estradiol and testosterone. The authors concluded: "Supplementation of a low-boron diet with an amount of boron commonly found in diets high in fruits and vegetables induces changes in postmenopausal women consistent with the prevention of calcium loss and bone demineralization" (5).

- Four men, nine postmenopausal women (five on estrogen therapy), and one premenopausal woman were fed a diet supplying 0.25 mg boron/2,000 calories for 63 days while living in a metabolic unit. They were then fed the same diet supplemented with 3 mg boron/day for 49 days. Women on estrogen therapy had significantly higher serum 17β-estradiol and plasma copper levels, specifically during the boron supplementation phase. Boron enhanced the effects of estrogen in women on estrogen therapy and mimicked some of these effects in men and postmenopausal women not taking estrogen. The authors suggested that because estrogen ingestion is beneficial for calcium metabolism, it may be beneficial for boron metabolism as well (6).

- Several animal studies have shown that boron deprivation has a negative effect on calcium and magnesium metabolism, and that the absorption and balance of these minerals improves when boron is supplemented (7).

Boron and Osteoarthritis

- A review article summarized evidence pointing to the potential beneficial role of boron in arthritis: (1) clinical evidence suggesting that subjects with arthritis have lower concentrations of boron in bone and synovial fluid than those without arthritis; (2) epidemiological evidence suggesting that in areas of the world where boron intakes are < 1.0 mg/day, the estimated arthritis incidence ranges from 20 percent to 70 percent, whereas where boron intakes are 3 mg to 10 mg/day, the incidence of arthritis is 0 percent to 10 percent (8). However, the author of the review has been criticized for basing his argument on "weak epidemiological evidence, hearsay and testimonials" (3). This article is included because it is cited to support claims that boron supplements benefit arthritis patients.

- In a double-blind, placebo-controlled pilot trial (not randomized), 20 subjects (17 women, mean age 65 y) with radiographically confirmed osteoarthritis were given 6 mg boron/day in the form of sodium tetraborate decahydrate or a placebo for five weeks. Twenty-five percent of the patients dropped out of the study. Boron supplementation improved symptoms in 5 out of 10 subjects, whereas only 1 of 10 subjects benefited in the placebo group. Statistical analyses were not performed because of small sample size (9). This study is included despite its limitations because it is cited to support to support claims that boron supplements benefit arthritis patients.

Boron and Body Building

- In a placebo-controlled (not blinded) study, 19 male body builders were randomly assigned to receive 2.5 mg boron/day or a placebo for seven weeks. There were no differences in testosterone levels, strength tests, or body mass between groups, indicating that boron supplementation was not beneficial in this study of young, male body builders (10).

Boron and Cognitive Function

- Three placebo-controlled, double-blind, randomized trials evaluated the effect of low vs high boron (0.25 mg vs 3.25 mg boron/2,000 calories) on a variety of cognitive and psychomotor tasks in healthy older adults (total n = 28 subjects) over a period of 105 days to 126 days. Low dietary boron resulted in significantly poorer performance than did higher boron intake on manual dexterity, eye-hand coordination, attention, perception, encoding, and short- and long-term memory tests. Electroencephalograms taken during boron depletion compared to those during high boron intake showed that low dietary boron depressed mental alertness (11).

SAFETY

- Boron has a low order of toxicity when consumed in amounts normally found in the diet (1, 3).
- Toxicity signs generally occur when boron intake exceeds 50 mg/day for an extended period of time. Symptoms include nausea, vomiting, fatigue, diarrhea, and dermatitis. High doses cause urinary riboflavin excretion (1).
- Large doses of boron (1,000 mg/kg) have been shown to interfere with gonad development in rats and cause testicular atrophy in dogs (3).

REFERENCES

1. Nielsen FH. Ultratrace minerals. In: Shils ME, Olson JA, Shike M, Ross AC, eds. *Modern Nutrition in Health and Disease.* 9th ed. Baltimore, Md: Williams & Wilkins; 1999:283–288.
2. Rainey CJ, Nyquist LA, Christensen RE, et al. Daily boron intake from the American Diet. *J Am Diet Assoc.* 1999;99:335–340.
3. Nielsen FH. Facts and fallacies about boron. *Nutr Today.* 1992;27:6–12.
4. Food and Nutrition Board, Institute of Medicine. *Dietary Reference Intakes: Vitamin A, Vitamin K, Arsenic, Boron, Chromium, Copper, Iodine, Iron, Manganese, Molybdenum, Nickel, Silicon, Vanadium, and Zinc.* Washington, DC: National Academy Press; 2001.
5. Nielsen FH, Hunt CD, Mullen LM, et al. Effect of dietary boron on mineral, estrogen, and testosterone metabolism in postmenopausal women. *FASEB J.* 1987;1:394–397.

6. Nielsen FH, Gallagher SK, Johnson LK, et al. Boron enhances and mimics some effects of estrogen therapy in postmenopausal women. *J Trace Elem Exp Med.* 1992;5:237–246.
7. Nielsen FH. Trace and ultratrace elements in health and disease. *Compr Ther.* 1991;17:20–26.
8. Newnham RE. Essentiality of boron for healthy bones and joints. *Environ Health Perspect.* 1994;102(suppl 7):83–85.
9. Travers RL, Rennie GC, Newnham RE. Boron and arthritis: the results of a double-blind pilot study. *J Nutr Med.* 1990;1:127–132.
10. Green NR, Ferrando AA. Plasma boron and the effects of boron supplementation in males. *Environ Health Perspect.* 1994;102(suppl 7):73–77.
11. Penland JG. Dietary boron, brain function, and cognitive performance. *Environ Health Perspect.* 1994;102(suppl 7):65–72.

Branched Chain Amino Acids (BCAA)

Branched-chain amino acids (isoleucine, leucine, and valine) are a group of essential amino acids that have been studied for their potential role in delaying central nervous system (CNS) fatigue, specifically in athletes. BCAA as ingested are not readily degraded by the liver but instead circulate and compete for uptake into the brain with the amino acid tryptophan. Tryptophan is a precursor to serotonin (5-hydroxytryptamine), which may depress the CNS and produce symptoms of fatigue. Research has shown that exercise increases the ratio of free tryptophan-BCAA, thus raising serotonin levels in the brain. There is also evidence that plasma BCAA levels decline during endurance exercise. Some researchers have proposed that supplementing with BCAA will lower this ratio and result in improved mental and physical performance, although the studies to date are inconclusive (1–3).

In addition to their purported benefits in athletes, BCAA have also been studied for their role in treating hepatic encephalopathy. BCAA circulate at unusually low levels in patients having liver failure compared to levels of the aromatic amino acids (phenylalanine, tyrosine, and tryptophan). Researchers have hypothesized that low levels of BCAA result in preferential brain uptake of the other amino acids, which are precursors to false neurotransmitters and may exacerbate encephalopathy (4). Although this theory has not been proven, BCAA are included in some enteral formulas specifically indicated for patients with liver diseases.

Media and Marketing Claims	Efficacy
Improves exercise performance by increasing stamina and mental concentration	↔
Builds muscle	NR

Advisory

Doses > 20 g may raise plasma ammonia to toxic levels and cause GI discomfort

Drug/Supplement Interactions

- No reported adverse interactions
- High doses of single amino acids could theoretically create imbalances of other amino acids in the body

KEY POINTS

- BCAA supplementation appears to lower the plasma free tryptophan to BCCA ratio and prevent the decline in plasma and muscle BCAA associated with exercise. However, ingestion of carbohydrates before, during, and after exercise also appears to have this effect on the blood and muscle, and is known to enhance exercise performance (1). Therefore, dietary carbohydrates are recommended to prolong exercise endurance because the ergogenic value of BCAA is still unproven.

- Field studies that have shown BCAA administration improves mental and physical performance have been criticized for the failure to control variables (exercise intensity, dietary intake), lack of matched controls, and subject bias. In general, controlled laboratory studies have not demonstrated any positive performance effect with BCAA supplementation, although some have shown improved mental performance.

- Preliminary studies in small numbers of subjects suggest that BCAA supplementation may attenuate muscle breakdown that occurs with exercise. More controlled research is needed in this area before conclusions can be made.

- Similarly, well-controlled research is needed to evaluate the potential effects of BCAA supplementation on body composition.

FOOD SOURCES

Leucine, isoleucine, and valine are amino acids found in protein-rich foods such as eggs, meat, poultry, fish, dairy products, and legumes.

Food	Isoleucine (mg)	Leucine (mg)	Valine (mg) (5)
Chicken breast (½)	1,409	2,002	1,324
Beef, ground, regular (3.5 oz)	1,022	1,797	1,106
Shrimp (3 oz)	862	1,411	836
Yogurt, nonfat (1 c)	711	1,310	1,076
Beans, pinto (1 c)	676	1,222	801
Egg (1)	343	538	384
Oatmeal (1 c)	248	459	335

Source: Data from Pennington (5)

DOSAGE INFORMATION/BIOAVAILABILITY

BCAA supplements are sold in pill and powder forms ranging from 7 g to 20 g per serving. BCAAs are also in some sports beverages with doses ranging from 1 g/L to 7 g/L.

RELEVANT RESEARCH

BCAA and Exercise Performance

- In a placebo-controlled (not blinded) study, 193 experienced runners were randomly assigned to drink 16 g BCAA in a 5 percent glucose beverage or a placebo (5 percent glucose drink) during a 30-km or 42.2-km race. The running performance, measured as time ratios for specific distances, was improved for the "slower runners" (3.05 hour to 3.30 hour) when BCAA were taken during the race. No improvement was seen in the faster runners (< 3.05 hour). A second part of this study examined the effects of 7.5-g BCAA on mental performance as measured by the Stroop Color and Word Test (CWT) during a 30-km cross-country race. Mental performance measured after the race was improved in runners supplemented with BCAA compared with mental performance measured before the 30-km (18.6-mile) race. In contrast, the CWT scores were similar when measured before and after the race in the placebo group (6). The authors concluded that BCAA ingestion during exercise improved both physical and mental performance, but other researchers have criticized choice of performance measures and lack of dietary control (1). In addition, the results should be viewed with caution because this study lacked blinding; thus, the potential for bias exists.

- In a double-blind, placebo-controlled study, 10 endurance-trained male athletes exercised to exhaustion on a cycle ergometer at 75 percent maximal power output. Subjects completed four cycling trials and received, at random, drinks containing (1) 6 percent sucrose (control); (2) 6 percent sucrose supplemented with 3 g tryptophan; (3) a low dose of BCAA (6 g); or (4) a high dose of BCAA (18 g). The rate of unidirectional tryptophan transport across the blood-brain barrier was calculated using an equation (Michaelis-Menten equation) that used the plasma concentrations of tryptophan and competing amino acids in the different treatments for kinetic parameters of transport of human brain capillaries *in vitro*. Plasma ammonia was increased at exhaustion in all four tests. However, the low and high BCAA-supplemented had significantly higher plasma ammonia levels compared to the control group. Both BCAA supplements were estimated to reduce brain tryptophan uptake by 8 percent to 12 percent, whereas tryptophan ingestion increased brain tryptophan uptake by an estimated 7- to 20-fold compared to the placebo. However, there were no differences in time to exhaustion between treatment groups, suggesting BCAA ingestion did not improve exercise performance (7).

- In a double-blind, placebo-controlled, randomized, crossover study, nine well-trained male cyclists were given a glucose solution alone, a glucose solution plus 18 g BCAA, or a placebo (water) during 100 km of cycling at maximal speed in a laboratory setting. Each trial was separated by one week. No difference in performance times was observed among the three trials, suggesting that BCAA had no effect on exercise performance in trained athletes (8).

- In a double-blind, crossover design study, seven endurance-trained male cyclists were given a 7 g BCAA solution or a placebo before cycling on a cycle ergometer for 1 hour at 70 percent maximal power output exercise followed by 20 minutes of maximal exercise. Every 10 minutes subjects rated their perceived exertion and mental fatigue on two scales. There were no differences in physical performance between the two trials. However, the ratings of perceived exertion and mental fatigue were significantly lower ($\downarrow$7 percent and $\downarrow$15 percent, respectively) when subjects were supplemented with the BCAA solution (9).

- In a double-blind, placebo-controlled, crossover design study, six female, well-trained soccer players were supplemented with 7.5 g BCAA in a carbohydrate solution or a carbohydrate solution alone (placebo) during two soccer games. Mental performance measured by the Stroop CWT was assessed 2 hours to 2.5 hours before the game and within 45 minutes after the end of the game. When subjects ingested BCAA drinks, mental performance on the Stroop CWT improved after as compared to before the game. No effect on mental performance was noted when subjects took placebos (10). The authors did not provide information on randomization, how the drink was administered, or whether beverage consumption was supervised.

- In a double-blind, placebo-controlled study, seven endurance-trained male cyclists performed exhaustive exercise with reduced muscle glycogen stores (measured by muscle biopsy) while ingesting BCAA in solution (90 mg BCAA/kg body weight in solution) or an isocaloric placebo. BCAA ingestion increased the muscle and plasma levels of BCAA by 135 percent and 57 percent, respectively, whereas the placebo trial resulted in no change in BCAA levels. In addition, there was a significant decrease in muscle glycogen during exercise in the placebo trial, whereas only a small decrease was found in the BCAA trial. The authors concluded that an increased supply of BCAA may have a sparing effect on muscle glycogen degradation during exercise (11).

- In a double-blind, placebo-controlled, crossover design study, 13 male and female subjects cycled at 40 percent VO_{2max} to exhaustion in the heat (34°C or 93°F, relative humidity 39 percent) while ingesting a BCAA drink or a placebo every 30 minutes. During the trial, female subjects consumed a total of 9.4 g BCAA in solution and male subjects consumed a total of 15.8 g BCAA. BCAA treatment increased plasma BCAA and decreased the plasma tryptophan:BCAA ratio. Compared to the placebo arm, BCAA ingestion resulted in significant improvement in cycle time to exhaustion compared to the placebo (153.1 ± 13.3 vs 137 ± 12.2 min). Cardiovascular responses (heart rate, mean arterial pressure) and thermoregulatory responses (skin and core body temperatures, sweat losses) and psychological measures of fatigue (rate of perceived exertion, ratings of perceived thermal sensations) were not different between treatments (12).

BCAA and Protein Degradation During Exercise

- In a placebo-controlled study, 58 male runners were supplemented with 7.5 g to 12 g BCAA in a carbohydrate drink or a placebo (carbohydrate drink without BCAA) during endurance races (26 subjects participated in a 30-km/18.6-mile cross country race; 32 participated in a 26.2-mile marathon race). In 17 of the subjects in the cross-country race and in 14 of the marathon runners, muscle biopsies were taken from the quadriceps one to two hours prior to the race and within 90 minutes (cross country) or 50 minutes (marathon) after the completion of the race. In the placebo group, both groups of runners experienced increases in muscle concentrations of the aromatic amino acids, tyrosine, phenylalanine, and the plasma levels of these amino acids were increased after the marathon. (Higher levels of tyrosine and phenylalanine may be markers of protein degradation because these amino acids are not taken up or metabolized by skeletal muscle.) However, BCAA-supplemented subjects experienced slower rates of increases in plasma and muscle levels of tyrosine and phenylalanine concentrations after both races. The authors proposed that an intake of BCAAs during exercise may prevent or decrease the net rate of protein breakdown caused by heavy exercise (13).

- In a controlled trial (not randomized or blinded), 16 male subjects were supplemented with 12 g BCAA or placebo daily for 14 days.

BCAA and Abdominal Fat

- In a controlled (not blinded) study, 25 competitive French wrestlers were randomly assigned to one of five diets for 19 days: (1) normocaloric diet—55 percent carbohydrate, 12 percent protein, 33 percent fat; (2) hypocaloric diet—55 percent carbohydrate, 12 percent protein, 33 percent fat; (3) hypocaloric diet enriched with 0.9 g/kg/day BCAA (51.9 g BCCA/100 g protein)—60 percent carbohydrate, 20 percent protein, 20 percent fat; (4) hypocaloric high-protein (6.1 g BCAA/100 g protein)—60 percent carbohydrate, 25 percent protein, 15 percent fat; or (5) hypocaloric low-protein diet—60 percent carbohydrate, 15 percent protein, 25 percent fat. The normocaloric diet provided 40 kcal/kg/day, whereas the other diets were isocaloric providing a daily energy intake 28 kcal/kg. All the meals were eaten in the same dining hall and subjects recorded their daily weighed-meals intake over seven successive days. A dietitian gave instructions about what to choose from the dining hall menu to obtain the desired diet. Activity levels were not controlled during the study. All subjects on the hypocaloric diets demonstrated reductions in body weight and body fat (measured by magnetic resonance imaging and skinfolds). However, subjects on hypocaloric diets taking BCAA supplements showed significant losses of abdominal visceral adipose tissue and preservation of lean body mass compared to the other diet groups. There were no differences in aerobic and strength tests between groups (14). The results of this study should be viewed with caution because it lacked blinding; thus, the potential for bias exists.

- In a placebo-controlled (not blinded) study, 24 subjects with type 2 diabetes (mean age = 45 y) were randomly assigned to one of four groups: (1) BCAA capsules providing 0.6 g BCAA/kg/day plus exercise (45 minutes cycling two times/week); (2) BCAA supplement without exercise; (3) isocaloric placebo and exercise; (4) placebo without exercise. All exercises were performed on a cycle ergometer supervised by researchers.

Food diaries were recorded by subjects daily for the first and last weeks of the study. After two months, BCAA supplementation had no effect on resting metabolic rate, VO_{2peak}; abdominal fat (measured by magnetic resonance imaging) and glucose metabolism were not altered by BCAA supplementation (15). Again, the results of this study should be viewed with caution because it lacked blinding; thus, the potential for bias exists.

SAFETY

- No long-term studies have assessed the safety of BCAA supplementation.

- Although no cases of toxicity occurred in any of the cited studies, one review article warned that large doses of BCAA (> 20 g) may increase plasma ammonia levels to toxic levels. Although acute ammonia toxicity is reversible, it may be serious enough to impair performance or induce central fatigue (1).

- Large doses of BCAA (> 20 g) may impair water absorption across the gut and cause gastrointestinal discomfort (1).

REFERENCES

1. Davis JM. Carbohydrates, branched-chain amino acids and endurance: the central fatigue hypothesis. *Int J Sport Nutr.* 1995;5:S29–S38.
2. Newsholme EA, Blomstrand E. The plasma level of some amino acids and physical and mental fatigue. *Experientia.* 1996;52:413–415.
3. Davis JM, Bailey SP. Possible mechanisms of central nervous system fatigue during exercise. *Med Sci Sports Exerc.* 1997;29:45–57.
4. Wolf L, Keutsch GT. Nutrition and infection. In: Shils ME, Olson JA, Shike M, Ross AC, eds. *Modern Nutrition in Health and Disease.* 9th ed. Baltimore, Md: Williams & Wilkins; 1999:1569–1588.
5. Pennington JAT. *Bowes & Church's Food Values of Portions Commonly Used.* 17th ed. Philadelphia, Pa: Lippincott-Raven Publishers; 1998.
6. Blomstrand E, Hassmen P, Ekblom B, et al. Administration of branched-chain amino acids during sustained exercise—effects on performance and on plasma concentration of some amino acids. *Eur J Appl Physiol.* 1991;63:83–88.
7. Van Hall G, Raaymakers J, Saris W, et al. Ingestion of branched-chain amino acids and tryptophan during sustained exercise in man: failure to affect performance. *J Physiol.* 1995; 486:789–794.
8. Madsen K, MacLean DA, Kiens B, et al. Effects of glucose, glucose plus branched-chain amino acids, or placebo on bike performance over 100 km. *J Appl Physiol.* 1996; 81:2644–2650.
9. Blomstrand E, Hassmen P, Ek S, et al. Influence of ingesting a solution of branched-chain amino acids on perceived exertion during exercise. *Acta Physiol Scand.* 1997; 159:41–49.

10. Blomstrand E, Hassmen P, Newsholme EA. Effect of branched-chain amino acid supplementation on mental performance. *Acta Physiol Scand.* 1991;143:225–226.

11. Blomstrand E, Ek S, Newsholme EA. Influence of ingesting a solution of branched-chain amino acids on plasma and muscle concentrations of amino acids during prolonged submaximal exercise. *Nutrition.* 1996;12:485–490.

12. Mittleman KD, Ricci MR, Bailey SP. Branched-chain amino acids prolong exercise during heat stress in men and women. *Med Sci Sports Exerc.* 1998;30:83–91.

13. Blomstrand E, Newsholme EA. Effect of branched-chain amino acid supplementation on the exercise-induced change in aromatic amino acid concentrations in human muscle. *Acta Physiol Scand.* 1992;146:293–298.

14. Mourier A, Bigard AX, de Kerviler E, et al. Combined effects of caloric restriction and branched chain amino acid supplementation on body composition and exercise performance parameters in elite wrestlers. *Int J Sports Med.* 1997;18:47–55.

15. Mourier A, Gautier JF, de Kerviler E, et al. Mobilization of visceral adipose tissue related to the improvement in insulin sensitivity in response to physical training in NIDDM: effect of branched-chain amino acid supplements. *Diabetes Care.* 1997;20:385–391.

Bromelain

Bromelain is the name that refers to proteases extracted from the stem and fruit of pineapple (*Ananas comosus*). In addition to its proteolytic fraction, bromelain also contains peroxidase, acid phosphatase, protease inhibitors, and calcium. It has been used throughout Japan, Europe, and South America to treat inflammation and edema resulting from burns, trauma, and athletic injuries. One of bromelain's proposed mechanisms of action is generally believed to be through direct or indirect effects on inflammatory mediators. Specifically, bromelain breaks down fibrin, an activator of pro-inflammatory prostaglandins responsible for clot formation and fluid accumulation. It may also stimulate the conversion of plasminogen to plasmin, causing an increase in fibrinolysis (1–3).

Media and Marketing Claims	Efficacy
Good for respiratory infections and enhances action of antibiotics	↔
Anti-inflammatory—speeds healing from surgery and sports injuries	NR
Reduces angina, lowers blood pressure, and improves other cardiovascular conditions	NR
Anticancer agent	NR
Digestive aid	NR
Reduces diarrhea	NR

Advisory

- No reported serious adverse effects
- Should be monitored by physician if individual is taking anticoagulant medications
- Should be avoided prior to surgery due to potential blood-thinning effects

Drug/Supplement Interactions

- May increase bleeding when taken with other blood-thinning drugs or supplements (ie, coumadin, warfarin, garlic, ginger, ginkgo biloba, vitamin E, flaxseed, bromelain, dong quai, fish oil, aspirin); should be monitored by a physician
- May increase blood levels of antibiotics (amoxicillin, erythromycin, penicillin)

KEY POINTS

- There is preliminary evidence from trials in the 1960s that bromelain has a beneficial effect on some, but not all, symptoms of sinusitis. In addition, some studies have suggested that bromelain may potentiate the action of antibiotics. However, there is not enough quality research to make therapeutic claims. Updated, well-designed clinical trials are needed.

- Insufficient evidence exists to support the anti-inflammatory properties of bromelain. The positive results reported in a few human studies from the 1960s need to be replicated in well-designed and adequately controlled trials.

- There is currently no valid scientific evidence in humans that bromelain intake has beneficial effects on factors that contribute to cardiovascular disease. Well-designed, controlled clinical human trials are needed.

- At this time, there is no evidence from controlled human trials that bromelain prevents and/or treats cancer. In preliminary *in vitro* studies, bromelain and pancreatin in combination with other enzymes appear to slow tumor growth. These enzymes also appear to increase host defense in healthy individuals. Additional controlled research in humans is needed to verify its potential therapeutic benefit.

- Bromelain contains proteolytic enzymes, like those found in pancreatin, and may be useful in treating clinically documented pancreatic insufficiency. However, the effect of bromelain in digestive function of healthy individuals has not been tested in controlled clinical trials (*see* Pancreatin).

- There is preliminary evidence from *in vitro* and animal studies that bromelain inhibits diarrhea-causing bacteria. Controlled research is needed in humans.

FOOD SOURCES

Concentrated amounts are found in pineapple stems, and smaller amounts of bromelain are also found in the flesh of the fruit.

B

DOSAGE INFORMATION/BIOAVAILABILITY

Bromelain is sold individually or in combination with other enzymes (pancreatin, papain, betaine, lactase, cellulase). There has been no scientific agreement on how to measure the proteolytic activity of bromelain. Several different designations are used to describe the proteolytic activity of bromelain. Proteases in bromelain are tested to determine how fast they dissolve a protein such as gelatin or casein. Three common measures of activity include: Rorer units (ru), gelatin-dissolving units (gdu), and milk-clotting units (mcu). One gram of bromelain standardized to 2,000 mcu activity is approximately equivalent to 1 g with 1,200 gdu of activity or 8 g with 100,000 ru of activity) (3). Manufacturers recommend taking anywhere from 500 mg/day to 2,000 mg/day divided into three or four doses. However, because proteolytic activity is measured differently in various products, it is difficult to obtain a consistent, standard dose. Highly purified bromelain may have no activity (4).

There is limited research on the absorption and bioavailability of bromelain in humans. In one study completed in 1964, 60 mg bromelain in enteric-coated tablets increased the ability of serum to digest casein, which the authors indicated was a measure of intestinal absorption of bromelain (5). In a rat study, bromelain was absorbed from the gastrointestinal tract after oral administration and was observable in serum after one hour of ingestion (6).

RELEVANT STUDIES

- Note: Many of the human studies on bromelain were completed in the 1960s and 1970s and lacked proper control, randomization, and appropriate statistical analysis. Some of these poorly designed trials are reported here because they are frequently cited to support media and marketing claims.

Bromelain and Sinusitis/Bronchitis Infections

- In a double-blind, placebo-controlled study completed in 1967, 49 patients with sinusitis (ages 9 y to 74 y) selected from one physician's private practice were randomized to receive 160 mg bromelain (400,000 ru of proteolytic activity) or a placebo for six days. All patients received standard, prescribed antibiotic medication for six days. Severity of symptoms was measured by the physician before and after treatment. There was a significant improvement in sinusitis symptoms (nasal discomfort, breathing difficulty, and pain), the mean duration of standard therapy required in patients (9.9 days vs 16.5 days), and the overall clinical rating among the bromelain-treated subjects compared to the placebo. However, there were no statistical differences between groups for the resolution of edema and inflammation of the nasal mucosa or headache relief. There were no reported adverse effects (7).

- In a double-blind, placebo-controlled study completed in 1967, 48 patients with moderate to severe sinusitis symptoms (ages 9 y to 70 y) were given bromelain (400,000 ru of proteolytic activity) or a placebo for six days. Randomization of subjects to treatment was not indicated. All patients were given standard therapy for sinusitis. Patients were evaluated by a physician before, during, and at the end of the study. There were no differences between groups in symptoms of nasal discharge, breathing difficulty, headache, and overall clinical rating. However, bromelain-treated subjects (83 percent) had a significant reduction in nasal mucosal inflammation compared to the placebo (52 percent). Among patients not taking antibiotics, there was a significant difference in complete resolution of nasal mucosal inflammation in the bromelain group (85 percent) compared to the placebo (40 percent), but no other significant differences were noted in the other parameters measured (8).

Bromelain and Antibiotic Activity

- Some studies have reported that bromelain increases the absorption of antibiotics as documented by higher blood, tissue, and urine levels of medication (9–11), although one study failed to report this effect (12).

Bromelain and Inflammation/Sports Injuries/Surgery

- Researchers induced muscle injury in 75 hamsters after which they were orally administered 10 mg bromelain/kg daily or no treatment for 14 days. The degree of muscle injury was evaluated using a measure of functional status—the maximum isometric tetanic force (P_o). The maximal force (P_o) of injured muscles returned to control levels in bromelain-treated hamsters but not in untreated animals. No negative side-effects of bromelain were observed in noninjured skeletal muscle. The authors suggested that bromelain may have worked by inhibiting pro-inflammatory prostaglandins, the inflammatory mediator bradykinin, and oxygen free radicals, but these possibilities were not tested (13).

- In a double-blind, placebo-controlled study completed in 1960, 146 amateur boxers with bruises to the face and hematomas of the eye orbits, lips, ears, chest, and arms received 160 mg bromelain divided into four doses, or a placebo for 14 days. At day 4, 78 percent of the bromelain treated subjects were completely cleared of bruising compared to 15 percent in the placebo group. Statistical significance was not tested (14). Because statistical analyses were not performed, it is impossible to assess the degree to which the findings were likely attributable to chance alone.

- In a double-blind, controlled study completed in 1966, 154 surgical patients (76 of 154 subjects were children ages 4 y to 12 y) were randomized to receive 400 mg bromelain divided into four doses/day (proteolytic activity not specified) or no treatment (control). Bromelain was administered one day before, and four days after, facial plastic surgery. The type of surgical procedures, and gender and age of adult subjects were not described. Surgeons evaluated postoperative edema/swelling on the first through the fourth postoperative day. There were no significant differences between groups on the number of postoperative infections, hematomas, or other complications that could affect swelling. Bromelain did not affect the average rate of postoperative edema as assessed by surgeons when compared to controls (15).

- Two other studies completed in the 1960s reported that oral administration of bromelain reduced the degree and duration of swelling and pain with oral surgery (16, 17). However, one trial did not perform statistical analyses and the other was neither controlled nor blinded, making these studies difficult to evaluate.

Bromelain and Cardiovascular Disease

- *In vitro* and animal studies have shown that bromelain decreases platelet aggregation (2, 4, 18, 19).

- In a double-blind, placebo-controlled trial completed in 1969, 73 patients hospitalized (ages 25 y to 70 y) for acute thrombophlebitis were randomized to receive eight tablets of enteric-coated bromelain (1 tablet = 50,000 ru of proteolytic activity) or a placebo daily for eight days in addition to standard medication. Patients were examined daily and impressions were recorded of the severity of inflammation. Symptoms of inflammation (pain, edema, redness, tenderness, elevated skin temperature, and disability) were also evaluated. At the end of the trial, a clinician rated each patient's overall condition. Although there was a trend toward mean improvement in all symptoms of inflammation in the bromelain group, only the symptom of redness reached statistical significance. The observer's overall evaluation of improvement with respect to inflammation was better in the bromelain group than the group using the placebo; however, statistical analyses were not reported for this measure. No adverse effects were reported (20).

Bromelain (and Other Proteases) and Cancer

- In an *ex vivo* study, blood samples from healthy volunteers (n = 44) who were given single oral doses of a commercial preparation of combined proteolytic enzymes (33 mg pancreatin, 15 mg bromelain, 20 mg papain [papaya enzyme], 8 mg trypsin, and 0.3 mg chymotrypsin) were assessed. The polyenzyme preparation containing bromelain stimulated the production of tumor necrosis factor-α (TNF-α), interleukin-1β, and interleukin-6 in peripheral-blood mononuclear cells of healthy donors. TNF-α has been identified as a stimulator of immune defense against tumor cells, but oral ingestion of this cytokine has been associated with toxicity (21).

- In a placebo-controlled study (not double-blind or randomized), 28 healthy subjects were given 10 to 20 tablets (dose not specified) of a commercial preparation of proteolytic enzymes (pancreatin, bromelain, papain, trypsin, and chymotrypsin), 8 subjects received placebo, and 16 subjects served as controls. Blood samples were drawn at 0, 2, 4, 6, and 8 hours after treatment. Enzyme treatment resulted in a time-dependent, significant increase in the release of reactive oxygen species (ROS) in polymorphonuclear neutrophils, the functional significance of which is unknown; however, ROS may mediate tumorcidal activity. (Note: ROS may also damage healthy tissues; however, this effect was not tested.) In the placebo and control subjects, there was no elevation of ROS production. In an *in vitro* experiment in the same study, enzymes stimulated the cytotoxic capacity of polymorphonuclear cells against tumor cells (22).

- Mice with implanted Lewis lung cancer cells had decreased lung metastasis with bromelain administration compared to controls (23, 24). In one study, the antimetastatic action was demonstrated by active and inactive bromelain preparations, suggesting that bromelain's action may be caused by components other than the proteolytic fractions (25).

Bromelain and Antibacterial Properties

- In an *in vitro* experiment, bromelain demonstrated antisecretory properties against *Vibrio cholerae* and *Escherichia coli* (26). Studies in piglets and a rabbit model of diarrhea reported that oral intake of enteric-coated bromelain inhibited enterotoxigenic *E coli* receptor activity in the small intestine and protected animals against diarrhea and diarrhea-induced death (27, 28).

SAFETY

- Doses of up to 10 g/kg of bromelain in mice and rats had no teratogenic or carcinogenic effects. Dogs administered 750 mg bromelain/kg body weight daily for six months showed no toxic effects (2, 3).
- Bromelain may increase blood levels of antibiotics such as tetracycline if administered at the same time (9–11).
- Though preliminary evidence suggests bromelain may decrease platelet activity (29), there is no evidence that it increases bleeding time (2). Additional research is needed to thoroughly investigate this possibility. However, as a precaution, individuals on anticoagulant therapy without pancreatic insufficiency should not take bromelain supplements without the advice of their physician.
- Occupational exposure to bromelain resulted in asthma and rhinitis in a 58-year-old pharmaceutical worker. Bromelain was reported to induce IgE-mediated respiratory and gastrointestinal allergic reactions in sensitive individuals with positive RAST and skin tests to bromelain and papain (papaya enzyme) (30).
- According to a review, dietary fiber interferes with the activity of enzymes *in vitro* and *in vivo* (31). The effect of high-fiber foods coingested with bromelain is uncertain.

REFERENCES

1. Taussig SJ, Yokoyama MM, Chinen A, et al. Bromelain: a proteolytic enzyme and its clinical application. A review. *Hiroshima J Med Sci.* 1975;24:185–193.
2. Taussig SJ, Batki S. Bromelain, the enzyme complex of pineapple (Annas comosus) and its clinical application. An update. *J Ethnopharmacol.* 1988;22:191–203.
3. Anonymous. Bromelain. *Altern Med Rev.* 1998;3:302–305.
4. Taussig SJ. The mechanism of the physiological action of bromelain. *Med Hypotheses.* 1980;6:99–104.
5. Miller JM, Opher AW. The increased proteolytic activity of human blood serum after the oral administration of bromelain. *Exp Med Surg.* 1964;22:277–280.
6. White RR, Crawley EH, Vellini M, et al. Bioavailability of ^{125}I-bromelain after oral administration to rats. *Biopharm Drug Dispos.* 1988;9:397–403.
7. Seltzer AP. Adjunctive use of bromelains in sinusitis: a controlled study. *Eye Ear Nose Throat Mon.* 1967;46:1281–1288.

B

8. Ryan RE. A double-blind clinical evaluation of bromelains in the treatment of acute sinusitis. *Headache.* 1967;7:13–17.

9. Tinozzi S, Venegoni A. Effect of bromelain on serum and tissue levels of Amoxycillin. *Drugs Exp Clin Res.* 1978;4:39–44.

10. Luerti M, Vignali ML. Influence of bromelain on penetration of antibiotics in uterus, salpinx, and ovary. *Drugs Exp Clin Res.* 1978;4:45–48.

11. Rimoldi R, Ginesu F, Giura R. The use of bromelain in pneumological therapy. *Drugs Exp Clin Res.* 1978;4:55–66.

12. Bradbrook ID, Morrison PJ, Rogers HJ. The effect of bromelain on the absorption of orally administered tetracycline. *Br J Clin Pharmacol.* 1978;6:552–554.

13. Walker JA, Cerny FJ, Cotter JR, et al. Attenuation of contraction-induced skeletal muscle injury by bromelain. *Med Sci Sports Exerc.* 1992;24:20–25.

14. Blonstein JL. Control of swelling in boxing injuries. *Practitioner.* 1964;193:334.

15. Gylling U, Rintala A, Taipale S, et al. The effect of a proteolytic enzyme combinate (bromelain) on the postoperative oedema by oral application. A clinical and experimental study. *Acta Chir Scand.* 1966;131:193–196.

16. Tassman GC, Zafran JN, Zayon GM. Evaluation of a plant proteolytic enzyme for the control of inflammation and pain. *J Dent Med.* 1964;19:73–77.

17. Tassman GC, Zafran JN, Zayon GM. A double-blind crossover study of a plant proteolytic enzyme in oral surgery. *J Dent Med.* 1965;20:51–54.

18. Metzig C, Grabowska E, Eckert K, et al. Bromelain proteases reduce human platelet aggregation *in vitro,* adhesion to bovine endothelial cells, and thrombus formation in rat vessels in vivo. *In Vivo.* 1999;13:7–12.

19. Heinicke RM, Van der Wal M, Yokoyama MM. Effect of bromelain (Ananase) on human platelet aggregation. *Experientia.* 1972;28:844–845.

20. Seligman B. Oral bromelains as adjuncts in the treatment of acute thrombophlebitis. *Angiology.* 1969;20:22–26.

21. Desser L, Rehberger A, Kokron E, et al. Cytokine synthesis in human peripheral blood mononuclear cells after oral administration of polyenzyme preparations. *Oncology.* 1993;50:403–407.

22. Zavadova E, Desser L, Mohr T. Stimulation of reactive oxygen species production and cytotoxicity in human neutrophils in vitro and after oral administration of a polyenzyme preparation. *Cancer Biother.* 1995;10:147–152.

23. Batkin S, Taussig SJ, Szekerczes J. Modulation of pulmonary metastasis (Lewis lung carcinoma) by bromelain, an extract of the pineapple stem. *Cancer Invest.* 1988;6:241–242.

24. Taussig SJ, Szekerczes J, Batkin S. Inhibition of tumor growth in vitro by bromelain, an extract of the pineapple plant (Ananas comosus). *Planta Med.* 1985;6:538–539.

25. Batkin S, Taussig SJ, Szekerezes J. Antimetastatic effect of bromelain with or without its proteolytic and anticoagulant activity. *J Cancer Res Clin Oncol.* 1988;114:507–508.

26. Mynott TL, Guandalini S, Raimondi F, et al. Bromelain prevents secretion caused by *Vibrio cholerae* and *Escherichia coli* enterotoxins in rabbit ileum in vitro. *Gastroenterology.* 1997;113:175–184.

27. Mynott TL, Luke RKJ, Chandler DS. Oral administration of protease inhibits entero-

toxigenic Escherichia coli (ETEC) receptor activity in piglet small intestine. *Gut.* 1996;38:28–32.

28. Chandler DS, Mynott TL. Bromelain protects piglets from diarrhea caused by oral challenge with K88-positive enterotoxigenic *Escherichia coli. Gut.* 1998;43:196–202.

29. Felton GE. Fibrinolytic and antithrombotic action of bromelain may eliminate thrombosis in heart patients. *Med Hypotheses.* 1980;6:1123–1133.

30. Baur X, Fruhmann G. Allergic reactions, including asthma, to the pineapple protease bromelain following occupational exposure. *Clin Allergy.* 1979;9:443–450.

31. Leng-Peschlow E. Interference of dietary fibres with gastrointestinal enzymes *in vitro. Digestion.* 1989;44:200–210.

Calcium

Calcium is well known for its structural role in bones and teeth. Ninety-nine percent of the calcium in the body is found in the skeleton, with the remaining one percent in the blood, lymph, and other body fluids. As part of every cell, calcium also acts as a messenger directing cell function, hormone action, and nerve impulses. In order to consistently provide the calcium ions necessary for these functions, serum calcium levels are closely regulated by calcitonin, parathyroid hormone, and vitamin D, which affect calcium transport in the intestine, bone, and kidney (1).

Bone density (calcium deposition) increases during the first 25 y to 30 y of life, and gradually declines with age. In 1993, the FDA reviewed research demonstrating the benefit of supplemental calcium and approved the health claim for food and supplement labels stating that calcium reduces the risk of osteoporosis (2). The recent revisions by the Food and Nutrition Board of the National Academy of Sciences (NAS) increased calcium recommendations close to those set by the National Institutes of Health (NIH) Consensus Development Conference on Optimal Calcium Intake in 1994 (3). Under the new dietary reference intakes (DRIs), the Adequate Intake (AI) for calcium for young adults (9 y to 18 y), adults aged 19 to 50, and adults over 50 years is 1,300 mg, 1,000 mg, and 1,200 mg, respectively (4).

Media and Marketing Claims	Efficacy
Prevents osteoporosis	↑
Reduces blood pressure	↑?
Decreases colon cancer risk	↔
Helps reduce symptoms of PMS	↔

Advisory

- Tolerable Upper Intake Level for adults = 2,500 mg/day
- Supplementation not advisable for patients with absorptive hypercalciuria, primary hyperthyroidism, or sarcoidosis

- Doses > 4,000 mg may increase blood calcium levels and cause renal damage and milk alkali syndrome

Drug/Supplement Interactions

- May interfere with absorption of the following drugs: salicylates; biphosphates; tetracyclines; thyroid hormones (synthroid, levothyroid); fluoroquinolones (ciprofloxacin)
- Users of thiazide diuretics are at increased risk of developing milk alkali syndrome from high doses of calcium
- Calcium competes for absorption with the following nutrients: fluoride, iron, zinc, magnesium
- Calcium depletion may occur with chronic use of corticosteroids and laxatives (magnesium salts)

KEY POINTS

- There is significant evidence linking calcium supplementation to increased bone mineral density in the elderly and adolescent population. This relationship has been recognized by the NIH, NAS, and the FDA. According to one review article, the increase in BMD from calcium supplementation could reduce fracture rates by as much as 50 percent (5).

- There may be a small reduction in systolic blood pressure, but not diastolic blood pressure with calcium supplementation according to two meta-analyses. However, a greater blood pressure reduction (systolic and diastolic) was apparent in the DASH study where subjects consumed a 25 percent fat diet (low in saturated fat) rich in low-fat dairy products, fruits and vegetables, and whole grains. The average daily dietary calcium intake in the DASH study was 1,265 mg/day.

- The relationship between calcium supplements and colon cancer has not been adequately determined. One large study found a reduced risk of developing recurrent adenomas in subjects supplemented with calcium. Uncontrolled trials have demonstrated a reduction in colon cancer cell proliferation rates, whereas other larger, controlled trials have produced conflicting reports.

- There is preliminary evidence that calcium supplementation may improve symptoms associated with PMS. Although more research is needed, the amount of calcium supplemented in these studies would be beneficial for women to consume whether or not it affects PMS.

- Individuals should be encouraged to meet their calcium requirements with dietary sources when possible. However, because it can be difficult for some people to consume enough calcium to meet the AI (particularly preadolescent and adolescent girls, the elderly, or those with lactose intolerance), supplements may be needed.

FOOD SOURCES

Food	Calcium (mg)
Milk, nonfat (1 c)	302
Juice, orange (calcium-fortified) (6 oz)	200
Milk, whole (1 c)	291
Yogurt, low-fat (1 c)	314
Cheese, mozzarella, part skim (1 oz)	183
Tofu, raw (calcium-precipitated) (½ c)	130
Almonds, dry roasted (1 oz)	80
Kale, (½ c)	47
Beans, garbanzo (½ c)	40
Broccoli, (½ c)	36
Beans, kidney (½ c)	25
Egg (1)	25

Source: Data from Pennington (6)

DOSAGE INFORMATION/BIOAVAILABILITY

Calcium supplements are available in multivitamin/mineral supplements or in single preparations. Calcium is found in the form of calcium carbonate (the form used in antacids), citrate, citrate malate, phosphate, gluconate, lactate, calcium from dolomite (calcium magnesium carbonate), or bone meal. In 1981, the FDA issued a warning against using dolomite, bone meal or oyster shell calcium because of the presence of high levels of lead (7). Supplements typically provide 250 mg to 1,000 mg elemental calcium, often with added vitamin D and magnesium. If labels do not express calcium as "elemental," assume the elemental calcium is 40 percent, 21 percent, 13 percent, and 9 percent from carbonate, citrate, lactate, and gluconate, respectively (2) (i.e., a label that states it supplies 1,000 mg calcium carbonate actually contains 400 mg elemental calcium).

In one study, subjects with achlorhydria absorbed calcium citrate more efficiently than carbonate supplements when taken on an empty stomach, but both were equally absorbed when taken with a meal (8). Similarly, in healthy women, calcium citrate supplements were more bioavailable than carbonate when taken on an empty stomach (9,10). The NIH Consensus Statement reported that calcium absorption is most efficient at individual doses of 500 mg or less and when taken between meals in the form of calcium citrate (4). Homebound, institutionalized, or other individuals who lack exposure to the sun may require supplemental vitamin D to ensure adequate calcium absorption (3).

Calcium absorption can be affected by a variety of food factors. Foods high in oxalates (spinach) or phytates (wheat bran) have less available calcium than foods without these constituents (1). High-protein and/or high-sodium diets increase urinary calcium excretion (for each 50 g increment in dietary protein, 60 mg calcium is excreted in urine) (1).

RELEVANT RESEARCH

Calcium and Bone Mineral Density (BMD)/Osteoporosis

- In a double-blind, placebo-controlled study, 240 postmenopausal women were randomized to receive 1,000 mg elemental calcium as calcium carbonate plus 560 IU vitamin D_3 or a placebo for two years. There was a significant increase in the bone mass density (BMD) of the lumbar spine in calcium-supplemented subjects at one and two years. An insignificant trend of greater hip BMD was seen with calcium. There were no significant changes from baseline values noted in the BMD of the distal forearm in either group. The authors concluded: "A positive effect on BMD was demonstrated, even in a group of early postmenopausal women, with a fairly good initial calcium and vitamin D status" (11).

- Researchers reviewed clinical trials that measured BMD of postmenopausal women to evaluate whether calcium supplementation influenced the efficacy of estrogen therapy on bone mass change. Of the 31 estrogen trials, 20 used a supplement or modified the diet (total 1,183 mg calcium/day), and 11 did not (total 563 mg calcium/day). The mean BMD of the lumbar spine, femoral neck, and forearm were significantly greater in studies providing calcium with estrogen therapy compared to estrogen alone (12).

- In a placebo-controlled study, 60 older postmenopausal women were randomized to receive one of three treatments for two years: (1) milk supplementation (4 cups— mean calcium intake = 1,028 mg/day); (2) 1,000 mg calcium carbonate divided into two doses (mean calcium intake = 1,633 mg/day); or (3) a placebo (mean dietary calcium intake = 683 mg/day). The placebo subjects had significant losses in their greater trochanteric (hip) BMD, whereas the calcium-supplemented group had no bone loss and showed a significant increase in spinal and femoral neck BMD. The dietary group sustained minimal losses from the greater trochanteric BMD, but this did not reach statistical significance. In all groups, serum 25-OH vitamin D levels declined during the winter and parathyroid hormone (PTH) levels increased. The authors concluded: "Calcium supplementation prevents bone loss in elderly women by suppressing bone turnover during the winter when serum 25-OH vitamin D declines and serum PTH increases" (13).

- In a double-blind, placebo-controlled study, two groups of elderly women (> 60 y), one with prevalent fractures (n = 94) and the other without (n = 103) were randomized to receive 1,200 mg calcium as calcium carbonate or a placebo for an average of four years. Annual lateral spine radiographs and semiannual forearm bone density were obtained during 4.3 years. The subjects with fractures supplemented with calcium (15 of 53) had significantly fewer incident fractures than the subjects with fractures using the placebo (21 of 41). Calcium supplementation did not reduce the rate of incident fractures in the subjects without fractures. In subjects with fractures, calcium-supplemented subjects had significantly greater forearm bone mass than did placebo subjects. There were no statistical differences in subjects without fractures The authors concluded that in elderly, postmenopausal women with spinal fractures and self-selected calcium intakes of < 1,000 mg/day, a calcium supplement may reduce the incidence of spinal fractures and halt bone loss (14).

- In a placebo-controlled study, 389 subjects > 65 years were randomized to receive 500 mg calcium plus 700 IU vitamin D_3/day or a placebo for three years. In calcium plus vitamin D-supplemented subjects, there was a significantly greater BMD at the femoral neck and spine and total-body BMD after one year compared to placebo, which remained significant for total body BMD in the following two years after cessation of the intervention. Of the 37 subjects who experienced nonvertebral fractures during the study, significantly more were in the placebo group (n = 26) than the supplemented group (n = 11) (15).

- To determine whether BMD gains remained when calcium supplements were discontinued, subjects from the above study were followed for two years. In the female subjects, there were no lasting benefits in total body BMD or at any bone site. In the male subjects, supplement-induced increases in spinal and femoral neck BMD were lost during the two years of stopping calcium supplementation. However, small benefits in total body BMD remained (16).

- In a double-blind, placebo-controlled trial, 84 elderly women (54 y to 74 y) more than 10 years post-menopause were randomized to receive 1,000 mg elemental calcium or a placebo daily for four years. BMD was assessed using dual-energy X-ray absorptiometry at two and four years. In the treatment group, 49 subjects declined to continue after the first two years ("noncompliant"), and only 14 took the supplements for the entire duration of the study. The control group (mean calcium = 952 mg/day) lost significantly more bone than the calcium-supplemented group (mean calcium = 1,988 mg/day) at all sites of the hip and ankle. After two years, the noncompliant group lost significantly more bone at the ankle than the supplement group. No overall bone loss in the spine was seen in any group during the four years (17).

- In a double-blind, placebo-controlled study of adolescent twins, one twin in each pair (42 female twin pairs, mean age = 14 y) was randomized to receive 1,000 mg calcium or a placebo daily for 12 to 18 months. Compliance was similar in both groups (85 percent placebo, 83 percent calcium). At the end of the first six months, there was a significant within pair difference at the spine and hip, which stabilized throughout the remainder of the study. Compared to placebo, calcium-supplemented subjects had a significant increase in BMD at the spine after 18 months (18).

Calcium and Hypertension

- According to a meta-analysis on 22 randomized clinical trials testing the effect of calcium supplements (500 mg to 2,000 mg) on blood pressure in hypertensive and normotensive subjects (n = 1,231), pooled estimates showed a significant decrease in systolic blood pressure (—1.68 mm Hg) with calcium supplementation for hypertensive patients. There was also a significant decrease in systolic blood pressure for the overall sample of normotensive and hypertensive subjects. There was no significant effect on diastolic blood pressure in either subgroup. The authors concluded: "The effect was too small to support the use of calcium supplementation for preventing or treating hypertension" (19).

- A separate meta-analysis was conducted on 33 randomized, controlled trials (n = 2,412) lasting at least two weeks that tested the effect of calcium supplementation (800 mg to 2,000 mg) on blood pressure in normotensive and hypertensive subjects. The pooled analysis showed a significant reduction in systolic blood pressure and an insignificant reduction in diastolic blood pressure. The authors concluded: "Calcium supplementation may lead to a small reduction in systolic but not diastolic blood pressure. The results do not exclude a larger, important effect of calcium on blood pressure in subpopulations. In particular, further studies should address the hypothesis that inadequate calcium intake is associated with increased blood pressure that can be corrected with calcium supplementation" (20).

- In a double-blind, placebo-controlled study, 193 male and female subjects (aged 30 y to 74 y) were randomized to receive 1 to 2 g/day of elemental calcium or placebo daily for four months (for cholesterol determinations) and six months (for blood pressure data). Serum total cholesterol, HDL cholesterol, and systolic and diastolic blood were measured. There was no change in blood pressure until six months, when the mean systolic and diastolic blood pressure dropped by a half percent, but this was not statistically significant. There was also a trend toward a two to four percent reduction in total cholesterol, but this was not statistically significant (21).

- In a randomized, multicenter trial (Dietary Approaches to Stop Hypertension—DASH), 459 subjects with systolic blood pressure < 160 mm Hg and diastolic blood pressures of 80 mm Hg to 95 mm Hg were randomized to one of three diets for eight weeks: (1) control diet—low in fruits and vegetables and low-fat dairy, and a fat content typical of the average diet in the U.S. (dietary fat = 37 percent; average dietary calcium intake = 443 mg); (2) diet rich in fruits and vegetables (dietary fat = 37 percent fat; average calcium intake = 534 mg); or (3) combination diet rich in fruits and vegetables and low-fat dairy products and with reduced saturated fat and total fat (dietary fat = 25 percent; average calcium intake = 1,265 mg). Subjects consumed lunch or dinner on site on weekdays and picked up all other meals from the preparation site. Prior to the study, all subjects were fed control diets for three weeks. Sodium intake and body weight were maintained at constant levels. The combination diet resulted in a significant reduction in systolic (-5.0 mm Hg) and diastolic (-3.0 mm Hg) blood pressure compared to subjects on the control diet. The fruits and vegetable diet resulted in a significant reduction of systolic (-2.8 mm Hg) and diastolic (-1.1 mm Hg) compared to the control diet. Among the 133 subjects with hypertension, the combination diet significantly reduced systolic and diastolic pressure by 11.4 and 5.5 mm Hg more, respectively, than did the control diet. Subjects without hypertension who consumed the combination diet also experienced significant reductions of systolic and diastolic blood pressure by 3.5 mm Hg and 2.1 mm Hg. The authors concluded that a diet rich in fruits, vegetables, and low-fat dairy foods and with reduced saturated and total fat can substantially lower blood pressure (22). They found similar results when data were

C

analyzed by subgroups (race, sex, age, BMI, years of education, income, physical activity, alcohol intake, and hypertension status) (23).

- One review of nine controlled studies and a meta-analysis of six controlled studies concluded that calcium supplementation during pregnancy appears to reduce the risk of pregnancy-induced hypertension, especially in women at high risk and in those with low dietary calcium intakes (24, 25). There was no overall effect of calcium supplements on the risk of preterm delivery, although there was a significant reduction in risk in women classified as high risk for developing hypertension. Also, there was no evidence of any effect of calcium supplements on stillbirth or death before discharge from hospital (25).

Calcium and Colon Cancer

- In a double-blind, placebo-controlled study, 930 subjects (mean age = 61 y) with a recent history of colorectal adenomas were randomized to receive 1,200 mg elemental calcium as calcium carbonate or a placebo daily, with follow-up colonoscopies one and four years after qualifying examinations. Risk ratios for adenoma recurrence were adjusted for age, sex, lifetime number of adenomas prior to the study, clinical center, and length of surveillance period. Calcium-supplemented subjects had a significantly lower risk of recurrent adenomas compared to placebo subjects. The adjusted risk ratio of the average number of adenomas in the calcium group compared to that in the placebo group was 0.76. The effect of calcium was independent of initial dietary fat and calcium intake (26).

- In a review of five uncontrolled, and nine small-scale and three large-scale randomized trials, the authors concluded that it is unlikely that calcium supplementation can substantially lower colorectal epithelial cell proliferation rates (biomarker for increased risk of colon cancer) in humans, but it may normalize the distribution of proliferating cells within colon crypts. All of the uncontrolled trials indicated significant decreases in cancer cell proliferation rates, whereas the controlled studies reported conflicting results (27).

Calcium and PMS

- In a prospective, double-blind, placebo-controlled study, 466 premenopausal women (18 y to 45 y) were randomly assigned to receive 1,200 mg elemental calcium/day (carbonate) or a placebo for three menstrual cycles. Subjects recorded symptoms and adverse effects daily, and underwent routine blood and urine analysis. The primary outcome measure was a 17-parameter symptom complex score. There were no differences in age, weight, height, oral contraceptive use, or menstrual length between groups. There were also no differences in the initial screening symptom complex score of the luteal, menstrual, or intermenstrual phase between groups. During the luteal phase of the treatment cycle, there was a significantly lower mean symptom complex score in the calcium group for the third menstrual cycles. The authors concluded: "Calcium supplementation is a simple and effective treatment in premenstrual syndrome, resulting in a major reduction in overall luteal phase symptoms" (28).

- In a double-blind, placebo-controlled, crossover study, 33 women with a history of recurrent PMS symptoms received in random order 1,000 mg calcium carbonate (400 mg elemental calcium) or a placebo daily for three months each. Efficacy was determined prospectively by measuring changes in daily symptom scores throughout a six-month period and retrospectively by an overall global assessment. There was a significant reduction in daily PMS scores during calcium treatment during the luteal and menstrual phase, but not during the intermenstrual phase. Premenstrual factors (negative affect, water retention, pain) and pain during menstruation were significantly improved by calcium. When subjects were asked to assess effectiveness retrospectively, 73 percent reported fewer symptoms with calcium, 15 percent reported fewer symptoms with the placebo, and 12 percent reported no differences between treatments (29).

SAFETY

- Under the dietary reference intakes (DRIs), the tolerable upper intake level (UL) of calcium for adults is 2,500 mg/day (4). Constipation and bloating have been reported as a side-effect in controlled studies. Doses exceeding 4,000 mg have been associated with increased blood calcium levels, severe renal damage, and ectopic calcium deposition (milk-alkali syndrome) (3). Users of thiazide diuretics and patients with renal dysfunction are at increased risk of developing milk-alkali syndrome with high-dose calcium (30).

- Patients with absorptive or renal hypercalciuria, primary hyperthyroidism, or sarcoidosis may need to avoid calcium supplements (1, 3).

- Most researchers agree that high calcium intakes do not promote kidney stone formation in healthy people. Although calcium restriction has previously been recommended to patients with calcium oxalate stone disease, some research suggests that a dietary calcium restriction could actually increase the risk of stone formation (31). However, there may be an increased risk of stones in patients having absorptive hypercalciuria who take supplements (25). One article suggested that patients with a history of kidney stones should be screened for this disorder before beginning supplements. Calcium citrate has been suggested as the form to be used by individuals at risk for stone formation (9).

- Calcium supplements may interfere with the absorption of drugs such as atenolol, salicylates, biphosphates (used to treat osteoporosis), fluoride, iron, and tetracyclines (9).

- Calcium competes with iron for absorption. In one study of 61 healthy women, 600-mg calcium supplements (citrate and phosphate) inhibited absorption of an iron supplement (18 mg) and dietary nonheme iron when taken with food. For better iron absorption, calcium supplements ideally should not be taken at the same time as iron supplements or with iron-rich meals (32).

- High-calcium diets generally do not interfere with magnesium status in healthy individuals. However, adverse effects of high doses of calcium may occur in populations with poor renal function or in conditions of magnesium depletion (diabetes, alcoholism, malabsorption). A calcium supplement providing 100 mg magnesium for every 500 mg calcium has been suggested for these conditions (30).

REFERENCES

1. Weaver CM, Heaney RP. Calcium. In: Shils ME, Olson JA, Shike M, Ross AC, eds. *Modern Nutrition in Health and Disease.* 9th ed. Baltimore, Md: Williams & Wilkins; 1999:141–155.

2. Food and Drug Administration. Food labeling: health claims; calcium and osteoporosis. *Fed Regist.* 1993;58:2665–2681.

3. National Institutes of Health. Optimal calcium intake. *NIH Consens Statement.* 1994;12:1–31.

4. Food and Nutrition Board, Institute of Medicine. *Dietary reference Intakes: Calcium, Phosphorus, Magnesium, Vitamin D, and Fluoride.* Washington, DC: National Academy Press; 1997.

5. Reid IR. The roles of calcium and vitamin D in the prevention of osteoporosis. *Endocrinol Metab Clin North Am.* 1998;27:389–398.

6. Pennington JAT. *Bowes and Church's Food Values of Portions Commonly Used.* 17th ed. Philadelphia, Pa: Lippincott-Raven Publishers; 1998.

7. Whiting SK, Wood R, Kim K. Calcium supplementation. *J Am Acad Nurse Pract.* 1997;9:187–192.

8. Recker RR. Calcium absorption and achlorhydria. *N Engl J Med.* 1985;313:70–73.

9. Harvey JA, Kenny P, Poindexter J, et al. Superior calcium absorption from calcium citrate than calcium carbonate using external forearm counting. *J Am Coll Nutr.* 1990;9:583–587.

10. Levenson DI, Bockman RS. A review of calcium preparations. *Nutr Rev.* 1994;52:221–232.

11. Baeksgaard L, Andersen KP, Hyldstrup L. Calcium and vitamin D supplementation increases spinal BMD in healthy, postmenopausal women. *Osteoporos Int.* 1998;8:255–260.

12. Nieves JW, Komar L, Cosman F, et al. Calcium potentiates the effect of estrogen and calcitonin on bone mass: a review and analysis. *Am J Clin Nutr.* 1998;67:18–24.

13. Storm D, Eslin R, Porter ES, et al. Calcium supplementation prevents seasonal bone loss and changes in biochemical markers of bone turnover in elderly New England women: a randomized placebo-controlled trial. *J Clin Endocrinol Metab.* 1998;83:3817–3825.

14. Recker RR, Hinders S, Davies KM, et al. Correcting calcium nutritional deficiency prevents spine fractures in elderly women. *J Bone Miner Res.* 1996;11:1961–1966.

15. Dawson-Hughes B, Harris SS, Krall EA, et al. Effect of calcium and vitamin D supplementation on bone density in men and women 65 years of age or older. *N Engl J Med.* 1997;337:670–676.

C

16. Dawson-Hughes B, Harris SS, Krall EA, et al. Effect of withdrawal of calcium and vitamin D supplements on bone mass in elderly men and women. *Am J Clin Nutr.* 2000;72:745–750.

17. Devine A, Dick IM, Heal SJ, et al. A 4-year follow-up study of the effects of calcium supplementation on bone density in elderly postmenopausal women. *Osteoporos Int.* 1997;7:23–28.

18. Nowson CA, Green RM, Hopper JL, et al. A co-twin study of the effect of calcium supplementation on bone density during adolescence. *Osteoporos Int.* 1997;7:219–225.

19. Allender PS, Cutler JA, Follman D, et al. Dietary calcium and blood pressure: a meta-analysis of randomized clinical trials. *Ann Intern Med.* 1996;124:825–831.

20. Bucher HC, Cook RJ, Guyatt GH, et al. Effects of dietary calcium supplementation on blood pressure. A meta-analysis of randomized controlled trials. *JAMA.* 1996;275:1016–1022.

21. Bostick RM, Fosdick L, Grandits GA, et al. Effect of calcium supplementation on serum cholesterol and blood pressure. A randomized, double-blind, placebo-controlled, clinical trial. *Arch Fam Med.* 2000;9:31–39.

22. Appel LJ, Moore TJ, Obarzanek E, et al. A clinical trial of the effects of dietary patterns on blood pressure. DASH Collaborative Research Group. *N Engl J Med.* 1997;336:1117–1124.

23. Svetkey LP, Simons-Morton D, Vollmer VM, et al. Effects of dietary patterns on blood pressure: subgroup analysis of the Dietary Approaches to Stop Hypertension (DASH) randomized clinical trial. *Arch Intern Med.* 1999;159:285–293.

24. Villar J, Belizan JM. Same nutrient, different hypotheses: disparities in trials of calcium supplementation during pregnancy. *Am J Clin Nutr.* 2000;71:1375S—1379S.

25. Atallah AN, Hofmeyr GJ, Duley L. Calcium supplementation during pregnancy for preventing hypertensive disorders and related problems. *Cochrane Database Syst Rev.* 2000;2:CD001059.

26. Baron JA, Beach M, Mandel JS, et al. Calcium supplements for the prevention of colorectal adenomas. Calcium Polyp Prevention Study Group. *N Engl J Med.* 1999;340:101–107.

27. Bostick RM. Human studies of calcium supplementation and colorectal epithelial cell proliferation. *Cancer Epidemiol Biomarkers Prev.* 1997;6:971–980.

28. Thys-Jacobs S, Starkey P, Bernstein D, et al. Calcium carbonate and the premenstrual syndrome: effects on premenstrual and menstrual symptoms. Premenstrual Syndrome Study Group. *Am J Obstet Gynecol.* 1998;179:444–452.

29. Thys-Jacobs S, Ceccarelli S, Bierman A, et al. Calcium supplementation in premenstrual syndrome: a randomized crossover trial. *J Gen Intern Med.* 1989;4:183–189.

30. Heaney RP. Calcium supplements: practical considerations. *Osteoporos Int.* 1991;1:65–71.

31. Curhan GC. Dietary calcium, dietary protein, and kidney stone formation. *Miner Electrolyte Metab.* 1997;23:261–264.

32. Cook JD, Dassenko SA, Whittaker P. Calcium supplementation: effect on iron absorption. *Am J Clin Nutr.* 1991;53:106–111.

Carnitine (L-Carnitine)

Synthesized in the body from lysine and methionine, L-carnitine is a short-chain carboxylic acid containing nitrogen. It plays a central role in fatty acid metabolism by transporting long-chain fatty acids into mitochondria for beta-oxidation. L-carnitine also affects the metabolism of acetyl-coenzyme-A. Approximately 95 percent of the body's carnitine stores are located in skeletal and cardiac muscle. Carnitine has not been considered essential because low dietary intakes are compensated for by increased synthesis and limited renal clearance. Although not essential in healthy individuals, carnitine becomes conditionally essential when an impairment in carnitine function exists as in congenital deficiency, defects in liver or kidney function, or increased catabolism. Carnitine deficiency is associated with muscle weakness, cardiomyopathy, and fatty acid accumulation (1). Different molecules of carnitine have been studied. L- and propionyl-L-carnitine have been examined for their effects on the heart while acetyl-L-carnitine has been investigated for its potential neurological effects.

Media and Marketing Claims	Efficacy
Improves symptoms of cardiovascular disease	↑?
Improves aerobic power	↓
May improve neurological function—help for Alzheimer's disease	↔
Improves immune function	NR
Provides extra energy	NR
Burns fat to aid weight loss	NR

Advisory

- No reported serious adverse effects with doses ranging from 0.5 g to 6.0 g/day
- Larger doses have been associated with nausea and diarrhea

Drug/Supplement Interactions

Some drugs may deplete body stores of L-carnitine, including valproic acid (anticonvulsant), pivalic acid-containing drugs (antibiotic), doxorubicin (chemotherapeutic agent), and AZT for HIV infection

KEY POINTS

- Preliminary studies suggest a possible benefit of L-carnitine for some cardiovascular disorders such as ischemia, myocardial infarction, peripheral vascular disease, congestive heart failure, and arrhythmias. Most researchers agree that more studies are needed before the role of L-carnitine in the management of these conditions can be precisely defined.

- Athletes do not appear to have increased needs for carnitine and are not at risk for carnitine deficiency. The small studies that have been published have reported no improvements in exercise performance.

- There is preliminary evidence that acetyl-L-carnitine (an ester of L-carnitine) may slow the deterioration of some aspects of cognitive impairment/dementia in patients with Alzheimer's disease. However, not all studies have reported benefits. Before using acetyl-L-carnitine supplements, patients should consult with their physician.

- Studies suggest that AIDS patients often present with carnitine deficiency. Preliminary trials suggest that L-carnitine may improve some parameters of immune function in AIDS patients. Several open trials (not discussed here) have reported patient improvements. At this time, no studies have tested the effects of carnitine supplements on the morbidity and/or mortality in these patients.

- Supplemental carnitine only "provides extra energy" if a true clinical carnitine deficiency exists. Deficiency is associated with muscle weakness, cardiomyopathy, and dysfunctional fat metabolism. There is no evidence that L-carnitine supplementation in healthy individuals improves energy or enhances fat loss. However, in patients suffering from chronic fatigue syndrome (CFS) there is some evidence that reduced serum carnitine levels are related to symptoms, and one preliminary study suggested that carnitine supplementation may be beneficial to CFS patients. Additional research is needed to verify these findings.

- The limited research on carnitine and body weight does not support using the supplement for weight loss.

FOOD SOURCES

Carnitine is found mainly in meat—specifically, red meats—and dairy products. Very small amounts are found in fruits, vegetables, grains, and eggs. The average nonvegetarian diet provides approximately 100 mg to 300 mg carnitine/day.

Food	Carnitine (mg/Serving)*
Beef, ground, raw (4 oz)	106
Milk, whole (1 c)	8
Codfish (3 oz)	4.7
Chicken breast, raw (½ breast)	3.3
Ice cream (½ c)	2.5
Cheese, American (2 oz)	2.1
Asparagus (½ c)	0.1
Bread, whole wheat (1 slice)	0.1

Serving sizes calculated from values from Reference 1.

DOSAGE INFORMATION/BIOAVAILABILITY

Carnitine is sold in capsules or tablets in the form of L-carnitine or propionyl-L-carnitine. An esterified form, acetyl-L-carnitine, is also sold as a supplement. Carnitine is also available as a prescription drug for the treatment of carnitine deficiency resulting from clinically diagnosed metabolic disorders. Most studies used 2 g to 4 g L-carnitine divided into two or three doses. Supplemental carnitine raises plasma levels but also increases renal clearance of carnitine (1). The bioavailability/absorption of a 2-g dose is approximately 16 percent of the oral dose and decreases as the dosage increases (2). Muscle carnitine content is raised after long-term supplementation, but not with supplementation lasting less than two weeks (3). There is preliminary evidence that supplemental choline maintains carnitine status by reducing urinary carnitine excretion (4). In contrast, valproic acid (anticonvulsant) and pivalic acid-containing drugs (antibiotic) negatively affect carnitine status in humans (1).

RELEVANT RESEARCH

Carnitine and Cardiovascular Disorders

- Animal studies and clinical trials have suggested that carnitine supplementation may have potential benefits in various cardiovascular disorders, including ischemia, myocardial infarction, peripheral vascular disease, congestive heart failure, arrhythmias, and cardiotoxicity associated with anthracycline therapy. In patients with systemic carnitine deficiency, carnitine administration has been shown to reverse cardiomyopathy (5, 6).

- In a double-blind, placebo-controlled study, 245 patients with intermittent claudication were randomized to receive 1 g propionyl-L-carnitine or a placebo for six months. Only 187 subjects completed the study (87 in the carnitine group and 102 in the placebo group) because of lack of compliance and other unspecified reasons. The study was preceded by a two-week run-in period to assess maximal walking distance and allow for washout of medications for claudication. Quality of life (physical, emotional, social) as measured by the McMaster Health Index Questionnaire revealed a small, but statistically significant, improvement with carnitine compared to placebo. In patients with a maximal walking distance < 250 m at baseline, physical function was significantly improved but not in patients walking > 250 m at baseline (7). One review article criticized this study for failing to use intention-to-treat analysis and for the high dropout rate of subjects (8).

- In a double-blind, placebo-controlled study, 155 patients with claudication were randomized to receive 2 g propionyl-L-carnitine or a placebo daily for six months. Subjects were assessed at baseline, and months 3 and 6 using a graded treadmill test and a questionnaire on functional status. Subjects treated with carnitine significantly increased their maximal walking time by 54 percent as compared to a 25 percent increase for those taking the placebo. Carnitine also significantly improved walking distance and walking speed, and enhanced functional status compared to the placebo (9).

- In a double-blind, placebo-controlled trial, 101 patients with suspected myocardial infarction were randomized to receive 2 g L-carnitine or a placebo daily for 28 days. There were no differences at baseline between the groups regarding the extent of cardiac disease, cardiac enzymes, and lipid peroxides. When compared to the placebo group, carnitine-supplemented subjects had a significant reduction in average infarct size, assessed by cardiac enzymes and electrocardiographic tests, serum aspartate transaminase and lipid peroxides, and lactate dehydrogenase (day 6 postinfarction). Angina pectoris, heart failure plus left ventricular enlargement, and total arrhythmias were significantly less in the carnitine group. The authors concluded: "It is possible that L-carnitine supplementation in patients with suspected acute myocardial infarction may be protective against cardiac necrosis and complications during the first 28 days" (10).

- In a double-blind, placebo-controlled, parallel-design study, 37 patients with angina (> 2 attacks/week) were randomized to receive 1,500 mg L-propionyl-carnitine or a placebo for six weeks. The incidence of angina attacks and total consumption of nitroglycerin were not affected in either group. Carnitine significantly increased the time to 0.1 mV ST-segment depression (electrocardiogram reading that measures ischemic changes). The authors summarized: "It is of question whether in these patients this form of metabolic treatment will achieve great benefit, although in some, improvement can be expected" (11).

- Eighty patients with heart failure caused by dilated cardiomyopathy were randomly assigned to receive 2 g L-carnitine or a placebo daily for about three years. There were no statistical differences between groups at baseline examination or in hemodynamic parameters, exercise tests, peak oxygen intake, arterial and pulmonary blood pressure, or cardiac output. After a mean of 33.7 months, 70 subjects were in the study (33 in the placebo group, 37 in the carnitine). At the time of analysis, 63 patients were alive (six deaths occurred in the placebo group and one death in the carnitine group). Survival analysis showed that survival was significant in favor of the carnitine supplement subjects (12).

Carnitine and Exercise Performance

- The following theories have been put forward regarding the potential for carnitine to improve physical performance: An increase in carnitine from dietary supplements may increase fatty acid oxidation, thus sparing glycogen and glucose. L-carnitine may affect the acetyl CoA/CoA ratio by enhancing conversion of pyruvate to acetyl CoA. This would decrease lactic acid production, thereby improving exercise performance (3).

- In a double-blind, placebo-controlled, crossover study, seven trained subjects were given 2 g L-carnitine tablets or a placebo two hours before the start of a marathon and again after 20 km of the race. Blood samples and the respiratory exchange ratio were obtained one hour before, at the end of the run, and the next morning. There was a month washout period between treatments. Supplementation significantly raised plasma carnitine concentrations, but it had no effect on marathon running time, respiratory exchange ratio, plasma concentrations of carbohydrate or fat metabolites (glucose, lactate, pyruvate, free fatty acids, glycerol, β-hydroxybutyrate), hormone levels (insulin, glucagon, cortisol), or enzyme activities (creatine kinase, lactate dehydrogenase). There was also no difference in performance on a submaximal exercise test the morning after the run. The authors concluded: "Acute administration of L-carnitine did not affect the metabolism or improve the performance of the endurance-trained athletes during the run and did not alter their recovery" (13)

- In a double-blind, placebo-controlled, crossover study, 14 healthy male subjects were randomized to receive an acute dose of intravenous carnitine (185 µmol/kg) or a placebo two hours before starting three different bicycle ergometer protocols, separated by one-month washout periods. Each exercise protocol was performed twice in randomized order, once with the placebo and once with carnitine. Carnitine administration had no effect on muscle carnitine content, respiratory exchange ratio, muscle lactate accumulation, plasma lactate concentration, muscle glycogen utilization, or plasma β-hydroxybutyrate concentration during exercise. The authors concluded that muscle carnitine is segregated from large shifts in the plasma carnitine pool, and that short-term administration of carnitine has no significant effect on fuel metabolism during exercise (14).

- In a randomized, double-blind, placebo-controlled, crossover study, 20 collegiate swimmers completed a control trial of swim sprints, followed by a week of daily supplementation with 4 g L-carnitine in a citrus drink or a placebo drink. After the week of supplementation, subjects completed a second sprint trial. The treatment group had elevated serum carnitine levels and free and short-chain serum carnitine fractions compared to the placebo but no differences in blood pH, lactate, or base excess. There were no differences between trials or between groups on sprint performance time. The authors concluded: "L-carnitine supplementation does not provide an ergogenic benefit during repeated bouts of high-intensity anaerobic exercise in highly-trained swimmers" (15).

- In a single-blind, placebo-controlled study, six untrained subjects were given a placebo for three weeks. A week later, subjects were given 3 g L-carnitine for three more weeks. Each subject performed a 20-minute eccentric step test on the first day of weeks 3 (after placebo) and 7 (after carnitine), inverting the order of the exercising limb. Eight months later, a second set of step tests was performed without supplementation. For four days after each exercise test, subjects noted daily the intensity of perceived soreness. The day before, the day of, and immediately after the test, and every 24 hours after the test for 4 days, subjects underwent measurement of pain thresholds to mechanical and electrical stimulation of the quadriceps. L-carnitine resulted in a significant reduction in pain, tenderness, and creatine kinase (CK) release after eccentric effort compared to the placebo. There was no significant difference between the two tests without supplementation, suggesting subjects did not improve because of a training effect. The authors concluded that L-carnitine has a protective effect against pain and damage from eccentric exercise of the quadriceps. They attributed this effect to the vasodilation effects of L-carnitine, which could improve oxygen supply and enhance removal of metabolites that contribute to delayed onset muscle soreness (16).

Acetyl-L- Carnitine and Alzheimer's Disease (AD)

- In a double-blind, placebo-controlled study, 431 subjects > 50 y with mild to moderate probable AD were randomized to receive 3 g acetyl-L-carnitine hydrochloride or a placebo divided into three doses daily for one year. Eighty-three percent of the subjects completed the entire trial. The Alzheimer's Disease Assessment Scale cognitive component and the Clinical Dementia Rating Scale were used to assess participants every three months. Overall, both treatments were associated with the same rate of decline on tests. However, subanalysis (comparing early-onset patients aged 65 or younger to late-onset patients older than 66) revealed an insignificant trend for early-onset patients taking carnitine to decline more slowly than early-onset patients on placebo. Early-onset patients as a whole tended to decline more rapidly than did older patients in the placebo group. Conversely, late-onset/older patients supplemented with carnitine tended to decline more rapidly than did early-onset patients on carnitine. The authors concluded: "A subgroup of AD patients aged 65 or younger may benefit from treatment with acetyl-L-carnitine, whereas older individuals may do more poorly" (17).

- In a double-blind, placebo-controlled trial, 30 patients with mild to moderate probable AD were randomized to receive acetyl-L-carnitine hydrochloride (2.5 g/day for three months, followed by 3 g/day for three months) or a placebo. Subjects were given tests of memory, language, visuospatial, and constructional abilities, and the level of carnitine was measured in cerebrospinal fluid. After six months, there was significantly less deterioration in timed cancellation tasks and Digit Span and an insignificant trend toward less deterioration in the timed verbal fluency task in patients taking carnitine. No differences were found in any other neurological tests. A subgroup with the lowest baseline scores receiving carnitine had significantly less deterioration on the verbal memory test and a significant increase in cerebrospinal fluid levels of carnitine compared to the placebo group. The authors concluded: "Acetyl L-carnitine may retard the deterioration in some cognitive areas in patients with AD" (18).

- In a double-blind, placebo-controlled, multicenter study, 130 patients diagnosed with AD were randomized to receive 2 g acetyl-L-carnitine divided into four doses or a placebo daily for one year. Fourteen outcome measures were used to assess functional and cognitive impairment. After one year, both groups worsened, but the carnitine treated group showed a slower rate of deterioration in 13 of the 14 outcome measures, reaching statistical significance for the Blessed Dementia Scale, logical intelligence, ideomotor and buccofacial apraxia, and selective attention. After results were adjusted for initial scores, the carnitine subjects showed better scores on all outcome measures compared to placebo subjects, reaching statistical significance for the Blessed Dementia Scale, logical intelligence, verbal critical abilities, long-term verbal memory, and selective attention (19).

- In a double-blind, placebo-controlled study, 229 subjects aged 45 y to 65 y with a diagnosis of probable AD were randomized to receive 3 g acetyl-L-carnitine or a placebo divided into three doses daily for one year. Primary outcome measures were the

Alzheimer's Disease Assessment Scale (ADAS) and the Clinical Dementia Rating Scale. Overall, there were no significant differences between groups on the change from baseline to endpoint. There were no differences in incidence of adverse effects between groups. (20)

Carnitine and Immune Function/AIDS

- Reduced levels of serum carnitines have been reported in AIDS patients treated with zidovudine (21).

- In a randomized, placebo-controlled study, 20 male patients with advanced AIDS and normal serum levels of carnitine were treated with 6 g L-carnitine or a placebo daily for two weeks. Serum and peripheral blood mononuclear cell (PBMC) carnitine levels, CD4 cell counts, serum triglycerides, and lymphocyte proliferation to mitogen stimulation were measured at baseline and at the end of the study. Concentrations of total carnitine in PBMC from AIDS patients were lower than levels in healthy controls. Carnitine supplementation resulted in a significant increase in cellular carnitine content and improved lymphocyte proliferative responsiveness to mitogens compared to baseline. There was also a significant reduction in serum triglycerides compared to baseline (22).

Carnitine and Chronic Fatigue Syndrome

- Decreased carnitine levels have been reported in patients with CFS (23, 24). One study of 35 CFS patients reported significantly lower serum total carnitine, free carnitine, and acylcarnitine levels. Higher serum carnitine levels correlated with better functional capacity. Dietary intake of carnitine was not assessed (25). However, another study reported no differences in carnitine levels between 25 women with CFS and 25 healthy women (26).

- In a parallel-design, crossover (not blinded) study, 30 clinically diagnosed CFS patients were given in random order 3 g L-carnitine or 100 mg amantadine (medication used to treat fatigue in multiple sclerosis patients) for two months each, with a two-week washout period. Patients were assessed before, during, and after treatment. All patients underwent detailed clinical evaluation including the Fatigue Severity Scale (FSS), the Beck Depression Inventory (BDI), the Symptom Checklist 90-R consisting of multiple psychological test categories and general summary scales (SCL-90-R), and the CFS Impairment Index (CFS-II), which consists of physical and mental subsets. The degree of improvement in each of the psychometric parameters studies (total of 18) was calculated by subtracting the baseline results from the eight-week results. Amantadine was poorly tolerated (only 50 percent of the subjects could complete all eight weeks). One patient in the L-carnitine group did not complete treatment because of diarrhea. In those who completed eight weeks of amantadine treatment, there was no significant change in any of the clinical parameters measured. After four weeks of L-carnitine treatment, 5 of 18 outcome measures showed a significant improvement. After eight weeks, L-carnitine treatment resulted in a significant clinical improvement in 12 of the 18 studied parameters. No statistical comparison between L-carnitine and amantadine was performed (27).

Carnitine and Weight Loss

- In a double-blind, placebo-controlled study, 36 moderately overweight pre-menopausal women were pair-matched for body mass index and randomly assigned to receive 4 g L-carnitine (divided into two doses) or placebo daily for eight weeks. All subjects walked for 30 minutes at 60 percent to 70 percent maximum heart rate four days per week. Body composition, resting energy expenditure (REE), and substrate utilization were estimated before and after treatment. There were no significant changes in mean total body mass, fat mass, and resting lipid utilization. REE increased significantly for all subjects, but no difference was observed between treatments. Five of the carnitine subjects experienced nausea and diarrhea and consequently dropped out of the study (28).

SAFETY

- No serious adverse effects have been reported with carnitine doses ranging from 0.5 g/day to 6 g/day. Larger doses have been associated with nausea and diarrhea (29).
- In the cited studies, only L-carnitine, propionyl L-carnitine, and acetyl L-carnitine hydrochloride were used. The safety, bioavailability, and efficacy of other forms of L-carnitine available as dietary supplements may differ with form. The D or D,L-carnitine forms may be associated with impaired exercise performance (30).

REFERENCES

1. Rebouche CJ. Carnitine. In: Shils ME, Olson JA, Shike M, Ross AC, eds. *Modern Nutrition in Health and Disease.* 9th ed. Baltimore, Md: Williams & Wilkins; 1999:505–512.
2. Harper P, Elwin CE, Cederblad G. Pharmacokinetics of intravenous and oral bolus doses of L-carnitine in healthy subjects. *Eur J Clin Pharmacol.* 1988;35:555–562.
3. Kanter MM, Williams MH. Antioxidants, carnitine, and choline as putative ergogenic aids. *Int J Sport Nutr.* 1995;5:S120–S131.
4. Dodson WL, Sachan DS. Choline supplementation reduces urinary carnitine excretion in humans. *Am J Clin Nutr.* 1996;63:904–910.
5. Atar D, Spiess M, Mandinova A, et al. Carnitine—from cellular mechanisms to potential clinical applications in heart disease. *Eur J Clin Invest.* 1997;27:973–976.
6. Pepine CJ. The therapeutic potential of carnitine in cardiovascular disorders. *Clin Ther.* 1991;13:2–21.
7. Brevetti G, Perna S, Sabba C, et al. Effect of propionyl-L-carnitine on quality of life in intermittent claudication. *Am J Cardiol.* 1997;79:777–780.
8. Deckert J. Propionyl-L-carnitine for intermittent claudication. *J Fam Pract.* 1997;44:533–534.
9. Hiatt WR, Regensteiner JG, Creager MA, et al. Propionyl-L-carnitine improves exercise performance and functional status in patients with claudication. *Am J Med.* 2001;110:616–622.

10. Singh RB, Niaz MA, Agarwal P, et al. A randomized, double-blind, placebo-controlled trial of L-carnitine in suspected acute myocardial infarction. *Postgrad Med J.* 1996;72:45–50.

11. Bartels GL, Remme WJ, den Hartog RF, et al. Additional antiischemic effects of long-term L-propionylcarnitine in anginal patients treated with conventional antianginal therapy. *Cardiovasc Drugs Ther.* 1995;9:749–753.

12. Rizos I. Three-year survival of patients with heart failure caused by dilated cardiomyopathy and L-carnitine administration. *Am Heart J.* 2000;139:S120–S123.

13. Colombani P, Wenk C, Kunz I, et al. Effects of L-carnitine supplementation on physical performance and energy metabolism of endurance-trained athletes: a double-blind crossover field study. *Eur J Appl Physiol.* 1996;73:434–439.

14. Brass EP, Hoppel CL, Hiatt WR. Effect of intravenous L-carnitine on carnitine homeostasis and fuel metabolism during exercise in humans. *Clin Pharmacol Ther.* 1994;55:681–692.

15. Trappe SW, Costill DL, Goodpaster B, et al. The effects of L-carnitine supplementation on performance during interval swimming. *Int J Sports Med.* 1994;15:181–185.

16. Giamberardino MA, Dragani L, Valente R, et al. Effects of prolonged L-carnitine administration on delayed muscle pain and CK release after eccentric effort. *Int J Sports Med.* 1996;17:320–324.

17. Thal LJ, Carta A, Clarke WR, et al. A one-year multicenter placebo-controlled study of acetyl-L-carnitine in patients with Alzheimer's disease. *Neurology.* 1996;47:705–711.

18. Sano M, Bell K, Cote L, et al. Double-blind parallel design pilot study of acetyl levocarnitine in patients with Alzheimer's disease. *Arch Neurol.* 1992;49:1137–1141.

19. Spagnoli A, Lucca U, Menasce G, et al. Long-term acetyl-L-carnitine treatment in Alzheimer's disease. *Neurology.* 1991;41:1726–1732.

20. Thal LJ, Calvani M, Amato A, et al. A one year controlled trial of acetyl-L-carnitine in early onset Alzheimer's disease. *Neurology.* 2000;55:805–810.

21. Mintz M. Carnitine in Human Immunodeficiency Virus Type 1 Infection/Acquired Immune Deficiency Syndrome. *J Child Neurol.* 1995;10(suppl 2):S40–S44.

22. De Simone C, Famularo G, Tzantzoglou S, et al. Carnitine depletion in peripheral blood mononuclear cells from patients with AIDS: effect of oral L-carnitine. *AIDS.* 1994;8:655–660.

23. Kuratsune H, Yamaguti K, Lindh G, et al. Low levels of serum acylcarnitine in chronic fatigue syndrome and chronic hepatitis C, but not seen in other diseases. *Int J Mol Med.* 1998;2:51–56.

24. Kuratsune H, Yamaguti K, Takahashi M, et al. Acylcarnitine deficiency in chronic fatigue syndrome. *Clin Infect Dis.* 1994;18(suppl 1):S62—S67.

25. Plioplys AV, Plioplys S. Serum levels of carnitine in chronic fatigue syndrome: clinical correlates. *Neuropsychobiology.* 1995;32:132–138.

26. Soetekouw PM, Wevers RA, Vreken P, et al. Normal carnitine levels in patients with chronic fatigue syndrome. *Neth J Med.* 2000;57:20–24.

27. Plioplys AV, Plioplys S. Amantadine and L-carnitine treatment of chronic fatigue syndrome. *Neuropsychobiology.* 1997;35:16–23.

28. Villani RG, Gannon J, Self M, et al. L-carnitine supplementation combined with aerobic exercise does not promote weight loss in moderately obese women. *Int J Sport Nutr Exerc Metab.* 2000;10:199–207.

29. Wiseman LR, Brogden RN. Propionyl-L-carnitine. *Drugs Aging.* 1998;12:243–248.

30. Watanabe S, Ajisaka R, Masuoka T, et al. Effects of L- and DL-carnitine on patients with impaired exercise tolerance. *Jpn Heart J.* 1995;36:319–331.

C

Chitosan

Chitosan is an amino polysaccharide that has a chemical structure similar to the dietary fiber cellulose. It differs from other fibers in that it contains an amino group. Chitosan is derived by the deacetylation of chitin that is naturally found in the exoskeleton of insects and crustaceans and in the cell walls of fungi. Chitosan cannot be hydrolyzed by human digestive enzymes. When solubilized in acid environments like the gastrointestinal tract, chitosan has a positive charge and binds with negatively charged molecules such as fat and bile. Because of its ability to bind with lipids, chitosan has been promoted in dietary supplements as a weight loss aid and cholesterol-lowering agent. It has also been investigated as a food and feed additive, a cationic agent for waste or water treatment, and for use in biomedical and pharmaceutical materials (1–4).

Media and Marketing Claims	Efficacy
Traps fat—promotes weight loss	↔
Lowers total cholesterol	↑?

Advisory

- Could cause allergic reaction in individuals with allergies to shellfish
- Not for use by individuals with malabsorption disorders
- Long-term use may cause nutrient deficiencies
- Raised triglyceride levels in one study

Drug/Supplement Interactions

- Decreases absorption of fat soluble vitamins and calcium
- May interfere with absorption of medications that bind with dietary fibers

KEY POINTS

- Animal studies have demonstrated chitosan reduces body weight. A meta-analysis of five Italian trials reported a pooled result of significant weight loss when chitosan was supplemented while subjects consumed low-calorie diets for one month. However, another controlled study did not report weight loss with chitosan supplementation in subjects not following a diet regimen. More efficacy and safety data from controlled trials that last longer than 28 days are needed to determine the effect of chitosan on weight control.

- Preliminary data from animal and human studies suggest a cholesterol-lowering effect of chitosan. However, in one human study, chitosan lowered LDL cholesterol, had no effect on HDL cholesterol, and raised triglyceride levels. More information is needed to determine the exact effect that chitosan may have on lipid control, and whether it is safe for long-term use.

- Chitosan interferes with the absorption of some vitamins and minerals. Therefore, the long-term consequences of supplementing chitosan on bone health, nutrient deficiencies, growth, and malabsorption syndromes need to be determined.

FOOD SOURCES

None in significant quantities (derived from exoskeleton of shellfish)

DOSAGE INFORMATION/BIOAVAILABILITY

Chitosan is sold in capsules providing about 500 mg of chitosan with manufacturers recommending a dose of 1,500 mg per day. Labels suggest taking chitosan with meals, especially fatty foods.

RELEVANT RESEARCH

Chitosan and Weight Loss

- In a meta-analysis, researchers summarized data from five randomized, double-blind, placebo-controlled trials examining chitosan supplementation for weight loss. None of the studies was cited in searchable databases, but all were retrieved by contacting one manufacturer. All of the studies were performed in Italy, had nearly identical designs, and were published in the same Italian peer-reviewed journal during a two-year period. Each study administered chitosan or a placebo in addition to a hypocaloric diet for 28 days, and all reported significantly greater weight loss with chitosan. Content of chitosan tablets was not described; the study noted only that four tablets per day were supplemented. Pooled results from these trials suggest a significant and clinically relevant reduction of body weight in overweight individuals on a hypocaloric diet. In addition, in three of the trials, chitosan was associated with reductions in blood lipids. However, the authors of the meta-analysis raised some concerns about the study designs and potential bias (all studies were not cited in databases but were provided by one manufacturer). The researchers concluded that the clinical effectiveness of chitosan for weight control needs to be confirmed by independent, rigorous trials (5).

- In a double-blind, placebo-controlled study, 34 overweight subjects (28 women, 6 men) were randomized to receive eight capsules of chitosan (1,000 mg) or a placebo daily for 28 days. Subjects were told to maintain their normal diet and keep a detailed food diary. Measurements (weight, height, blood pressure, blood samples, and quality of life) were taken at baseline, at day 14, and at day 28 of the study. Fat-soluble vitamins and B-carotene were assessed using high performance liquid chromatography. Four subjects withdrew from the study. Baseline characteristics did not differ between groups. At the end of the study, there were no significant differences between groups on weight, body mass index, blood pressure, total cholesterol, triglycerides, serum beta-carotene, vitamin A, vitamin D_3, or vitamin E. However, subjects taking chitosan had significantly higher serum vitamin K levels than the placebo group. However, the authors noted that these higher vitamin K values are not abnormal for healthy people. Six subjects receiving chitosan complained of constipation compared to two in the placebo group. An analysis of the chitosan capsules was performed and revealed that they contained 42 percent chitosan, less than the 71 percent (250 mg) stated by the distributor (6).

- Chitosan added to the diets of mice fed a high-fat diet for nine weeks prevented the increase of body weight, hyperlipidemia, and fatty liver (7).

Chitosan and Cholesterol

- In a double-blind, placebo-controlled study in Finland, 51 healthy obese women with normal cholesterol levels were randomized to receive microcrystalline chitosan containing 800 mg chitosan (Novamic™) or a placebo just before meals for eight weeks. Weight, serum lipids, and safety laboratory parameters were measured before the trial and at weeks 4, 6, and 8 of treatment. Subjects were told to maintain their normal eating habits. One subject in the chitosan group and three subjects in the placebo group reported that they had changed their eating habits during the study. No reductions in weight were observed in any of the treatment groups. After four weeks (but not after eight weeks), there was a significant decrease in LDL cholesterol in the chitosan-treated subjects compared to the placebo group. There was no significant difference between groups in serum total or HDL cholesterol. However, chitosan-treated subjects had a significant increase in serum triglycerides compared to the placebo group. The authors note that similar increases in triglycerides have been reported with bile acid-binding resin (cholesterolyamine). When a subset of subjects with a body mass index $\geq$ to 30 who had not changed their eating habits was analyzed separately, serum LDL levels were decreased significantly at weeks 4 and 8 in the chitosan group compared to the placebo group. There were no serious adverse events or changes in serum fat-soluble vitamins A and E, and serum Fe ++ and transferrin (8).

- Forty Chinese subjects with type 2 diabetes and hypercholesterolemia who were taking oral hypoglycemics were recruited in a two-part study. In part A, 19 subjects underwent a mixed meal test for eight hours. Subjects received 450 mg chitosan three times per day or a placebo. Blood samples were drawn hourly to determine blood glucose and triglyceride concentrations. No differences in blood values were seen between the two groups. In part B of the study, 33 of 40 subjects completed a randomized, double-blind, placebo-controlled, crossover study lasting 16 weeks. Patients were randomly assigned to receive either 450 mg chitosan three times daily or a placebo daily and were crossed over to the other treatment after eight weeks. Plasma total cholesterol and LDL cholesterol levels were significantly lower in the chitosan recipients than those in the placebo group, with no other differences in triglycerides, HDL cholesterol, ratio of total to HDL cholesterol, hemoglobin A_{1c}, or fasting glucose values between subjects (9).

- Studies in chickens have demonstrated that high doses of chitosan (15 g to 30 g/kg body weight) added to feed appears to have a hypolipidemic effect (10–12).

- Chitosan intake in rats (7.5 percent of diet) on cholesterol enriched diets prevented increases in plasma cholesterol and liver weight and reduced the liver cholesterol content (3).

- In one study of apolipoprotein E-deficient mice with atherosclerosis, diets containing 5 percent chitosan lowered serum cholesterol and inhibited atherogenesis compared to control diets (13).

SAFETY

- There are no long-term controlled trials in humans testing the safety of chitosan supplements at this time. The long-term consequences of supplementing chitosan on bone health, nutrient deficiencies, growth, and malabsorption syndromes need to be determined.

- Although chitosan is a fiber, it is plausible that a residual protein could remain in a product derived from shellfish. Therefore, it may be prudent for individuals with allergies to shellfish to avoid chitosan products.

- Chitosan binds with fat and may reduce the absorption of fat-soluble vitamins and calcium. In one study of rats fat a high fat diet with large amounts of chitosan for two weeks, chitosan caused a decrease in mineral absorption and bone mineral content compared to rats fed high-fat diets containing cellulose or glucosamine. Chitosan also reduced serum vitamin E levels in this study (14). In another study, rats fed a 5 percent chitosan diet had increased urinary excretion of calcium when compared to control rats fed 5 percent cellulose diets (15).

- Individuals with malabsorption disorders should avoid using chitosan because it may aggravate symptoms and could potentially exacerbate nutrient deficiencies (16)

- In one study, use of 800 mg chitosan raised serum triglycerides in normocholesterolemic obese subjects (8).

- In one study, mice fed a 5 percent chitosan diet had a decreased number of *Bifidobacterium* and *Lactobacillus* (protective bacteria) in normal flora of the intestinal tract (17). Because of this effect, a possible adverse effect of long-term intake of chitosan is that it may negatively alter the normal intestinal flora, thus affecting lipid and bile acid metabolism and promoting the growth of intestinal pathogens (16).

- Because chitosan is a fiber, as with any plant fiber, it can interfere with the absorption of other nutrients and some medications. In addition, adequate fluid is necessary to prevent constipation.

REFERENCES

1. Omrod DJ, Holmes CC, Miller TE. Dietary chitosan inhibits hypercholesterolemia and atherogenesis in the apolipoprotein E-deficient mouse model of atherosclerosis. *Atherosclerosis.* 1998;138:329–334.
2. Illum L. Chitosan and its use as a pharmaceutical excipient. *Pharm Res.* 1998;15:1326–1321.
3. LeHoux JG, Grondin F. Some effects of chitosan on liver function in the rat. *Endocrinology.* 1993; 132: 1078–1084.
4. Hirano S. Chitin biotechnology applications. *Biotechnol Annu Rev.* 1996;2:237–258.
5. Ernst E, Pittler MH. "A meta-analysis of chitosan for body weight reduction. *Perfusion.* 1998;11:461–465.
6. Pittler HM, Abbot NC, Harkness EF, et al. Randomized, double-blind trial of chitosan for body weight reduction. *Eur J Clin Nutr.* 1999; 53: 379–381.
7. Han LK, Kimura Y, Okuda H. Reduction in fat storage during chitin-chitosan treatment in mice fed a high-fat diet. *Int J Obes Relat Metab Disord.* 1999; 2: 174–179.
8. Wuolijoki E, Hirvela T, Ylitalo P. Decrease in serum LDL cholesterol with microcrystalline chitosan. *Methods Find Exp Clin Pharmacol.* 1999; 21: 257–361.
9. Tsai-Sung, T, Sheu WHH, Lee WJ, et al. Effect of chitosan on plasma lipoprotein concentrations in type 2 diabetic subjects with hypercholesterolemia [letter]. *Diabetes Care.* 2000;23:1703–1704.
10. Razdan A, Pettersson D. Hypolipidemic, gastrointestinal and related responses of chickens to chitosans of different viscosity. *Br J Nutr.* 1996;76: 387–397.
11. Razdan A, Pettersson D. Effect of chitin and chitosan on nutrient digestibility and lipid concentrations in broiler chickens. *Br J Nutr.* 1994; 72: 277–288.
12. Razdan A, Pettersson D, Pettersson J. Broiler chicken body weights, feed intakes, plasma lipid and small intestinal bile acid concentrations in response to feeding of chitosan and pectin. *Br J Nutr.* 1997;78:283–291.
13. Omrod DJ, Holmes CC, Miller TE. Dietary chitosan inhibits hypercholesterolemia and atherogenesis in the apolipoprotein E-deficient mouse model of atherosclerosis. *Atherosclerosis.* 1998;138:329–334.
14. Deuchi K, Kanauchi O, Shizukuishi M, et al. Continuous and massive intake of chitosan affects mineral and fat-soluble vitamin status in rats fed on a high-fat diet. *Biosci Biotechnol Biochem.* 1995; 59: 1211–1216.
15. Wada M, Nishimura Y, Watanabe Y, et al. Accelerating effect of chitosan intake on urinary calcium excretion by rats. *Biosci Biotechnol Biochem.* 1997;61:1206–1208.
16. Koide SS. Chitin-chitosan: properties, benefits and risks. *Nutr Res.* 1998;18:1091–1101.
17. Tanaka Y, Tanioka S, Tanaka M, et al. Effects of chitin and chitosan particles on BALB/c mice by oral and parenteral administration. *Biomaterials.* 1997; 18: 591–595.

Chondroitin Sulfate

Chondroitin sulfate (CS) is the most abundant glycosaminoglycan in articular cartilage. (Glycosaminoglycans are the ground substance in which collagen fibers are embedded in cartilage.) CS is made endogenously and consists of repeating disaccharide units of glucuronic acid and galactosamine sulfate. Chondroitin appears to inhibit degradative enzymes that break down the cartilage matrix and synovial fluid. Normally secreted by the cells that form cartilage (chondrocytes), chondroitin provides elasticity to joints by drawing fluid into cartilage tissue. Because of these effects, CS supplements have been investigated for their potential role in treating osteoarthritis (1–3).

Media and Marketing Claims	Efficacy
Relieves osteoarthritis pain	↑?
Protects joints and tendons from sports injuries	NR

Advisory

No reported serious adverse effects

Drug/Supplement Interactions

No reported adverse interactions

KEY POINTS

- Preliminary evidence suggests that CS reduces pain associated with osteoarthritis of the knee compared to placebo. However, the potential for confounding by concomitant use of nonsteroidal anti-inflammatory drugs (NSAID) make the studies difficult to interpret. Currently, a large, long-term, multicenter trial of glucosamine and CS is underway in the United States to further determine the efficacy, dosage, and safety of these supplements in treatment of osteoarthritis.

- At the present time, the Arthritis Foundation does not recommend glucosamine or chondroitin in the treatment of osteoarthritis. Instead, patients are encouraged to continue a regimen of exercise, weight control, proper use of medications, joint protection, and application of heat and cold.

- Although preliminary studies suggest that CS decreases pain and improves joint function in knee osteoarthritis, there are currently no clinical trials in humans specifically testing the role of CS supplements in protecting joints from sports injuries.

- *See also* the summary for Glucosamine.

FOOD SOURCES

None (derived from bovine trachea)

DOSAGE INFORMATION

CS is typically sold in 250-mg to 750-mg capsules, often along with glucosamine (*see* Glucosamine) and mucopolysaccharides, which are also promoted for their potential role in joint protection. Most products suggest taking 1,200 mg CS/day. The CS in supplements is usually derived from bovine trachea or shark cartilage. Intestinal absorption of CS can depend on the chain length. Despite the high molecular mass and charge density, there is evidence that CS is effectively absorbed in the human intestine (1, 4). In one study, the absolute bioavailability was 12 percent in humans, with peak levels reached in one to four hours (4). Labeled CS administered orally in humans was found to be distributed to the synovial fluid and cartilage (4). In contrast, another study reported that neither intact nor depolymerized chondroitin sulfate administered orally raised serum glycosaminoglycans (5).

RELEVANT RESEARCH

Chondroitin Sulfate and Osteoarthritis

- In a double-blind, parallel multicenter study, 127 patients (> 45 y) with knee osteoarthritis were randomly assigned to receive one of three treatments for three months: (1) 1,200 mg CS gel in one dose; (2) 1,200 mg CS capsules divided into three doses; or (3) a placebo. Patients were assessed at days 0, 14, 42, and 91. Patients were permitted to take authorized nonsteroidal anti-inflammatory drugs (NSAIDs) if needed, and daily ingestion was recorded. In both CS groups, the Lesquesne's Index (assessment of functional status and quality of life) and spontaneous joint pain measured by a visual analogue scale (VAS) showed a significant decrease in clinical symptoms. In the placebo group, there was a significant reduction on the VAS, but not for Lequesne's Index. There were no differences in the efficacy of single vs multiple doses of CS on clinical parameters. CS was rated by physicians and patients as significantly more effective than the placebo. There was an insignificant trend toward less NSAID use in the CS groups compared to the placebo (6).

- In a double-blind, placebo-controlled study (at two centers), 85 patients (ages 39 y to 83 y) with knee osteoarthritis were randomized to receive 800 mg CS/day divided into two doses or a placebo for six months. Five patients dropped out of the study for reasons unrelated to treatment. Patients were assessed at months 0, 1, 3, and 6. Patients were permitted to take paracetamol (analgesic) as needed. Consumption was recorded as total number of tablets taken during the study. In the CS group, the Lesquesne's Index and spontaneous joint pain significantly decreased. In the CS group, walking time of a 20-m walk showed a significant reduction at six months. Global assessment of efficacy by physicians and patients was significantly in favor of CS compared to the placebo. There was an insignificant trend for CS patients to consume less paracetamol for pain than placebo subjects (7).

- In a double-blind, placebo-controlled study, 60 patients (ages 35 y to 78 y) with knee osteoarthritis were randomized to receive 800 mg CS (divided into two doses daily) or a placebo for one year. Eighteen patients (equal number of dropouts in both groups) did not complete the study. Patients were assessed at months 0, 3, 6, and 12 and were given free access to paracetamol as a rescue medication, but use was not recorded. There were no significant differences in knee pain between groups at baseline. At month 12, joint pain and overall mobility were significantly improved in the CS group. In CS patients, the metabolism of bone and joints (assessed by various biochemical markers in serum) was normalized, whereas it remained abnormal in patients taking placebo. The authors hypothesized that CS may have an effect on the subchondral bone by inhibiting the degradation of the collagen. They concluded: "Further trials, including more patients and over longer periods of time, are definitely necessary to confirm the possible structure-modifying properties of CS" (8).

- In a double-blind, parallel-group study, 146 patients (ages 40 y to 75 y) with knee osteoarthritis were randomized to receive either diclofenac sodium (NSAID) or 400 mg CS three times a day for one month. In months 2 and 3, the diclofenac group was given only a placebo, whereas the chondroitin group continued taking CS. During months 4 through 6, both groups received a placebo. Subjects taking diclofenac showed immediate reduction of symptoms, which reappeared at the end of treatment. Subjects taking chondroitin had a delay in therapeutic improvement, but it lasted for up to three months after the end of treatment. At the end of the four- to six-month period, the Lesquesne's Index score was 64.4 percent lower than baseline levels in the chondroitin group, whereas in the diclofenac group this value was 29.7 percent lower than the baseline. The difference between groups was significant. At days 10 and 20, reduction of paracetamol consumption was more evident in the diclofenac group than in the chondroitin group (significant). At day 30, the reduction in paracetamol consumption was not different between groups. At the end of treatment with CS (day 90), there was an 88 percent reduction in paracetamol use compared to baseline values, whereas the reduction with diclofenac was 37.8 percent; the difference between groups was significant (9).

SAFETY

- There are currently no long-term studies of more than one year testing the safety of CS supplementation. More information will be available when a three-year, three-arm multicenter study (n = 1,000) of glucosamine and CS supplements funded by the National Institutes of Health is completed.

- In the above study, CS was well-tolerated with no serious adverse effects.

REFERENCES

1. Conte A, Volpi N, Palmieri L, et al. Biochemical and pharmacokinetic aspects of oral treatment with chondroitin sulfate. *Arzneimittelforschung.* 1995;45:918–925.
2. Paroli E, Antonilli L, Biffoni M. A pharmacological approach to glycosaminoglycans. *Drugs Exp Clin Res.* 1991;17:9–20.

3. Hardingham T. Chondroitin sulfate and joint disease. *Osteoarthritis Cartilage*. 1998; 6(suppl A):3–5.

4. Ronca F, Palmieri L, Panicucci P, et al. Anti-inflammatory activity of chondroitin sulfate. *Osteoarthritis Cartilage*. 1998;6(suppl A):14–21.

5. Baici A, Horler D, Moser B, et al. Analysis of glycosaminoglycans in human serum after oral administration of chondroitin sulfate. *Rheumatol Int*. 1992;12:81–88.

6. Bourgeois P, Chales G, Dehais J, et al. Efficacy and tolerability of chondroitin sulfate 1,200 mg/day vs chondroitin sulfate 3 × 400 mg/day vs placebo. *Osteoarthritis Cartilage*. 1998;6(suppl A):25–30.

7. Bucsi L, Poor G. Efficacy and tolerability of oral chondroitin sulfate as a symptomatic slow-acting drug for osteoarthritis (SYSADOA) in the treatment of knee osteoarthritis. *Osteoarthritis Cartilage*. 1998;6(suppl A):31–36.

8. Uebelhart D, Thonar EJ, Dlemas PD, et al. Effects of oral chondroitin sulfate on the progression of knee osteoarthritis: a pilot study. *Osteoarthritis Cartilage*. 1998;6(suppl A):39–46.

9. Morreale P, Manopulo R, Galati M, et al. Comparison of the anti-inflammatory efficacy of chondroitin sulfate and diclofenac sodium in patients with knee osteoarthritis. *J Rheumatol*. 1996;23:1385–1391.

Chondroitin Sulfate and Glucosamine Combinations and Osteoarthritis

See Glucosamine.

Chromium

Chromium is an essential trace mineral that, in the form of a low-molecular-weight chromium binding substance, potentiates insulin, which influences carbohydrate, lipid, and protein metabolism (1). It has been suggested that chromium in its biologically active form stimulates insulin receptor protein tyrosine kinase activity after the receptor is activated by insulin. Because of its potential effect on metabolism by potentiating insulin, chromium has been promoted as a weight-loss aid and muscle builder.

Media and Marketing Claims	Efficacy
Helps control diabetes	↑?
Lowers cholesterol	↔
Eliminates body fat and builds muscle	↓
Promotes protein anabolism—a safe alternative to steroids	↓

Advisory

- Tolerable Upper Intake Level not established
- Long-term effects of high doses not known

Drug/Supplement Interactions

- Vitamin C and aspirin may increase chromium absorption
- Antacids may decrease chromium absorption
- In theory, chromium could enhance the blood glucose-lowering effects of diabetes medications and injected insulin

KEY POINTS

- According to national consumption surveys, the average American diet meets the new Adequate Intake (AI) amounts set by the Food and Nutrition Board. A varied diet, consisting of foods rich in chromium is recommended to meet the AI chromium status, may also be maximized by choosing a diet low in simple sugars and rich in whole, unprocessed foods.

- According to one study, high-dose chromium supplements (1,000 μg) may be beneficial for individuals with types 1 and 2 diabetes presenting with a low chromium status by improving glycosylated hemoglobin, glucose, insulin, and cholesterol levels. Long-term research is needed to determine the safety and efficacy of high-dose supplements, and whether chromium supplements have a beneficial effect on retinopathy, nephropathy, and mortality associated with diabetes.

- Preliminary evidence suggests that chromium positively affects blood lipids, specifically HDL cholesterol and triglycerides. However, various studies reported little consistency concerning which blood lipids were affected. There are currently no studies investigating the effects of chromium supplements on morbidity or mortality associated with cardiovascular disease.

- There is little evidence from well-designed studies that chromium increases lean body mass or decreases body fat.

- Although it has been hypothesized that athletes may require additional chromium in their diets due to increased losses from exercise, there is currently no evidence that supplements are anabolic or have other benefits for healthy athletes.

FOOD SOURCES

Brewer's yeast, black pepper, mushrooms, broccoli, dried beans, seeds, wine, and beer are good sources of chromium. Refining wheat removes chromium found in the germ and bran. It is estimated that the average American diet provides 15 μg/1,000 calories (2, 3). The chromium content of foods varies widely, and a significant portion of chromium present in foods may be introduced externally during growing processing, preparation, fortification, and handling (4).

Food	Chromium (µg/Serving)
Broccoli (1 c)	22.0
Ham (3 oz)	3.6
Potatoes, mashed (1 c)	2.7
Beans, green (1 c)	2.2
Turkey breast (3 oz)	1.7
Apple (1 medium)	1.4
Rice, white (1 c)	1.2
Banana (1 medium)	1.0
Bread, whole wheat (1 slice)	0.98

Source: Data from Anderson RA, Brydn NA, Polansky MM (4)

DOSAGE INFORMATION/BIOAVAILABILITY

Chromium in the form of chromium picolinate, nicotinic acid, or chloride is sold in doses ranging from 50 µg to 600 µg. Chromium is also found in smaller amounts in multivitamin/mineral supplements. Chromium picolinate (tripicolinate) and nicotinic acid and chromium from brewer's yeast (organic complexes) are apparently absorbed and retained better than the chromium chloride form (inorganic complex) (5). Chromium absorption appears to vary with dosage. A dietary intake of 10 µg chromium had a 2 percent absorption rate, whereas a dietary intake of 40 µg had an absorption rate of 0.5 percent (6). Vitamin C and aspirin may enhance absorption, whereas antacids may decrease absorption of chromium (3, 7).

The Food and Nutrition Board recently set Adequate Intakes (AI) for chromium but did not set an RDA due to insufficient evidence (8). The new AI for men is 35 µg and 25 µg/day for men and women aged 19y to 50 y, respectively. For ages > 51 y, the AI is is 30 µg and 20 µg daily for men and women, respectively. These values differ from the previous Estimated Safe and Adequate Daily Dietary Intake (ESADDI) of 50 µg to 200 µg for people aged seven and older (9). However, the newer research suggests that the actual chromium requirements for healthy adults is substantially less than originally thought, which was based on dietary intake data from the early 1980s when methods of chromium analysis in foods were less accurate (2, 10). The World Health Organization recommended a basal chromium intake of 25 µg/day to prevent pathological symptoms of deficiency, and a daily intake of 33 µg to maintain desirable tissue storage concentrations (3, 10).

RELEVANT RESEARCH

Chromium Metabolism

- Diets high in simple sugars (35 percent simple sugars, 15 percent complex carbohydrates) increase urinary chromium excretion compared to diets low in sugar (15 percent simple sugars, 35 percent complex carbohydrates). This may be a result of elevated chromium use in response to the increase in glucose metabolism (11–13).

- Strenuous exercise and physical trauma may also increase urinary excretion of chromium (14–16). However, urinary chromium losses with exercise have been associated with accompanying increases in chromium absorption (17).

Chromium and Diabetes

- In a double-blind, placebo-controlled study, 180 patients with type 2 diabetes were randomized among three groups to be supplemented with: (1) a placebo; (2) 200 µg chromium picolinate (100 µg elemental chromium) divided into two doses; or (3) 1,000 µg chromium picolinate (500 µg elemental chromium) divided into two doses. Subjects maintained their usual diet and medication throughout the four-month study. Glycosylated hemoglobin values significantly improved after two months in the high-dose chromium group, and were lower in both chromium groups after four months compared to placebo. Fasting and two-hour insulin values were significantly lower in both chromium groups at two and four months. However, only the subjects taking high-dose chromium had significantly lower two-hour glucose values and lower plasma total cholesterol (18).

- In a double-blind, placebo-controlled study, crossover study, 78 type 2 diabetes patients in Saudi Arabia received in random order Brewer's yeast (23 µg chromium) and 200 µg chromium from chromium chloride for four weeks each. In all subjects there were four, 8 week phases in the study. Each phase of chromium supplementation was followed by a placebo administration for eight weeks. At the beginning and end of each phase, weight, diet, drug usage, and blood and urine glucose and lipids were recorded. Both forms of chromium resulted in a significant decrease in levels of mean glucose (fasting and two hour post-glucose load), fructosamine, and triglycerides. Mean HDL-cholesterol and serum and urinary chromium levels were all increased during chromium intake. After either chromium phase, mean drug dosage tended to decrease, but was not significant, except with the drug Glibenclamide. There was no change in dietary intakes or body mass index. Overall, Brewer's yeast was associated with chromium retention and greater positive effects than the chromium chloride form (19).

- In a prospective double-blind, placebo-controlled, crossover study, 28 subjects having type 2 diabetes received in random order 200 µg chromium picolinate or a placebo for two months each, with a two-month washout. There was no change in fasting glucose control, plasma HDL or LDL cholesterol concentrations. However, during chromium supplementation, mean triglyceride concentrations were reduced significant by 17.4 percent. The authors acknowledged that long-term studies are needed to determine whether the short-term change in triglycerides can be sustained (20).

- In a review, researchers examined 15 studies on chromium supplementation (picolinate and chloride forms) and concluded: (1) Overt chromium deficiency results in insulin resistance; (2) insulin resistance due to chromium deficiency can be improved with chromium supplementation; (3) chromium deficiency, although rare, may be a cause of insulin resistance in deficient populations (21).

- According to another review, consumption of low chromium diets (< 20 µg) by healthy controls does not appear to affect blood glucose or insulin variables. In addition, control subjects with good glucose tolerance (90-minute glucose = 5.6 mmol/L following a glucose challenge) on low-chromium diets do not show signs of deficiency and supplementation of 200 μg elemental chromium daily for five weeks is without effect on glucose or insulin variables (10).

Chromium and Cardiovascular Disease

- In a double-blind, placebo-controlled study, 72 male subjects using beta-blockers were randomized to receive 600 μg chromium picolinate (300 μg elemental chromium) daily divided into three doses or a placebo for eight weeks. Fasting lipid values were taken before and after treatment, and eight weeks after the completion of the study. There was a significant increase in mean HDL cholesterol concentrations in the chromium-supplemented group after adjusting for baseline HDL and total cholesterol concentrations, age, and weight change. There were no differences in total cholesterol, triglycerides, or body weight between groups (22).

- In a placebo-controlled (not blinded) study, 76 patients with atherosclerosis (25 of the subjects had stable type 2 diabetes) were randomized to receive 250 μg chromium as chromium chloride or a placebo daily for 7 to 16 months. Blood samples were taken at the beginning, at three months, and at the end of the study. There was a significant increase in serum chromium and decreased triglyceride concentrations at three and six months in the chromium group compared to placebo. At six months only, there was a significant increase in serum HDL cholesterol concentrations in the chromium group compared to the placebo group. Chromium supplements had no effect on blood glucose or total cholesterol levels (23). The results of this study would be strengthened if the study were conducted in a double-blind design.

- In a double-blind, placebo-controlled, crossover study, 14 healthy subjects and 5 type 2 diabetics received in random order 200 μg elemental chromium as chromium nicotinic acid or a placebo for eight weeks each. There were no significant changes on plasma insulin, glucose, or lipid concentrations among subjects taking chromium following an oral glucose tolerance test. In the subjects with diabetes, however, there was an insignificant trend toward lower fasting plasma total and LDL cholesterol, triglycerides, glucose, and 90-minute postprandial glucose concentrations (24).

- In a double-blind, placebo-controlled, crossover study, 28 healthy subjects received in random order 200 μg elemental chromium as chromium picolinate or a placebo daily for 42 days. Chromium supplements resulted in a significant decrease in total cholesterol and LDL cholesterol. Apolipoprotein A-I (the principal protein in HDL) was increased during the chromium supplementation phase, although the HDL level was not raised significantly (25).

Chromium and Obesity

- In double-blind, placebo-controlled study, 43 obese female subjects were randomly assigned into one of four groups for nine weeks, undergoing treatment with: (1) chromium picolinate (400 μg elemental chromium/day) with no exercise, (2) chromium with exercise, (3) placebo with exercise, or (4) chromium nicotinate supplementation (400 µg elemental chromium/day) with exercise. Chromium picolinate supplementation without exercise resulted in a statistically significant weight gain but no statistical change in body fat, fat free mass, or fat mass as assessed by hydrostatic weighing. The chromium nicotinate group experienced significant weight loss and a lowered insulin response to an oral glucose loading test. The authors speculated that the high dose of chromium picolinate used (double the amount in most of the earlier studies) may have caused the weight gain, although they did not attempt to explain the possible mechanism of action. Although their sample size was small, the authors concluded that the chromium picolinate may be contraindicated in nonexercising, young, obese women (26).

- In a double-blind, placebo-controlled study, 95 overweight Navy personnel subjects were randomly assigned to receive 400 µg chromium picolinate (200 µg elemental chromium) or a placebo daily for 16 weeks. Subjects completed 30 minutes of exercise training (unsupervised) at least three times per week during the study. Chromium had no effect on the percent of body fat (computed from body circumference and height), body weight, or increased lean body mass compared to placebo. The authors concluded: "Chromium picolinate was ineffective in enhancing body fat reductions in this group and could not be recommended as an adjuvant to Navy weight-loss programs in general" (27).

Chromium for Strength Training and Body Mass

- In a double-blind, placebo-controlled study, 36 male weight-trained subjects were randomized to receive 170 µg to 180 µg chromium (as chromium picolinate or chromium chloride), or a placebo daily during an eight-week resistance training program. Both chromium supplements increased serum and urinary chromium concentrations. However, chromium had no effect on strength, mesomorphy, or body composition (X-ray absorptiometry, skinfolds) compared to the placebo (28).

- In a double-blind, placebo-controlled study, 16 untrained men were pair- matched for strength and then randomly assigned to receive 200 µg chromium as chromium picolinate or a placebo daily during a 12-week weight-training program. Diet analysis of food records estimated an average dietary intake of 36 µg chromium/day. At the end of 12 weeks, both groups had increased muscular strength; however, there was no change in body weight, percent body fat, lean body mass (hydrostatic weighing), and skinfold thickness in the chromium-supplemented group compared to the placebo group. The chromium group had significantly greater urinary chromium excretion than did the placebo group (29).

- In a double-blind, placebo-controlled study, 59 college students were enrolled in a 12-week weight lifting program and were randomized to receive 200 µg chromium as chromium picolinate or a placebo. No treatment effects of chromium were seen on strength (one-repetition maximum for the squat and bench press), skinfold, and circumference measures. However, chromium picolinate resulted in a significant increase in body weight in female weight-lifters, but resulted in no change in the male weight-lifters. It was not clear whether the weight gain was fat or lean body mass, although the authors hypothesized the gain was muscle mass because of a insignificant decrease in skinfold measures (30).

- In a double-blind, placebo-controlled study, 38 football players were randomized to receive 200 μg chromium as chromium picolinate or a placebo daily for nine weeks. Subjects were assessed for strength and body composition measured by hydrostatic weighing pre-, mid-, and posttreatment. There was no change in body composition or strength (maximal isometric actions for each muscle group) during intensive weight-training compared to the placebo group. Chromium-supplemented subjects increased urinary chromium excretion 5-fold compared to the placebo group (31).

- A review article concluded: (1) Athletes may be at risk for negative chromium balance and may have increased chromium requirements because of increased urinary and sweat losses, and (2) anabolic steroid-like muscle mass increases following chromium supplementation are very unlikely (32).

SAFETY

- The long-term effects of increased cellular concentrations of chromium in the body are not known. It has been hypothesized that five years of consuming 600 μg of chromium picolinate (300 μg elemental chromium) could possibly lead to an accumulation in some tissues similar to levels that caused DNA damage observed in animals and *in vitro* studies (3, 33).

- Researchers investigating the safety of chromium supplements (picolinate or chloride) found that supplementing rats with several thousand times the equivalent of the upper limit of the ESSADI for humans resulted in no toxicity. Rats were fed 0, 5, 25, 50, or 100 mg of chromium per kilogram. There were no differences in body weight, organ weights, or blood glucose, cholesterol, triglycerides, BUN, lactic acid dehydrogenase, transaminases, or total protein and creatinine among study groups. However, animals consuming the picolinate form had several-fold higher chromium concentrations in the liver and kidney than rats fed the chromium chloride, suggesting that the picolinate form had an increased absorption rate (34).

- However, one review article on the genotoxicity of chromium stated that sublethal doses of chromium cannot produce tissue levels high enough to cause clastogenic damage *in vivo* and that "dietary supplementation with trivalent chromium in reasonable amounts is unlikely to carry any genotoxic risk" (35).

- There have been reports of headaches, sleep disturbances, and mood swings with chromium supplements (36).

- Chromium exists in two forms: trivalent (occurs mainly in nature) and hexavalent (occurs mainly in industrial settings). The hexavalent form is a synthetic compound that is very toxic and carcinogenic (3).

- One review cautioned that chromium may compete with iron for serum protein binding sites and questioned the safety of picolinate. The authors state the need for further research on the safety of long-term chromium supplementation at elevated levels (32).

- A dose of 1,200 µg to 2400 µg chromium picolinate daily for 5 months resulted in liver dysfunction and renal failure in one 33 year old woman taking the supplement for weight loss (37).

REFERENCES

1. Davis CM, Vincent JB. Chromium oligopeptides activates insulin receptor tyrosine kinase activity. *Biochemistry.* 1997;36:4382–4385.
2. Stoecker BJ. Chromium. In: Shils ME, Olson JA, Shike M, Ross AC, eds. *Modern Nutrition in Health and Disease.* 9th ed. Baltimore, Md: Williams & Wilkins; 1999:277–282.
3. Nielsen FH. Controversial chromium. *Nutr Today.* 1996;31:226–233.
4. Anderson RA, Bryden NA, Polansky MM. Dietary chromium intake: freely chosen diets, institutional diets, and individual foods. *Biol Trace Elem Res.* 1992;32:117–121.
5. Olin KL, Stearns D, Armstrong W, et al. Comparative retention/absorption of ^{51}chromium (^{51}Cr) from ^{51}Cr chloride, ^{51}Cr nicotinate, and ^{51}Cr picolinate in a rat model. *J Trace Electrolytes Health Dis.* 1994;11:182–186.
6. Anderson RA, Kozlovsky AS. Chromium intake, absorption, and excretion of subjects consuming self-selected diets. *Am J Clin Nutr.* 1985;41:1177–1183.
7. Seaborn CD, Stoecker BJ. Effects of antacid or ascorbic acid on tissue accumulation and urinary excretion of ^{51}chromium. *Nutr Res.* 1990;10:1401–1407.
8. Food and Nutrition Board, Institute of Medicine. *Dietary Reference Intakes For Vitamin A, Vitamin K, Arsenic, Boron, Chromium, Copper, Iodine, Iron, Manganese, Molybdenum, Nickel, Silicon, Vanadium, and Zinc.* Washington, DC: National Academy Press; 2001.
9. Food and Nutrition Board, National Research Council. *Recommended Dietary Allowances.* 10th ed. Washington, DC: National Academy Press; 1989.
10. Anderson RA. Nutritional factors influencing the glucose/insulin system: chromium. *J Am Coll Nutr.* 1997;16:404–410.
11. Kozlovsky AS, Moser PB, Reiser S, et al. Effects of diets high in simple sugars on urinary chromium losses. *Metabolism.* 1986;35:515–518.
12. Anderson RA, Bryden NA, Polansky MM, et al. Urinary chromium excretion and insulinogenic properties of carbohydrates. *Am J Clin Nutr.* 1990;51:864–868.
13. Anderson RA, Polansky MM, Bryden NA, et al. Urinary chromium excretion of human subjects: effects of chromium supplementation and glucose loading. *Am J Clin Nutr.* 1982; 36: 1184–1193.
14. Anderson RA, Bryden NA, Polansky MM, et al. Exercise effects on chromium excretion of trained and untrained men consuming a constant diet. *J Appl Physiol.* 1988;64:249–252.
15. Campbell WW, Anderson RA. Effects of aerobic exercise and training on the trace minerals chromium, zinc, and copper. *Sports Med.* 1987;4:9–18.
16. Borel JS, Majerus TC, Polansky MM, et al. Chromium intake and urinary chromium excretion of trauma patients. *Biol Trace Elem Res.* 1984;6:317–326.
17. Rubin MA, Miller JP, Ryan AS, et al. Acute and chronic resistive exercise increase uri-

nary chromium excretion in men as measured with an enriched chromium stable isotope. *J Nutr.* 1998;128:73–78.

18. Anderson RA, Cheng N, Bryden NA, et al. Elevated intakes of supplemental chromium improve glucose and insulin variables in individuals with Type II diabetes. *Diabetes.* 1997;46:1786–1791.

19. Bahijiri SM, Mira SA, Mufti AM, et al. The effects of inorganic chromium and brewer's yeast supplementation on glucose tolerance, serum lipids, and drug dosage in individuals with type 2 diabetes. *Saudi Med J.* 2000;21:831–837.

20. Lee NA, Reasner CA. Beneficial effect of chromium supplementation on serum triglyceride levels in NIDDM. *Diabetes Care.* 1994;17:1449–1452.

21. Mertz W. Chromium in human nutrition: a review. *J Nutr.* 1993;123:626–633.

22. Roeback JR, Hla KM, Chambless LE, et al. Effects of chromium supplementation on serum high-density-lipoprotein cholesterol levels in men taking β-blockers. A randomized, controlled trial. *Ann Intern Med.* 1991;115:917–924.

23. Abraham AS, Brooks BA, Eylath U. The effect of chromium supplementation on serum glucose and lipids in patients with and without non-insulin-dependent diabetes. *Metabolism.* 1992;41:768–771.

24. Thomas VL, Gropper SS. Effect of chromium nicotinic acid supplementation on selected cardiovascular disease risk factors. *Biol Trace Elem Res.* 1996;55:297–305.

25. Press RI, Geller J, Evans GW. The effect of chromium picolinate on serum cholesterol and apolipoprotein fractions in human subjects. *West J Med.* 1990;152:41–45.

26. Grant KE, Chandler RM, Castle AL, et al. Chromium and exercise training: effect on obese women. *Med Sci Sports Exerc.* 1997;29:992–998.

27. Trent LK, Thieding-Cancel D. Effects of chromium picolinate on body composition. *J Sports Med Phys Fitness.* 1995;35:273–280.

28. Lukaski HC, Bolonchuk WW, Siders WA, et al. Chromium supplementation and resistance training: effects on body composition, strength, and trace element status of men. *Am J Clin Nutr.* 1996;63:954–965.

29. Hallmark MA, Reynolds TH, DeSouza CA, et al. Effects of chromium and resistive training on muscle strength and body composition. *Med Sci Sports Exerc.* 1996;28:139–144.

30. Hasten DL, Rome EP, Franks BD, et al. Effects of chromium picolinate on beginning weight training students. *Int J Sport Nutr.* 1992;2:343–350.

31. Clancy SP, Clarkson PM, DeCheke ME, et al. Effects of chromium picolinate supplementation on body composition, strength, and urinary chromium loss in football players. *Int J Sport Nutr.* 1994;4:142–153.

32. Lefavi RG, Anderson RA, Keith RE, et al. Efficacy of chromium supplementation in athletes: emphasis on anabolism. *Int J Sport Nutr.* 1992;2:111–122.

33. Stearns DM, Belbruno JJ, Wetterhahn KE. A prediction of chromium (III) accumulation in humans from chromium dietary supplements. *FASEB J.* 1995;9:1650–1657.

34. Anderson RA, Bryden NA, Polansky MM. Lack of toxicity of chromium chloride and chromium picolinate in rats. *J Am Coll Nutr.* 1997;16:273–279.

35. McCarty MF. Subtoxic intracellular trivalent chromium is not mutagenic: implications for safety of chromium supplementation. *Med Hypotheses.* 1997;49:263–269.

C

36. Schrauzer GN, Shrestha KP, Arce MF. Somatopsychological effects of chromium supplementation. *J Nutr Med.* 1992;3:42–48.
37. Cerulli J, Grabe DW, Gauthier I, et al. Chromium picolinate toxicity. *Ann Pharmacother.* 1998;32:428–431.

Cobalamin

See Vitamin B_{12} (Cobalamin).

Coenzyme Q_{10}

Coenzyme Q_{10} (CoQ$_{10}$) or ubiquinone is an electron and proton carrier supporting ATP synthesis in the lipid phase of the mitochondria membrane. It is synthesized endogenously within the intracellular environment throughout the body, specifically in the heart, liver, kidney, and pancreas. The CoQ$_{10}$ content of human tissue appears to be related to age, peaking at age 20, and subsequently declining (1). CoQ$_{10}$ has demonstrated antioxidant activity in experimental studies (2–4). Because of its potential antioxidant role and involvement in mitochondrial function, CoQ$_{10}$ has been investigated in cardiovascular disease, exercise performance, cancer, AIDS/HIV, and neurodegenerative diseases.

Media and Marketing Claims	Efficacy
Improves symptoms of cardiovascular disease	↑?
Enhances exercise performance	↓
Reduces breast cancer risk	NR
Supports immune function in HIV-positive individuals	NR
Helpful in neurological disorders—Parkinson's disease	NR
Slows aging process	NR

Advisory

- No reported serious adverse effects with 200 mg CoQ$_{10}$ daily for one year and 100 mg daily for up to six years
- Potential side-effects may include mild gastrointestinal distress

Drug/Supplement Interactions

- HMG-CoA reductase inhibitor drugs (statins) used for cholesterol reduction may deplete blood coenzyme Q_{10} levels
- Endogenous synthesis of coenzyme Q_{10} is dependent upon adequate vitamin B_6 status

KEY POINTS

- Some evidence from controlled human studies suggests that CoQ$_{10}$ supplementation may improve the symptoms and outcome of cardiac surgery, myocardial infarction, and congestive heart failure. However, not all research has reported benefits resulting from CoQ$_{10}$ supplementation. More studies are needed to determine the dosage, timing, and safety of supplementation in this population.

- Controlled trials do not support CoQ$_{10}$ supplementation for athletes because it does not appear to enhance exercise performance or reduce oxidative stress induced by exercise.

- Although blood CoQ$_{10}$ concentrations appear to be depressed in patients with breast cancer, controlled trials are lacking to support the claim that CoQ$_{10}$ prevents or treats cancer. Case reports and uncontrolled studies suggesting remission of cancer with CoQ$_{10}$ administration do not provide adequate information to determine the potential role of CoQ$_{10}$ supplements in cancer patients.

- Likewise, controlled research is lacking and is needed to determine the potential role of CoQ$_{10}$ supplements in immune function in AIDS. Case studies and uncontrolled trials suggesting a beneficial effect of CoQ$_{10}$ supplements in AIDS patients and healthy subjects do not provide adequate information to make recommendations for this population.

- Controlled clinical trials are lacking and are necessary to determine the potential role of CoQ$_{10}$ supplements in neurodegenerative diseases.

- Although blood CoQ$_{10}$ concentrations appear to decline with age, there is currently no evidence suggesting that supplements slow the human aging process.

FOOD SOURCES

An analysis of the CoQ$_{10}$ content of the Danish diet (U.S. data not available) revealed an average intake of 3 to 5 mg/day mainly from meat and poultry. Frying foods destroys 14 percent to 34 percent of the CoQ$_{10}$ content, whereas boiling causes no detectable destruction (5).

Food	CoQ$_{10}$ (mg) *
Beef (3 oz)	2.6
Chicken (3 oz)	1.4
Pork chop (3 oz)	1.2
Trout (3 oz)	0.9
Salmon (3 oz)	0.4
Orange (1 medium)	0.4
Broccoli (½ c)	0.2

Source: Data from Weber C, Bysted A, Holmer G (5)
*Serving sizes calculated from values from Reference 5.

C

DOSAGE INFORMATION/BIOAVAILABILITY

Because CoQ_{10} is not an essential nutrient, no RDA has been set. CoQ_{10} is sold in capsules and tablets in dosages ranging from 10 mg to 130 mg per capsule. One study found that CoQ_{10} in both food and dietary supplement sources significantly raised serum concentrations (6). Another study found a new soluble form of CoQ_{10} was absorbed more efficiently than were other commercially available forms, and therefore lower doses of that form could be used to raise serum levels (7).

RELEVANT RESEARCH

Tissue and Blood Concentrations of CoQ_{10} in Cardiovascular Disease

- A review article cited several studies suggesting that CoQ_{10} concentrations are reduced in heart tissue measured from biopsies obtained during catheterization in patients with cardiovascular disease. The lowest tissue levels were observed in patients with advanced heart failure (8).

- In a cross-sectional study of 94 hospital patients, subjects with very low serum CoQ_{10} levels had a significant increased risk of dying or having congestive heart failure and/or myalgia (9).

- Several studies have reported decreased blood concentrations of CoQ_{10} in patients treated with HMG-CoA reductase inhibitors (cholesterol-lowering medications such as pravastatin) (10–12), although not all studies have been consistent (13).

CoQ_{10} Supplements and Cardiovascular Disease

- In a double-blind, placebo-controlled, crossover study, 30 patients with ischemic or idiopathic dilated cardiomyopathy and chronic left ventricular dysfunction were randomized to receive CoQ_{10} or a placebo for three months each. Right heart pressures, cardiac output, echocardiographic left ventricular volumes, and quality of life measured using the Minnesota "Living with Heart Failure" questionnaire were assessed at baseline and after each treatment. Plasma levels of CoQ_{10} increased to more than twice basal values. There were no significant differences between treatments in left ventricular ejection fraction, cardiac volumes, hemodynamic indices, or quality of life measures (14).

- In a double-blind, placebo-controlled trial, 144 patients with acute myocardial infarction were randomized to receive 120 mg CoQ_{10} or a placebo daily for 28 days starting within 3 days after infarction. The extent of cardiac disease, elevation in cardiac enzymes and oxidative stress were similar between groups at baseline. After treatment, angina pectoris, total arrhythmias, and poor left ventricular function were significantly improved in the CoQ_{10} group compared with the placebo group. Total cardiac events, including cardiac deaths and nonfatal infarction, were also significantly reduced in the CoQ_{10} group compared with the placebo group (15.0 vs 30.9 percent). The authors concluded that further studies in larger number of patients and long-term follow-up are needed to confirm their results (15).

- A meta-analysis of eight clinical trials of CoQ$_{10}$ in patients with congestive heart failure (CHF) found that supplemental treatment of CHF was consistent with a significant improvement in stroke volume, ejection fraction, cardiac output, cardiac index, and diastolic volume index (16).

- In a double-blind, placebo-controlled study, 322 patients with chronic congestive heart failure were randomly assigned to receive 2 mg CoQ$_{10}$/kg/day or a placebo for one year. The number of episodes of pulmonary edema or cardiac asthma were significantly less in the CoQ$_{10}$ group than in the placebo group. In addition, CoQ$_{10}$-supplemented subjects had significantly fewer hospitalizations (17).

- In a double-blind, placebo-controlled study, 20 high-risk cardiac surgery patients were randomly assigned to receive 100 mg CoQ$_{10}$ or a placebo for 2 weeks prior to and 30 days following surgery. In both groups there were low blood CoQ$_{10}$ concentrations (< 0.6 micrograms/mL), low cardiac index, and low left ventricular ejection fraction (LVEF) before treatment. Myocardial tissue (atria muscle) samples were collected during cardiac catheterization, in the operating room during cardiac cooling, and after cardiac warming and reperfusion. CoQ$_{10}$ supplementation significantly raised blood and myocardial CoQ$_{10}$ and myocardial ATP compared to the control group. Among patients treated with CoQ$_{10}$, cardiac function did not improve before surgery. However, after surgery improvement was statistically significant. Patients treated with CoQ$_{10}$ maintained blood and tissue levels of CoQ$_{10}$ after cardiac cooling, rewarming, and reperfusion and recovered sooner (3 days to 5 days) as assessed by cardiac function. Patients taking placebos had depressed CoQ$_{10}$ levels after surgery and a longer recovery period (15 days to 30 days) (18).

- In a double-blind, placebo-controlled study, 20 coronary artery-bypass grafting surgery candidates were randomly assigned to receive 600 mg CoQ$_{10}$ or a placebo 12 hours before surgery. There were no differences in CoQ$_{10}$ levels prior to surgery, and levels fell postsurgery in both groups. Outcome was assessed based on clinical events, electrocardiographic changes, and biochemical markers of myocardial injury. Supplementation of CoQ$_{10}$ did not improve myocardial protection in patients undergoing coronary revascularization. The authors note that supplementation in their study was given the night before surgery as opposed to one to two weeks prior to the procedure as in other studies (19).

- In a double-blind, placebo-controlled study, 55 patients with congestive heart failure were randomly assigned to receive 200 mg CoQ$_{10}$ or a placebo daily for six months. Cardiac performance (ventricular ejection fraction), peak oxygen consumption, and exercise duration were measured at baseline and at study's end. Subjects receiving CoQ$_{10}$ supplements had higher serum concentrations of CoQ$_{10}$, but there were no differences in any of the parameters measured when compared to the placebo (20).

CoQ$_{10}$ and Exercise Performance

- In a placebo-controlled study, 18 male endurance cyclists and triathletes were given 1 mg CoQ$_{10}$/kg/day or a placebo for 28 days. Subjects were evaluated during and following graded cycling to exhaustion, which was completed before and after the trial.

Although CoQ_{10} supplements significantly raised plasma concentrations, there was no effect on submaximal or maximal performance measures (oxygen uptake, anaerobic and respiratory compensation thresholds, blood lactate, glucose and triglyceride levels, heart rate, and blood pressure). The authors noted that these results do not preclude the possibility that supplemental CoQ_{10} may be beneficial to athletes with a preexisting cellular CoQ_{10} deficiency (21).

- In a double-blind, placebo-controlled study, 18 subjects were given 120 mg CoQ_{10}/day or a placebo for 22 days. The first week included normal physical activity, followed by four days of high-intensity anaerobic training, with a seven-day recovery period. There was a significantly greater increase in anaerobic performance in the placebo group compared to the CoQ_{10} group. There were no significant differences between groups in VO_{2max}, submaximal and peak VO_2, perceived exertion, respiratory quotient, blood lactate, or heart rate (22).

- In a single-blind, placebo-controlled study, 15 middle-aged men received either 150 mg CoQ_{10}/day or a placebo for two months. Whereas blood CoQ_{10} levels increased and subjective perception of vigor increased in the CoQ_{10} treatment group, there was no effect on aerobic capacity (VO_{2max}, lactate threshold) as measured on the cycle ergometer (23). The lack of randomization and single-blind design weaken the findings of this study.

- In a double-blind, placebo-controlled trial, 10 trained cyclists performed graded cycle ergometry before and after being given 100 mg CoQ_{10}/day or a placebo for eight weeks. Although supplementation increased serum CoQ_{10} levels, CoQ_{10} supplements did not improve cycling performance, maximal oxygen uptake, submaximal physiological parameters, or lipid peroxidation (24).

- In a double-blind, placebo-controlled study, 37 moderately-trained male marathon runners were randomized to receive 90 mg CoQ_{10} plus 13.5 mg alpha-tocopherol or a placebo daily for three weeks before a marathon. Just before the run, there was a significant 282 percent increase in plasma CoQ_{10} and a 16 percent increase in plasma vitamin E in subjects supplemented with treatment compared to the placebo group. Also, the proportion of plasma ubiquinol of total CoQ_{10}, an indication of plasma redox status *in vivo*, was significantly higher in supplemented subjects. Additionally, the susceptibility of the VLDL plus LDL fraction, to *ex vivo* copper-induced oxidation, was significantly reduced after CoQ_{10} and vitamin E supplementation compared to placebo. The marathon race increased lipid peroxidation in both groups. However, supplementation of CoQ_{10} plus vitamin E had no effect on lipid peroxidation or on the muscular damage (increase in serum creatine kinase activity or in plasma lactate levels) induced by the marathon race (25).

CoQ_{10} and Cancer

- Observational studies of women diagnosed with breast cancer have reported reduced blood CoQ_{10} concentrations (26). In one study, 200 women aged 18 y to 65 y hospitalized for the biopsy and/or ablation of a breast tumor had significantly reduced plasma CoQ_{10} levels compared to blood samples from 253 healthy controls aged 18 y to 65 y. There was no difference in plasma CoQ$_{10}$ reduction between patients with malignant tumors (n = 80) and nonmalignant lesions (n = 120). There was also no correlation between age and CoQ$_{10}$ levels (27).

- In an uncontrolled study, 32 patients with metastasized breast cancer were supplemented with a combination of antioxidants (vitamin C, selenium, beta-carotene, and essential fatty acids) that included 90 mg CoQ$_{10}$. After 18 months, the authors reported partial remission in six subjects (28). An article by the same researchers reported regression of metastases in 10 breast cancer patients supplemented with 390 mg CoQ$_{10}$ daily during three to five years (29). However, these results should be viewed with caution because it is impossible to evaluate the efficacy of CoQ$_{10}$ from case studies and uncontrolled trials. They are included here because they are often cited to support marketing claims.

CoQ$_{10}$ for Immunity and HIV/AIDS

- One study reported that AIDS patients had reduced CoQ$_{10}$ blood concentrations compared to control subjects (30).

- Three uncontrolled trials in small numbers of healthy subjects and cancer patients supplemented with CoQ$_{10}$ reported improvement in immune parameters (30–33). These studies are included, despite their methodological flaws, because they are often cited to support marketing claims.

CoQ$_{10}$ and Neurodegenerative Disease

- One researcher hypothesized that CoQ$_{10}$ may play a role in the pathogenesis of neurodegenerative conditions by: (1) increasing ATP concentrations as a result of improved mitochondrial energetics, or (2) providing antioxidant protection in the brain (34).

- In one study, platelet mitochondrial CoQ$_{10}$ concentrations were significantly lower in 17 patients with Parkinson's disease compared to age- and sex-matched controls (35). However, in another study, serum levels of CoQ$_{10}$ were not correlated with duration or phase of Parkinson's disease (36).

- In an uncontrolled pilot study, 15 subjects (ages 54 y to 70 y) with Parkinson's disease were supplemented with one of three doses of CoQ$_{10}$ plus 400 IU vitamin E. Subjects 1 through 5 were given 400 mg/d CoQ$_{10}$, subjects 6 through 10 were given 600 mg/d CoQ$_{10}$, and subjects 11 through 15 were given 800 mg/day CoQ$_{10}$ for one month. Plasma CoQ$_{10}$ levels increased with all doses. CoQ$_{10}$ plus vitamin E did not change the mean score on the motor portion of the Unified Parkinson's Disease Rating Scale. There was a trend toward an increase in complex I activity of the mitochondrial electron-transport chain (reduced in the platelets and substatia niagra of patients with Parkinson's disease). The authors noted that any symptomatic effect caused by CoQ$_{10}$ would likely have been overshadowed by the effect of medication that the patient continued to take during the study. In two of the five subjects supplemented with 800 mg CoQ$_{10}$, at the final visit, mild, transient changes in the urine (trace protein and hyaline casts) were observed, the clinical significance of which was unclear. No abnormality was observed on follow-up urinalyses after discontinuation of CoQ_{10}. The authors suggested that if CoQ_{10} is supplemented at doses > 600 mg/day it would be prudent to periodically monitor renal function. Because CoQ_{10} and vitamin E were administered together it is impossible to ascribe the effects to CoQ_{10} alone (37).

SAFETY

- In the cited studies, 200 mg/d CoQ_{10} has been apparently well tolerated for up to one year and 100 mg/d for up to six years with no reported serious adverse events (38). Some subjects have reported mild gastrointestinal distress.

- In a small study of patients with Parkinson's disease, 800 mg/d CoQ_{10} plus vitamin E for one month resulted in mild changes in urine, the clinical significance of which was unclear. The authors suggested that if CoQ_{10} is supplemented at doses > 600 mg/day, it would be prudent to periodically monitor renal function (37).

REFERENCES

1. Kalen A, Appelkvist EL, Dallner G. Age-related changes in the lipid composition of rat and human tissue. *Lipids.* 1989;24:579–584.
2. Mordente A, Martorana GE, Santini SA, et al. Antioxidant effect of coenzyme Q on hydrogen peroxide-activated myoglobin. *Clin Investig.* 1993;71:S92–S96.
3. Ernster L, Forsmark-Andree P. Ubiquinol: an endogenous antioxidant in aerobic organisms. *Clin Investig.* 1993;71:S60–S65.
4. Weber C, Sejersgard Jakobsen T, Mortensen SA, et al. Antioxidative effect of dietary coenzyme Q_{10} in human blood plasma. *Int J Vitam Nutr Res.* 1994;64:311–315.
5. Weber C, Bysted A, Holmer G. The coenzyme Q_{10} content of the average Danish diet. *Int J Vitam Nutr Res.* 1997;67:123–129.
6. Weber C, Bysted A, Holmer G. Coenzyme Q_{10} in the diet–daily intake and relative bioavailability. *Mol Aspects Med.* 1997;18:S251–S254.
7. Chopra RK, Goldman R, Sinatra ST, et al. Relative bioavailability of coenzyme Q_{10} formulations in human subjects. *Int J Vitam Nutr Res.* 1998;68:109–113.
8. Mortensen SA. Perspectives on therapy of cardiovascular diseases with coenzyme Q_{10} (ubiquinone). *Clin Investig.* 1993:71:S116–S123.
9. Jameson S. Statistical data support prediction of death within 6 months on low levels of coenzyme Q_{10} and other entities. *Clin Investig.* 1993;71:S137–S139.
10. Appelkvist EL, Edlund C, Low P, et al. Effects of inhibitors of hydroxymethylglutaryl coenzyme A reductase on coenzyme Q and dolichol biosynthesis. *Clin Investig.* 1993;71:S97–S102.
11. De Pinieux G, Chariot P, Ammi-Said M, et al. Lipid-lowering drugs and mitochondrial function: effects of HMG-CoA reductase inhibitors on serum ubiquinone and blood lactate/pyruvate ratio. *Br J Clin Pharmacol.* 1996;42:333–337.
12. Bargossi AM, Battino M, Gaddi A, et al. Exogenous CoQ_{10} preserves plasma ubiquinone

levels in patients treated with 3-hydroxy-3methylglutaryl coenzyme A reductase inhibitors. *Int J Clin Lab Res.* 1994;24:171–176.

13. Laaksonen R, Jokelainen K, Sahi T, et al. Decreases in serum ubiquinone concentrations do not result in reduced levels in muscle tissue during short-term simvastatin treatment in humans. *Clin Pharmacol Ther.* 1995;57:62–66.

14. Watson PS, Scalia GM, Galbraith A, et al. Lack of effect of coenzyme Q on left ventricular function in patients with congestive heart failure. *J Am Coll Cardiol.* 1999;33:1549–1552.

15. Singh RB, Wander GS, Rastogi A, et al. Randomized, double-blind, placebo-controlled trial of coenzyme Q_{10} in patients with acute myocardial infarction. *Cardiovasc Drugs Ther.* 1998;12:347–353.

16. Soja AM, Mortensen SA. Treatment of congestive heart failure with coenzyme Q_{10} illuminated by meta-analyses of clinical trials. *Mol Aspects Med.* 1997;18:S159–S168.

17. Morisco C, Trimarco B, Condorelli M. Effect of coenzyme Q_{10} therapy in patients with congestive heart failure: a long-term multicenter randomized study. *Clin Investig.* 1993;71:S134–S136.

18. Judy WV, Stogsdill WW, Folkers K. Myocardial preservation by therapy with coenzyme Q_{10} during heart surgery. *Clin Investig.* 1993;71:S155–S161.

19. Taggart DP, Jenkins M, Hooper J, et al. Effects of short term supplementation with coenzyme Q_{10} on myocardial protection during cardiac operations. *Ann Thorac Surg.* 1996;61:829–833.

20. Khatta M, Alexander BS, Krichten CM, et al. The effect of coenzyme Q_{10} with congestive heart failure. *Ann Intern Med.* 2000;132:636–640.

21. Weston SB, Zhou S, Weatherby RP, et al. Does exogenous coenzyme Q_{10} affect aerobic capacity in endurance athletes? *Int J Sport Nutr.* 1997;7:197–206.

22. Malm C, Svensson M, Ekblom B, et al. Effects of ubiquinone-10 supplementation and high intensity training on physical performance in humans. *Acta Physiol Scand.* 1997;161:379–384.

23. Porter DA, Costill DL, Zachwieja JJ, et al. The effect of oral coenzyme Q_{10} on the exercise tolerance of middle-aged, untrained men. *Int J Sports Med.* 1995;16:421–427.

24. Braun B, Clarkson PM, Freedson PS, Kohl RL. Effects of coenzyme Q_{10} supplementation on exercise performance, VO_{2max}, and lipid peroxidation in trained cyclists. *Int J Sport Nutr.* 1991;1:353–365.

25. Kaikkonen J, Kosonen L, Nyyssonen K, et al. Effect of combined coenzyme Q_{10} and d-alpha-tocopherol acetate supplementation on exercise-induced lipid peroxidation and muscular damage: a placebo-controlled, double-blind study in marathon runners. *Free Radic Res.* 1998;29:85–92.

26. Folkers K, Osterborg A, Nylander M, et al. Activities of vitamin Q_{10} in animal models and a serious deficiency in patients with cancer. *Biochem Biophys Res Commun.* 1997;234:296–299.

27. Jolliet P, Simon N, Barre J, et al. Plasma coenzyme Q_{10} concentrations in breast cancer: prognosis and therapeutic consequences. *Int J Clin Pharmacol Ther.* 1998;36:506–509.

28. Lockwood K, Moesgaard S, Hanioka T, et al. Apparent partial remission of breast can-

cer in 'high risk' patients supplemented with nutritional antioxidants, essential fatty acids and coenzyme Q_{10}. *Mol Aspects Med.* 1994;15:S231–S240.

29. Lockwood K, Moesgaard S, Yamamoto T, et al. Progress on therapy of breast cancer with vitamin Q_{10} and the regression of metastases. *Biochem Biophys Res Commun.* 1995;212:172–177.

30. Folkers K, Langsjoen P, Nara Y, et al. Biochemical deficiencies of coenzyme Q_{10} in HIV-infection and exploratory treatment. *Biochem Biophys Res Commun.* 1988;153:888–896.

31. Folkers K, Hanioka T, Xia LJ, et al. Coenzyme Q_{10} increases T4/T8 ratios of lymphocytes in ordinary subjects and relevance to patients having the AIDS related complex. *Biochem Biophys Res Commun.* 1991;176:786–791.

32. Folkers K, Morita M, McRee J. The activities of coenzyme Q_{10} and vitamin B_6 for immune responses. *Biochem Biophys Res Commun.* 1993;193:88–92.

33. Folkers K, Brown R, Judy WV, et al. Survival of cancer patients on therapy with coenzyme Q_{10}. *Biochem Biophys Res Commun.* 1993;192:241–245.

34. Beal MF, Matthews RT. Coenzyme Q_{10} in the central nervous system and its potential usefulness in the treatment of neurodegenerative diseases. *Mol Aspects Med.* 1997;18:S169–S179.

35. Shults CW, Haas RH, Passov D, et al. Coenzyme Q_{10} levels correlate with the activities of complexes I and II/III in mitochondria from parkinsonian and nonparkinsonian subjects. *Ann Neurol.* 1997;42:261–264.

36. Jimenez-Jimenez FJ, Molina JA, de Bustos F, et al. Serum levels of coenzyme Q_{10} in patients with Parkinson's disease. *J Neural Transm.* 2000;107:177–181.

37. Shults CW, Beal MF, Fontaine D, et al. Absorption, tolerability, and effects on mitochondrial activity of oral coenzyme Q_{10} in parkinsonian patients. *Neurology.* 1998;50:793–795.

38. Overvad K, Diamant B, Holm L, et al. Coenzyme Q_{10} in health and disease. *Eur J Clin Nutr.* 1999;53:764–770.

Colostrum/Bovine Colostrum

Colostrum is the premilk fluid secreted from the mammary glands during the first few days after birth. In addition to supplying both macro- and micronutrients to the newborn, colostrum is a source of several growth and immune factors that contribute to the neonate's development and immune defense. Both bovine and human colostrum contain a variety of peptide growth factors, including insulin-like growth factors (IGF-1, IGF-2), insulin, transforming growth factor –α and –β, and epidermal growth factor (EGF). IGF-1 and -2 are heat and acid stable growth factors that are involved in cellular growth, development, and differentiation in mammals. TGF –α and –β have many functions including wound repair and maintaining gut integrity. EGF may play a role in preventing bacterial translocation and stimulating gut growth in newborns (1, 2, 3).

Colostrum also contains several antimicrobial compounds, including immunoglobulins, lactoferrin, lysozyme, and lactoperoxidase. Immunoglobulins are largely responsible for the antimicrobial activity of bovine colostrum. IgG1 is the most abundant type of immunoglobulin in colostrum, whereas IgG2, IgM, and IgA are found at much lower levels. At birth, calves have very low serum levels of immunoglobulins because these antibodies are not passed through the placenta. Immunoglobulins from colostrum play an important role in protecting newborn calves from infectious enteric and respiratory diseases. Lactoferrin, an iron-binding glycoprotein, is another antimicrobial compound found in colostrum. It has been shown to inhibit the growth of a number of microbes and has also demonstrated antiviral activity *in vitro* against herpes simplex virus type-I, human immunodeficiency virus, and human cytomegalovirus. Lactoferrin may also play a role in intestinal iron absorption and neonatal gut growth. Lysozyme and lactoperoxidase are antibacterial enzymes found in colostrum that have been shown to be toxic to gram-positive and gram-negative bacteria (1–3).

Researchers have discovered that hyperimmunizing cows with repeated injections of vaccines can increase the immunoglobulin content of the milk (1). The resulting product is referred to as "hyperimmune colostrum" and contains high amounts of specific antibodies against the microbes in the vaccines. Although a number of studies have examined hyperimmune colostrum and/or its individual antibodies, it is important to note that this product differs from commercially available colostrum and it is not sold as a dietary supplement in the United States.

Because of its unique composition, bovine colostrum has been marketed as a dietary supplement for gut health, immunity, weight loss, skin health, and other conditions. Research from *in vitro*, animal, and clinical trials suggests that hyperimmune colostrum and/or its individual fractions might be useful for treating a number of gastrointestinal disorders, including short-bowel syndrome, NSAID (nonsteroidal anti-inflammatory drug) injury, chemotherapy-induced mucositis, inflammatory bowel diseases, and infective diarrhea (2, 3).

Media and Marketing Claims	Efficacy
Beneficial for digestive system (hyperimmune colostrum)	↑?
Beneficial for digestive system (nonimmune colostrum)	NR
Supports immune function in individuals with HIV+	NR
Builds muscle and reduces fat	NR

Advisory

- No reported serious adverse effects
- Must not be contaminated (potential risk with supplements derived from cows due to bovine spongiform encephalopathy/mad cow disease)
- Avoid if allergic to cow's milk

Drug/Supplement Interactions

- No reported adverse interactions
- Colostrum taken may have a beneficial effect on the gut when taken with NSAIDs (nonsteroidal anti-inflammatory drugs)

C

KEY POINTS

- There is a theoretical basis that bovine colostrum and its individual components may be helpful in intestinal illnesses. *In vitro* animal and some human evidence that bovine colostrum may be beneficial for infectious diarrhea. Preliminary data suggest that colostrum might help reduce NSAID-induced gut injury, but this association needs to be tested in long-term clinical trials. Overall, most of the research to date has been conducted in small trials. Many studies used colostrum from hyperimmunized cows, and this is currently not commercially available as a dietary supplement in the United States. Large-scale, controlled clinical trials of nonimmune colostrum are needed to determine its efficacy for use with intestinal diseases.

- Although a number of uncontrolled trials have suggested that bovine colostrum may be helpful for patients with AIDS-related diarrhea, controlled trials are needed to determine efficacy for this population.

- Much more data collection and analysis are necessary to determine the effect of bovine colostrum supplements on body composition and exercise training.

FOOD SOURCES

Not a constituent of food besides human breast milk
Regular cow's milk contains negligible amounts of the immune and growth factors found in bovine colostrum.

DOSAGE INFORMATION/BIOAVAILABILITY

Colostrum sold in supplements is typically collected during the first 72 hours after a cow gives birth. Supplements may either be pasteurized at minimum heat after filtration and homogenization or sterilized through microfiltration and vacuum packaging (4). Ideally, colostrum products should be taken from a pool of pasture-fed cows to insure a wide spectrum of antibodies and growth factors. Colostrum is available in capsules, chewable tablets, powders, liquid, energy bars and protein powders, and in topical skin creams and lotions. Manufacturers suggest taking 2,000 to 5,000 mg of colostrum (about 8 to 10 capsules) daily, although some studies have used 20 g dosages.

The biochemical makeup of colostrum may provide inherent protection against proteolytic digestion in the gut, whereas isolated growth factors may be digested when administered orally (2). Infants and children have greater gut permeability and, therefore, absorb the immune and growth factors in colostrum better than adults (1). In one small study of six subjects, nearly 50 percent of orally ingested 2.1 g bovine colostral immunoglobulins were recovered in ileal fluid and the activity of the immunoglobulins against *C difficile* toxins was retained (5). In another study of seven healthy adults, 19 percent of orally ingested IgG and IgM, but 0 percent of IgA, was still immunologically active after passing the ileum (6). In a study of 105 preschoolers supplemented with hyperimmune colostrum from cows immunized with rotavirus (rotavirus causes infectious diarrhea), colostral antibodies survived passage through the gut and remained active (7).

RELEVANT RESEARCH

Colostrum and Intestinal Disorders

- In a double-blinded, placebo-controlled study, 27 patients (aged 1 mo to 18 y) with *E. coli* associated diarrhea were randomized to receive 7,000 mg bovine colostrum (from nonimmunized cows) or placebo daily for two weeks. Stool frequency and fecal excretion of the infecting strains were assessed. At the end of therapy, subjects treated with colostrum had significantly reduced stool frequency (from three stools to one). Placebo-treated subjects had no change in stool frequency. However, colostrum had no effect on the carriage of pathogens in feces (8).

- Other controlled clinical trials using colostrum from hyperimmunized cows have reported improvements in diarrhea infection in children infected with rotavirus (9, 10) and in healthy adults challenged with *Cryptosporidium parvum* infection (11).

Colostrum and NSAID-Induced Gut Injury

- In a placebo-controlled, crossover trial, seven healthy male subjects received in random order 375 mL bovine colostrum (nonimmune) or isocaloric placebo daily for seven days each. There was a two-week washout period between treatments. For the last five days of each study arm, subjects also took indomethacin (50 mg × 3). At the beginning and end of each test period, intestinal permeability was assessed by quantifying absorption of lactulose, rhamnose, and mannitol sugars. Gut permeability is a method of testing small intestinal injury. There were no significant differences in baseline permeability values. However, permeability significantly increased about three-fold in response to indomethacin in the placebo subjects, but not the colostrum-treated subjects. This pilot study was not blinded, and therefore the results should be viewed with caution (12).

- A second study was performed by the same researchers in 15 subjects who had regularly been taking a stable, substantive dose of a nonselective NSAID for at least a year. Patients in a double-blind, crossover design were randomized to receive 375 mL bovine colostrum or placebo daily for seven days each, with a two-week washout period. All subjects continued to take their NSAID therapies. Intestinal permeability was assessed at baseline and at the end of the study. Baseline permeability levels were significantly lower than those of the healthy subjects on short-term NSAID therapy in study 1 (above). At the study's end, colostrum had no significant effect on gut permeability (12)

- Bovine colostrum reduced intestinal injury associated with NSAID medication in rats (13).

Colostrum and AIDS-Related Diarrhea

- There is some evidence from small, uncontrolled trials that hyperimmune and/or non-immune colostrum may benefit patients with AIDS infected with the parasite *Cryptosporidium parvum*. In one *in vitro* study, hyperimmune colostrum inhibited *C parvum* infection in human intestinal cells, whereas nonimmune colostrum did not (14).

■ In an open study of 24 AIDS patients with severe diarrhea, 21 days of hyperimmune colostrum treatment reduced stool weight (from 1,158 to 595 g/day at study's end) and stool frequency (from 6.6 to 5.4 bowel movements/day at study's end) (15). Because this study was not controlled, the results should be viewed with caution.

■ In a double-blind, comparative pilot study, five AIDS patients with diarrhea due to *C parvum* were randomized to receive either hyperimmune colostrum or nonimmune colostrum by continuous nasogastric infusion for 10 days. One of three patients treated with hyperimmune colostrum had a reduction in diarrhea and in the stool concentration of *C parvum* oocytes. Two patients receiving nonimmune colostrum had decreases in diarrhea volume, but no change in oocytes excreted (16). The small sample size in this study did not allow for statistical analysis and therefore, the results are difficult to interpret.

■ There are also case reports of clinical improvement with hyperimmune colostrum in two patients with AIDS and diarrhea secondary to *C parvum* (17, 18).

Colostrum and Body Weight

■ In a double-blind, placebo-controlled study, 22 resistance and aerobically trained subjects were randomized to receive 20 g colostrum in powder form or placebo (whey protein) daily for eight weeks. (The 20 g dose of colostrum contained 71 calories, 16 g protein, 4 g carbohydrate, and 0.2 g fat.) Subjects were instructed not to change their current diet and exercise level. Body composition was assessed by dual x-ray absorptiometry (DEXA). Treadmill time to exhaustion, one repetition maximum strength during bench press, and the total number of repetitions performed during one set to exhaustion at a submaximal load for bench press were assessed. There were no significant differences in baseline measures of age, height, weight, body composition, performance measures, or exercise training frequency between groups. Each subject performed aerobic and weight training exercise at least three times per week. The whey protein group experienced a significant increase in body weight, but no change in lean body mass (LBM), whereas the colostrum group had a significant increase in LBM (mean gain of 1.5 kg), but no significant change in body weight. However, the authors noted that the coefficient of variation for DEXA may be as high as 3.1 percent, which could account for the 1.5 kg increase. There were no other differences in any other parameter measured. The authors hypothesized that if colostrum does increase lean body mass, the mechanism of action may be due to an increase in circulating IGF-1 levels (although this was not measured) (19).

■ In a double-blind, placebo-controlled, crossover study, nine male, active sprinters and jumpers received in random order the following treatments for eight days each: (1) 125 mL colostrum drink (67 µg/L insulin-like growth factors-1 (IGF-1) and 0.39 g/liter IgG); (2) 25 mL colostrum drink (13.5 µg/liter IGF-1 and 0.12 g/liter IgG); or (3) isocaloric placebo (whey). Each treatment was separated by a 13-day washout period. All subjects were trained according to the same program starting at four weeks before treatment and continuing through the study. On the sixth day of each test period, subjects performed a 90-minute strenuous exercise session and a jump test before and after the 90 minutes. Blood and saliva samples of IGF-1, IgG, amino acids, and hormones were collected before and after the test training sessions. Both the low- and high-dose colostrum produced a significant increase in IGF-1 concentrations, whereas the placebo did not. However, the placebo group did have higher IGF-1 levels at baseline. Serum IgG, hormone, amino acid and saliva IgA were not different between groups. The authors concluded that in this small study, bovine colostrum raised serum IGF-1 levels (IGF stimulates protein synthesis) in athletes during strength and speed training. This study did not evaluate the effect of colostrum on exercise performance or body composition (20).

SAFETY

- No serious adverse effects have been reported with hyperimmune or nonimmune colostrum products.

- Products need to be properly processed by pasteurization or microfiltration. Colostrum suppliers need to certify that products are free of bovine spongiform encephaplopathy (mad cow disease) and other bovine diseases. Additionally, products should be tested for the presence of heavy metals, pesticides, herbicides, and pathogens, and tested to verify that the final product is biologically active.

- Colostrum could cause mild gastrointestinal discomfort in the lactose-intolerant patient, because the products do contain a small amount of lactose. Individuals with a true cow's milk allergy should avoid colostrum.

REFERENCES

1. Pakkanen R, Aalto J. Growth factors and antimicrobial factors of bovine colostrum. *Int Dairy J.* 1997;7:285–297.
2. Playford RJ, Macdonald CE, Johnson WS. Colostrum and milk-derived peptide growth factors for the treatment of gastrointestinal disorders. *Am J Clin Nutr.* 2000;72:5–14.
3. Lilius EM, Marnila P. The role of colostral antibodies in prevention of microbial infections. *Curr Opin Infec Dis.* 2001;14:295–300.
4. Maher TJ. *Bovine Colostrum Continuing Education Module.* Boulder, Colo: New Hope Institute of Retailing; 2000.
5. Warny M, Fatimi A, Bostwick EF, et al. Bovine immunoglobulin concentrate-clostridium difficile retains *C difficile* toxin neutralizing activity after passage through the human stomach and small intestine. *Gut.* 1999;44:212–217.
6. Roos N, Mahe S. Benamouzig R, et al. 15-N labeled immunoglobulins from bovine colostrum are partially resistant to digestion in human intestine. *J Nutr.* 1995;125:1238–1244.
7. Pacyna J, Siwek K, Terry SJ, et al. Survival of rotavirus antibody activity derived from

bovine colostrum after passage through the human gastrointestinal tract. *J Pediatr Gastroenterol Nutr.* 2001;32:162–167.

8. Huppertz HI, Rutkowski S, Busch DH, et al. Bovine colostrum ameliorates diarrhea in infection with diarrheagenic *Escherichia coli*, shiga toxin-producing *E. coli*, and *E. coli* expressing intimin and hemolysin. *J Pediatr Gastroenterol Nutr.* 1999;29:452–456.

9. Sarker SA, Casswall TH, Mahalanabis D, et al. Successful treatment of rotavirus diarrhea in children with immunoglobulin from immunized bovine colostrum. *Pediatr Infect Dis J.* 1998;17:149–154.

10. Mitra Ak, Mahalanabis D, Ashraf H, et al. Hyperimmune cow colostrum reduces diarrhea due to rotavirus: a double-blind, controlled clinical trial. *Acta Paediatr.* 1995;84:996–1001.

11. Okhuysen PC, Chappell CL, Crabb J, et al. Prophylactic effect of bovine anti-*Cryptosporidium* hyperimmune colostrum immunoglobulin in healthy volunteers challenged with *Cryptosporidium*. *Clin Infec Dis* 1998;26:1324–1329.

12. Playford RJ, MacDonald CE, Calnan DP, et al. Co-administration of the health food supplement, bovine colostrum, reduces the acute non-steroidal anti-inflammatory drug-induced increase in intestinal permeability. *Clin Sci (Lond).* 2001;100:627–633.

13. Playford RJ, Floyd DN, Macdonald CE, et al. Bovine colostrum is a health food supplement which prevents NSAID induced gut damage. *Gut.* 1999;44:653–658.

14. Flanigan T, Marshall R, Redman D, et al. In vitro screening of therapeutic agents against Crytosporidium: hyperimmune cow colostrum is highly inhibitory. *J Protozol.* 1991;38:225S–227S.

15. Greenberg PD, Cello JP. Treatment of severe diarrhea caused by *Cryptosporidium parvum* with oral bovine immunoglobulin concentrate in patients with AIDS. *J Acquir Immune Defic Syndr Hum Retrovirol.* 1996;13:348–354.

16. Nord J, Ma P, DiJohn D, et al. Treatment with bovine hyperimmune colostrum of cryptosporidial diarrhea in AIDS patients. *AIDS.* 1990;4:581–584.

17. Shield J, Melville C, Novelli V, et al. Bovine colostrum immunoglobulin concentrate for cryptosporidiosis in AIDS. *Arch Dis Child.* 1993;69:451–453.

18. Ungar BL, Ward DJ, Fayer R, et al. Cessation of Cryptosporidium-associated diarrhea in an acquired immunodeficiency syndrome patient after treatment with hyperimmune bovine colostrum. *Gastroenterology.* 1990;98:486–489.

19. Antonio J, Sanders MS, Van Gammeren D. The effect of bovine colostrum supplementation on body composition and exercise performance in active men and women. *Nutrition.* 2001;17:243–247.

20. Mero A, Miikkulainen H, Riski J, et al. Effects of bovine colostrum supplementation on serum IGF-I, IgG, hormone and saliva IgA during training. *J Appl Physiol.* 1997;83:1144–1151.

Conjugated Linoleic Acid

Conjugated linoleic acid (CLA) is a term used to describe a group of linoleic acid isomers in which the double bonds are conjugated at carbons 10 and 12 or 9 and 11 in the *cis* and *trans* configurations. Nine different isomers of CLA have been identified. CLA is a class of fatty acids produced naturally by microorganisms associated with digestion, particularly certain microorganisms in the rumen of cattle. It is found in low concentrations in human blood and tissues. Although linoleic acid has been found to have a stimulatory effect on some types of cancer in animals, preliminary evidence suggests CLA may have the opposite effect. Researchers have not determined the mechanism behind the potential anticarcinogenic activity of CLA. CLA has also recently been investigated for its effect on body composition. A specific CLA isomer (*trans*10, *cis*12) may be responsible for this by inhibiting a number of biochemical factors associated with lipid uptake. Some theorize that CLA inhibits heparin-releasable lipoprotein lipase, which cleaves triglycerides so that free fatty acids are absorbed into cells (1–3).

Media and Marketing Claims	Efficacy
Enhances weight loss and reduces appetite	↓?
Stimulates immune system	NR
Protects against cancer	NR
Reduces risk of cardiovascular disease	NR
Improves glucose tolerance	NR

Advisory

No reported serious adverse effects

Drug/Supplement Interactions

No reported adverse interactions

KEY POINTS

- Studies in animals suggest that CLA supplementation reduces body fat and increases lean body mass. Preliminary human research suggests that CLA does not seem to have the same favorable effects on body composition. One study completed in a metabolic unit showed no positive effect of CLA supplementation on weight loss, lean body mass, or appetite. More research in larger groups of subjects is needed before CLA can be used as adjunctive therapy for weight management.

- Although CLA appears to enhance immune function in animal models, one study reported no immune enhancement in healthy women. More human research is needed.

- Preliminary animal and *in vitro* studies suggest CLA has anticarcinogenic properties. However, to date, there are no human studies. One review article speculated that if the cancer protective efficacy of CLA can be characterized further and its mechanism of action delineated, there is a possibility that CLA-enriched food products may become available (2).

- There is preliminary evidence from animal studies that CLA may reduce atherosclerosis and blood lipids. However, CLA had no effect on blood cholesterol (total, LDL,

HDL), triglyceride levels, platelet function or blood coagulation in healthy women with normal cholesterol levels, and had no effect on blood lipids in obese men. At this time, there are no controlled studies testing the effects of CLA supplements on cardiovascular disease endpoints in humans.

- There is preliminary research indicating that CLA may benefit prediabetic fatty rats. However, limited evidence from human trials (published in peer review journals) suggests that CLA does not significantly impact glucose or insulin levels in healthy or obese subjects. More research is needed to determine the effects of CLA on diabetic control.

FOOD SOURCES

CLA is primarily found in the milk and meat of ruminant animals. The CLA content of dairy products ranges from 2.3 to 11.3 mg/g of fat of which the majority is in the *cis*-9, *trans*-11 isomer form. Beef fat contains 3.1 mg/g to 8.5 mg/g fat with the same isomer predominating. Cooking has been shown to increase the CLA content of meat. Food products from non-ruminant animals and plant oils have a CLA content of 0.6 mg/g to 0.9 mg/g fat. The estimated CLA content of the U.S. diet is approximately 1 g/day (1), although another study suggested a much lower daily intake of approximately 150 mg to 200 mg CLA (2).

Food	CLA (mg/Serving) (4)*
Lamb, uncooked (4 oz)	137
Beef, ground, uncooked (4 oz)	130
Butter (1 tbsp)	54
Yogurt, low-fat (1 c)	16.7
Peanut butter (2 tbsp)	3.3
Chicken, uncooked (½ chicken)	3.2
Oil, olive (1 tbsp)	2.7
Shrimp, uncooked (3 oz)	0.9
Yogurt, nonfat (1 tbsp)	0.7

Serving sizes calculated from values from Reference 4.

DOSAGE INFORMATION/BIOAVAILABILITY

CLA produced synthetically from sunflower oil is sold in capsules providing about 60 percent to 80 percent CLA. Manufacturers typically recommend 1 g to 4 g CLA/day. Many products contain the patented CLA formula Tonalin or Clarinol used in some research studies. These products contain the biologically active CLA isomers (*cis* 9, *trans* ll and *trans* 10, *cis* 12). The amount of CLA in human adipose tissue and serum is significantly related to dietary milk fat intake (5, 6).

RELEVANT RESEARCH

CLA and Body Composition

- In a double-blind, placebo-controlled study, 60 overweight or obese subjects were randomized into five groups receiving a placebo (9 g olive oil) or 1.7, 3.4, 5.1, or 6.8 g CLA/day for 12 weeks. Dual-energy x-ray absorptiometry measured body composition at baseline, and at weeks 6 and 12. Forty-seven subjects completed the study. CLA reduced body fat mass compared to the placebo, with significant reductions observed in the 3.4-g and 6.8-g CLA groups. However, there were no differences among groups in lean body mass, body mass index, blood safety variables, or blood lipids. There were no differences among groups regarding adverse events (7).

- In a randomized, controlled study, the effect of CLA (3 g/day for 64 days) vs. a placebo (sunflower oil) was investigated in 17 healthy women confined to a metabolic suite for 94 days where diet and activity were controlled and held constant. Subjects entered the metabolic suite for a control period lasting 30 days just prior to treatment. CLA supplementation had no effect on fat-free mass, fat mass, and percent body fat compared to the placebo. In addition, CLA did not change exercise or resting baseline, four-week or eight-week measures of energy expenditure (kcal/min), fat oxidation, respiratory exchange ratios (8).

- In another report of the same subjects, the effects of CLA on circulating leptin levels, appetite, insulin, glucose, and lactate concentrations were examined. CLA supplementation caused a transient decrease in mean circulating leptin levels for seven weeks, but then returned to baseline over the last two weeks of the study. Appetite parameters measured during the time when the greatest decreases in leptin levels were observed showed no significant effect of CLA compared to the placebo. There was a nonsignificant trend for mean insulin levels to increase toward the end of supplementation period in CLA-treated subjects. No effects were seen on plasma glucose or lactate levels (9).

- In a randomized, double-blind, placebo-controlled trial (reported as an abstract), 80 male and female obese subjects (mean age = 41 y) were randomized to receive 2.7 g CLA or a placebo daily for six months. Subjects were instructed in diet, exercise, and lifestyle modification, and participants were asked to reduce their caloric intake by 500 kcal from the baseline. Subjects were asked to exercise three times weekly for at least 30 minutes. Seventy-one subjects completed the trial. Overall, there were no differences in weight loss (CLA subjects lost 12.8 kg vs 10.8 kg for the placebo), fat mass or fat-free mass between groups. When researchers examined a subpopulation of subjects who gained fat-free mass (10 in the CLA group, 5 in the placebo group), they found that fat mass decreased by 4.8 kg in the CLA group, but increased by 9.2 kg in the placebo group, this difference did not reach statistical significance. Of 10 subjects who gained both fat mass and fat free mass (CLA = 6, placebo = 4), 74 percent of the gain was fat in the placebo group vs 55 percent in the CLA group, and this difference was statistically significant. The authors suggested that this result may indicate that CLA preferentially causes deposition of lean body mass rather than fat mass in obese individuals in an anabolic state. Overall, however, they concluded that CLA had no impact on enhancing weight or fat loss in calorie-restricted obese subjects (10). This study is included here although it has not been published in a peer review journal because it has been reported in the media and in testimonials for CLA.

- Several studies in mice have reported that CLA diets (0.25 percent to 5 percent) decrease fat deposition when fed high fat diets, reduce energy intake, and increase lean body mass (11–15). In one of these studies, *trans*-10, *cis*-12 CLA isomer, but not the *trans*-9, *trans*-11 isomer, had a favorable effect on body composition (14).

CLA and Immunity

- In a double-blind, placebo-controlled study, 17 women (aged 20 y to 41 y) participated in a 93-day study confined to a metabolic research unit where exercise and diet were strictly controlled. Seven subjects were fed the basal diet (19, 20, and 51 percent energy from protein, fat, and carbohydrate, respectively). The remaining subjects were fed the basal diet for the first 30 days, followed by 3.9 g CLA daily for the next 63 days. Indices of immune response (number of circulating white blood cells, granulocytes, monocytes, lymphocytes, and their subsets) were tested at weekly intervals, and delayed type hypersensitivity (DTH) to a panel of six antigens was tested on days 30 and 90. All subjects were immunized with an influenza vaccine on day 65, with antibody titers collected on day 65 and day 92. CLA feeding had no effect on any of the parameters of immune status tested (16).

CLA and Cancer

- According to a review article that summarized animal model and cell culture studies of CLA and cancer, CLA inhibited proliferation in all cell lines such as human malignant melanoma, colorectal, breast, and lung cancer. CLA also reduced the incidence of chemically induced mouse skin and forestomach cancers; and CLA inhibited chemically induced rat mammary tumors independent of the amount or type of fat in the diet (17).

CLA and Cardiovascular Disease

- In a controlled study of 17 healthy, normolipidemic female subjects confined to a metabolic research unit, subjects were randomized to receive 3.9 g CLA or a placebo (equivalent amount of sunflower oil) for 63 days, following a 30-day stabilization period of no treatment. Subjects were fed a low-fat diet (30 percent fat) consisting of natural foods meeting the RDA for all known nutrients. Fasting blood was drawn at baseline, midpoint (day 60), and at the end of the study (day 93). Adipose tissue samples were taken at baseline and at day 93. The plasma CLA increased significantly in subjects taking CLA, with the 9 *cis*-, 11 *trans*-isomer predominating. However, CLA in adipose tissue was not influenced by supplementation. CLA had no significant effects on plasma cholesterol (total, LDL, and HDL), or triglyceride levels (18). Another report of the same subjects also reported that CLA had no effect on platelet aggregation, or blood clotting parameters (19).

- In a double-blind, placebo-controlled study, 25 abdominally obese men (ages 39 y to 64 y) were randomized to receive 4.2 g CLA/day or a placebo for four weeks. The main endpoints were differences between the two groups in sagittal abdominal diameter (SAD), serum cholesterol, low-density lipoprotein, high-density lipoprotein, triglycerides, free fatty acids, glucose, and insulin. At baseline, there were no significant differences between groups in anthropometric or metabolic variables. At the study's end, there was a significant decrease in SAD (cm) in the CLA group compared to the placebo. However, there were no other differences in measurements of anthropometry or metabolism (20).
- Animal studies of rabbits and hamsters fed CLA containing diets reported reductions in lipoprotein levels, triglycerides, and atherosclerotic lesions of the aorta (21, 22).

CLA and Diabetes

- In non-diabetic subjects, CLA had no significant effect on insulin or glucose levels (9, 20).
- A 1.5 percent CLA diet inhibited the development of impaired glucose tolerance and hyperinsulinemia in prediabetic Zucker fatty rats. CLA also lowered serum triglycerides, free fatty acids, and leptin (23).

SAFETY

- CLA (3.9 g/day) had no adverse effects in a study lasting 93 days; however, long-term safety of CLA supplements has not been tested.
- A dose of 4.2 g CLA daily for one month caused lipid peroxidation in obese men. The authors noted that the consequences of the increased peroxidation are unknown. (24)
- A toxicology study of rats on 1.5 percent CLA diets for 36 weeks showed no treatment-related effects to organs or significant differences in hematological analysis of cardiac blood when compared to controls. The amount of CLA intake by rats was 50-fold greater than the 90th percentile of CLA intake of teenage boys (25).

REFERENCES

1. Decker EA. The role of phenolics, conjugated linoleic acid, carnosine, and pyrroloquinoline quinone as nonessential dietary antioxidants. *Nutr Rev.* 1995;53:49–58.
2. Ip C, Scimeca JA, Thompson HJ. Conjugated linoleic acid. A powerful anticarcinogen from animal fat sources. *Cancer.* 1994;74:1050–1054.
3. Terpstra AH. Differences between humans and mice in efficacy of the body fat lowering effect of conjugated linoleic acid: role of metabolic rate. *J Nutr.* 2001;131:2067–2068.
4. Rizenthaler KL, McGuire MK, Falen R, et al. Estimation of conjugated linoleic acid intake by written dietary assessment methodologies underestimates actual intake evaluated by food duplicate methodology. *J Nutr.* 2001;131:1548–1554.
5. Chin SF, Liu W, Storkson JM, et al. Dietary sources of conjugated dienoic isomers of

linoleic acid, a newly recognized class of anticarcinogens. *J Food Comp Analysis.* 1992;5:185–197.

6. Jiang J, Wolk A, Vessby B. Relation between the intake of milk fat and the occurrence of conjugated linoleic acid in human adipose tissue. *Am J Clin Nutr.* 2000;70:21–27.

7. Blankson H, Stakkestad JA, Fagertun E, et al. Conjugated linoleic acid reduces body fat mass in overweight and obese humans. *J Nutr.* 2000;130:2943–2948.

8. Zambell KL, Keim NL, Van Loan MD, et al. Conjugated linoleic acid supplementation in humans: effects on body composition and energy expenditure. *Lipids.* 2000;35:777–782.

9. Medina EA, Horn WF, Keim NL, et al. Conjugated linoleic acid supplementation in humans: effects on circulating leptin concentrations and appetite. *Lipids.* 2000;35:783–788.

10. Atkinson RL. Conjugated linoleic acid for altering body composition and treating obesity. In: Yurawecz MP, Mossoba MM, Kraner JGK, et al. eds. *Advances in Conjugated Linloeic Acid Research, Volume 1.* Champaign, Ill: American Oil Chemists' Society Press; 1999:348–353.

11. DeLany JP, Blohm F, Truett AA, et al. Conjugated linoleic acid rapidly reduces body fat content in mice without affecting energy intake. *Am J Physiol.* 1999;276(pt 2):R1172–R1179.

12. West DB, DeLany JP, Camet PM, et al. Effects of conjugated linoleic acid on body fat and energy metabolism in the mouse. *Am J Physiol.* 1998;275(pt 2):R667–R672.

13. Park Y, Albright KJ, Liu W, et al. Effect of conjugated linoleic acid on body composition in mice. *Lipids.* 1997;32:853–858.

14. Park Y, Storkson JM, Albright KJ, et al. Evidence that the trans-10, cis-12 isomer of conjugated linoleic acid induces body composition changes in mice. *Lipids.* 1999;34:235–241.

15. Kelley DS, Taylor PC, Rudolph IL, et al. Dietary conjugated linoleic acid did not alter immune status in young healthy women. *Lipids.* 2000;35:1065–1071.

16. Park Y, Albright KJ, Storkson JM, et al. Changes in body composition in mice during feeding and withdrawal of conjugated linoleic acid. *Lipids.* 1999;34:243–248.

17. Parodi PW. Cow's milk fat components as potential anticarcinogenic agents. *J Nutr.* 1997;127:1055–1060.

18. Benito P, Nelson GJ, Kelley DS, et al. The effect of conjugated linoleic acid on plasma lipoproteins and tissue fatty acid composition in humans. *Lipids.* 2001;36:229–236.

19. Benito P, Nelson GJ, Kelley DS, et al. The effect of conjugated linoleic acid on platelet function, platelet fatty acid composition, and blood coagulation in humans. *Lipids.* 2000;36:221–227.

20. Riserus U, Berglund L, Vessby B. Conjugated linoleic acid (CLA) reduced abdominal adipose tissue in obese middle-aged men with signs of the metabolic syndrome: a randomised controlled trial. *Int J Obes Relat Metab Disord.* 2001;25:1129–1135.

21. Lee KN, Kritchevsky D, Pariza MW. Conjugated linoleic acid and atherosclerosis in rabbits. *Atherosclerosis.* 1994;108:19–25.

22. Nicolosi RJ, Rogers EJ, Kritchevsky D, et al. Dietary conjugated linoleic acid reduces

plasma lipoproteins and early aortic atherosclerosis in hypercholesterolemic hamsters. *Artery*. 1997;22:266–277.

23. Houseknecht KL, Vanden Heuvel JP, Moya-Camarena SY, et al. Dietary conjugated linoleic acid normalizes impaired glucose tolerance in the Zucker diabetic fatty fa/fa rat. *Biochem Biophys Res Commun*. 1998;244:678–682.

24. Basu S, Riserus U, Turpeinen A, et al. Conjugated linoleic acid induces lipid peroxidation in men with abdominal obesity. *Clin Sci (Colch)*. 2000;99:511–516.

25. Scimeca JA. Toxicological evaluation of dietary conjugated linoleic acid in male Fischer 344 rats. *Food Chem Toxicol*. 1998;36:391–395.

Cranberry Extract

The cranberry (*Vaccinium macrocarpon*) is one of the few fruits native to North America. Cranberries get their name from Dutch and German settlers who called them "crane berries" since the vines and flowers resemble the head of a crane. Later, the name was shortened into cranberry. Native Americans used cranberries to help preserve food, as a dye, and in poultices to draw poison from arrow wounds. In the last century, cranberry juice was a folk remedy used to prevent urinary tract infections (UTI). Early research from the 1920s through the 1970s proposed that cranberry helped UTIs by acidifying urine. Cranberry juice contains quinic acid, which was thought to cause excretion of hipurric acid in the urine acting as an antibacterial agent. However, more recent data suggest that cranberry juice contains proanthocyanidins (tannins) that appear to block *Escherichia coli* bacteria from attaching to the bladder or kidney walls. Proanthocyanidins in blueberries also appear to have this effect. It has been shown that the fructose in cranberries interferes with *E coli* adhesion. Because of the potential positive effects of cranberry juice on the urinary tract, supplements containing cranberry juice extract have become available and are marketed for urinary tract health (1–5).

Media and Marketing Claims	Efficacy
Prevents urinary tract infections (cranberry juice)	↑?
Treats urinary tract infections	NR

Caution

Not a substitute for antibiotic treatment during urinary tract infection

Drug/Supplement Interactions

No reported adverse interactions

KEY POINTS

- There is some evidence that drinking cranberry juice (about 10 ounces daily) may reduce the incidence of urinary tract infections. However, many of the studies on cranberries have been criticized for poor design, high dropout rates, and small sample sizes.

- More evidence is needed to determine the efficacy of cranberry extract supplements. One very small study reported positive benefits with cranberry juice extract pills. However, the amount of the active ingredient (proanthocyanidin) needed to produce an antibacterial effect is unknown for the supplemental form. Because of this variability, some researchers recommend using the juice rather than pills. If the sugar content is a concern, sugar-free cranberry juice is available.

- There is currently no evidence that cranberry juice or pills treat an existing urinary tract infection. Individuals who think they may have an infection should consult their health care provider for treatment to avoid serious kidney infection.

FOOD SOURCES

Fresh or frozen cranberries, cranberry juice, dried cranberries
Approximately 4,400 cranberries make one gallon of juice (687 cranberries make 10 ounces of juice, the serving size used in the clinical trials) (1).

DOSAGE INFORMATION/BIOAVAILABILITY

Cranberry extract is available in pills and capsules with manufacturers recommending doses ranging from 400 mg to 2,400 mg daily (3 to 6 capsules/day). Many products are standardized to 5 percent proanthocyanidins, though the amount needed to have an antibacterial effect in the urinary tract is unknown. Some products are prepared from spray dried cranberry juice, and these most closely resemble the juice product.

Bioavailability of the proposed active components of cranberry (proanthocyanidins/tannins) is currently being tested in humans. There is an *in vivo* animal study demonstrating that proanthocyanidins are absorbed and excreted in mouse urine, and that the urine prevented adhesion of P-fimbriated *E coli* bacteria (6)

RELEVANT RESEARCH

Cranberry and UTIs

- A systematic review of controlled trials using cranberry in the prevention of UTIs in susceptible populations summarized the results of five trials that met inclusion criteria (total subjects = 304). Four of the studies compared cranberry juice to placebo juice or water, and one used cranberry capsules vs a placebo. Data from two out of the five trials indicated that cranberries were effective for symptomatic or asymptomatic UTIs, but this result was not obtained in an intention-to-treat analysis. The overall quality of the trials was considered to be poor, the sample sizes small, and number of dropouts high. The authors noted that the large number of dropouts (20 percent to 55 percent) may indicate that juice may not be acceptable for long-term use. They concluded that further properly designed trials are needed to determine whether cranberry juice can prevent UTIs, and the dose, formulation, and duration need to be clarified (7).

C

- A systematic review of controlled trials using cranberry to treat UTIs could not locate any trials that fulfilled all of the inclusion criteria for analysis. Two trials were excluded because they did not have any relevant outcomes. After searching all English and non-English databases, the authors concluded: "No randomized trials which assessed the effectiveness of cranberry juice for the treatment of UTIs were found. Therefore, there is no good quality evidence to suggest that it is effective for the treatment of UTIs" (8).

- In a double-blind, placebo-controlled, multi-center study, 192 elderly women were randomized to receive 300 mL cranberry juice cocktail (sweetened with saccharin) or a placebo beverage (identical in taste, appearance, and vitamin C content) daily for six months. Baseline and monthly urine samples were analyzed for bacteriuria and the presence of white blood cells. Thirty-nine subjects dropped out of the study, leaving 60 participants in the cranberry group and 60 in the placebo group. Cranberry-treated subjects had odds of bacteriuria with pyuria that were only 42 percent of the odds in the placebo group, and this difference was statistically significant. Furthermore, the odds of remaining bacteriuric-pyuric were 27 percent of the odds in the placebo group. There was no evidence that cranberry lowered the pH of the urine, indicating that urinary acidification was not responsible for the antibacterial effect. The study did not examine the effect of cranberry juice on UTI incidence. The authors concluded the cranberry drink appeared to be bacteriostatic in the bladder, but that longer controlled trials are needed in different populations to determine whether a cranberry drink prevents or reduces symptoms of symptomatic infection, and specifically whether cranberry juice plus antibiotics is superior to antibiotics alone (9).

- In a double-blind, placebo-controlled, crossover study, 19 subjects with a history of recurring UTIs (four UTIs in the past year or one UTI in the last three months) were recruited to participate. Subjects received in random order either cranberry extract or placebo after developing a UTI episode which was treated with standard antibiotics. The exact dosage of cranberry was not specified. Subjects took each treatment for three months before switching to the other for another three months. Only 10 subjects completed the six-month study (nine dropped out due to pregnancy). In total, 21 UTIs were recorded among the 10 remaining subjects during the study. Only six UTIs occurred during cranberry ingestion compared to 15 UTIs during placebo intake, and this difference was statistically different (10).

- An *in vitro* study was undertaken to determine if cranberry juice inhibits encrustation and blockage of urethral catheters. Researchers assigned 24 healthy volunteers to drink cranberry juice (2 × 500 mL during eight hours) or equivalent amount of water (placebo). Urine was collected, then incubated for 24 or 48 hours in laboratory models of the catheterized bladder that were inoculated with *Proteus mirabilis* (a typical pathogen that causes encrustation and blockage in catheters). The amount of calcium and magnesium recovered from catheters did not differ between the two groups. However, there was significantly less encrustation on catheters in subjects who drank the water compared to juice drinkers. The authors concluded that drinking large volumes of cranberry juice did not result in the excretion of factors into urine that inhibit encrustation (11).

SAFETY

- Cranberry juice or supplements are not a substitute for treatment with antibiotics during acute urinary tract infections.

- Conflicting values have been published on the oxalate content of cranberry juice; but recent advances in analytical techniques have revealed the level to be 0.52 mg oxalic acid/100 g of cranberry juice (12). There have been some reports that high intakes of cranberry juice (1 L or more daily) may stimulate oxalate and uric acid stones forming in acidic urine (13). However, others have found that cranberry juice contained low amounts of oxalate and is safe for patients with calcium kidney stones (14).

- Five healthy subjects were administered cranberry tablets for seven days according to manufacturers' recommended dosage. Twenty-four hour urine collection was obtained on the seventh day. Urinary oxalate levels significantly increased by an average of 43 percent compared to baseline. Urinary calcium, phosphate, and sodium increased (all potential promoters of stone formation) while magnesium and potassium also rose (inhibitors of stone formation). The authors cautioned patients at risk for kidney stones against using cranberry dietary supplements (15). However, the results from this small study are confounded by the fact that vitamin C and calcium intakes, which can contribute to urinary oxalate concentrations, were not monitored.

REFERENCES

1. Ocean Spray Cranberries. About Cranberries. Available at http://www.oceanspray.com. Accessed July 3, 2002.
2. Howell AB, Vorsa N, Der Marderosian A, et al. Inhibition of the adherence of P-fimbriated *Escherichia coli* to uroepithelial-cell surfaces by proanthocyanidin extracts from cranberries. *N Engl J Med.* 1998;339:1085–1086.
3. Foo LY, Lu Y, Howell AB, et al. A-type proanthocyanidin trimers from cranberry that inhibit adherence of uropathogenic P-fimbriated *Escherichia coli. J Nat Prod.* 2000;63:1225–1228.
4. Kerr KG. Cranberry juice and prevention of recurrent urinary tract infection. *Lancet.* 1999;353:673.
5. Avorn J, Monane M, Gurwitz JH, et al. Reduction of bacteruria and pyuria after ingestion of cranberry juice. *JAMA.*1994;271:751–754.
6. Howell AB, Leahy M, Kurowska E, et al. In vivo evidence that cranberry proanthocyanidins inhibit the adherence of p-fimbriated *E coli* bacteria to uroepithelial cells. *Fed Am Soc Exp Biol J.* 2001;15:A284.
7. Jepson RG, Mihaljevic L, Craig L. Cranberries for preventing urinary tract infections. *Cochrane Database Syst Rev.* 2001;3:CD001321.
8. Jepson RG, Mihaljevic L, Craig J. Cranberries for treating urinary tract infections. *Cochrane Database Syst Rev.* 2001;2:CD001322.
9. Avorn J, Monane M, Gurwitz JH, et al. Reduction of bacteriuria and pyuria after ingestion of cranberry juice. *JAMA.* 1994;271:751–754.

10. Walker EB, Barney DP, Mickelsen JN, et al. Cranberry concentrate: UTI Prophylaxis [letter to editor]. *J Fam Practice.* 1997;45:167–168.

11. Morris NS, Stickler DJ. Does drinking cranberry juice produce urine inhibitory to the development of crystalline, catheter-blocking *Proteus mirabilis* biofims? *BJU Int.* 2001;88:192–197.

12. Leahy M, Roderick R, Brilliant K. The cranberry-promising health benefits, old and new. *Nutrition Today.* 2001;36:254–265.

13. Rogers J. Clinical: Pass the cranberry juice. *Nurs Times.* 1991;27:36–37.

14. Massey L, Roman-Smith H, Sutton RAL. Effect of dietary oxalate and calcium on urinary oxalate and risk of formation of calcium oxalate kidney stones. *J Am Diet Assoc.* 1993;93:901–906.

15. Terris MK, Issa MM, Tacker JR. Dietary supplementation with cranberry concentrate tablets may increase the risk of nephrolithiasis. *Urology.* 2001;57:26–29.

Creatine

Creatine is synthesized from amino acids (glycine, arginine, methionine) in the liver, pancreas, and kidneys at a rate of approximately 1 g/day. Skeletal muscle holds 95 percent of the 120 g to 140 g creatine found in the body. In the muscle, creatine is converted into phosphocreatine necessary for ATP production. Studies suggest that consuming 20 g to 25 g creatine/day (for two to six days) increases muscle creatine by 20 to 30 percent, of which 20 percent is in the phosphocreatine form. The availability of phosphocreatine is believed to become a limiting factor during short bouts of high-intensity exercise (phosphocreatine is the major source of muscle energy during exercise lasting 2 to 30 seconds). Therefore, it is thought that if more phosphocreatine is available via creatine supplementation, there will be a faster recovery of ATP, which would improve high-power activity that is dependent on the ATP-phosphocreatine energy system. In the past decade, numerous studies have tested the effects of supplemental creatine on exercise performance (1–4).

Media and Marketing Claims	Efficacy
Increases muscular strength	↑?
Delays fatigue, and allows for harder training to achieve greater muscle gains	NR
Helps burn fat and increases muscle mass	NR
Increases strength in the elderly	NR
Increases strength in patients with muscular diseases	↑?
Increases strength in patients with heart disease	NR

Advisory

- Not for use by patients with renal disease or insufficiency
- Do not exceed maintenance dose (2 g to 5 g/day)
- May cause weight gain/water retention

Drug/Nutrient Interactions

- Possible negative interaction when taken with ma huang (ephedra)
- Caffeine may decrease ergogenic effect of creatine
- Should not be used long-term with nephrotoxic drugs (nonsteroidal antiinflammatories, cyclosporin, ACE inhibitors)

KEY POINTS

- There is some evidence that creatine supplementation may increase muscular strength/power during short bouts of exercise. One reviewer summarized: "Some, but not all, studies suggest that creatine supplementation may enhance performance in high-intensity, short-term exercise tasks that are dependent primarily on phosphocreatine (ie, < 30 seconds), particularly laboratory tests involving repeated exercise bouts with limited recovery time between repetitions; additional corroborative research is needed regarding its ergogenic potential in actual field exercise performance tasks dependent on phosphocreatine. Creatine supplementation has not been consistently shown to enhance performance in exercise tasks dependent on anaerobic glycolysis, but additional laboratory and field research is merited" (2).

- Additional research is needed to determine whether chronic creatine supplementation during training enhances overall competitive performance in actual sport activities. If creatine does enable subjects to train more intensely, that could cause greater muscular gains than without supplementation.

- There is no evidence that creatine increases fat metabolism, although in some studies, creatine in conjunction with resistance exercise has demonstrated an increase in lean body mass in males. Several studies did not determine the composition of weight gain (ie, whether it was because of water retention or actual muscle mass). Additional research is needed to confirm the effect of creatine on body composition and field performance.

- In sum, although many studies have claimed an ergogenic effect of creatine in the laboratory, the overall relevance of supplementation to specific sports activities relying on short bouts of high-power exercise (football, hockey, tennis, skiing, soccer, wrestling, body building, sprint aspect of running—100-yard dash, swimming—25-yard swim, cycling) needs to be determined.

- A preliminary study in the elderly reported no benefit with creatine supplementation. Controlled, clinical trials of sufficient sample sizes are needed to verify claims that creatine increases strength in this population. Elderly patients choosing to supplement with creatine should be assessed for renal function because of potential adverse effects.

- There is preliminary evidence that creatine may improve strength in patients with neuromuscular diseases. More controlled research is needed in this population.

- There is preliminary evidence from one study that creatine supplementation may improve strength in patients with congestive heart failure. Again, more controlled research is needed.

- There is a tendency for athletes to consume higher doses of creatine than manufacturers recommend. Because the long-term effects of these doses are unknown, health professionals should assess athletes for dietary supplement use (including creatine) and discourage the practice of exceeding recommended dosages.

FOOD SOURCES

A mixed diet provides approximately 1 g creatine/day (1). Most dietary creatine comes from animal products with only trace amounts found in plant foods.

Food	Creatine (mg/Serving)*
Herring, raw (3 oz)	553–850
Pork, raw (3 oz)	425
Salmon, raw (3 oz)	383
Beef, raw (3 oz)	383
Cod, raw (3 oz)	255
Milk (1 c)	24

Serving sizes calculated from values from Reference 1.

DOSAGE INFORMATION/BIOAVAILABILITY

Creatine is produced endogenously, so there are no set dietary requirements. Creatine is available as creatine monohydrate in pills, powders and beverages, often with other supplements such as HMB (Beta-hydroxy Beta-Methylbutyrate), amino acids, and carnitine. Studies have reported that the maximal muscle storage of creatine is achieved by supplementing 5 g creatine monohydrate four times/day for five to six days, followed by a maintenance phase of 2 g/day to replace daily turnover (2, 4, 5). In one study, consuming carbohydrates with creatine supplements further enhanced intramuscular creatine uptake and glycogen deposition (6). Caffeine appears to inhibit phosphocreatine resynthesis during recovery from exercise; therefore, caffeine may interfere with any ergogenic effect of creatine (7). Vegetarians have lower muscle stores of creatine and absorb more from supplements than nonvegetarians with higher stores (8).

RELEVANT RESEARCH

- Note: Because of the large number of studies only the more recent trials are discussed. Refer to reference 2 for a detailed review.

Creatine and High-Intensity Exercise (Phosphocreatine-ATP System) in Laboratory Setting

- In a double-blind, crossover study, 12 subjects were either creatine loaded (25 g/day for 5 days); or were creatine loaded plus ingested creatine (5 g/hour) during an exercise test; or received placebo on three occasions separated by five-week washout periods. Each subject underwent a 2.5-hour standardized endurance protocol on their own bicycles mounted to an electromagnetically braked roller system, where they cycled to exhaustion. Immediately after, subjects performed five maximal 10-second sprints on a cycle ergometer, separated by 2-minute recovery periods. Creatine loading for five days, but not creatine loading plus an acute dose before exercise, resulted in a statistically significant increase in peak and mean sprint power output (8 percent to 9 percent greater) for all five sprints compared to the placebo. Endurance time to exhaustion was not affected by either creatine dose (9).

- In a double-blind, crossover design study, eight active, untrained men performed a 20-second maximal sprint on a cycle ergometer after five days of supplementing in random order 30 g creatine plus 30 g dextrose/day or a placebo (30 g dextrose). Each trial was separated by a four-week washout period. Muscle and blood samples were taken at rest, after exercise and two minutes after recovery. Although the creatine supplementation significantly increased muscle creatine, there was no improvement in sprint performance. In addition, there were no changes in measures of muscle degradation (adenine nucleotides, phosphocreatine) and plasma metabolites (lactate, ammonia) during exercise or recovery (10).

- In a double-blind, placebo-controlled study, nine male subjects underwent three randomly ordered tests following ingestion of 20 g/day creatine monohydrate, placebo, or control for three days. Tests were performed 14 days apart on a monarch ergometer adjusted for immediate resistance loading. Needle biopsies were taken from the vastus lateralis (in quadriceps muscle) at the end of each treatment and before the exercise test. There were no significant differences among conditions on peak, mean 10-second, and mean 30-second power output, percent fatigue, or postexercise blood lactate concentration. There were no differences in muscle levels of ATP, phosphocreatine, or total creatine; however, the total creatine to ATP ratio was higher in the creatine condition than in the placebo or control. The authors concluded: "Findings suggest that three days of oral creatine supplementation does not increase resting muscle phosphocreatine concentration and has no effect on performance during a single short-term maximal cycling task" (11).

- In a double-blind, randomized study, 25 collegiate football players (NCAA division IA) were matched-paired by total body weight and assigned to supplement their diet during off-season weight training for 28 days with a placebo (glucose-taurine-electrolyte mixture) or 15.75 g creatine monohydrate (plus glucose-taurine-electrolyte mixture)/day. Before and after supplementation, subjects performed a maximal repetition test on the isotonic bench press, squat, and power clean (Olympic weight-lifting exercise); and performed a sprint test on the cycle ergometer (12 × 6 sprints with 30-second rest recovery). Body weight, body water and composition by X-ray absorptiometry) were also determined. Gains in bench press lifting volume, the sum of weight lifted during the bench press, squat, and power clean exercises and total work performed during the first five six-second sprints resulted in a significant increase in the creatine-supplemented group compared to placebo. Creatine-supplemented subjects also had significant greater gains in total body weight and fat/bone-free mass, whereas no differences were observed in total body water (12).

- In a placebo-controlled study, 16 elite male rowers were randomized to receive 20 g creatine plus 4 g glucose (divided into four doses) for five days or a placebo. Subjects performed three maximal kayak ergometer tests of 90, 150, and 300 seconds duration before supplementation (control). The same kayak ergometer tests were performed after supplementation, after a four-week washout period, and after a second supplementation period. There was a significant increase in work in all three tests completed by creatine subjects compared to placebo or control. Creatine subjects also had a statistically significant increase in total body mass (body composition not determined), whereas the control and placebo groups remained stable (13).

- In a placebo-controlled study, two matched groups of 19 competitive rowers each were given a placebo or 0.25 g creatine/kg body weight for five days before completing a 1,000-m simulated race. The control group showed no change in rowing performance, whereas 16 of 19 supplemented subjects improved performance times that did not reach statistical significance (14).

- In a double-blind, placebo-controlled study, 14 weight-trained male subjects were matched based on weight-lifting ability and body mass, and randomly assigned to receive creatine or a placebo. On three occasions (T1, T2, T3) separated by six days, both groups completed a bench-press exercise protocol (five sets to exhaustion using subject's predetermined 10-repetitions maximum) and a jump squat exercise protocol (five sets of 10 repetitions using 30 percent of each subject's 1-repetition maximum squat). Before T1, both groups received no supplementation. From T1 to T2, both groups received a placebo. From T2 to T3, the creatine group ingested 25 g creatine monohydrate/day and the placebo group ingested placebos. There were no changes in lifting performance on either exercise protocol after placebo ingestion. Creatine supplementation resulted in a statistically significant improvement in peak power output during all five sets of jump squats and during all five sets of bench presses. After creatine, postexercise lactate concentrations were significantly higher after the bench press but not the jump squat. The authors hypothesized the increased lactate was because of the higher total repetitions performed (approximately eight more repetitions) after creatine supplementation. A significant increase in body mass (1.4 kg) occurred after one week of creatine ingestion, which the authors attributed to an increase in total body water, although body composition was not determined. The sum of seven skinfold measurements was not different at any point within the creatine and placebo groups (15).

- Several other studies have shown significant improvement in short bouts of activities that require high levels of strength and power (knee extensions, bench press, running, and cycling sprints) (2, 16–21). However, other studies failed to show any benefit (2, 22–24). The studies of endurance have generally not reported an ergogenic benefit (1, 2, 25).

Creatine and High-Intensity Exercise in Field Studies

- In a double-blind, placebo-controlled study, 18 highly trained subjects (male soccer players and female field hockey players) completed two testing sessions of three 60-m distance running trials (control and postsupplement) one week apart. Subjects were pair-matched on gender and running speed. Run sessions were videotaped with high-speed cameras. Speed velocities were determined at 10 m to 30 m, 40 m to 50 m, and 50 m to 60 m. After the control session, subjects were randomized to receive 20 g creatine plus 5 g glucose or a placebo (5 g glucose only) divided into five doses daily for seven days, followed by the second 60-m sprint. There were no statistically significant main or interaction effects on velocity between groups (26).

- In a double-blind, placebo-controlled study, 12 competitive male runners completed two maximal 700-meter running bouts 60 minutes apart on an outdoor track. Subjects were then assigned to receive 20 g creatine monohydrate or a placebo for five days prior to a second identical trial. There were no significant differences between groups by trial or trial × time for running time, postexercise blood lactate levels, or body weight. The authors concluded: "Creatine supplementation does not enhance performance of single or twice-repeated maximal running bouts lasting 90 to 120 seconds" (27).

- In a double-blind, placebo-controlled study, 14 elite male swimmers performed a single 50-yard sprint and repeated sprint set (8 × 50 yards at 1.5-minute intervals) before and after supplementing 9 g creatine or a placebo for five days. Mean times for the single sprint were not affected by creatine. Mean times during repeated sprints increased for all subjects. However, the percentage of decline in performance times for repeated sprints was significantly reduced in the creatine group. There were no differences in blood lactate or pH levels between groups. The authors summarized: "Our results suggest that ingesting 9 g creatine per day for five days can improve swimming performance in elite competitors during repeated sprints, but appears to have no effect on a single 50-yard sprint" (28).

- In a double-blind, placebo-controlled study, 32 elite swimmers were tested on two occasions separated by one week (50-m and 100-m maximal effort sprints with 10 minutes active recovery and a 10-second maximal leg ergometry test). Swimmers were divided into two groups matched for gender, stroke, and sprint time and randomly assigned to 20 g creatine monohydrate (divided into four doses) or a placebo daily for five days prior to the second exercise trial. There were no significant differences between the group means for sprint times or between maximal leg ergometry power and work. The authors concluded: "This study does not support the hypothesis that creatine supplementation enhances single-effort sprint ability of elite swimmers" (29).

- In a double-blind, placebo-controlled study, 20 highly trained male and female swimmers were tested for blood ammonia and lactate concentrations after 25-, 50-, and 100-m performance in their best stroke on two occasions seven days apart. After the first trial, subjects were randomized to receive 20 g creatine divided into four doses or a placebo (20 g lactose) for five days. There were no significant differences in performance times between trials. There was no effect on postexercise blood lactate levels. Postexercise blood ammonia decreased in the 50- and 100-m trials in the creatine group, and in the 50-m trial in the placebo group. The authors concluded: "Creatine supplementation cannot be considered as an ergogenic aid for sprint performance in highly trained swimmers after five days of creatine ingestion" (30).

Creatine and Body Composition

- Several studies in male subjects reported an increase in body mass averaging 0.7 to 2.0 kg following short-term creatine intake (20 g to 25 g creatine/day for 5 days to 14 days) (2, 5, 12, 13, 15, 18, 19, 21, 23). It is controversial whether the weight gain is because of water retention or actual muscle mass because most studies did not measure lean body mass (1, 2). Some new research indicates that the increase in body mass is indeed fat-free mass (31, 32)

Creatine and the Elderly

- In a double-blind, placebo-controlled study, 32 male and female elderly subjects (aged 67 y to 80 y) were randomly assigned to one of four groups for eight weeks: (1) no exercise plus creatine, (2) no exercise plus placebo, (3) strength-training program plus creatine, and (4) strength-training program plus placebo. The strength program was performed three days per week for eight weeks. The supplementation regimen consisted of 20 g creatine monohydrate plus 8 g glucose for five days, followed by 3 g of creatine plus 2 g glucose for the remainder of the study. Body mass, body fat, lower-limb muscular volume, 1- and 12-repetition maximums, and isometric intermittent endurance tests for leg press, leg extension, and chest press were measured before and after the study. There were no statistically significant changes in anthropometric measurements in all groups. The strength-trained subjects (both creatine and placebo groups) experienced significant increases in repetition maximums compared to control subjects. The authors concluded: "Oral creatine supplementation does not provide additional benefits for body composition, maximal dynamical strength, and dynamical and isometric endurances of healthy elderly subjects, whether or not it is associated with an effective strength training" (33).

Creatine and Muscular Disease

- In a double-blind, placebo-controlled, crossover study, seven male and female subjects with mitochondrial cytopathies were randomized to receive creatine monohydrate (10 g daily for 14 days, followed by 4 g daily for 7 days) or a placebo for 21 days each. (Patients with mitochondrial cytopathies have defects in mitochondrial function that are often accompanied by various symptoms, including exercise intolerance, lactic acidosis, stroke, seizure, and cardiomyopathy.) Measurements included: activities of daily living; ischemic isometric handgrip strength; basal and postischemic exercise lactate; evoked and voluntary contraction strength of the dorsiflexor muscles; nonischemic, isometric, dorsiflexion torque (NIDFT); and aerobic cycle ergometry with pre- and postlactate measurements. Creatine resulted in a significant increase in handgrip strength, and postexercise lactate, with no changes in the other variables. The authors concluded: "Creatine monohydrate increased the strength of high-intensity anaerobic and aerobic type activities in patients with mitochondrial cytopathies but had no apparent effects upon lower intensity aerobic activities" (34).

- In a pilot study, 81 subjects with neuromuscular diseases were given 10 g creatine monohydrate for five days and 5 g daily for another five days. The authors then performed a second study after finding improvements in strength. In the second study, 21 subjects from the open trial were entered into a single-blinded, placebo-controlled trial of creatine (same dosage). The authors did not specify the reason for not employing a double-blind design. Body weight, handgrip, dorsiflexion, and knee extensor strength were measured before and after treatment. Creatine resulted in a significant increase in all measurements in both pilot studies (35).

Creatine and Congestive Heart Failure

- In a double-blind, placebo-controlled study, 20 male patients (mean age = 63 y) with congestive heart failure were assigned to receive 20 g creatine divided into four doses or a placebo for five days. Before and after supplementation, subjects performed hand-grip exercises, five-second contraction followed by five-second rest for five minutes at 25 percent, 50 percent, and 75 percent of maximum voluntary contraction or until exhaustion. Blood was taken at rest and zero and two minutes after exercise to measure lactate and ammonia. After 30 minutes the procedure was repeated with fixed workloads. There was a significant increase in contractions until exhaustion at 75 percent maximum voluntary contraction after creatine treatment, but no effect in the placebo group. There was a significant fall in ammonia levels per contraction at 75 percent maximum voluntary contraction compared to placebo, but no significant effect on lactate concentrations. The authors concluded: "Creatine supplementation in chronic heart failure augments skeletal muscle endurance and attenuates the abnormal skeletal muscle metabolic response to exercise" (36).

SAFETY

- The FDA has advised consumers to consult a physician before they use creatine because of reports of deaths caused by dehydration in wrestlers who were purportedly using creatine. However, further investigation by the Centers for Disease Control revealed that creatine was not the cause of death. Nevertheless, there is a concern that athletes in weight-controlled sports may resort to extreme weight-loss methods to decrease the extra water gain that occurs with creatine ingestion. These athletes should be discouraged from using creatine (2, 37, 38).

- In a survey of 52 collegiate athletes supplementing with creatine, 16 reported diarrhea, 13 reported muscle cramping, and 7 reported dehydration (39). Theoretically, increased intramuscular water content could dilute electrolytes causing cramping and intracellular swelling, which could result in muscle tightness (2, 37). Patients choosing to supplement with creatine may need to increase fluid intake to prevent dehydration.

- In the same survey of 52 collegiate athletes, 39 exceeded the maintenance dose of 2 g/day to 5 g/day. Individuals choosing to supplement with creatine must not exceed recommended doses because of potential adverse effects (39).

- No serious adverse effects have been reported in the cited research; however, there are no controlled studies testing the safety of creatine supplementation for longer than eight weeks (2). Large, randomized, controlled studies are needed to evaluate the short- and long-term effects of creatine supplementation on the renal and hepatic systems, as well as the many other organ systems in which creatine may play a role (40).

- In a case report, a 20-year-old healthy man developed acute interstitial nephritis and focal tubular injury associated with dehydration, hypertension, and elevated serum creatinine after supplementing with 20 g creatine daily for four weeks. The patient had exceeded the recommended dosage, which advised taking 20 g/day for one week, followed by 5 g/day for maintenance (41).

- In another report, a patient with nephrotic syndrome who had been supplementing with creatine experienced a deterioration in renal function. Based on both these reports, creatine supplementation should be avoided, especially by patients with renal disease/insufficiency (42).

- It is not known whether supplementation suppresses endogenous creatine synthesis in humans (1).

- Some athletes, especially those competing in endurance events and weight-controlled sports, could potentially experience an impairment in performance because of weight gain associated with creatine supplementation (1, 2, 37).

REFERENCES

1. Balsom PD, Soderlund K, Ekblom B. Creatine in humans with special reference to creatine supplementation. *Sports Med.* 1994;18:268–280.
2. Williams MH, Branch JD. Creatine supplementation and exercise performance: an update. *J Am Coll Nutr.* 1998;17:216–234.
3. Greenhaff PL, Bodin K, Soderlund K, et al. Effect of oral creatine supplementation on skeletal muscle phosphocreatine resynthesis. *Am J Physiol.* 1994;266(pt 1):E725–E730.
4. Harris RC, Soderlund K, Hultman E. Elevation of creatine in resting and exercised muscle of normal subjects by creatine supplementation. *Clin Sci (Colch).* 1992;83:367–374.
5. Greenhaff PL. Creatine and its application as an ergogenic aid. *Int J Sport Nutr.* 1995;5:S100–S110.
6. Green AL, Sewell DA, Simpson L, et al. Creatine ingestion augments muscle creatine uptake and glycogen synthesis during carbohydrate feeding in man. *J Physiol.* 1996;491:63.
7. Vandenberghe K, Gillis N, Van Leemputte M, et al. Caffeine counteracts the ergogenic action of muscle creatine loading. *J Appl Physiol.* 1996;80:452–457.
8. Delanghe J, De Slypere JP, De Buyzere J, et al. Normal reference values for creatine, creatinine, and carnitine are lower in vegetarians. *Clin Chem.* 1989;35:1802–1803.
9. Vandebuerie F, Vanden Eynde B, Vandenberghe K, et al. Effect of creatine loading on endurance capacity and sprint power in cyclists. *Int J Sports Med.* 1998;19:490–495.
10. Snow RJ, McKenna MJ, Selig SE, et al. Effect of creatine supplementation on sprint exercise performance and muscle metabolism. *J Appl Physiol.* 1998;84:1667–1673.
11. Odland LM, MacDougall JD, Tarnopolsky MA, et al. Effect of oral creatine supplementation on muscle [PCr] and short-term maximum power output. *Med Sci Sports Exerc.* 1997;29:216–219.
12. Kreider RB, Ferreira M, Wilson M, et al. Effect of creatine supplementation on body composition, strength, and sprint performance. *Med Sci Sports Exerc.* 1998;30:73–82.
13. McNaughton LR, Dalton B, Tarr J. The effects of creatine supplementation on high-intensity exercise performance in elite performers. *Eur J Appl Physiol.* 1998;78:236–240.
14. Rossiter HB, Cannell ER, Jakeman PM. The effect of oral creatine supplementation on the 1,000-m performance of competitive rowers. *J Sports Sci.* 1996;14:175–179.
15. Volek JS, Kraemer WJ, Bush JA, et al. Creatine supplementation enhances muscular performance during high-intensity resistance exercise. *J Am Diet Assoc.* 1997;97:765–770.

16. Greenhaff PL, Casey A, Short AH, et al. Influence of oral creatine supplementation on muscle torque during repeated bouts of maximal voluntary exercise in man. *Clin Sci (Colch).* 1993;84:565–571.

17. Harris RC, Viru M, Greenhaff PL, et al. The effect of oral creatine supplementation on running performance during maximal short-term exercise in man. *J Physiol.* 1993;467:74P.

18. Balsom PD, Ekblom B, Soderlund K, et al. Creatine supplementation and dynamic high-intensity intermittent exercise. *Scand J Med Sci Sports.* 1993;3:143–149.

19. Soderlund K, Balsom PD, Ekblom B. Creatine supplementation and high-intensity exercise: influence on performance and muscle metabolism. *Clin Sci.* 1994;87:S120–S121.

20. Birch R, Noble D, Greenhaff PL. The influence of dietary creatine supplementation on performance during repeated bouts of maximal isokinetic cycling in man. *Eur J Appl Physiol.* 1994;69:268–270.

21. Earnest CP, Snell PG, Rodriguez R, et al. The effect of creatine monohydrate ingestion on anaerobic power indices, muscular strength and body composition. *Acta Physiol Scand.* 1995;153:207–209.

22. Cooke WH, Grandjean PW, Barnes WS. Effect of oral creatine supplementation on power output and fatigue during bicycle ergometry. *J Appl Physiol.* 1995;78:670–673.

23. Earnest CP, Rash J, Snell AL, et al. Effect of creatine monohydrate ingestion on intermediate length treadmill running to exhaustion. *Med Sci Sports Exerc.* 1995;27:S14.

24. Mujika I, Chatard JC, Lacoste L, et al. Creatine supplementation does not improve sprint performance in competitive swimmers. *Med Sci Sports Exerc.* 1996;28:1435–1441.

25. Balsom PD, Harridge SD, Soderlund K, et al. Creatine supplementation per se does not enhance endurance exercise performance. *Acta Physiol Scand.* 1993;149:521–523.

26. Redondo DR, Dowling EA, Graham BL, et al. The effect of oral creatine monohydrate supplementation on running velocity. *Int J Sport Nutr.* 1996;6:213–221.

27. Terrillion KA, Kolkhorst FW, Dolgener FA, et al. The effect of creatine supplementation on two 700-m maximal running bouts. *Int J Sport Nutr.* 1997;7:138–143.

28. Peyrebrune MC, Nevill ME, Donaldson FJ, et al. The effects of oral creatine supplementation on performance in single and repeated sprint swimming. *J Sports Sci.* 1998;16:271–279.

29. Burke LM, Pyne DB, Telford RD. Effect of oral creatine supplementation on single-effort sprint performance in elite swimmers. *Int J Sport Nutr.* 1996;6:222–233.

30. Mujika I, Chatard JC, Lacoste L, et al. Creatine supplementation does not improve sprint performance in competitive swimmers. *Med Sci Sports Exerc.* 1996;28:1435–1441.

31. Becque MD, Lochmann JD, Melrose DR. Effects of oral creatine supplementation on muscular strength and body composition. *Med Sci Sports Exerc.* 2000;32:654–658.

32. Mihic S, MacDonald JR, McKenzie S, et al. Acute creatine loading increases fat-free mass, but does not affect blood pressure, plasma creatinine, or CK activity in men and women. *Med Sci Sports Exerc.* 2000;32:291–296.

33. Bermon S, Venembre P, Sachet C, et al. Effects of creatine monohydrate ingestion in sedentary and weight-trained older adults. *Acta Physiol Scand.* 1998;164:147–155.

34. Tarnopolsky MA, Roy BD, MacDonald JR. A randomized, controlled trial of creatine monohydrate in patients with mitochondrial cytopathies. *Muscle Nerve.* 1997; 20:1502–1509.

35. Tarnopolsky M, Martin J. Creatine monohydrate increases strength in patients with neuromuscular disease. *Neurology.* 1999;52:854–857.

36. Andrews R, Greenhaff P, Curtis S, et al. The effect of dietary creatine supplementation on skeletal muscle metabolism in congestive heart failure. *Eur Heart J.* 1998;19:617–622.

37. Feldman EB. Creatine: a dietary supplement and ergogenic aid. *Nutr Rev.* 1999; 57:45–50.

38. Andres LPA, Sacheck J, Tapia S. A review of creatine supplementation: side effects and improvements in athletic performance. *Nutr Clin Care.* 1999;2:73–81.

39. Juhn MS, O'Kane JW, Vinci DM. Oral creatine supplementation in male collegiate athletes: a survey of dosing habits and side effects. *J Am Diet Assoc.* 1999;99:593–595.

40. Juhn MS, Tarnopolsky M. Potential side effects of oral creatine supplementation: a critical review. *Clin J Sport Med.* 1998;8:298–304.

41. Koshy KM, Griswold E, Schneeberger EE. Interstitial nephritis in patient taking creatine. *N Engl J Med.* 1999;340:814–815.

42. Pritchard NR, Kalra PA. Renal dysfunction accompanying oral creatine supplements. *Lancet.* 1998;351:1252–1253.

Decosahexanoic Acid (DHEA)

See Fish Oil.

Dehydroepiandosterone (DHEA)

Dehydroepiandosterone (DHEA) is the most abundant hormone secreted by the adrenal glands. Dehydroepiandosterone-3-sulfate (DHEAS) is the metabolic precursor to DHEA, and they are interconvertable (1). In the peripheral tissues, both DHEA and DHEAS can be converted into active androgens and estrogens (2). Despite numerous studies investigating the potential role of DHEA in health and disease, little is known about the function of this hormone. Serum DHEA levels peak by 20 to 30 years of age, and decline thereafter with age (3).

Media and Marketing Claims	Efficacy
Slows aging	NR
Improves memory	NR
Enhances libido	NR
Enhances the immune system	↔
Improves cardiovascular health	↔
Anticancer aid	↔
Reduces symptoms of lupus	↔
Beneficial for AIDS patients	NR
Aids weight-loss	↔

Advisory

- May increase risk of breast, endometrial, or prostate cancer
- May promote masculine characteristics in females
- May decrease serum HDL cholesterol
- Self-supplementation not advised

Drug/Nutrient Interactions

May increase blood levels of triazolam (Halcion), a benzodiazepine used for insomnia, anxiety, and seizures

KEY POINTS

- DHEA levels decline with age; however, there is no evidence DHEA supplementation prevents aging or lengthens life span in humans.

- The role of serum DHEA levels in cognitive function in elderly subjects is unclear, although at this time epidemiological studies have not found a correlation between decreased DHEA levels and cognitive function. Although one controlled study showed an improvement in mood (but not libido), other studies showed no effect on mood or memory. There is not enough evidence to substantiate claims that DHEA improves mood, memory, and libido.

- The role of DHEA in immune function is conflicting, and even in the reports showing improved immune response, the magnitude of the effects in humans is modest (3).

- Epidemiological studies have provided conflicting reports on the role of DHEA levels and CVD. One review article concluded that whether DHEA in either maintenance or pharmacological doses has any cardiovascular benefit is still unknown (4). Although animal and some human studies have demonstrated that DHEA reduces platelet aggregation and may lower total cholesterol (including HDL), controlled clinical trials are needed to determine whether DHEA supplementation affects CVD morbidity and mortality.

- There is conflicting evidence from epidemiological and animal studies on the level of serum DHEA and DHEAS that may affect the risk of cancer. Because of a potential for increased risk of breast cancer associated with elevated DHEA levels, supplements should clearly be avoided by women at risk for breast or endometrial cancer. One researcher summarized the research: "There are nearly as many observations suggesting that DHEA promotes cancer as there are that it retards tumors. Indeed, these reports often use the same animal model, the same authors, and the very same dosage" (3). Because DHEA supplementation has not been tested in controlled clinical trials of cancer patients, the claim that it can have a beneficial effect on cancer is unsubstantiated at this time.

- Preliminary trials of DHEA supplements using patients having lupus have shown some reduction in disease activity. More controlled research is needed in this population.

- Although DHEA levels may decline with HIV infection, one uncontrolled trial of DHEA supplements using HIV-positive subjects showed no benefit. More research is needed before recommendations can be made in this population.

- DHEA supplements do not appear to have a beneficial effect on body composition or energy expenditure at either pharmacologic or physiologic replacement doses for one to three months. DHEA also has not been shown to alter insulin sensitivity (5).

- Overall, most of the effects of DHEA replacement have been extrapolated from epidemiological or animal model studies, and need to be investigated in humans (6). The long-term consequences of supplementing with DHEA are unknown, and the potential adverse effects may outweigh the possible benefits. Until more research is available on the safety, efficacy, and dosage of DHEA, self-supplementation with this hormone is not recommended.

FOOD SOURCES

None

DOSAGE INFORMATION/BIOAVAILABILITY

DHEA supplements are available in capsules or tablets ranging in doses from 25 mg to 50 mg. Some products also contain pregnenolone, a direct precursor to DHEA. Numerous studies have used doses ranging from 0.1 mg/kg body weight to 1,000 mg/kg body weight. In a study of 45 DHEA products, 53 percent contained DHEA at 85 percent to 95 percent of the declared amounts; only one had no trace of DHEA; and four exceeded 100 percent of the amount stated on the label (7).

An oral dose of DHEA (400 mg) reached maximal serum androgen levels within 180 minutes to 240 minutes in postmenopausal women. This dose also was reported to increase serum DHEA by 6-fold, testosterone by 2.5-fold, dihydrotestosterone by 15-fold, and androstenedione by 12-fold compared to the baseline. After four weeks of supplementation in the same subjects, estrone and estradiol levels increased 2-fold compared to baseline (8). However, in another study, a 50-mg dose did not raise estrone or estradiol (9). In another study, a single 200 mg dose increased DHEA concentrations by 5- to 6-fold in healthy subjects aged 65 y to 79 y. It also raised DHEA-S by 5-fold in men and by 21-fold in women (10).

RELEVANT RESEARCH

Serum DHEA Levels and Age

- In a prospective study of 614 free-living male and female adults, DHEA concentrations were assessed every 5 years for 15 years. Overall, the average decline in DHEA was 5.6 percent per year, and the rate of decline was directly related to age, but not gender, adiposity, or serum glucose. However, when analyzed by gender, DHEA levels were higher and decreased more rapidly in men aged 20 y to 49 y than in women. After 50 years of age, DHEA concentrations and rates of decline were similar in men and women. The average decline in DHEAS after age 50 y was 2 percent per year and was not related to age, gender, adiposity, or glucose (11).

DHEA and Aging, Memory, Libido, and Mood

- In a prospective cohort study (Rancho Bernardo Study), 437 subjects (men > 50 y and women > 55 y) from an upper-middle-class community had plasma obtained for DHEAS assays in 1972 to 1974. Subjects were screened for dementia in 1988 to 1991. (Mini-Mental Status Examination, Buschke selective reminding test, Trails B, category fluency, and Heaton Visual Reproduction Test were used.) DHEAS levels were higher in men than women, and decreased with age in both sexes. There were no significant differences in age-adjusted DHEAS levels in subjects having impaired performance on any cognitive test. Low baseline DHEAS levels were not associated with any record of dementia on death certificates (12).

- In a case-control study, 45 patients with Alzheimer's disease and cerebrovascular dementia had similar serum DHEA levels compared to healthy controls. However, DHEAS and DHEAS/DHEA ratio were reduced compared to controls. The authors concluded that the role of DHEA in dementia is unclear (13).

- In a double-blind, placebo-controlled, crossover study, 17 elderly, healthy, male subjects took 50 mg DHEA daily or a placebo for two weeks. Baseline DHEAS levels were lower compared to younger adults, but rose 5-fold after two weeks of supplementation with DHEA. After each treatment period, subjects underwent a series of memory tests (visual, spatial, and semantic) including an experiment using event-related potentials. Participants filled out a psychological assessment of mood, self-perceived changes, and physical complaints. DHEA had no effect on memory or mood. Subjects taking DHEA had changes in electrophysiological indices of central nervous system stimulus processing if the task was performed repeatedly. However, the authors concluded that DHEA did not appear to improve memory or mood (14).

- In a double-blind, placebo-controlled, crossover study, 30 healthy subjects aged 40 y to 70 y were randomized to receive in random order 50 mg DHEA or a placebo daily for three months each. At baseline, three months, and six months, fasting blood samples were taken. A subgroup of 13 subjects had several blood samples taken over a 24-hour period. Another subgroup of five subjects underwent a hyperinsulinemic euglycemic clamp. Subjects were instructed by a nutritionist to continue their current exercise and dietary regimens. A monthly food recall questionnaire revealed no significant changes in diet or exercise during the study period. Average DHEA and DHEAS serum levels reached levels normally seen in young adults within two weeks and were sustained for three months of treatment. DHEA had no effect on insulin sensitivity or body fat. There was a significant increase in serum insulin-like-growth-factor-I levels (IGF-I), a metabolic growth factor regulated by growth hormone. During DHEA supplementation, there was a significant increase in perceived physical and psychological well-being (increased energy, deeper sleep, improved mood, more relaxed feeling, better ability to handle stress), but no effect on libido (9).

- In a double-blind, placebo-controlled study, 280 healthy male and female subjects (aged 60 y to 79 y) were randomized to receive 50 mg DHEA or a placebo daily for one year. Subjects were tested at the baseline and at one year for bone turnover (assessed by dual-energy x-ray absorptiometry). Libido, quality of life, and psycho-affective state were assessed by the General Well Being scale of Dupuy. Muscular strength was measured by handgrip, and skin status was assessed by hydration, epidermal thickness, sebum production and pigmentation. DHEA increased DHEAS levels to normal young adult levels after month 6 and 12 in men, and after month 12 in women (for month 6 in women, DHEAS levels exceeded those of normal young women). DHEA supplementation significantly increased bone turnover and decreased osteoclastic activity only in women > 70 y compared to the placebo. A significant improvement in libido parameters was also noted in this subgroup, but not in the other subjects. In all subjects, DHEA was associated with a statistically signficant improvement in skin status (15).

- In a double-blind, placebo-controlled study, 60 perimenopausal women with complaints of altered mood and well-being were randomized to receive 50 mg DHEA/d or a placebo for three months. Changes in serum DHEA, DHEAS, and testosterone were significantly greater in the DHEA group than the placebo group. There were no differences between groups in the severity of perimenopausal symptoms, mood, dysphoria, libido, cognition, memory or well-being (16)

DHEA and Immunity

- In a single-blind, placebo-controlled study, nine healthy men (mean age = 63 y) were supplemented with a placebo for 2 weeks, followed by 50 mg DHEA for 20 weeks. Fasting blood samples were taken at four- to eight-week intervals for immune studies and hormone testing. Compared to baseline, levels of serum DHEAS increased three- to four-fold within two weeks and were sustained throughout the trial. DHEA stimulated immune function by significantly increasing the number of monocyte and B cells, stimulating T and B cell mitogenic response, interleukin-2 secretion, and the number and cytotoxicity of natural killer cells. The authors acknowledged that the results of this study were limited because posttreatment immune responses were not measured. They also stated: "It is premature to relate these findings to clinical applications" (17).

- In a double-blind, placebo-controlled study, 78 healthy, elderly subjects were randomized to receive DHEAS injection (7.5 mg) or a placebo coadministered with the influenza vaccine (consisting of three antigens: H1N1, H3N2, and B). Immune responses to vaccine after weeks 0, 2, and 4 of DHEA supplementation were measured by vaccine antigen-induced lymphoproliferation in peripheral mononuclear cells and serum antibody response to hemagglutination inhibition (HI). No significant differences were found for antibody responses to the H1N1 and B antigens or vaccine-antigen induced lymphoproliferation. There was an insignificant trend in subjects with lower DHEAs concentrations for enhanced specific HI antibody response to the H3N2 antigen. The authors concluded: "Although clinical implications of these findings for influenza vaccine are uncertain, these results suggest additional immunologic investigations on the role of DHEAs in the aging human immune response are warranted" (18).

- In a prospective, double-blind study, 71 apparently healthy, elderly subjects (ages 61 y to 89 y) were randomized to receive 50 mg DHEA or a placebo for four days (starting two days before receiving three strains of influenza vaccine). Antibody response against the strains of vaccine was measured before and 28 days after vaccination, and compared between previously vaccinated and nonvaccinated subjects. As expected, DHEA levels increased 5- to 10-fold in the treatment group but were not affected in the placebo group. DHEA did not enhance established immunity as measured by antibody levels (19).

DHEA and Cardiovascular Disease

- In a prospective cohort study, 1971 subjects aged 30 y to 88 y were followed for 19 years. After the first 12 years, high levels of plasma DHEAS were associated with a reduced risk of fatal cardiovascular disease (CVD) in men but an increased risk in women. After 19 years, DHEAS levels were not associated with CVD or ischemic heart disease (IHD) deaths when compared to controls without CVD or IHD. However, when compared to survivors of CVD, there was a significant, modestly reduced risk of fatal CVD in men with elevated DHEAS and an insignificant increased risk of fatal CVD in women (20). In a follow-up analysis, after adjusting for age, cholesterol, blood pressure, smoking, estrogen replacement, obesity, blood glucose, and family history of heart disease, higher DHEAS levels were unrelated to the risk of fatal CVD in women (21).

- In a double-blind, placebo-controlled, crossover study, six postmenopausal women with low endogenous DHEA and DHEAS received 1,600 mg DHEA or a placebo daily divided in four doses for 28 days each. Serum DHEA, androstenedione, dihydrotestosterone, and testosterone increased significantly compared to baseline. At two weeks and at the end of the trial, there was a significant decline in total and HDL cholesterol, and an insignificant downward trend for triglycerides, LDL, and VLDL cholesterol. There was no change in body weight and percent body fat as measured by underwater weighing (22).

- One review article reported on placebo-controlled human studies demonstrating inhibition of platelet aggregation and reduced plasminogen activator inhibitor type 1 with DHEA supplementation (900 mg/day and 150 mg/day, respectively). DHEA administration also reduced atherosclerosis in cholesterol-fed rabbits and reduced serum cholesterol in monkeys and dogs (3).

DHEA and Cancer

- In a prospective cohort study, 534 women aged 50 y to 79 y had plasma DHEAS levels obtained in 1972 to 1974 and were followed for 15 years. At the end of the study, there were 21 cases of breast cancer, 20 cases with earlier diagnosis, and 10 cases with unknown date of onset who were identified from death certificates only. After controlling for age, body mass index, estrogen use, and smoking, DHEAS levels were not associated with breast cancer (23).

- In a prospective, nested case-control study, 71 healthy postmenopausal subjects not on estrogen therapy when they donated blood and who were diagnosed with breast cancer up to 10 years later were compared to matched controls. Increased serum DHEA and the metabolite 5-androstene-3 beta, 17 beta-diol (ADIOL) levels were associated with a significant increase in incidence of breast cancer. Women whose serum DHEAS were in the highest quartile also had a significantly elevated risk. The authors concluded that the adrenal androgens, DHEA, DHEAS, and ADIOL may play a role in the etiology of breast cancer (24).

- An *in vitro* study reported that DHEAS, at physiological concentrations, had a high estrogenic activity in human breast cancer cell lines. The authors concluded: "DHEAS could contribute to the pool of compounds having estrogenic activities in human breast cancer hormone-dependent cell lines" (25).
- Several animal studies have shown both an inhibitory and stimulatory effect on tumors with DHEA administration (3). However, one reviewer noted that most of the animal research has been conducted in rodents which have little, if any, circulating DHEA, and therefore, results can not be extrapolated to humans (26).

DHEA and Lupus

- In a double-blind, placebo-controlled trial, 28 female patients with mild to moderate systemic lupus erythematosus (SLE) were randomized to receive 200 mg DHEA or a placebo daily for three months. There was an insignificant trend for DHEA-treated subjects to have greater improvement in SLE Disease Activity Index scores, physician's overall assessment of disease activity, and a reduction in the dosage of prednisone when compared to the placebo group. The difference between patient's assessment of disease activity between groups was significant. Mild acne was a frequent side-effect of DHEA (27).
- In an open study, 50 female patients with mild to moderate SLE were treated with 50 mg to 200 mg DHEA daily for 6 to 12 months. DHEA increased the serum levels of DHEA, DHEAS, and testosterone. DHEA therapy was associated with a significant decrease in disease activity (SLE Disease Activity Index score) and significant improvement in patient and physician global assessment compared to the baseline. Concurrent prednisone doses were reduced significantly. Mild acne occurred in 54 percent of the patients (28).

DHEA and HIV Infection

- Serum DHEA concentrations in HIV-positive patients appear to progressively decrease as infection advances (29).
- In an open, uncontrolled trial, 31 subjects with HIV disease were given 750 mg to 2,250 mg DHEA divided into three doses daily for 16 weeks. There were no sustained improvements in CD4 counts or decreases in serum p24 antigen or beta-2 microglobulin levels. Serum neopterin levels decreased transiently by 23 percent to 40 percent at week 8 compared with baseline in all dosing groups. The authors concluded that DHEA was well tolerated by patients with mild symptomatic HIV disease, but that randomized, controlled trials are needed to determine the efficacy of DHEA in HIV-related diseases (30).

DHEA and Body Composition

- In a double-blind, placebo-controlled, crossover study, eight healthy men were randomized to receive 1,600 mg DHEA or a placebo daily divided into four doses for four weeks each. DHEA raised mean plasma DHEAS concentrations 9-fold, but had no significant effect on body weight, lean body mass (total body water and total body potassium), or parameters of energy and protein metabolism (resting metabolic rate, total energy expenditure, leucine flux). Cholesterol, T3, and T4 were also unaffected by DHEA supplementation. The authors concluded that DHEA is not an important regulator of energy or protein metabolism in humans (31).

- In a double-blind, placebo-controlled trial, six obese men (aged 21 y to 37 y) were given placebos from day 1 to day 28, followed by 1,600 mg DHEA/day divided into four doses from day 29 to day 56. Diet and exercise were not controlled. Serum DHEAS levels rose significantly after DHEA administration compared to the baseline. Body fat mass assessed by three methods (hydrostatic weighing, impedance plethysmography, and skinfold measurements) was reduced in two of the six subjects; however, for the group as a whole body weight, body fat mass, and waist-hip ratio did not change significantly. There was also no effect on tissue insulin sensitivity or serum lipids (32).

- In a double-blind, placebo-controlled study, 10 healthy men were randomized to receive 1,600 mg DHEA or a placebo daily for 28 days. In the DHEA group after 28 days, serum DHEAS and androstenedione were elevated, but not testosterone, sex-hormone binding globulin, estradiol, or estrone levels. DHEA-supplemented subjects had a statistically significant mean decrease in body fat of 31 percent, with no changes in weight. DHEA treatment was also associated with a significant decrease in mean serum total that was almost entirely attributable to a 7.5 percent drop in LDL cholesterol. There were no changes in average anthropometric parameters or serum lipids in the placebo group. There were no differences between groups in insulin sensitivity as measured by the hyperinsulinemic-euglycemic clamp technique (33).

- Obese dogs on a low-fat diet treated with DHEA had increased rate of weight loss and cholesterol reduction compared to control dogs (34, 35).

SAFETY

- The safety of long-term administration of DHEA is unknown.

- Chronic supplementation of DHEA can alter levels of other hormones, which may have unknown adverse effects.

- Excess DHEA appears to increase levels of testosterone. In women this promotes masculinization (increased facial hair, stimulated acne, increased hair loss, deepening of the voice, menstrual irregularities). In men, it may increase the risk of prostate cancer (36).

- DHEA also has estrogenic activity and may increase the risk of hormone-stimulated cancers such as breast and endometrial cancer (24, 25).

- DHEA may decrease serum HDL cholesterol levels (22)

REFERENCES

1. Longcope C. Dehydroepiandrosterone metabolism. *J Endocrinol.* 1996;150:S125–S127.
2. Labrie F, Belanger A, Simard J, et al. DHEA and peripheral androgen and estrogen formation: intracrinology. *Ann N Y Acad Sci.* 1995;774:16–28.
3. Svec F, Porter JR. The actions of exogenous dehydroepiandrosterone in experimental animals and humans. *Proc Soc Exp Biol Med.* 1998;218:174–191.

4. Khaw KT. Dehydroepiandrosterone, dehydroepiandrosterone sulfate and cardiovascular disease. *J Endocrinol.* 1996;150:S149–S153.

5. Clore JN. Dehydroepiandrosterone and body fat. *Obes Res.* 1995;3(suppl 4):613S–616S.

6. Watson RR, Huls A, Araghinikuam M, et al. Dehydroepiandrosterone and diseases of aging. *Drugs Aging.* 1996;9:274–291.

7. Thompson RD, Carlson M. Liquid chromatographic determination of dehydroepiandrosterone (DHEA) in dietary supplement products. *J AOAC Int.* 2000;83:847–857.

8. Mortola JF, Yen SS. The effects of oral dehydroepiandrosterone on endocrine metabolic parameters in postmenopausal women. *J Clin Endocrinol Metab.* 1990;71:696–704.

9. Morales AJ, Nolan JJ, Nelson JC, et al. Effects of replacement dose of DHEA in men and women of advancing age. *J Clin Endocrinol Metab.* 1994;78:1360–1367.

10. Frye RF, Kroboth PD, Kroboth FJ, et al. Sex differences in the pharmacokinetics of dehydroepiandrosterone (DHEA) after single- and multiple dose administration in healthy older adults. *J Clin Pharmacol.* 2000;40:596–605.

11. Nafziger AN, Bowlin SJ, Jenkins PL, et al. Longitudinal changes in dehydroepiandrosterone concentrations in men and women. *J Lab Clin Med.* 1998;131:316–323.

12. Barrett-Connor E, Edelstein SL. A prospective study of dehydroepiandrosterone sulfate and cognitive function in an older population: the Rancho Bernardo Study. *J Am Geriatr Soc.* 1994;42:420–423.

13. Yanase T, Fukahori M, Taniguchi S, et al. Serum dehydroepiandrosterone (DHEA) and DHEA-sulfate (DHEA-S) in Alzheimer's disease and in cerebrovascular dementia. *Endocr J.* 1996;43(1):119–123.

14. Wolf OT, Naumann E, Hellhammer DH, et al. Effects of dehydroepiandrosterone replacement in elderly men on event-related potentials, memory, and well-being. *J Gerontol A Biol Sci Med Sci.* 1998;53:M385–M390.

15. Baulieu EE, Thomas G, Legrain S, et al. Dehydroepiandrosterone (DHEA), DHEA sulfate, and aging: contribution of the DHEAge Study to a sociobiomedical issue. *Proc Natl Acad Sci USA.* 2000;97:4279–4284.

16. Barnhart KT, Freeman E, Grisso JA, et al. The effect of dehydroepiandrosterone supplementation to symptomatic perimenopausal women on serum endocrine profiles, lipid parameters, and health-related quality of life. *J Clin Endocrinol Metab.* 1999;84:3896–3902.

17. Khorram O, Vu L, Yen SS. Activation of immune function by dehydroepiandrosterone (DHEA) in age-advanced men. *J Gerontol A Biol Sci Med Sci.* 1997;52(1):M1–M7.

18. Degelau J, Guay D, Hallgren H. The effect of DHEAS on influenza vaccination in aging adults. *J Am Geriatr Soc.* 1997;45:747–751.

19. Ben-Yehuda A, Danenberg HD, Zakay-Rones Z, et al. The influence of sequential annual vaccination and of DHEA administration on the efficacy of the immune response to influenza vaccine in the elderly. *Mech Ageing Dev.* 1998;102:299–306.

20. Barrett-Connor E, Goodman-Gruen D. The epidemiology of DHEAS and cardiovascular disease. *Ann N Y Acad Sci.* 1995;774:259–270.

21. Barrett-Connor E, Goodman-Gruen D. Dehydroepiandrosterone sulfate does not predict cardiovascular death in postmenopausal women. The Rancho Bernardo Study. *Circulation.* 1995;91:1757–1760.

22. Mortola JF, Yen SS. The effects of oral dehydroepiandrosterone on endocrine-metabolic parameters in postmenopausal women. *J Clin Endocrinol Metab.* 1990;71:696–704.

23. Barrett-Connor E, Friedlander NJ, Khaw KT. Dehydroepiandrosterone sulfate and breast cancer risk. *Cancer Res.* 1990;50:6571–6574.

24. Dorgan JF, Stanczyk FZ, Longcope C, et al. Relationship of serum dehydroepiandrosterone (DHEA), DHEA sulfate, and 5-androstene-3 beta, 17 beta-diol to risk of breast cancer in postmenopausal women. *Cancer Epidemiol Biomarkers Prev.* 1997;6(3):177–181.

25. Le Bail JC, Allen K, Nicolas JC, et al. Dehydroepiandrosterone sulfate estrogenic action at its physiological plasma concentration in human breast cancer cell lines. *Anticancer Res.* 1998;18:1683–1688.

26. Nestler JE. DHEA: a coming of age. *Ann NY Acad Sci.* 1995;774:ix–xi.

27. van Vollenhoven RF, Engleman EG, McGuire JL. Dehydroepiandrosterone in systemic lupus erythematosus. Results of a double-blind, placebo-controlled, randomized clinical trial. *Arthritis Rheum.* 1995;38:1826–1831.

28. van Vollenhoven RF, Morabito LM, Engleman EG, et al. Treatment of systemic lupus erythematosus with dehydroepiandrosterone: 50 patients treated up to 12 months. *J Rheumatol.* 1998;25:285–289.

29. Christeff N, Gherbi N, Mammes O, et al. Serum cortisol and DHEA concentrations during HIV infection. *Psychoneuroendocrinology.* 1997;22(suppl 1):S11–S18.

30. Dyner TS, Lang W, Geaga J, et al. An open-label, dose-escalation trial of oral dehydroepiandrosterone tolerance and pharmacokinetics in patients with HIV disease. *J Acquir Immune Defic Syndr.* 1993;6:459–465.

31. Welle S, Jozefowicz R, Statt M. Failure of dehydroepiandrosterone to influence energy and protein metabolism in humans. *J Clin Endocrinol Metab.* 1990;71:1259–1264.

32. Usiskin KS, Butterworth S, Clore JN, et al. Lack of effect of dehydroepiandrosterone in obese men. *Int J Obes.* 1990;14:457–463.

33. Nestler JE, Barlascini CO, Clore JN, et al. Dehydroepiandrosterone reduces serum low density lipoprotein levels and body fat but does not alter insulin sensitivity in normal men. *J Clin Endocrinol Metab.* 1988;66:57–61.

34. Kurzman ID, Panciera DL, Miller JB, et al. The effect of dehydroepiandrosterone combined with a low-fat diet in spontaneously obese dogs: a clinical trial. *Obes Res.* 1998;6:20–28.

35. MacEwen EG, Kurzman ID. Obesity in the dog: role of the adrenal steroid dehydroepiandrosterone (DHEA). *J Nutr.* 1991;121:S51–S55.

36. Anonymous. Dehydroepiandrosterone (DHEA). *Med Lett Drugs Ther.* 1996;38:91–92.

Dong quai (Angelica sinensis)

Dong quai, also known as dang guei or *Angelica sinensis,* is a medicinal herb used for more than 2,000 years in traditional Chinese medicine. It is produced from the plant's root, after the plant is grown for one year and then been harvested and dried. According to Chinese classification, dong quai is considered a "tonifying herb" that strengthens or supplements an area or body process that is insufficient or weakened. Dong quai is one of the most widely used herbs in China as part of a formula for gynecological ailments such as menstrual cramps, irregularity, irregular flow, and weakness during the menstrual period, and menopausal symptoms. In the United States, dong quai is most often used as a single-herb preparation, which some suggest to be less effective than when the plant is used in traditional Chinese multiple-herb formulas. Although the exact mechanism of action has not been determined, a few theories have been proposed on the how dong quai might affect menopause. Some speculate that dong quai might support endogenous estrogen production, might contain estrogenic compounds, or might alleviate signs of estrogen deficiency without altering estrogen levels (1, 2).

Media and Marketing Claims	Efficacy
Relieves symptoms of menopause	NR
Good for pre-menstrual syndrome, dysmenorrhea	NR

Advisory

- Not for use in patients with hormone sensitive cancers until mechanism of action is understood
- Long-term safety (beyond six months' use) not known

Drug/Supplement Interactions

May increase bleeding when taken with other blood-thinning drugs or supplements (eg, coumadin, warfarin, garlic, ginger, ginkgo, vitamin E, flaxseed, bromelain, fish oil, aspirin); should be monitored by a physician

KEY POINTS

- Limited controlled evidence exists to support using single preparations of dong quai to manage menopausal symptoms. In China, dong quai is typically used with four or more herbs that together have been reported to reduce hot flashes. However, most of this research is not available in English, and it consists of primarily *in vitro*, animal, and uncontrolled human studies. One controlled study reported no effect of dong quai on menopausal complaints. Clearly, much more controlled research is needed, using single and multiherb preparations to determine the efficacy and safety of dong quai.

- Though there is a long history of use in traditional Chinese medicine of dong quai for female complaints such as premenstrual syndrome and dysmenorrhea, controlled clinical trials are needed to support using dong quai for these conditions.

FOOD SOURCES

None

DOSAGE INFORMATION/BIOAVAILABILITY

Dong quai is available in capsules, tablets, tinctures, and teas. Dosage recommended is 1 g to 2 g or 10 to 40 drops of tincture three times daily (3 g to 6 g total). The extract is also used in many combination herbal supplements marketed for women's issues and it is often combined with black cohosh (*See* Black cohosh).

RELEVANT RESEARCH

Dong Quai and Menopause

- In a double-blind, placebo-controlled study, 71 postmenopausal women were randomized to receive 4.5 g donq quai root in capsules or a placebo daily for 24 weeks. The subjects had elevated follicle stimulating hormone (FSH) levels and complained of hot flashes. At the end of the study, endometrial thickness was measured by ultrasonography, vaginal cells were evaluated for cellular maturation, and menopausal symptoms were assessed by the Kupperman index and diary of vasomotor flushes. Though not significantly different, endometrial thickness increased 2.3 mm in the placebo group compared to 0.3 mm in the dong quai group, suggesting that dong quai had no estrogenic effects. The authors could not explain why endometrial thickness would have increased in the placebo group. There were also no significant differences in menopausal symptoms, or in the number of hot flashes (both groups reported significant improvements). Serum levels of estradiol, estrone, sex hormone-binding globulin, blood pressure, and weight did not differ between groups. The authors concluded that dong quai administered alone does not produce estrogen-like responses in vaginal cells or endometrial thickness and was no more helpful than placebo in relieving menopausal symptoms (2).

Dong Quai and PMS

- Research in Chinese medical journals (not available in English) has reported animal experiments using intravenous injection of water or alcohol extraction of dong quai root into female rabbits, cats, and dogs. All studies showed increased excitability of the uterus, and the contractive rhythm of smooth muscle of the uterus changed from fast, irregular, and weak to become slow, regular, and strong. One reviewer suggested that this is the pharmacological basis for using dong quai for dysmenorrhea (3).

SAFETY

- There are no controlled studies conducted for longer than 24 weeks testing the safety of dong quai supplementation in humans.
- Dong quai increased bleeding time in rabbits stabilized on warfarin (4). There is one case report of a 46-year-old woman with atrial fibrillation who had increased bleeding times while taking dong quai and warfarin for four weeks. Prothrombin times normalized one month after discontinuation of dong quai (5). Given these data,

combining dong quai with other blood-thinning medications or supplements (warfarin/Coumadin, heparin, aspirin, garlic, ginkgo, vitamin E, fish oil) is not recommended (6, 7).

- One case study reported the development of gynaecomastia (enlarged breasts) in a man after taking dong quai. The authors of this report suggested that the result may have been due to phytoestrogens contained within the herb (8).

- Although the exact mechanism underlying the efficacy of dong quai is not understood, some purport that the herb may have estrogenic effects. Because of this, some recommend that women with hormone sensitive conditions such as breast, uterine, and ovarian cancers, endometriosis, and uterine fibroids should not use this herb until more data on safety are available.

- Dong quai is not recommended during pregnancy due to potential stimulating effects on the uterus.

REFERENCES

1. Noe JE. Angelica sinensis: a monograph. *J Naturopathic Med.* 1997; 66–72.
2. Hirata JD, Swiersz LM, Zell B, et al.. Does dong quai have estrogenic effects in postmenopausal women? A double blind, placebo-controlled trial. *Fertility and Sterility.* 1997;68:981–986.
3. Zhu DP. Dong quai. *Am J Chinese Med.* 1987;15:117–125.
4. Lo ACT, Chan K, Yeung JHK, et al. Dang gui (*Angelica sinensis*) affects the pharmacodynamics but not the pharmacokinetics of warfarin in rabbits. *Eur J Drug Metab Pharmacokinet* 1995; 20: 55–60.
5. Page RL, Lawrence JD. Potentiation of warfarin by dong quai. *Pharmacotherapy.* 1999;19:870–876.
6. Fugh-Berman A. Herb-drug interaction. *Lancet.* 2000;355:134–138.
7. Heck AM, DeWitt BA, Lukes AL. Potential interactions between alternative therapies and warfarin. *Am J Health Syst Pharm.* 2000;57:221–227.
8. Goh SY, Loh KC. Gynaecomastia and the herbal tonic "Dong Quai." *Singapore Med J.* 2001;42:115–116.

Echinacea

The echinacea plant, known as the purple cone flower herb, was originally used by Native Americans to treat a variety of ailments. Although echinacea is indigenous to the United States, most clinical research on this plant has been completed in Germany. In Germany, *Echinacea purpurea* (above-ground parts) and *Echinacea pallida* (root) are approved by the government's expert committee, the German Commission E, for use as supportive therapy for colds and chronic infections of the respiratory and lower urinary tract. Commission E has not approved the above-ground parts of *E pallida* or any part (root or leaves) of *E angustifolia* because their efficacy has not been substantiated. Of the nine existing *Echinacea* species, the roots and the flowering leaves of *Echinacea purpurea, E pallida,* and *E angustifolia* are the most commonly used in supplements. Several polysaccharides, volatile oil, caffeic acid derivatives, isobutylamides, polynes, and polyines have been identified in the plant, although the active ingredient(s) are not entirely known (1–3).

Media and Marketing Claims	Efficacy
Boosts the immune system	?↑
Protects against the common cold and flu	↔

Advisory

- Not for use in patients with autoimmune disorders
- Potential allergic reaction in individuals having asthma or those sensitive to grass pollens

Drug/Supplement Interactions

- May decrease the effectiveness of immune-suppressing drugs (cyclosporine, corticosteroids)
- Potential negative interaction with hepatotoxic medications (anabolic steroids, amiodarone, methotrexate, ketoconazole)

KEY POINTS

- Animal and *in vitro* studies suggest that echinacea enhances immune system function. Human studies completed in Europe have also suggested immune modulation; however, many of these trials have been criticized for poor design.
- Clinical studies have reported conflicting results on the role of echinacea in preventing or reducing symptoms of upper respiratory infections. Additional well-controlled research is needed to verify the claim that echinacea protects the immune system against upper respiratory tract infections and influenza viruses.
- Because there are many varieties of echinacea with varying levels of potentially active compounds, future studies must control these variables to provide accurate information on the efficacy, dosage, administration, and preparation of supplements.

FOOD SOURCES

None

DOSAGE INFORMATION/BIOAVAILABILITY

Echinacea extract prepared from the fresh expressed juice of the flowering plant or root is available in tinctures, capsules, or tablets. It is also sold in herbal teas and throat lozenges. Most supplements provide echinacea from the fresh flower, roots, or a combination of the whole plant equivalent to 300 mg to 900 mg dried extract.

RELEVANT RESEARCH

Echinacea and Cellular Immunity

- *E purpurea* from fresh pressed juice and dried juice powder effectively induced cytokine production (Interleukin-1[IL-1], IL-6, IL-10, tumor necrosis factor-α) by human macrophages *in vitro* (4).

- Peripheral blood mononuclear cells from healthy individuals or patients with either chronic fatigue syndrome or AIDS were treated *ex vivo* with extracts of either *E purpurea* or *Panax ginseng*. Both echinacea and ginseng at concentrations > or = 0.1 or 10 μg/kg, respectively, resulted in a statistically significant enhancement of natural killer cell function and antibody-dependent cellular toxicity in all cells (5).

- In animal and *in vitro* studies, polysaccharides isolated from *E purpurea* enhanced immune function by activating macrophages and increased the resistance of immuno-compromised mice to the pathogens *Listeria monocytogenes* and *Candida albicans* (6, 7).

Echinacea and Immunity (Clinical Trials)

- In a double-blind, placebo-controlled study, 108 patients with a history of more than three colds or respiratory infections in the preceding year were randomized to receive 4 mL fluid extract of *E purpurea* (above-ground plant) or a placebo twice daily. The incidence and severity of colds and respiratory infections were determined during eight weeks of treatment, based on patient-reported symptoms together and findings on physical exam. During the study, 35 of 54 (65 percent) of patients in the echinacea group and 40 of 54 (70 percent) in the placebo group had at least one infection. There were no significant differences between groups in incidence, duration, or severity of colds and respiratory infection (8).

- In a double-blind, placebo-controlled study, 246 of 559 recruited healthy volunteers developed symptoms of a common cold and were randomized to one of four treatments daily: (1) 6.78 mg crude extract of *E purpurea* tablets (95 percent above-ground plant, 5 percent root); (2) 48.2 mg crude extract of *E purpurea* tablets (seven times higher concentration than group 1); (3) 29.6 mg crude extract of *E purpurea* radix (root) tablets; or (4) a placebo. Subjects were instructed to take preparations until they felt healthy again, but not longer than seven days. The primary endpoint was the relative reduction of the complaint index defined by 12 symptoms during common cold according to the physician's record. Sixty-five of 246 cases (27 percent) were excluded from analysis because of dropouts and protocol violations such as co-medication and late start of treatment. In regard to the relative reduction of the complaint index by the doctor's record, echinacea supplementation in groups 1 and 2 was significantly more effective than the echinacea root extract or a placebo. With respect to the complaint index according to the patient's diary, groups 1 and 2 were also significantly more effective than group 3 or the placebo. According to subjective assessments by the doctor and patients, groups 1 and 2 were judged as more effective than placebo. The frequency of adverse effects (mainly gastrointestinal symptoms) was similar for all groups (9).

- In a double-blind, placebo-controlled study, 95 subjects with early symptoms of cold or flu were randomly assigned to receive Echinacea Plus tea or a placebo in five to six cups daily over one to five days. The efficacy, number of days the symptoms lasted, and number of days before change was measured with a self-scoring questionnaire by subjects 14 days after beginning the program. There was a significant difference between the groups, with the Echinacea-treated subjects having more effective and faster relief of symptoms (10).

- A systematic review of 26 controlled clinical trials testing the effects of echinacea on the immune response rated the methodological quality of most studies as "modest." All of the original studies were published in German journals from 1961 to 1993. Of the studies reviewed, only 6 tested single preparations, 18 were randomized, and 11 were double-blinded. In general, statistical evaluations and baseline data were insufficient or poorly described. Despite the limitations, the authors concluded: "Existing controlled clinical trials indicate that preparations containing extracts of echinacea can be efficacious immunomodulators. However, the evidence is still insufficient for clear therapeutic recommendations as to which preparation to use and which dose to employ for a specific indication" (3).

- In a double-blind, placebo-controlled trial, 160 subjects with upper respiratory infections were randomized to receive 900 mg (or 90 drops) *E pallida* root extract or a placebo for 8 to 10 days. The presence of infection was confirmed by blood tests (raised differential lymphocyte count indicating viral infection and raised differential neutrophil count indicating a bacterial infection). Symptoms (weakness, sweating, tear flow, burning eyes, sore throat), were recorded at day 3 or 4 and at days 8 and 10 of the study. The duration of illness was significantly reduced from 13 to 9.8 days in bacterial infections and 9.1 days in viral infections with echinacea supplementation. The clinical findings correlated with the lymphocytosis and differential neutrophil count; as patients were treated, both of these fell back to normal, but at a faster rate in echinacea-treated subjects than in placebo-treated subjects (statistical significance not reported). There was a significant improvement in overall symptom scores with echinacea supplementation compared to the placebo (11).

- Five German, placebo-controlled, randomized studies (total n = 134 subjects) investigating the immunomodulatory activity of intravenous and oral echinacea extracts (*angustifolia, pallida,* and *purpurea*) in healthy volunteers were reviewed. Two studies supplying intravenous echinacea extract showed a significant increase in phagocytic activity of polymorphonuclear neutrophil granulocytes (PNG) compared to placebo. However, in the studies testing oral echinacea (950 mg dried *E purpurea* extract or 1,600 mg to 1,800 mg *E purpurea* extract in ethanol daily), no statistically significant immune response was observed. The author reported that results were difficult to interpret because of the different methods used for measuring phagocytosis, the small sample size, and failure to use standardized monopreparations of echinacea (12).

- In a double-blind, placebo-controlled trial, 180 patients visiting a general medicine clinic for flu-type or feverish infections of the upper respiratory tract were randomized to receive one of three treatments: (1) 450 mg (90 drops) of *Echinacea purpurea* radix in unstandardized liquid extract (1:5, 55 percent ethanol); (2) 900 mg (180 drops) *Echinacea purpurea* radix in unstandardized ethanol extract; (3) a placebo. Physician and patient assessments were obtained at the beginning of treatment, after 3 to 4 days, and after 8 to 10 days of treatment. The low-dose echinacea did not differ statistically from the placebo in relieving symptoms and duration of flu-like infections at all periods of measurement. Compared to the placebo, the 900-mg dose resulted in a significant improvement in symptoms (inflamed nose, frontal sensitivity, coated tongue) after 3 to 4 days, and after 8 to 10 days, only one symptom (inflamed nose) remained significant (13).

- The Bastyr University Research Institute has completed the first U.S. trial (double-blind, placebo-controlled, 26 weeks) testing *E purpurea* in 160 subjects having frequent respiratory tract infections. Treatment was given prior to infection. Preliminary reported results did not suggest a favorable effect of echinacea.

SAFETY

- Oral echinacea appears to be well-tolerated, although the safety of long-term use is unknown (3). Symptoms of immunostimulation (eg, shivering, fever, and muscle weakness) have been observed after parenteral administration, but not with oral use (14). German Commission E recommends taking echinacea orally no longer than eight weeks and parenterally no longer than three weeks.

- One review suggested that hepatotoxic effects may be associated with persistent echinacea use and therefore, it should not be taken with other known hepatotoxic drugs (eg, anabolic steroids, amidarone, methotrexate, or ketoconazole). However, the reviewer noted that the magnitude of liver toxicity has been questioned because echinacea lacks the compounds (1,2 unsaturated necrine ring system) associated with hepatotoxicity of pyrrolizidine alkaloids (13).

- Because echinacea appears to stimulate the immune system, it has been recommended that individuals having autoimmune and progressive systemic diseases (lupus, HIV, tuberculosis, multiple sclerosis, scleroderma) should not take echinacea supplements (2). It has also been suggested that individuals on immunostimulant medications such as corticosteroids and cyclosporine avoid supplementing with echinacea (13).

- According to a case report, one woman had an anaphylactic reaction after taking 5 mL of a commercial extract of echinacea (equivalent to 150 mg dry root of *E purpurea* and 3,825 mg dried extract *E angustifolia*). Hypersensitivity to the plant was confirmed by skinprick tests and RASTs. Patients with atopy or allergies to grass pollens should be cautioned about the risk of developing severe allergic reactions to echinacea (15).

- A case of recurrent erythma nodosum (hypersensitive reddening of the skin with subcutaneous nodules) was associated with echinacea use (16).

REFERENCES

1. Hobbs C. Echinacea: a literature review. *HerbalGram*. 1994;30:33–48.
2. Blumenthal M, ed. *The Complete German Commission E Monographs Therapeutic Guide to Herbal Medicines*. Austin, Tex: American Botanical Council; 1998.

3. Melchart D, Linde K, Worku R, et al. Immunomodulation with echinacea—a systematic review of controlled clinical trials. *Phytomedicine.* 1994;1:245–254.

4. Burger RA, Torres AR, Warren RP, et al. Echinacea-induced cytokine production by human macrophages. *Int J Immunopharmacol.* 1997;19:371–379.

5. See DM, Broumand N, Sahl L, et al. In vitro effects of echinacea and ginseng on natural killer and anti-body dependent cell cytotoxicity in healthy subjects and chronic fatigue syndrome or acquired immunodeficiency syndrome patients. *Immunopharmacology.* 1997;35:229–235.

6. Steinmuller C, Roesler J, Grottrup E, et al. Polysaccharides isolated from plant cell cultures of *Echinacea purpurea* enhance the resistance of immunosuppressed mice against systemic infections with *Candida albicans* and *Listeria monocytogenes. Int J Immunopharmacol.* 1993;15:605–614.

7. Roesler J, Emmendorffer A, Steinmuller C, et al. Application of purified polysaccharides from cell cultures of the plant *Echinacea purpurea* to test subjects mediates activation of the phagocyte system. *Int J Immunopharmacol.* 1991;13:931–941.

8. Grimm W, Muller HH. A randomized controlled trial of the effect of fluid extract of *Echinacea purpurea* on the incidence and severity of colds and respiratory infections. *Am J Med.* 1999;106:138–143.

9. Brinkeborn RM, Shah DV, Degenring FH. Echinaforce and other echinacea fresh plant preparations in the treatment of the common cold. A randomized, placebo-controlled, double-blind clinical trial. *Phytomedicine.* 1999;6:1–5.

10. Lindenmuth GF, Lindenmuth EB. The efficiacy of Echinacea compound herbal tea preparation on the severity and duration of upper respiratory and flu symptoms: a randomized, double-blind, placebo-controlled study. *J Altern Complement Med.* 2000;6:327–334.

11. Dorn M, Knick E, Lewith G. Placebo-controlled, double-blind study of *Echinacea pallidae* radix in upper respiratory tract infections. *Complement Ther Med.* 1997;3:40–42.

12. Melchart D, Linde K, Worku F, et al. Results of five randomized studies on the immunomodulatory activity of preparations of echinacea. *J Altern Complement Med.* 1995;1:145–160.

13. Braunig B, Dorn M, Limburg E, et al. *Echinacea purpureae* radix. For strengthening the immune response in flu-like infections [in German]. *Z Phytother.* 1992;13:7–12.

14. Miller LG. Herbal medicinals. Selected clinical considerations focusing on known or potential drug-herb interactions. *Arch Intern Med.* 1998;158:2200–2211.

15. Mullins RJ. Echinacea-associated anaphylaxis. *Med J Aust.* 1998;168:170–171.

16. Soon SL, Crawford RI. Recurrent erythma nodosum associated with Echinacea herbal therapy. *J Am Acad Dermatol.* 2001;44:298–299.

Eicosapentaenoic Acid (EPA)

See Fish Oil.

Enzymes

See Bromelain *and* Pancreatin.

Evening Primrose Oil (*Oenothera biennis*)

See Gamma Linolenic Acid.

Fish Oil

Fish consumption is associated with lower rates of coronary artery disease in many, but not all, epidemiological studies. Because fish oil is a rich source of the essential omega-3 (n-3) fatty acids eicosapentaenoic acid (EPA) and docosahexaenoic acid (DHA), this cardioprotective effect has been attributed to the omega-3 (n-3) fatty acids. N-3 fatty acids are essential polyunsaturated fatty acids necessary for normal growth and development.

There has been interest in fish oil because EPA and DHA are precursors to eicosanoids, which have antiatherogenic and anti-inflammatory effects. Specifically, n-3 fatty acids have beneficial effects on several precipitating factors involved in the development of cardiovascular and inflammatory diseases, including the production of thromboxane A_2, leukotriene B_4, and prostaglandin E_2 (PGE_2), interleukin 1, tumor necrosis factor, platelet-derived growth factor-like protein, triglycerides, lipoprotein (a), and fibrinogen. Additionally, fish oil has been shown to inhibit platelet aggregation, intimal hyperplasia, and monocyte and macrophage function, and to possibly lower blood pressure. Omega-3 fatty acids also increase the formation of protective factors including prostacyclin (PGI_3), leukotriene B_5, interleukin 2, endothelial-derived relaxing factor, fibrinolytic activity, red cell deformability, and HDL cholesterol (1–3).

In 2000, the FDA approved a limited health claim for labeling of n-3 fatty acid supplements regarding coronary heart disease (CHD). Supplement labels can state that the evidence is "suggestive, but not conclusive" and that it is not known if diets or Omega-3 fatty acids in fish reduce risk of CHD in the general population.

Media and Marketing Claims	Efficacy
Lowers triglycerides	↔
Improves lipids and glucose control in diabetes	↑?
Lowers blood pressure	↑?
Improves atherosclerosis	↔
Reduces risk of death from heart attack	↑?
Improves rheumatoid arthritis	↑?
Improves ulcerative colitis	↑?
Improves symptoms of psoriasis	↓
Beneficial in depression	NR

Advisory

Should not be used prior to surgery to avoid potential increase in bleeding

Drug/Supplement Interactions

In theory, fish oil may increase bleeding when taken with other blood-thinning drugs or supplements (coumadin, warfarin, garlic, ginger, ginkgo, vitamin E, flaxseed, bromelain, dong quai); should be monitored by a physician

KEY POINTS

- The typical American diet provides n-3 fatty acids in relatively low amounts. The amount of n-6 fatty acids in the diet has increased in the past 100 years, resulting in a much higher ratio of n-6 to n-3 fatty acids. A low intake of n-3 fatty acids has been hypothesized by some researchers to contribute to the etiology of many chronic diseases (3).

- Many studies have shown that intake of dietary fish oil appears to inhibit or decrease the risk of precipitating factors in the development of inflammatory and cardiovascular diseases.

- *Blood Lipids:* There is considerable evidence that fish oil (> 3 g n-3 fatty acids/day) reduces plasma triglycerides, which may be accompanied by an increase in total and LDL- cholesterol in patients having hypertriglyceridemia. Preliminary studies in small numbers of subjects reported that garlic administered with fish oil suppressed the rise in LDL that accompanies fish oil.

- *Blood Lipids and Glycemic Control in Diabetes:* A meta-analysis of studies in patients having diabetes reported favorable effects of fish oil on triglyceride levels, and on glucose and glycosylated hemoglobin in people having type 2 diabetes.

- *Blood Pressure:* A meta-analysis reported that fish oil may produce a small reduction in blood pressure, especially in hypertensive subjects.

- *Atherosclerosis:* Studies have not shown a clear pattern of reducing atherosclerosis or restenosis after angioplasty following supplementation.

- *Cardiovascular Disease Morbidity and Mortality:* There is evidence that low intakes fish oil (< 1 g n-3 fatty acids/day) may reduce the risk of myocardial infarction and death in patients with coronary heart disease.

- The American Heart Association (AHA) recognizes the benefits of consuming fish rich in omega-3 fatty acids for heart health, and recommends consuming fish two times per week. However, fish oil supplements are not recommended in the AHA 2000 dietary guidelines because they state that more compelling evidence is needed to show that supplements are beneficial to overall cardiovascular health.

- There is evidence that fish oil can have mild beneficial effects (reduction of tender joints and morning stiffness) on rheumatoid arthritis.

- There is evidence that fish oil provides modest improvements in patients having ulcerative colitis and Crohn's disease. More research is needed to determine the potential role of fish oil in inflammatory intestinal diseases.

- Although fish oil has documented anti-inflammatory effects in laboratory studies, controlled trials have not shown clinical improvements in patients having psoriasis. However, fish oil may reduce hypertriglyceridemia associated with retinoid therapy used to treat psoriasis. In addition, there is preliminary evidence that those with IgA nephropathy may benefit from fish oil supplements.

- There is some evidence that individuals with mood disorders have reduced n-3 fatty acid concentrations. Controlled trials are necessary to determine the role of fish oil supplements in depression, schizophrenia, bipolar disorder, dementia, and other psychiatric conditions. Clinical studies are currently being developed at Massachusetts General Hospital.

- Patients with conditions shown to benefit from n-3 fatty acid supplementation should discuss this option with their physicians. Eating two to three servings of fatty fish per week while limiting intake of high saturated fat foods will increase the n-3 fatty acid content of the diet. In addition, n-3 fatty acids may also be consumed in EPA and DHA-fortified foods such as eggs, margarine, milk, yogurt, and bread. (*See also* Flaxseed.)

FOOD SOURCES

Although not a direct source of EPA and DHA, foods such as flaxseed and walnuts are rich in alpha-linolenic acid, the precursors to EPA and DHA. (*See* Flaxseed.)

Consumption of an average serving of fatty fish two to three times per week provides approximately 3 g fish oil (3). Farm-raised fish contain a lower amount of omega-3 fatty acids than fish found in oceans, rivers, and lakes (3). The fattier the fish, the higher the content of omega-3 fatty acids. However, the lipid content can vary depending on water temperature and place and season of capture (1).

An excess of omega-6 fatty acids (vegetable oils) reduces the metabolism of long-chain omega-3 fatty acids (2).

Fish, Raw (3.5 oz or 100 g)	EPA (g)	DHA (g)
Mackerel	0.90	1.40
Salmon, Chinook	0.79	0.57
Herring	0.71	0.86
Anchovy	0.54	0.91
Tuna	0.28	0.89
Blue fish	0.25	0.52
Swordfish	0.11	0.53
Cod liver oil	6.90	10.97

Source: Data from Jones PJ, Kubow S (2)

DOSAGE INFORMATION/BIOAVAILABILITY

Fish oil supplements are usually derived from sardine, salmon, tuna, menhaden, or anchovy fish and are sold as liquid oil or in softgel capsules. Concentrated EPA and DHA are also available as supplements. Before packaging, oils must be refined to remove moisture, impurities, sulfur, halogen and nitrogen compounds, toxic metals, trace metals, sterols, and other contaminants. Supplements typically provide approximately 180 mg to 300 mg EPA and 120 mg to 200 mg DHA per capsule, with manufacturers suggesting a total intake ranging from 1 g to 10 g/day. In a bioavailability study, 4 g of highly purified EPA or DHA administered with a high-fat meal to healthy subjects increased EPA and DHA levels in chylomicrons peaking six hours after supplementation (4).

The United States has no guidelines for recommended levels of n-3 fatty acid intake. Canadian dietary guidelines specify a daily intake of 1.0 g to 1.5 g of n-3 fatty acids and 7 g to 9 g n-6 fatty acids for adults more than 25 years old (5). In the United States, the average estimated daily intake of 0.050 g EPA and 0.080 g DHA is far lower than recommended in the Canadian guidelines (3).

RELEVANT RESEARCH

Note: Because of the large number of studies of fish oil, only recent trials and review articles are discussed.

Fish Oil and Blood Lipids

- Numerous studies have reported that fish oil supplementation has a beneficial effect on plasma triglyceride levels, lowering them about 30 percent, and up to 50 percent in patients with severe hypertriglyceridemia (6). However, the triglyceride-lowering effects can be accompanied by increases in low-density-lipoprotein (LDL) cholesterol, especially in patients with low baseline LDL cholesterol levels (7, 8). It has been suggested that the increase in LDL cholesterol may not necessarily increase atherosclerosis risk in light of the antithrombotic, anti-inflammatory, and antivasoconstrictive actions of n-3 fatty acids (3). However, it remains unknown whether an increase in LDL cholesterol from fish oil is, in fact, atherogenic.

- According to one reviewer: "The effects of n-3 fatty acids on serum cholesterol concentrations are similar to those of other PUFAs. When n-3 fatty acids replace saturated fatty acids in the diet, they lower serum cholesterol concentrations. Omega-3 fatty acids have the added benefit of consistently lowering serum triglycerides concentrations, whereas the n-6 fatty acids do not and may even increase them" (3).

Fish Oil and Blood Lipids in Diabetes

- A meta-analysis of 26 trials testing fish oil administration (on lipid levels in patients with types 1 and 2 diabetes revealed a significant 25 percent to 30 percent decrease in mean triglyceride concentrations and a slight but statistically significant increase in serum LDL cholesterol. Both findings were more prominent in type 2 diabetes patients. Fasting blood glucose levels were significantly lower in type 1 diabetic participants but increased insignificantly in subjects with type 2 diabetes. When all studies were combined, there were no changes in glycosylated hemoglobin with fish oil. When the effects of EPA and DHA were analyzed separately, there was a statistically significant inverse relationship between EPA and DHA intake on triglyceride levels in both type 1 and type 2 diabetes patients. In patients with type 2 diabetes, positive relationships between EPA and glycosylated hemoglobin, and between DHA and fasting blood glucose and glycosylated hemoglobin were apparent. In contrast, there were no significant effects of EPA or DHA on these parameters in patients with type 1 diabetes. The authors concluded that overall: "The use of fish oil has no adverse effects on HbA_{1c} in diabetic subjects and lowers triglyceride levels effectively by almost 30 percent. However, this may be accompanied by a slight increase in LDL cholesterol concentration. Fish oil may be useful in treating dyslipidemia in diabetes" (9).

Fish Oil Combined with Garlic Supplements and Blood Lipids

- In a double-blind (single-blind for fish oil group because of the difficulty of masking fish odor), placebo-controlled study, 50 male subjects with moderate hypercholesterolemia were randomly assigned for 12 weeks to one of four groups who received one of the following: (1) 900 mg garlic plus placebo oil, (2) 12 g fish oil (3.6 g n-3 fatty acids), (3) both garlic and fish oil, or (4) a placebo. There was a significant reduction in mean group serum total cholesterol with garlic plus fish oil (−12.2 percent) and garlic alone (−11.5 percent), but not with fish oil alone. Mean LDL-cholesterol levels were significantly lower with garlic plus fish oil (−9.5 percent) and garlic alone (−14.2 percent), but again, were significantly increased (+8.5 percent) with fish oil alone. Mean triglyceride levels were significantly reduced with garlic plus fish oil (−34.3 percent) and with fish oil alone (−37.3 percent). The authors concluded that co-ingestion of garlic and fish oil apparently reversed the fish oil-induced rise in LDL-cholesterol (10).

- In a single-blind, placebo-controlled, crossover study, 40 subjects having hyperlipidemia were assigned to receive in random order fish oil/garlic capsules (2 g fish oil, 1.2 g garlic powder) or a placebo for four weeks each, with a four-week washout period between arms. Fish oil/garlic supplements resulted in a significant 11 percent decrease in cholesterol levels, 10 percent decrease in LDL levels, and 34 percent decrease in triglyceride levels. There was no change in HDL cholesterol (11).

Fish Oil and Blood Pressure

- A meta-analysis of 31 placebo-controlled trials (n = 1,356 subjects) reported a small but significant reduction in blood pressure (↓3.0 mm Hg systolic/↓ 1.5 mm Hg diastolic) associated with fish oil consumption. N-3 fatty acids (mean daily dose 4.2 g) had no effect on blood pressure in eight studies of healthy, normotensive subjects. Doses of 5.6 g/day resulted in a significant blood pressure lowering effect in studies of hypertensive and hypercholesterolemic patients. The authors concluded: "There is a dose response effect of fish oil on blood pressure of ↓0.66/↓0.35 mm Hg/g omega-3 fatty acids. The hypotensive effect may be strongest in hypertensive subjects and those with clinical atherosclerotic disease or hypercholesterolemia" (12).

- In a placebo-controlled, multicenter trial, 350 normotensive subjects (ages 30 y to 54 y) were randomly assigned to receive 6 g purified fish oil daily (3 g n-3 fatty acids) or a placebo for six months. At baseline, the mean differences in blood pressure changes between groups were not significant. There was no tendency for fish oil to lower blood pressure more in subjects with baseline blood pressure in the upper (132/87 mm Hg) versus lower quartile (114/75 mm Hg), or with low habitual fish consumption (0.4 vs 2.9 times/week), or with low baseline plasma n-3 fatty acids. Fish oil supplementation resulted in a significant increase in HDL cholesterol compared to the placebo. Subgroup analysis showed this effect to be significant in women but not in men (13).

Fish Oil and Atherosclerosis

- A meta-analysis of seven trials testing fish oil supplements in patients who underwent angioplasty reported that in the four studies using angiography there was a reduction in restenosis (reconstriction of blood vessels) with fish oil intake. In the three studies that used stress testing to evaluate restenosis, there was no benefit from fish oil consumption. There was a significant positive relationship between the dose and the absolute difference in restenosis rates (14).

- In a placebo-controlled study, 59 patients with angiographically documented coronary heart disease and normal plasma lipid levels were randomized to receive either fish oil capsules (6 g of n-3 fatty acids daily) or a placebo (olive oil) for an average of 28 months. As expected, lipid tissue EPA levels in the fish oil group were significantly higher than in the placebo group at the end of the trial. Fish oil resulted in a significant 30 percent reduction in triglyceride levels but had no effect on other plasma lipoprotein levels. There were no significant reductions in mean minimal diameter of atherosclerotic coronary arteries or percent stenosis between groups. The authors concluded: "Fish oil treatment for two years does not promote major favorable changes in the diameter of atherosclerotic coronary arteries" (15).

- In a controlled study, 610 patients undergoing coronary artery bypass grafting were randomly assigned to receive 4 g concentrated fish oil/day or no supplement (control) for one year. All patients in the fish oil and control groups were also assigned to antithrombotic treatment using either aspirin or warfarin. Compared to the control, the fish oil group had significantly fewer occluded vein grafts (16).

Fish Oil and Cardiovascular Morbidity or Mortality

- In a large-scale, open label, Italian study (GISSI Prevenzione Study), 11,324 patients surviving recent (≤ 3 months) myocardial infarction were randomly assigned to one of four groups for 3.5 years: (1) 1 g n-3 supplements; (2) 300 mg vitamin E; (3) both supplements; or (4) neither supplement. The main endpoint was the combined occurrence of death, nonfatal myocardial infarction, and nonfatal stroke. N-3 treatment significantly lowered the risk of the primary endpoint by 10 percent to 15 percent. Total mortality in patients treated with n-3 fatty acid supplements was 20 percent lower (a significant difference) than subjects not receiving n-3 fats. There was no additional benefit of the combined vitamin E and n-3 supplements. The results of this study would have been strengthened if it had been double-blinded (17).

- In a double-blind, placebo-controlled study in India, 360 patients with suspected myocardial infarction (MI) were randomized to receive fish oil (1.08 g EPA/day), or mustard oil (2.9 g alpha-linolenic acid/day), or placebo for one year. Treatments were administered approximately 18 hours after symptoms of MI in all three groups. The extent of cardiac disease, rise in cardiac enzymes, and levels of lipid peroxides were similar among the groups at entry. After one year, total cardiac events were significantly fewer in the fish oil and mustard oil groups compared to the group using the placebo (24.5 percent and 28 percent vs 34.7 percent, respectively). Nonfatal infarctions were also significantly fewer in the fish oil and mustard oil groups compared to the group using the placebo (13 percent and 15 percent vs 25.4 percent, respectively). Fish oil supplementation was significantly correlated with fewer cardiac deaths compared to use of the placebo (11.4 percent vs 22.0 percent). Mustard oil had no effect on total cardiac death rate. Both the fish oil and mustard oil groups showed a significant reduction in the incidence of total cardiac arrhythmias, left ventricular enlargement, and angina pectoris compared to the placebo group (18).

- In a population-based, case-control study, 334 case patients with primary cardiac arrest (aged 25 y to 74 y) and 493 randomly selected control cases matched for age and gender were assessed for dietary intake of n-3 fatty acids from seafood. Spouses of case patients and control subjects were interviewed to quantify n-3 fatty acid intake during the prior month. Blood specimens from 82 cases and 108 controls were analyzed to determine red blood cell membrane fatty acid composition, an indirect biomarker of n-3 intake. An intake of 5.5 g n-3 fatty acids/month (the mean of the third quartile and the equivalent of one fatty fish meal per week) was associated with a significant 50 percent reduction in the risk of primary cardiac arrest after adjustment for confounding variables when compared to no intake of n-3 fatty acids (odds ratio = 0.5, 95 percent CI, 0.4 to 0.8). Compared with a red blood cell membrane n-3 fatty acid level of 3.3 percent of total fatty acids (mean of the lowest quartile), a level of 5.0 percent (mean of the third quartile) was associated with a 70 percent reduction in the risk of primary cardiac arrest (odds ratio = 0.3, 95 percent CI, 0.2 to 0.6) (19).

- According to one review, n-3 fatty acid supplementation has been shown to prevent ischemia-induced ventricular fibrillation and arrhythmias in animal studies (20).

Fish Oil and Rheumatoid Arthritis

- A meta-analysis of 10 double-blind, placebo-controlled, randomized trials (total n = 395 subjects, mean age = 54 y) reported that fish oil supplemented for three months was associated with a significant reduction in occurrence of subjective assessment of joint tenderness and morning stiffness as compared to use of placebo oils, but no significant improvements in joint swelling, grip strength, patient and physician assessment, or erythrocyte sedimentation rate (marker of inflammation). A mega-analysis of the data using primary data from each study (the previous meta-analysis used only summary data), confirmed the results. The doses of fish oil used in the studies were not given. The authors noted that most of the studies did not report disease duration, rheumatoid factor seropositivity, and functional status of subjects (21).

- In a double-blind, placebo-controlled study, 66 rheumatoid arthritis patients were randomized to receive 130 mg/kg/day n-3 fatty acids (~ 9 g fish oil/day) or a placebo (corn oil) while taking diclofenac for pain. Placebo diclofenac was substituted at week 18 or 22, and fish oil supplements were continued for eight weeks (week 26 or 30). In subjects taking fish oil, there was a significant decrease from baseline in the mean number of tender joints, duration of morning stiffness, physician's and patient's evaluation of global arthritis activity, and physician's evaluation of pain. Subjects taking the placebo had no differences from baseline. Interleukin-1 beta (a marker of inflammation) decreased significantly from the baseline through weeks 18 and 22 in patients consuming fish oil. The authors concluded: "Some patients who take fish oil are able to discontinue NSAIDs without experiencing a disease flare" (22).

- In a double-blind, placebo-controlled study, 50 subjects with rheumatoid arthritis whose background diets were naturally low in n-6 fatty acids (< 10 g/day) were randomized to receive fish oil supplements (40 mg/kg) or placebo daily for 15 weeks. Clinical evaluations—consisting of tender joint count, swollen joint count, duration of early morning stiffness, visual analog scale of pain, patient and physician global assessment of arthritis activity, and Health Assessment Questionnaire, erythrocyte sedimentation rate(ESR), C-reactive protein (CRP)—were assessed at baseline and at weeks 4, 8, and 15. Twenty-four hour food recalls at each clinical assessment were used to monitor subjects background diet of < 10 g n-6 fatty acids per day. Plasma and monocyte EPA levels rose significantly in the fish oil treated subjects. There were no differences between groups at week 4 or 8. By week 12, subjects receiving supplements achieved a significant change from baseline in all clinical variables except total joint count, ESR, CRP. The control group had no significant changes from the baseline (23).

Fish Oil and Inflammatory Bowel Disease

- In a double-blind, placebo-controlled trial, 78 patients with Crohn's disease in remission who had a high risk of relapse were randomized to receive nine fish-oil capsules (2.7 g n-3 fatty acids) or nine placebo capsules daily for one year. A special coating protected the capsules against gastric acidity for at least 30 minutes. Patients in the fish oil group had significantly fewer relapses than patients receiving the placebo (28 percent vs 69 percent). Fifty-nine percent of the subjects treated with fish oil remained in remission compared to 26 percent of the subjects in the placebo group; this difference was statistically significant. Logistic-regression analysis revealed that fish oil, but not gender, age, previous surgery, duration of disease, or smoking status affected the incidence of relapse (24).

- In a double-blind, placebo-controlled trial, 87 patients with ulcerative colitis were randomized to receive 20 ml EPA concentrated fish oil (4.5 g EPA) or a placebo (olive oil) daily for one year in addition to standard drug therapy. Fish oil use resulted in a significant increase in EPA content of rectal mucosa (at six months) and increased synthesis of leukotriene B_5, and suppression of leukotriene B_4 synthesis by ionophore-stimulated neutrophils (at two months). For patients entering the trial in relapse (n = 53), there was a significant reduction in corticosteroid requirements after one and two months of fish oil supplementation. There was an insignificant trend toward achieving remission (off the use of steroids) faster with fish oil. For patients in remission (n = 69) at entry or during the trial, there were no significant differences in rate of relapse. The authors concluded: "Fish oil supplementation produces a modest corticosteroid-sparing effect in active disease, but there is no benefit in maintenance therapy" (25).

- In a double-blind, placebo-controlled, crossover trial, 18 patients with ulcerative colitis received 18 fish oil capsules (3.24 g EPA, 2.16 g DHA) or an isocaloric placebo daily each in random order for four months, with a one-month washout period. Monthly assessments of clinical symptoms, sigmoidocoscopies and biopsies, and rectal dialysates for leukotriene B_4 were measured at the baseline and at the end of each treatment. Fish oil supplementation resulted in a statistically significant increase in weight gain, improved histology, and a decline in rectal dialysate leukotriene B_4 levels. In contrast, there were no differences from baseline during placebo administration. The mean Prednisone dose decreased during fish oil ingestion, but this change did not reach statistical significance (26).

- In a double-blind, placebo-controlled, crossover study, 11 patients with ulcerative colitis received fish oil capsules (2.7 g EPA, 1.8 g DHA) or a placebo daily in random order for three months each, with a two-month washout period. Patients were assessed monthly on a disease activity index measuring frequency of bowel movements, bleeding, sigmoidoscopic appearance, and a physician assessment. Rectal and colonic mucosal biopsies were taken. Colonic mucosal levels of leukotriene B_4 were also measured. Compared to the baseline, there was a significant decrease in the disease activity index with intake of fish oil. There were no changes in frequency of diarrhea, colonic mucosal leukotriene B_4 levels, or histopathologic scores between treatments (27).

Fish Oil and Psoriasis

- In a double-blind, placebo-controlled study, 38 patients with psoriatic arthritis were randomized to receive a combination of fish oil and evening primrose oil (total of 12 capsules/day) or a placebo for nine months. All patients received placebo capsules for a further three months. At month 3, patients were asked to reduce their NSAID intake and maintain this level if tolerable. Clinical assessments were performed at baseline and every three months thereafter. All measures of skin and joint disease activity including severity, percentage of body affected, and itch were not changed by fish and evening primrose oil supplementation. There was also no difference in NSAID requirements between groups or arthritis activity as measured by morning stiffness, Ritchie articular index, and number of active joints. However, in the subjects who had been taking fish oil/primrose oil, a significant rise in thromboxane B_2 was observed during the three months of placebo treatment. In addition, a significant fall in leukotriene B_4 production occurred during fish oil/evening primrose treatment followed by a rise during the three months of placebo treatment, which the authors noted as suggestive of an anti-inflammatory effect. They concluded that fish oil/evening primrose oil supplements may alter prostaglandin metabolism in patients with psoriatic arthritis, although it did not produce a clinical improvement and did not allow reduction in NSAID requirement (28). This study design does not address whether the effects on prostaglandin metabolism resulted from fish oil, evening primrose oil, or a combination of both.

- In a double-blind, placebo-controlled, multicenter study, 145 patients having moderate to severe psoriasis were randomized to receive 6 g highly purified fish oil (5 g EPA and DHA) or an isocaloric placebo (corn oil) for four months. All patients were advised to reduce their saturated fat intake. In the fish oil group, there was a statistically significant increase in n-3 fatty acids in serum phospholipids and statistically significant decreases in the ratio of arachidonic acid to EPA, the level of n-6 fatty acids, and serum triglyceride levels. In the corn oil-supplemented group, only DHA in serum phospholipids increased significantly. The score on the Psoriasis Area and Severity Index, as evaluated by the physicians, did not change in either group. The subjective score also did not change, but a selected area of skin in the corn oil group showed a significant reduction in clinical signs. There were no notable differences in clinical manifestations between groups. In the fish oil group, an increase in the concentration of n-3 fatty acids in serum phospholipids was not accompanied by clinical improvement, whereas in the corn oil group there was a statistically significant correlation between clinical improvement and an increase in EPA and total n-3 fatty acids. The authors concluded: "Dietary supplementation with very-long-chain n-3 fatty acids was no better than corn oil supplementation in treating psoriasis" (29).

- A review article cited research suggesting that fish oil (1.5 g/day) may minimize the increase in triglycerides associated with retinoid therapy for psoriasis (30).

Fish Oil and Mental Illness

- Individuals experiencing major depression appear to have significantly lower levels of n-3 fatty acids (specifically DHA) in erythrocyte phospholipids compared to healthy controls. However, whether low levels of n-3 causes depression is unclear (31–33).

- Review articles note that there is some evidence that n-3 fatty acids may be beneficial in patients with bipolar disorder and in patients with schizophrenia, but that more controlled studies are needed (31–33).

Fish Oil and Nephropathy

- In a placebo-controlled, multicenter trial, 106 patients with IgA nephropathy with persistent proteinuria were randomized to receive 12 g fish oil (3.6 g n-3 fatty acids) or a placebo (olive oil) daily for two years. Serum creatinine concentrations (elevated in 68 percent of the patients at baseline) and creatinine clearance were measured during the study. The primary endpoint was an increase of 50 percent or more in the serum creatinine concentration at the end of the study. Three patients in the fish oil group and 14 patients in the placebo group had serum creatinine increases = 50 percent; this difference was significant. After four years, there was a significantly greater percentage of patients who died or had end-stage renal disease in the placebo group (40 percent) than in the fish oil group (10 percent) (34).

SAFETY

- The safety of n-3 fatty acids from Menhaden oil was reviewed by the U.S. Food and Drug Administration (FDA) in 1997. After evaluating more than 2,600 articles, the FDA concluded that dietary intakes of up to 3 g of EPA and DHA from Menhaden oil/day were "Generally Recognized as Safe" (GRAS). This conclusion was reached after addressing three major concerns: (1) the rise in LDL cholesterol in hypertriglyceridemic patients (2) prolonged bleeding times, and (3) worsening glycemic control in patients with type 2 diabetes. The FDA determined that none of these effects presented any danger to consumers when fish oil was consumed in amounts less than 3 g of EPA and DHA daily (35).

- Because some fish oils (halibut and shark liver oils) contain high levels of vitamin A, pregnant women should avoid fish oil supplements high in vitamin A because of that vitamin's teratogenic effects (36, 37). However, most commercial fish oil products do not contain vitamin A.

- Fish oils, specifically EPA, prolong bleeding time and decrease thromboxane A_2 production (1). It has been suggested that patients undergoing surgery avoid fish oil supplements (38). However, no clinically significant bleeding was observed in coronary artery bypass patients given 4.3 g n-3 fatty acids for 28 days before surgery (39). In addition, patients taking anticoagulant medication or with clotting disorders should be monitored while using fish oil. Individuals taking other dietary supplements that may prolong bleeding time (garlic, *Gingko biloba*, vitamin E) should also be cautioned about a possible synergistic effect, although direct evidence that such effects occur is not available.

- Some have expressed concern that fish oil is highly susceptible to lipid peroxidation, even more so than vegetable oils. One study reported that the addition of vitamin E protected against lipid peroxidation (40), whereas another study supplementing 900 IU vitamin E did not suppress oxidation (41).

- In a long-term, open, prospective study, consumption of 10 mL to 20 mL refined fish oil providing 1.8 g to 3.6 g EPA/day for seven years was not associated with any serious adverse affects in 295 subjects aged 18 y to 76 y (42).

- Some individuals may experience fishy-smelling belches with fish oil supplements.

REFERENCES

1. Uauy-Dagach R, Valenzuela A. Marine oils: the health benefits of n-3 fatty acids. *Nutr Rev.* 1996;54(11 pt 2):S102–S108.
2. Jones PJ, Kubow S. Lipids, Sterols, and Their Metabolites. In: Shils ME, Olson JA, Shike

F

M, Ross AC, eds. *Modern Nutrition in Health and Disease.* 9th ed. Baltimore, Md: Williams & Wilkins; 1999:67–94.

3. Simopoulos AP. Omega-3 fatty acids in health and disease and growth and development. *Am J Clin Nutr.* 1991;54:438–463.

4. Hansen JB, Grimsgaard S, Nilsen H, et al. Effects of highly purified eicosapentaenoic acid and docosahexaenoic acid on fatty acid absorption, incorporation into serum phospholipids and postprandial triglyceridemia. *Lipids.* 1998;33:131–138.

5. Scientific Review Committee. *Nutrition Recommendations.* Ottawa: Minister of National Health and Welfare, Canada; 1990.

6. Harris WS, Ginsberg HN, Arunakul N, et al. Safety and efficacy of Omacor in severe hypertriglyceridemia. *J Cardiovasc Risk.* 1997;4:385–392.

7. Harris WS. N-3 fatty acids and serum lipoproteins: human studies. *Am J Clin Nutr.* 1997;65:1645S–1654S.

8. Kris-Etherton PM, Etherton TD, Yu S. Efficacy of multiple dietary therapies in reducing cardiovascular disease risk factors. *Am J Clin Nutr.* 1997;65:560–561.

9. Friedberg CE, Janssen MJ, Heine RJ, et al. Fish oil and glycemic control in diabetes. A meta-analysis. *Diabetes Care.* 1998;21:494–500.

10. Adler AJ, Holub BJ. Effect of garlic and fish-oil supplementation on serum lipid and lipoprotein concentrations in hypercholesterolemic men. *Am J Clin Nutr.* 1997;65:445–450.

11. Morcos NC. Modulation of lipid profile by fish oil and garlic combination. *J Natl Med Assoc.* 1997;89:673–678.

12. Morris MC, Sacks F, Rosner B. Does fish oil lower blood pressure? A meta-analysis of controlled trials. *Circulation.* 1993;88:523–533.

13. Sacks FM, Hebert P, Appel LJ, et al. The effect of fish oil on blood pressure and high density lipoprotein-cholesterol levels in phase I of the Trials of Hypertension Prevention. Trials of Hypertension Prevention Collaborative Research Group. *J Hypertens Suppl.* 1994;12:S23–S31.

14. Gapinski JP, VanRuiswyk JV, Heudebert GR, et al. Preventing restenosis with fish oils following coronary angioplasty. A meta-analysis. *Arch Intern Med.* 1993;153:1595–1601.

15. Sacks FM, Stone PH, Gibson CM, et al. Controlled trial of fish oil for regression of human coronary atherosclerosis. HARP Research Group. *J Am Coll Cardiol.* 1995;25:1492–1498.

16. Eritsland J, Arnesen H, Gronseth K, et al. Effect of dietary supplementation with n-3 fatty acids on coronary artery bypass graft patency. *Am J Cardiol.* 1996;77:31–36.

17. Gruppo Italiano per lo Studio della Sopravvivenza nell'Infarto Miocardico. Dietary supplementation with n-3 polyunsaturated fatty acids and vitamin E after myocardial infarction: results of the GISSI-Preventzione trial. *Lancet.* 1999;354:447–455.

18. Singh RB, Niaz MA, Sharma JP, et al. Randomized, double-blind, placebo-controlled trial of fish oil and mustard oil in patients with suspected acute myocardial infarction: the Indian experiment of infarct survival–4. *Cardiovasc Drugs Ther.* 1997;11:485–491.

19. Siscovick DS, Raghunathan TE, King I, et al. Dietary intake and cell membrane levels of long-chain n-3 polyunsaturated fatty acids and the risk of primary cardiac arrest. *JAMA.* 1995;274:1363–1367.

20. Leaf A, Kang JX. Prevention of cardiac sudden death by n-3 fatty acids: a review of the evidence. *J Intern Med*. 1996;240:5–12.

21. Fortin PR, Lew RA, Liang MH, et al. Validation of a meta-analysis: the effects of fish oil in rheumatoid arthritis. *J Clin Epidemiol*. 1995;48:1379–1390.

22. Kremer JM, Lawrence DA, Petrillo GF, et al. Effects of high-dose fish oil on rheumatoid arthritis after stopping nonsteroidal antiinflammatory drugs. Clinical and immune correlates. *Arthritis Rheum*. 1995;38:1107–1114.

23. Volker D, Fitzgerald P, Major G, et al. Efficacy of fish oil concentrate in the treatment of rheumatoid arthritis. *J Rheumatol*. 2000;27:2305–2307.

24. Belluzzi A, Brignola C, Campieri M, et al. Effect of an enteric-coated fish-oil preparation on relapse in Crohn's disease. *N Engl J Med*. 1996;334:1557–1560.

25. Hawthorne AB, Daneshmend TK, Hawkey CJ, et al. Treatment of ulcerative colitis with fish oil supplementation: a prospective 12 month randomized controlled trial. *Gut*. 1992;33:922–928.

26. Stenson WF, Cort D, Rodgers J, et al. Dietary supplementation with fish oil in ulcerative colitis. *Ann Intern Med*. 1992;116:609–614.

27. Aslan A, Triadafilopoulos G. Fish oil fatty acid supplementation in active ulcerative colitis: a double-blind, placebo-controlled, crossover study. *Am J Gastroenterol*. 1992;87:432–437.

28. Veale DJ, Torley HI, Richards IM, et al. A double-blind placebo controlled trial of Efamol Marine on skin and joint symptoms of psoriatic arthritis. *Br J Rheumatol*. 1994;33:954–958.

29. Soyland E, Funk J, Rajka G, et al. Effect of dietary supplementation with very-long-chain n-3 fatty acids in patients with psoriasis. *N Engl J Med*. 1993;328:1812–1816.

30. Frati C, Bevilacqua L, Apostolico V. Association of etretinate and fish oil in psoriasis therapy. Inhibition of hypertriglyceridemia resulting from retinoid therapy after fish oil supplementation. *Acta Derm Venereol Suppl (Stockh)*. 1994;186:151–153.

31. Mischoulon D, Fava M. Docosahexanoic acid and omega-3 fatty acids in depression. *Psychiatr Clin North Am*. 2000;23:785–794.

32. Maidment ID. Are fish oils effective therapy in mental illness—an analysis of the data. *Acta Psychiatr Scand*. 2000; 102:3–11.

33. Freeman MP. Omega-3 fatty acids in psychiatry: a review. *Ann Clin Psychiatry*. 2000;12:159–165.

34. Donadio JV, Bergstralh EJ, Offord KP, et al. A controlled trial of fish oil in IgA nephropathy. Mayo Nephrology Collaborative Group. *N Engl J Med*. 1994;331:1194–1199.

35. FDA Final Rule. Substances Affirmed as Generally Recognized as Safe: Menhaden Oil. *Fed Regist*. 1997;62:30,751–757.

36. Anonymous. Increasing fish oil intake—any net benefits? *Drug Ther Bull*. 1996;34:60–62.

37. Rothman KJ, Moore LL, Singer MR, et al. Teratogenicity of high vitamin A intake. *N Engl J Med*. 1995;333:1369–1373.

38. Petry JJ. Surgically significant nutritional supplements. *Plast Reconstr Surg*. 1996;97:233–240.

39. DeCaterina R, Gianessi D, Mazzone A, et al. Vascular prostacyclin is increased in patients

F

ingesting omega-3 polyunsaturated fatty acids before coronary artery bypass graft surgery. *Circulation.* 1990;82:428–438.

40. Harris WS. Fish oils and plasma lipid and lipoprotein metabolism in humans: a critical review. *J Lipid Res.* 1989;30:785–807.

41. Allard JP, Kurian R, Aghdassi E, et al. Lipid peroxidation during n-3 fatty acid and vitamin E supplementation in humans. *Lipids.* 1997;32:535–541.

42. Saynor R, Gillott T. Changes in blood lipids and fibrinogen with a note on safety in a long term study on the effects of n-3 fatty acids in subjects receiving fish oil supplements and followed for seven years. *Lipids.* 1992;27:533–538.

Flaxseed

Cultivated for more than 5,000 years, flaxseed originated in Central Asia and is now found throughout North America, Asia, and Europe. Flaxseed is 35 percent fat, 28 percent to 30 percent protein, 35 percent fiber, and 6 percent ash. The theory behind supplementing the diet with flaxseed products is because of compounds found in the seed: omega-3 fatty acids and lignans.

α-Linolenic Acid (Omega-3)

It has been suggested that humans evolved on diets providing a linoleic (n-6) to linolenic (n-3) fatty acid ratio of 1:1 to 2:1. However, because of changes in the food supply and production, the typical U.S. diet currently provides a much higher ratio of 10:1 to 30:1 (1). The essential fatty acid ratio is important because it affects the type of prostaglandins formed in the body. More than half of the fat content of flaxseed is α-linolenic acid as opposed to some other oils that compose only 1 percent to 11 percent of the total (2). Biochemically, some of the α-linolenic acid from flaxseed can be converted into eicosapentaenoic acid (EPA), and to a lesser extent, docosahexaenoic acid (DHA) (3, 4). Diets rich in linoleic acid (n-6) or high in saturated fats reduce the conversion of α-linolenic acid to its long chain metabolites. Because increased cellular levels of EPA and DHA are precursors to anti-inflammatory and antiatherogenic prostaglandins, flaxseed has been studied for its potential preventive role in heart disease and inflammatory disorders.

Lignans

Flaxseed contains 100 to 800 times more plant lignans (a type of phystoestrogen) than do other major seeds (2).Lignans are digested by colonic bacteria to mammalian lignans, enterolactone, and enterodiol, which enter hepatic circulation (5). These lignans are thought to be protective against cancer because of their antimitotic, antioxidant, antitumor, and antiestrogenic properties (6). Mammalian lignans are hypothesized to bind to estrogen receptors to prevent the cancer promoting effects of estrogen. Additionally, lignans may regulate sex-hormone-binding globulin, a protein that binds estrogen, lowering its bioavailability.

Media and Marketing Claims	Efficacy
Reduces cholesterol	↔
Reduces risk of stroke and heart attack	NR
May help prevent cancer	NR
Alleviates arthritis pain	NR
Improves symptoms of lupus, multiple sclerosis, eczema, and psoriasis	NR

Advisory

- Doses > 45 g of flaxseed have a laxative effect
- Flaxseed oil not to be used in high-temperature cooking because of its low smoke point

Drug/Supplement Interactions

- The fiber content of ground flaxseed can interfere with the absorption of other nutrients and some medications that are affected by fiber intake (Digoxin, Lovastatine, and Metformin)
- Theoretically, flaxseed may increase bleeding when taken with other blood-thinning drugs or supplements (ie, coumadin, warfarin, garlic, ginger, ginkgo biloba, vitamin E, flaxseed, bromelain, dong quai, fish oil, aspirin); should be monitored by a physician.

KEY POINTS

- At this time, there is insufficient research to support the claim that flaxseed reduces the risk of stroke and heart attack. Flaxseed raises cellular EPA levels under certain conditions but has not consistently lowered cholesterol and triglycerides. Alternatively, it may have antiatherogenic benefits by inhibiting platelet aggregation. Larger controlled human trials are needed to delineate the effects of flaxseed supplementation in cardiovascular disease.

- There is some evidence from experimental studies in animals that flaxseed inhibits tumor growth, specifically mammary tumors. Flaxseed supplementation appears to increase urinary excretion of estrogen metabolites associated with a reduced breast cancer risk in postmenopausal women. Long-term trials are needed to determine whether flaxseed can prevent or slow the progression of cancer in humans.

- Although flaxseed has been shown to inhibit mediators of inflammation, clinical trials are needed to determine the effects of flaxseed on rheumatoid arthritis and other inflammatory disorders such as psoriasis, multiple sclerosis, and lupus.

- Although the efficacy of flaxseed for certain disorders has not been confirmed, consumption of flaxseed products can increase the fiber (ground flaxseed) and omega-3 fatty acid (ground flaxseed and/or oil) content of the diet.

- Several researchers have suggested that the low ratio of n-3 to n-6 fatty acids in the average American diet creates an imbalance that is linked to several conditions, including coronary heart disease, hypertension, and inflammatory disorders. Consuming flaxseed products is one way to increase the omega-3 content of the diet. Other n-3 food sources include walnuts, soybean and canola oil (not partially hydrogenated), fatty fish (salmon, swordfish, mackerel, herring), and eggs from hens fed special diets rich in flaxseed.

- Individuals supplementing with flaxseed oil while following a weight-controlled diet should allow for approximately 140 calories and 14 g fat found in 1 tablespoon of oil.

FOOD SOURCES

Whole flaxseed, flaxseed oil, margarine made from flaxseed oil, cereals, and breads made with ground flaxseed flour

DOSAGE INFORMATION/BIOAVAILABILITY

Flaxseed is available in liquid, capsule, or powder form. Flaxseed oil and powder supplements are unstable and must be refrigerated in airtight, opaque containers and consumed before the expiration date. The oil should not be used in high-temperature cooking because it is easily oxidized. Manufacturers suggest one tablespoon of oil daily, which provides approximately 7 grams of α-linolenic acid and 2 grams linoleic acid. In the U.S., there are no specific recommendations on for the intake of omega-3 fatty acids. Canadian dietary guidelines recommend a daily intake of 1.0 g to 1.5 g of omega-3 fatty acids and 7 g to 9 g of omega-6 FAs for 25 to 74 year olds.

A study testing the bioavailability of 50 g flaxseed flour and 20 g flaxseed oil in healthy subjects found plasma n-3 fatty acids were raised only after two and four weeks of supplementation, respectively (7). Furthermore, it has been reported that a diet rich in linoleic acid may negatively affect the conversion of α-linolenic acid in flaxseed to EPA (8). In one study, EPA levels were maximized by reducing intake of n-6 from vegetable oils and increasing intake of n-3 rich flaxseed oil (8). Consumption of raw ground flaxseed (5 g to 25 g) for seven days raised urinary lignan (enterolactone and enterodiol) levels in a dose-dependent manner in healthy, young women. There were no differences in total urinary lignan excretion with the raw compared to the processed forms of flaxseed at an intake of 25 g (9). To increase the availability of lignans to the gut microflora, flaxseed should be consumed freshly ground (not whole). Note: the lignans are only found in the fiber portion of the plant, not the oil.

RELEVANT RESEARCH

Flaxseed and Cardiovascular Disease

- There is evidence from animal studies that flaxseed reduces the development of atherosclerosis but does not affect serum cholesterol levels (10).
- In a double-blind, comparative, crossover study, 29 hyperlipidemic subjects received in random order muffins that contributed approximately 20 g fiber/day from either flaxseed (50 g partially defatted flaxseed/day) or wheat bran (control) for three weeks each while they consumed self-selected National Cholesterol Education Program Step

II diets. Treatment phases were separated by a two-week washout period. Partially defatted flaxseed significantly reduced total cholesterol by 4.6 percent, LDL cholesterol by 7.6 percent, apolipoprotein B by 5.4 percent, and apolipoprotein A-I by 5.8 percent, but it had no effect on serum lipoprotein ratios at week 3 compared to the control. There were no significant effects after either treatment on serum HDL cholesterol, serum protein carbonyl content, or *ex vivo* androgen or progestin activity. Defatted flaxseed significantly reduced serum protein thiol groups compared to control. The authors suggested that the decrease in protein thiol groups is a possible indicator of increased oxidative activity. They concluded that further studies are needed to determine whether this potential pro-oxidant effect has any physiological significance (11).

- In a double-blind, comparative study, 32 healthy subjects were initially supplemented with 35 mg olive oil (run-in period) and then randomly assigned to receive 35 mg flaxseed oil or 35 mg fish oil from capsules for three months each. According to the authors, these low doses were chosen to reflect amounts of omega-3 fatty acids easily attainable in the diet by certain food selections. Although flaxseed supplementation raised the linolenic content (but not EPA levels) of all lipoproteins, it had no effect on plasma triglycerides, total, or LDL or HDL cholesterol levels. The authors concluded that flaxseed intake in this study may not have been great enough to produce sufficient EPA or the conversion of linolenic acid to EPA was limited (12).

- In a double-blind, placebo-controlled, crossover study, 11 patients with well-controlled type 2 diabetes were supplemented with flaxseed oil or fish oil capsules (35 mg FA/kg body weight) for three months each in random order, after an initial three months of placebo (olive oil). Subjects continued their routine medications and diabetic meal plans and were counseled to maintain isocaloric diets during the study. Fasting blood samples were taken after each three-month period. There were no significant differences in body weight, glycemic control, cholesterol values (total, LDL, and HDL), or insulin sensitivity with either type of oil. Fish oil was associated with a significant decrease in triglycerides (13).

- Eleven healthy male subjects were randomly assigned to consume 40 g flaxseed oil or sunflower oil for 23 days. Subjects were instructed to follow a low-fat, low-polyunsaturated-fat diet. The percent of energy from fat increased from 23 percent (run-in diet) to 33 percent for the flaxseed oil group and from 27 percent to 40 percent in the sunflower oil group. Polyunsaturated fatty acid intake did not differ between groups. EPA in platelet lipids more than doubled in the flaxseed group, but was not affected in the sunflower group. A significant decrease in platelet aggregation response to collagen was seen in flaxseed oil-supplemented subjects, but not in sunflower oil-supplemented subjects. The authors noted that the higher fat percentage of energy in the sunflower group could have skewed the overall results. Despite this limitation, the authors concluded that consumption of α-linolenic acid-rich oils may offer protective effects against cardiovascular disease over linoleic acid-rich oils via their ability to decrease the tendency of platelets to aggregate (14).

- Nine lupus nephritis patients were given 15 g, 30 g, and 45 g of flaxseed powder/day sequentially for four weeks at a time, followed by a final five-week period of no treatment. This study was not blinded or randomized. One subject dropped out of the study for reasons unrelated to treatment. Compared to the baseline, there was a significant reduction of total cholesterol of 11 percent and LDL cholesterol of 12 percent as well as blood viscosity with the 30 g dose. This effect was sustained over the four weeks of the 45-g dose (9 percent for total and 10 percent for LDL cholesterol) and during the final five weeks of no treatment (7 percent for total and 11 percent for LDL). *In vitro* platelet aggregation was inhibited by all doses. There was no effect on blood pressure, scores on Systemic Lupus Erythematous Disease Activity Index, or immune parameters. Subjects experienced significant decreases in proteinuria and serum creatine, and improved creatine clearance. Three of the subjects experienced difficulty after ingesting 45 g flaxseed powder due to increased laxation. These results should be viewed with caution because of the small number of subjects and lack of randomization and blinding (15).

Flaxseed and Cancer

- Several animal studies have shown flaxseed inhibits tumor growth in experimentally induced mammary cancer (16–18). and melanoma (19).

- In a randomized, crossover design trial, 28 postmenopausal women were studied for three seven-week feeding periods. Subjects ate their usual diets plus ground flaxseed (0 g, 5 g, or 10 g/day). Urinary excretion of estrogen metabolites 2-hydroxyestrogen and 16 alpha-hydroxyetrone, as well as their ratio (2:16alpha-OHE1 ratio) were measured (biomarkers for breast cancer risk). Flaxseed supplementation significantly increased urinary 2-hydroxyestrogen and the 2:16alpha-OHE1 ratio in a dose-response way. Women with elevated ratios of these metabolites are believed to have a decreased risk of breast cancer, and the authors hypothesized that flaxseed may have chemoprotective effects (20). A similar study by the same researchers compared flaxseed to wheat bran use, and found that flaxseed significantly increased the 2:16alpha-OHE1 ratio, but that wheat bran had no effect (21).

- In a cross-sectional study of 121 French breast cancer patients, low breast tissue levels of α-linolenic acid were associated with a significant increased risk of metastases but not tumor size or mitotic index. The authors hypothesized that flaxseed supplementation in breast cancer patients to replenish n-3 fatty acids in adipose stores might delay or even prevent the appearance of tumors (22).

- Several animal studies indicate flaxseed supplementation inhibits chemically induced colon cancer, which has been attributed to the lignan portion of the plant (23, 24). Researchers acknowledge it is difficult to distinguish whether the potential benefits are due to the fiber or the lignans in flaxseed.

Flaxseed and Inflammatory Disorders

- In a parallel group study, 30 healthy male subjects were instructed to consume a diet low in n-6 fatty acids by using flaxseed oil in food preparation or a diet high in n-6 fatty acids by using sunflower oil (control) for two months. At one month, all subjects took fish oil capsules (9 g/day). Subject's diet diaries indicated that dietary α-linolenic acid was 13.7 (± 5.5) g/day in the flaxseed group and 1.1 (± 0.5) g/day in the sunflower group. The total fat intake was not different between the two groups and had a mean of 29.4 percent of total energy intake. There were no significant differences in BMI during the course of the study. Unlike sunflower oil, flaxseed oil increased cellular EPA concentrations, which were further raised following fish oil intake. Proinflammatory markers (tumor necrosis factor alpha (TNF-α) and interleukin 1β (IL-1β) were significantly decreased by 30 percent in the flaxseed group compared to the sunflower group. These markers are hypothesized to aggravate the pathology occurring in rheumatoid arthritis and atherosclerosis (25).

- In a double-blind, placebo-controlled study, 22 patients with rheumatoid arthritis were randomized to receive 30 g flaxseed powder or 30 g sunflower oil powder (prepared identical in taste and appearance) for three months. Patients were instructed not to change their dietary habits or antirheumatic medication during the study. At the study end, the flaxseed group showed an increased bleeding time but no effect on the clinical, subjective (global assessment, classification of functional status, joint score index, visual analogue scale, pain tenderness score) and laboratory parameters. Despite serum increases in α-linolenic acid, there was no change in AA, EPA, or DHA concentrations. The authors suggested that the low conversion of α-linolenic acid to EPA and DHA, together with a low α-linolenic acid:linoleic acid body ratio, may explain the lack of clinical benefit (26).

SAFETY

- Flaxseed contains cyanogenic glycosides, a naturally occurring toxicant found in foods such as almonds, peaches, apricots, cherries, and plums. Baking was found to eliminate these compounds from muffins made with flaxmeal. A letter to the editor of *Lancet* questioned the safety of cyanogenic glycosides from high doses (> 60 g) of ground flaxseed, which could theoretically increase blood thiocyanate levels (27).

- Doses above 45 g flaxseed powder are associated with laxative effects (16, 28).

- The fiber from high doses of flaxseed, as with any plant food, can interfere with the absorption of other nutrients and some medications, such as Digoxin, Lovastatine, and Metformin. Because of the high fiber content, adequate fluid intake is necessary when consuming flaxseed supplements. German Commission E lists ileus of any origin as a contraindication for flaxseed (29).

- Because n-3 fatty acids favor production of the prostaglandins that increase bleeding time, it may be advisable for individuals undergoing surgery or patients with clotting disorders to avoid consuming flaxseed.

- To avoid consuming rancid oil, flaxseed oil cannot be used in high-temperature cooking or beyond the expiration date on the label. It can be added to hot foods after cooking (ie, soups, casseroles). In addition, freshly ground flaxseed or flaxseed powders should also be refrigerated to prevent oxidation of fatty acids (2).

REFERENCES

1. Simopoulos AP. Essential fatty acids in health and chronic disease. *Am J Clin Nutr.* 1999;70:560S–569S.
2. Carter JF. Potential of flaxseed and flaxseed oil in baked goods and other products in human nutrition. *Cereal Foods World.* 1993;10:753–759.
3. Mantzioris E, James MJ, Gibson RA, et al. Differences exist in the relationships between dietary linoleic and alpha-linolenic acids and their respective long-chain metabolites. *Am J Clin Nutr.* 1995;61:320–324.
4. Gerster H. Can adults adequately convert alpha-linolenic acid (18:3n-3) to eicosapentaenoic acid (20:5n-3) and docosahexaenoic acid (22:6n-3)? *Int J Vitam Nutr Res.* 1998;68:159–173.
5. Lampe JW, Martini MC, Kurzer MS, et al. Urinary lignan and isoflavonoid excretion in premenopausal women consuming flaxseed powder. *Am J Clin Nutr.* 1994;60:122–128.
6. Serraino M, Thompson LU. The effect of flaxseed supplementation on early risk markers for mammary carcinogenesis. *Cancer Lett.* 1991;60:135–142.
7. Cunnane SC, Ganguli S, Menard C, et al. High α-linolenic acid flaxseed (*Linum usitatissimum*): some nutritional properties in humans. *Br J Nutr.* 1993;69:443–453.
8. Mantzioris E, James MJ, Gibson RA, et al. Dietary substitution with alpha-linolenic acid-rich vegetable oil increases eicosapentaenoic acid concentrations in tissues. *Am J Clin Nutr.* 1994;59:1304–1309.
9. Nesbitt PD, Lam Y, Thompson LU. Human metabolism of mammalian lignan precursors in raw and processed flaxseed. *Am J Clin Nutr.* 1999;69:549–555.
10. Prasad K. Dietary flax seed in prevention of hypercholesterolemic atherosclerosis. *Atherosclerosis.* 1997;132:69–76.
11. Jenkins DJ, Kendall CW, Vidgen E, et al. Health aspects of partially defatted flaxseed, including effects on serum lipids, oxidative measures, ex vivo androgen, and progestin activity: a controlled crossover trial. *Am J Clin Nutr.* 1999;69:395–402.
12. Layne KS, Goh YK, Jumpsen JA, et al. Normal subjects consuming physiological levels of 18:3 (n-3) and 20:5 (n-3) from flaxseed or fish oils have characteristic differences in plasma lipid and lipoprotein fatty acid levels. *J Nutr.* 1996;126:2130–2140.
13. McManus RM, Jumpson J, Finegood DT. A comparison of the effects of n-3 fatty acids from linseed oil and fish oil in well-controlled type II diabetes. *Diabetes Care.* 1996;19:463–467.
14. Allman MA, Pena MM, Pang D. Supplementation with flaxseed oil versus sunflower seed oil in healthy young men consuming a low-fat diet: effects on platelet composition and function. *Eur J Clin Nutr.* 1995;49:169–178.
15. Clark WF, Parbtani A, Huff MW, et al. Flaxseed: a potential treatment for lupus nephritis. *Kidney Int.* 1995;48(2):475–480.
16. Serraino M, Thompson LU. The effect of flaxseed supplementation on the initiation and promotional stages of mammary tumorigenesis. *Nutr Cancer.* 1992;17:153–159.
17. Thompson LU, Rickard SE, Orcheson LJ, et al. Flaxseed and its lignan and oil components reduce mammary tumor growth at a late stage of carcinogenesis. *Carcinogenesis.* 1996;17(6):1373–1376.

18. Thompson LU, Seidl MM, Rickard SE, et al. Antitumorigenic effect of a mammalian lignan precursor from flaxseed. *Nutr Cancer.* 1996;26:159–165.
19. Yan L, Yee JA, Li D, et al. Dietary flaxseed supplementation and experimental metastasis of melanoma cells in mice. *Cancer Lett.* 1998;124:181–186.
20. Haggans CJ, Hutchins AM, Olson BA, et al. Effect of flaxseed consumption on urinary estrogen metabolites in postmenopausal women. *Nutr Cancer.* 1999;33:188–195.
21. Haggans CJ, Travelli EJ, Thomas W, et al. The effect of flaxseed and wheat bran consumption on urinary estrogen metabolites in premenopausal women. *Cancer Epidemiol Biomarkers Prev.* 2000;9:719–725.
22. Bougnoux P, Koscielny S, Chajes V, et al. Alpha-linolenic acid content of adipose breast tissue: a host determinant of the risk of early metastasis in breast cancer. *Br J Cancer.* 1994;70:330–334.
23. Serraino M, Thompson LU. Flaxseed supplementation and early markers of colon carcinogenesis. *Cancer Lett.* 1992;63:159–165.
24. Jenab M, Thompson LU. The influence of flaxseed and lignans on colon carcinogenesis and beta-glucuronidase activity. *Carcinogenesis.* 1996;17:1343–1348.
25. Caughey GE, Mantzioris E, Gibson RA, et al. The effect on human tumor necrosis factor alpha and interleukin 1 beta production of diets enriched in n-3 fatty acids from vegetable oil or fish oil. *Am J Clin Nutr.* 1996;63:116–122.
26. Nordstrom DC, Honkanen VE, Nasu Y, et al. Alpha-linolenic acid in the treatment of rheumatoid arthritis. A double-blind placebo controlled and randomized study: flaxseed vs safflower seed. *Rheumatol Int.* 1995;14:231–234.
27. Rosling H. Cyanide exposure from linseed [letter]. *Lancet.* 1993;341:177.
28. Cunnane SC, Hamadeh MJ, Liede AC, et al. Nutritional attributes of traditional flaxseed in healthy young adults. *Am J Clin Nutr.* 1995;61:62–68.
29. Blumenthal M, ed. *The Complete German Commission E Monographs Therapeutic Guide to Herbal Medicines.* Austin, Tex: American Botanical Council; 1998.

Folate/Folic Acid

Folate is the general term used to refer to a group of compounds structurally similar to folic acid. Folic acid, also referred to as pteroylmonoglutamate, is formed by the linkage of pteridine and para-aminobenzoic acid (PABA) conjugated to a molecule of glutamic acid. Folic acid is the synthetic form of the vitamin. Natural food forms of folate are chemically reduced, frequently have one-carbon substitutions in the pteridine ring, and may have up to 10 additional glutamate residues linked to the proximal glutamic acid moiety. Folates function in the body as a coenzyme in reactions involving the transfer of one-carbon units. In this role, folate is involved in amino acid and purine metabolism, and in nucleic acid synthesis. About half of the total body folate is stored as polyglutamate by the liver. When it functions as a coenzyme in various reactions, it is reduced to the active form tetrahydrofolic acid (THFA) (1).

A dietary deficiency or inadequate absorption of folate impairs DNA synthesis and cell division, and results in megaloblastic anemia among other clinical symptoms. In 1996, because of significant evidence showing that folic acid intake reduces the risk of neural tube defects (NTDs), the FDA mandated that all breads, pastas, rice, and cereal products be fortified with folic acid at levels ranging from 0.43 mg to 1.4 mg per pound of food (or 95 µg/100 g to 309 µg/100 g) beginning in June 1998 (2). Folic acid is also being investigated for its potential role in cardiovascular disease, particularly its effect on reducing homocysteine levels.

Media and Marketing Claims	Efficacy
Prevents birth defects	↑
Helps prevent heart disease	↑?
Protects against colon cancer	NR
Protects against cervical cancer	↔
Wards off depression	NR

Advisory

- Usually safe below the Tolerable Upper Intake Level (UL)—1,000 µg/day for adults
- Doses > 400 µg/d may mask pernicious anemia in individuals with B_{12} deficiency

Drug/Supplement Interactions

- Doses > 5,000 µg/day interfere with anticonvulsant medications (eg, diphenyhdantoin, carbamazepine, valproic acid, phenytoin)
- Some drugs interfere with the absorption or activity of folate. including oral contraceptives, aspirin, indomethacin (NSAID), methotrexate (chemotherapeutic), famotidine/pepcid AC (antacid), and some antibiotics (tetracycline, isoniazid, cycloserine, erythromycin, sulfonamides)

KEY POINTS

- There is compelling evidence that folic acid supplements administered to women periconceptually reduce the risk of NTDs. The FDA mandates fortification of certain food products and permits these foods and dietary supplements containing folic acid to carry a health claim acknowledging this protective effect apparent for NTDs in conjunction with a varied diet. NAS recommends that all women of childbearing age consume 400 µg of folic acid from fortified foods and/or supplements in addition to eating folate-rich food from a varied diet (4).

- There is also compelling evidence that folic acid supplements reduce blood homocysteine concentrations, considered by some researchers as a risk factor for cardiovascular disease. However, it is of note that the American Heart Association currently does not recognize an elevated level of homocysteine as an independent risk factor for CVD. Large-scale, controlled trials are needed to determine more clearly whether folic acid supplements have a protective effect against cardiovascular disease and stroke.

- Although epidemiological studies show an inverse relationship of folic acid supplements to colon cancer, controlled trials are needed to provide more definitive evidence that folate confers a protective effect.

- Studies testing the efficacy of supplemental folic acid in women with cervical dysplasia are conflicting. The relationship between human papilloma virus (associated with cervical cancer risk) and folate status must also be explored. Additional research is needed before any recommendations can be made.

- Poor folate status has been reported in a few studies of patients having depression. However, controlled clinical trials are needed to determine whether supplementation improves depressive symptoms.

- A dietary assessment is recommended to assess folic acid intake, particularly for women of childbearing age. If intake does not meet the RDA, individuals should be encouraged to increase food and supplemental sources of folic acid.

FOOD SOURCES

Food	µg Folate
Spinach (raw, 1 c)	108
Orange (1)	44
Romaine lettuce (1 c)	38
Peanut butter (2 tbsp)	29
Milk, nonfat (1 c)	13
Beef, ground (3.5 oz)	9
Raisin bran cereal (1 c)	181

Note: Approximately 50 percent to 95 percent of folate is destroyed during food processing such as canning (1).
Source: Data from Pennington, JAT (3)

DOSAGE INFORMATION/BIOAVAILABILITY

The National Academy of Sciences Food and Nutrition Board raised the RDA for adults from 180 µg to 400 µg dietary folate equivalents/day in 1998 (4). The RDA during pregnancy is 600 µg dietary folate equivalents. The NAS report recommended that women of childbearing age consume 400 µg as synthetic folic acid from supplements and/or fortified foods in addition to intake of food from the diet. The Tolerable Upper Intake Level for adults is set at 1,000 µg/day of folic acid, exclusive of food folate. Folic acid supplements are available in single preparations or multivitamin/mineral supplements providing up to 400 µg per serving. Prenatal vitamins available by prescription only may contain up to 1,000 µg.

According to the Food and Nutrition Board, dietary folate equivalents (DFE) adjust for nearly 50 percent lower bioavailability of food folate compared with that of synthetic folic acid: 1 µg food folate = 0.5 µg of folic acid taken on an empty stomach = 0.6 µg folic acid with meals (4). Food folate is absorbed less efficiently because it is primarily in the polyglutamate form and requires intestinal enzymes to split off excess glutamates before absorption can occur. In contrast, folic acid (supplemental form) is in the monoglutamate form and does not require hydrolysis to be absorbed (1).

RELEVANT RESEARCH

Folate and Neural Tube Defects

- In 1996, the FDA reviewed numerous studies showing a relationship between folic acid intake and NTDs. The FDA concluded that there was substantial research to permit foods and supplements containing folic acid to carry the health claim: "Healthful diets with adequate folic acid may reduce a woman's risk of having a child with a brain or spinal cord birth defects." Prior to this, the Centers for Disease Control and Prevention issued guidelines in 1992 recommending daily consumption of a 400 µg folic acid supplement by all women of childbearing age to reduce the risk of NTDs (5).

- In 1998, the National Academy of Sciences recommended that to reduce the risk of NTDs, all women capable of becoming pregnant should consume 400 µg of synthetic folic acid daily from fortified foods and/or supplements, in addition to consuming food folate from a varied diet (4).

- A national study examining the occurrence of NTDs before and after folic acid food fortification reported a 19 percent reduction in the incidence of NTDs after fortification (37.8 cases per 100,000 live births compared to 30.5 cases per 100,000 live births) (6).

Folate and Cardiovascular Disease

- In a prospective cohort study, 80,082 women from the Nurses' Health Study with no history of cardiovascular disease (CVD), cancer, hypercholesterolemia, or diabetes were followed from 1980 to 1994. After 14 years, 658 cases of nonfatal myocardial infarction (MI) and 281 cases of fatal coronary heart disease occurred. After controlling for cardiovascular risk factors, vitamin E, saturated, polyunsaturated, and trans fat intake, the relative risk of developing CHD was 0.55 (45 percent risk reduction) among women in the highest quintile of both folate and vitamin B_6 intake compared with the lowest quintiles. The risk of CHD was lower among women who regularly used multivitamins, the primary source of folate and vitamin B_6. After excluding vitamin users, CHD risk was also reduced among subjects with higher dietary intakes of folate and vitamin B_6 (7).

- A meta-analysis of 12 randomized trials (n = 1,114 subjects) assessed the effects of folic acid supplements on blood homocysteine concentrations. Reductions in blood homocysteine produced by folic acid supplements were greater at higher pretreatment blood homocysteine concentrations and at lower pretreatment blood folate concentrations. Researchers found that dietary folic acid significantly reduced blood homocysteine by 25 percent, with similar effects in the range of 0.5 mg to 5 mg folic acid daily. The authors concluded that large-scale randomized trials of folic acid supplementation in high-risk populations are needed to determine whether lowering blood homocysteine reduces the risk of vascular disease (8).

- In a meta-analysis of 27 studies relating homocysteine to vascular disease and 11 studies of folic acid effects on homocysteine levels, researchers reported that increased folic acid intake (approximately 200 µg/day) reduced homocysteine levels and that elevated homocysteine levels were considered an independent graded risk factor for arteriosclerotic vascular disease. The authors estimated that 13,500 to 50,000 deaths could be avoided annually by increasing dietary and supplemental folate (9).

- In a retrospective cohort study, 5,056 subjects with no history of coronary heart disease (CHD) had their serum folate levels measured between 1970 and 1972, and were assessed retrospectively through 1985. A total of 165 CHD deaths occurred after 15 years. There was a significant association between low serum folate levels and risk of fatal CHD, but no association between dietary folate (estimated by 24-hour food recall) and fatal CHD. Folic acid from supplements was not measured. The authors noted the limitations of using a food recall questionnaire to classify subjects because of within-individual variation in diet (10).

- In a double-blind, placebo-controlled, crossover trial, 18 healthy subjects with elevated homocysteine levels (> 13 αmol/L at entry) received in random order 5 mg folic acid daily and a placebo daily for six weeks each, with a six-week washout period in the middle. Endothelial function was assessed by comparing endothelium-dependent vasodilatation in response to flow (induced by release of a wrist cuff following a period of hand ischemia) with endothelial-independent response to sublingual glyceryl trinitrate (GTN). Folic acid significantly lowered plasma homocysteine by 28 percent compared to the placebo. Folic acid significantly enhanced endothelium dependent vascular responses, but endothelium-independent (GTN) responses were not changed. The authors concluded that folate improves brachial artery flow-mediated vasodilatation, and thus demonstrates an improvement in endothelial function that may have beneficial cardiovascular effects (11).

Folate and Colon Cancer

- In a prospective cohort study, 88,756 women from the Nurses' Health Study who were free of cancer in 1980 were followed until 1994. A total of 442 new cases of colon cancer were reported during the 14-year period. The study controlled for age, family history of colon cancer, aspirin use, smoking, body mass, physical activity, and intakes of red meat, alcohol, methionine, and fiber. A higher energy-adjusted folate intake (> 400 μg vs < 200 μg from food and supplements) assessed by food-frequency questionnaires in 1980 was related to a lower risk of colon cancer. Women who used multivitamins containing folic acid for more than 15 years had a significantly lower risk of developing colon cancer compared to users of supplements for 14 years or less. There was no benefit associated with 4 years or less of supplement use, and only an insignificant trend toward reduced colon cancer risk with supplement use for 5 years to 14 years. Folate from diet alone was related to a modest reduction in colon cancer risk (12).

- In a prospective cohort study, 751 patients with at least one recent large-bowel adenoma underwent colonoscopy one year and four years after their qualifying colon exam. A food-frequency questionnaire was administered at the beginning and end of the study. After adjusting for caloric intake, estimated dietary folate had a significant protective association with the risk of recurrence of adenoma. However, this effect was diminished after adjusting for fiber and fat intake. Reported use of folic acid supplements was not associated with a reduction in risk (13).

- In a relatively small retrospective cohort study, the records of 98 patients with ulcerative colitis who had the disease for a minimum of eight years were reviewed. Of the patients, 29.6 percent developed neoplasia and 40.2 percent took folate supplements. The adjusted relative risk of neoplasia for patients taking folate was 0.72. The authors concluded: "Although not statistically significant, the RR for folate supplementation on the risk of neoplasia is < 1 and shows a dose-response effect consistent with previous studies. Daily folic acid supplementation may protect against the development of neoplasia in ulcerative colitis" (14).

- In a double-blind, placebo-controlled, *ex vivo* study, 24 patients with ulcerative colitis (in remission for at least one month) were randomized to receive 15 mg folinic acid (as calcium folate) or placebo for three months. Cell proliferation was analyzed in rectal biopsies before and after treatment. Compared to the baseline, subjects treated with supplements had a significant reduction in the frequency of occurrence of labeled cells (measure of cell proliferation) in the upper 40 percent of the crypts (area typically associated with the development of colon cancer). No significant changes were seen in the placebo group. The authors concluded: "These results suggest that folate supplementation contributes to regulating rectal cell proliferation in patients with long-standing ulcerative colitis. These findings may be significant for chemoprevention of colon cancer in these patients" (15).

- Twenty subjects with adenomas were randomized to receive 5 mg folic acid or placebo daily one year after polypectomy. At baseline, 6 months, and one year, systemic and colonic measures of folate status were obtained, along with biomarkers of colon cancer (DNA methylation and DNA strand breaks in exons 5–8 of the p53 gene of the colonic mucosa). Serum, red blood cell, and colonic mucosal folate levels were significantly increased in subjects receiving folate, but not the placebo. Folic acid significantly increased the extent of genomic DNA methylation and reduced DNA strand breaks at six months and one year. Significant effects on these molecular markers were also observed in the placebo group, but only at the one year mark. The authors noted that improvement in the placebo group indicated that confounding factors other than folate supplementation were involved (16).

Folate and Cervical Cancer

- In a placebo-controlled study, 235 subjects with cervical dysplasia were randomly assigned to receive 10 mg folic acid or a placebo daily for six months. Clinical status, human papillomavirus Type 16 infection, and blood folate levels were monitored every two months. The baseline incidence of human papillomavirus infection was significantly greater among subjects in the lower tertile of red blood cell folate. However, there were no significant differences among the groups regarding dysplasia status, biopsy results, or prevalence of human papillomavirus. The authors concluded: "Folate deficiency may be involved as a cocarcinogen during the initiation of cervical dysplasia, but folic acid supplements do not alter the course of established disease" (17).

- In a double-blind, placebo-controlled trial, 47 women using oral contraceptives with mild or moderate cervical dysplasia were given 10 mg folic acid or a placebo daily for three months. Mean biopsy scores from folate supplemented subjects were significantly better (rated by a single observer without knowledge of treatment status using a scoring system) than those of placebo subjects. Final vs initial cytology scores were also significantly improved in supplemented subjects and unaffected in the placebo group. Compared to controls, mean red cell folate concentrations were lower and morphological features of megaloblastosis were seen in subjects with dyplasia. The authors concluded: "These studies indicate that either a reversible, localized derangement in folate metabolism may sometimes be misdiagnosed as cervical dysplasia, or else such a derangement is an integral component of the dysplastic process that may be arrested or in some cases reversed by oral folic acid supplementation" (18).

Folate and Depression

- Several studies suggest an association between low serum folate and red cell folate levels and depression (19, 20). One study found low folate levels were linked to poorer response to antidepressant treatment (21). One review article reported that low folate status has been detected in 15 percent to 38 percent of adults diagnosed with depressive disorders (22).

- In a placebo-controlled, multicenter trial, 127 male and female patients with major depression were randomized to receive 500 µg folic acid or a placebo daily in addition to treatment with the antidepressant fluoxetine for 10 weeks. Depressive symptoms were assessed using the Hamilton Rating Scale (HRS) at baseline and at weeks 2, 4, 6, and 10. Folic acid significantly increased plasma folate in all subjects, and homocysteine levels were reduced significantly only in female subjects. Overall, there was a significant improvement in depressive symptoms with folic acid supplements. However, when subjects were divided by gender, only in female subjects receiving folic acid and fluoxetine were responders. The authors concluded that folic acid is a simple method that may enhance the action of antidepressants, and that doses should be given in amounts sufficient to decrease plasma homocysteine. They also noted that the men may require a higher dose of folic acid to achieve this decrease than women (23).

SAFETY

- Doses up to 15 mg (15,000 µg) folic acid in healthy humans without convulsive disorders have not been associated with any reported serious, adverse effects (1).

- The Tolerable Upper Intake Level (UL) is 1 mg (1,000 µg) in adults older than 19 years (4).

- Supplementation with folic acid at levels exceeding 400 µg/day can mask pernicious anemia caused by a B_{12} deficiency, which could lead to permanent nerve damage (1). Some researchers have suggested that adding 0.5 mg to 1.0 mg of vitamin B_{12} to folic acid supplements would prevent this potential problem (12, 24).

- High doses of folic acid (> 5 mg) may interfere with anticonvulsant medications (eg, Diphenylhydantoin) used to treat epilepsy (1).

- There have been some studies suggesting that high intakes of folic acid negatively affect zinc status (1). However, other studies show no adverse effects (25, 26).

REFERENCES

1. Herbert V. Folic acid. In: Shils ME, Olson JA, Shike M, Ross AC, eds. *Modern Nutrition in Health and Disease.* 9th ed. Baltimore, Md: Williams & Wilkins; 1999:433–446.

2. Food and Drug Administration. Food standards: amendment of standards of identity for enriched grain products to require addition of folic acid. *Fed Regist.* 1996;61:8781–8807.

3. Pennington JAT. *Bowes and Church's Food Values of Portions Commonly Used.* 17th ed. Philadelphia, Pa: Lippincott-Raven Publishers; 1998.

4. Institute of Medicine Food and Nutrition Board. *Dietary Reference Intakes for Thiamin, Riboflavin, Niacin, Vitamin B-6, Folate, Vitamin B-12, Pantothenic Acid, Biotin, and Choline.* Washington, DC: National Academy Press; 1998.

5. Centers for Disease Control and Prevention. Recommendations for the use of folic acid to reduce the number of cases of spina bifida and other neural tube defects. *MMWR Morb Mortal Wkly Rep.* 1992;41(RR-14):1–7.

6. Honein MA, Paulozzi LJ, Mathews TJ, et al. Impact of folic acid fortification on the US food supply on the occurrence of neural tube defects. *JAMA.* 2001;285(23):2981–2986.

7. Rimm EB, Willett WC, Hu FB, et al. Folate and vitamin B_6 from diet and supplements in relation to risk of coronary heart disease among women. *JAMA.* 1998;279:359–364.

8. Collaboration HLT. Lowering blood homocysteine with folic acid-based supplements: meta-analysis of randomized trials. *BMJ.* 1998;316:894–898.

9. Boushey CJ, Beresford SA, Omenn GS, et al. A quantitative assessment of plasma homocysteine as a risk factor for vascular disease. Probable benefits of increasing folic acid intakes. *JAMA.* 1995;274:1049–1057.

10. Morrison HI, Schaubel D, Desmeules M, et al. Serum folate and risk of fatal coronary heart disease. *JAMA.* 1996;275:1893–1896.

11. Bellamy MF, McDowell IF, Ramsey MW, et al. Oral folate enhances endothelial function in hyperhomocysteinaemic subjects. *Eur J Clin Invest.* 1999;29:659–662.

12. Giovannucci E, Stampfer MJ, Colditz GA, et al. Multivitamin use, folate, and colon cancer in women in the Nurse's Health Study. *Ann Intern Med.* 1998;129:517–524.

13. Baron JA, Sandler RS, Haile RW, et al. Folate intake, alcohol consumption, cigarette smoking, and risk of colorectal adenomas. *J Natl Cancer Inst.* 1998;90:57–62.

14. Lashner BA, Provencher KS, Seidner DL, et al. The effect of folic acid supplementation on the risk for cancer or dysplasia in ulcerative colitis. *Gastroenterology.* 1997;112:29–32.

15. Biasco G, Zannoni U, Paganelli GM, et al. Folic acid supplementation and cell kinetics of rectal mucosa in patients with ulcerative colitis. *Cancer Epidemiol Biomarkers Prev.* 1997;6:469–471.

16. Kim YI, Baik HW, Fawaz K, et al. Effects of folate supplementation on two provisional molecular markers of colon cancer: a prospective, randomized trial. *Am J Gastroenterol.* 2001;96:184–194.

17. Butterworth CE, Hatch KD, Soong SJ, et al. Oral folic acid supplementation for cervical dysplasia: a clinical intervention trial. *Am J Obstet Gynecol.* 1992;166:803–809.
18. Butterworth CE, Hatch KD, Gore H, et al. Improvement in cervical dysplasia associated with folic acid therapy in users of oral contraceptives. *Am J Clin Nutr.* 1982;35:73–82.
19. Ortega RM, Manas LR, Andres P, et al. Functional and psychic deterioration in elderly people may be aggravated by folate deficiency. *J Nutr.* 1996;126:1992–1999.
20. Wesson VA, Levitt AJ, Joffe RT. Change in folate status with antidepressant treatment. *Psychiatry Res.* 1994;53:313–322.
21. Fava M, Borus JS, Alpert JE, et al. Folate, vitamin B$_{12}$, and homocysteine in major depressive disorder. *Am J Psychiatry.* 1997;154:426–428.
22. Alpert JE, Fava M. Nutrition and depression: the role of folate. *Nutr Rev.* 1997;55:145–149.
23. Coppen A, Bailey J. Enhancement of the antidepressant action of fluoxetine by folic acid: a randomized, placebo-controlled trial. *J Affect Disord.* 2000;60:121–130.
24. Herbert V, Bigaouette J. Call for endorsement of a petition to the Food and Drug Administration to always add vitamin B$_{12}$ to any folate fortification or supplement. *Am J Clin Nutr.* 1997;65:572–573.
25. Kauwell GP, Bailey LB, Gregory JF, et al. Zinc status is not adversely affected by folic acid supplementation and zinc intake does not impair folate utilization. *J Nutr.* 1995;125:66–72.
26. Keating JN, Wada L, Stokstad EL, et al. Folic acid: effect on zinc absorption in humans and in the rat. *Am J Clin Nutr.* 1987;46:835–839.

F

Fructooligosaccharides (FOS)

Fructoligoosaccharides (FOSs) are a class of oligosaccharides made up of glucose linked to multiple fructose units. Depending on their chain length, FOSs are classified as oligofructose—OF (2, 3, or 4 fructose units) or inulin (3 to 60 units). The chemical structure of FOSs does not permit digestion by intestinal enzymes. Instead, FOSs travel past the upper gastrointestinal tract and are selectively used as fuel by beneficial bacteria in the colon (see Acidophilus/*Lactobacillus Acidophilus* [LA]). Once fermented by bacteria, the energy value remaining for the host ranges between 1.5 kcal to 2.4 kcal per g FOS ingested. Because they selectively stimulate the growth and activity of beneficial colonic bacteria (*Bifidobacterium, Lactobacillus*), FOSs are termed "prebiotics" and have been investigated for their potential role in intestinal health (1–3).

Media and Marketing Claims	Efficacy
Supports a healthy digestive tract (reduces constipation)	↑?
May reduce risk of colon cancer	NR
Helps diabetics lower blood sugar level	NR
Lowers cholesterol	NR

Advisory

Doses > 50 g /day associated with bloating, cramping, and diarrhea; some of these side-effects were noted with lesser doses

Drug/Supplement Interactions

- No reported adverse interactions
- FOSs may enhance calcium absorption

KEY POINTS

- Eating a minimum of five servings of fruits and vegetables daily (focusing on the foods lists in Food Sources) will help increase FOS consumption in the diet.
- FOS supplementation appears to specifically increase bifidobacterium in the colon, which is beneficial to intestinal health. An increase in bifidobacteria is accompanied by a reduction in the number of bacteria reported to have pathogenic potential. This may have application in intestinal pathologies, although one study showed no benefits in patients with irritable bowel syndrome.
- FOSs appear to have stool bulking properties that may help prevent constipation. Further controlled clinical trials are needed in humans to test the role of FOSs on intestinal conditions and diseases.
- Some preliminary animal studies suggest that FOSs may have anticarcinogenic properties in the colon. However, there are no human studies testing FOS supplementation in the prevention and treatment of colon cancer, nor are there reliable data on the influence of FOSs on biomarkers or enzymes involved in colon carcinogenesis.
- More research is needed on the role of FOSs in reducing blood glucose and lipid levels in healthy, diabetic, and hyperlipidemic subjects. Preliminary trials do not suggest a beneficial effect on blood sugars and serum lipids.

FOOD SOURCES

FOSs are found naturally in onions, asparagus, Jerusalem artichokes, garlic, bananas, tomatoes, wheat, rye, honey, beer, chicory root, and leeks. Because of their mild sweetness and stability, FOSs are used in commercial confections and pastries (3). FOS concentrations in foods tend to vary depending on harvest time and storage time. The average American diet provides 2 g to 8 g FOS/day (4).

Food	FOS (mg/Serving)*
Artichoke, Jerusalem (½ c)	4,380
Onion powder (1 tbsp)	293
Banana, ripe (1 medium)	236
Chicory root, raw (½ c)	189
Shallot (1 tbsp)	85
Peach (½ c)	34
Garlic (1 clove)	12

Serving sizes calculated from values from Reference 4.

DOSAGE/BIOAVAILABILITY

FOS supplements are sold in powders and capsules. On a commercial scale, FOSs are produced from sucrose using a fungal enzyme or by partial hydrolysis using endoglycosidases made from chicory inulin (5). Labels suggest starting with 1 g (¼ tsp) and gradually increasing up to 4 g/day. In the powdered form, it can be used to mildly sweeten cereals, fruit, and drinks. Other products combine FOSs with probiotic bacteria (see Acidophilus/*Lactobacillus Acidophilus* [LA]). FOSs are also included in some enteral formulas. In one study, approximately 90 percent of a 20-g dose of FOSs was not absorbed and none was excreted in the stools, indicating that FOSs were completely fermented by colonic flora (1).

RELEVANT RESEARCH

FOSs and Intestinal Health

- In a double-blind, placebo-controlled, multicenter trial, 119 patients with diagnosed irritable bowel syndrome (IBS) were randomly assigned to receive 20 g FOS powder or placebo daily for 12 weeks. Before the study, all subjects received a placebo for a two-week, single-blind phase to wash out any effects of medication or dietary supplements previously used for IBS symptoms. Efficacy (based on patients' overall response to treatment and severity of abdominal distension, rumbling, pain and abnormal flatulence), tolerability, and compliance were assessed at baseline (end of first two weeks) and weeks 4, 6, 8, and 12. Twenty-three patients dropped out of the study (14 patients in the FOS group and 9 patients in the placebo group). After weeks 4 and 6, there was a nonsignficant trend toward a greater improvement in IBS symptoms in the placebo group, but not the FOS group. By weeks 8 and 12, there were no differences in symptoms between the groups. The authors concluded that although symptoms worsened at the onset of FOS ingestion, continuous treatment resulted in no deterioration of IBS symptoms (6).

- Eight subjects were fed a controlled diet while living in a metabolic unit for 15 days, followed by 15 g oligofructose (OF)/day for 15 days in place of dietary sucrose, followed by a final 15 days on the control diet again. This was followed by 5 days on a free diet for stool collection. Four subjects completed an additional study of 15 g inulin/day for 15 days. OF and inulin were administered with breakfast in free form, with the remaining 10 g given in biscuits. Both OF and inulin resulted in a significant increase in bifidobacteria in the stool compared to the sucrose control periods. There was a significant increase in stool wet matter and nitrogen excretion with OF compared to sucrose controls. The numbers of potentially pathogenic bacteria (*bacteroides, clostridia,* and *fusobacteria*) were significantly lowered in subjects fed OF. The authors concluded: "Small changes in diet can alter the balance of colonic bacteria towards a potentially healthier microflora" (7).

- In an animal study, 15 rats were fed a control diet or a diet supplemented with one of four oligosaccharides (FOSs, OF, cellulose, or xylooligosaccharides [XOS]). FOSs, OF, and XOS at 6 percent of the diet resulted in a greater production of short chain fatty acids than the control or cellulose diets. The authors noted that the potential clinical significance of an increase in short chain fatty acids (butyrate) that are the preferred energy source for colonic cells is that the reduction in colonic pH may inhibit pathogenic bacteria. The authors concluded that "providing these oligosaccharides as ingredients in nutritional formulas could benefit the health of the gastrointestinal tract" (8).

FOSs and Cancer

- In a double-blind, placebo-controlled study, 20 healthy subjects were supplemented with 12.5 g FOS/day or a placebo in addition to their usual diet for 12 days. Although colonic bifidobacteria increased with FOS supplementation, there were no changes in fecal pH, concentrations of bile acids and neutral sterols. Furthermore, there was no reduction in bacterial enzymes such as nitroreductase, azoreductase, and Acircumflex-glucuronidase, which are potential indices of colon carcinogenesis (9).

- A study of mice with intramuscularly implanted tumors reported that a 15 percent FOS diet inhibited tumor growth compared to a control diet (10).

- Preneoplastic lesions (aberrant crypt foci [ACF]) were chemically induced in the colons of male rats prior to feeding a control diet or OF- or inulin-supplemented diets. OF and inulin significantly inhibited ACF formation and the crypt multiplication in the colon, although inulin had a more pronounced effect. The authors hypothesized that this result may be caused by butyrate production by fermentation of FOSs and that butyrate may have anticarcinogenic properties (11).

Effects of FOSs on Blood Glucose and Cholesterol

- In a single-blind, placebo-controlled, crossover study, 20 patients with type 2 diabetes were randomized to receive 15 g FOS/day or a placebo (4 g glucose/day) for 20 days each. Average daily intakes of energy, macronutrients, and fiber were similar with both treatments. FOSs had no significant effects on total, HDL, and LDL cholesterol, serum triglycerides, serum free fatty acids, serum acetate, or blood glucose (12).

- In a double-blind, crossover design study, 12 healthy male subjects were randomly assigned to ingest 20 g FOS/day or a placebo in cookies for four weeks at a time, with a two-week washout period. There was a significant decrease in basal hepatic glucose during FOS intake; however, there was no change in insulin-stimulated glucose metabolism, serum triglycerides, total and HDL cholesterol, apolipoproteins A-I and B, or lipoprotein (A) (13). In a follow-up double-blind, placebo-controlled, crossover study, the same researchers investigated the effects of 20 g FOS powder/day in 12 patients with type 2 diabetes. After four weeks, FOS had no effect on fasting plasma glucose or insulin concentrations or basal hepatic glucose production. There was also no change in serum lipids or plasma glucose response to a fixed insulin bolus (14).

- Some animal studies have shown that FOSs reduce serum triglycerides and VLDL (15, 16). One article suggested that oligofructose has this effect by reducing de novo fatty acid synthesis in the liver, but this hypothesis requires further exploration (14).

SAFETY

- The effects of long-term, concentrated, daily use of FOSs have not been evaluated.

- One study testing the safety of 15 g/day FOS in enteral formulas for 14 days in healthy subjects reported no clinically significant differences in serum plasma compared to the placebo (17).

- Several researchers have given doses up to 20 g/day of FOSs with few side-effects other than mild flatulence (1). Doses exceeding 50 g/day have been associated with bloating, cramps, and osmotic diarrhea (18).

- Supplemental FOSs (15 g) did not interfere with calcium and nonheme-iron absorption in healthy, male subjects (19). Several animal studies have reported that FOSs positively affect calcium absorption (20–22).

F

REFERENCES

1. Gibson GR, Roberfroid MB. Dietary modulation of the human colonic microbiota: introducing the concept of prebiotics. *J Nutr.* 1995;125:1401–1412.
2. Oku T. Oligosaccharides with beneficial health effects: a Japanese perspective. *Nutr Rev.* 1996;54(11 pt 2):S59–S66.
3. Molis C, Flourie B, Ouarne F, et al. Digestion, excretion and energy value of fructooligosaccharides in healthy humans. *Am J Clin Nutr.* 1996;64:324–328.
4. Campbell JM, Bauer LL, Fahey GC, et al. Selected fructooligosaccharide (1-Kestose, Nystose, and 1^F-β-Fructofuranosylnystose) composition of foods and feeds. *J Agric Food Chem.* 1997;45:3076–3082.
5. Roberfroid MB. Health benefits of non-digestible oligosaccharides. *Adv Exp Med Biol.* 1997;427:211–219.
6. Olesen M, Gudmand-Hoyer E. Efficacy, safety, and tolerability of fructooligosaccharides in the treatment of irritable bowel syndrome. *Am J Clin Nutr.* 2000;72:1570–1575.
7. Gibson GR, Beatty ER, Wang X, et al. Selective stimulation of bifidobacteria in the human colon by oligofructose and inulin. *Gastroenterology.* 1995;108:975–982.
8. Campbell JM, Fahey GC, Wolf BW. Selected indigestible oligosaccharides affect large bowel mass, cecal and fecal short-chain fatty acids, pH, and microflora in rats. *J Nutr.* 1997;127:130–136.
9. Bouhnik Y, Flourie B, Riottot M, et al. Effects of fructo-oligosaccharides ingestion on fecal bifidobacteria and selected metabolic indexes of colon carcinogenesis in healthy humans. *Nutr Cancer.* 1996;26:21–29.
10. Taper HS, Delzenne NM, Roberfroid MB. Growth inhibition of transplantable mouse tumors by nondigestible carbohydrates. *Int J Cancer.* 1997;71:1109–1112.
11. Reddy BS, Hamid R, Rao CV. Effect of dietary oligofructose and inulin on colonic preneoplastic aberrant crypt foci inhibition. *Carcinogenesis.* 1997;18:1371–1374.
12. Alles MS, de Roos NM, Bakx JC, et al. Consumption of fructooligosaccharides does not favorably affect blood glucose and serum lipid concentrations in patients with type 2 diabetes. *Am J Clin Nutr.* 1999;69:64–69.

13. Luo J, Rizkalla SW, Alamowitch C, et al. Chronic consumption of short-chain fructooligosaccharides by healthy subjects decreased basal hepatic glucose production but had no effect on insulin-stimulated glucose metabolism. *Am J Clin Nutr.* 1996;63:939–945.

14. Luo J, Van Yperselle M, Rizkalla SW, et al. Chronic consumption of short-chain fructooligosaccharides does not affect basal hepatic glucose production or insulin resistance in type 2 diabetes. *J Nutr.* 2000;130:1572–1577.

15. Kok N, Roberfroid M, Robert A, et al. Involvement of lipogenesis in the lower VLDL secretion induced by oligofructose in rats. *Br J Nutr.* 1996;76:881–890.

16. Fiordaliso M, Kok N, Desager JP, et al. Dietary oligofructose lowers triglycerides, phospholipids and cholesterol in serum and very low density lipoproteins of rats. *Lipids.* 1995;30:163–167.

17. Garleb KA, Snook JT, Marco MJ, et al. Effect of fructooligosaccharide containing enteral formulas on subjective tolerance factors, serum chemistry profiles, and fecal bifidobacteria in healthy adult male subjects. *Microbial Ecology Health Dis.* 1996;9:279–285.

18. Briet F, Achour L, Flourie B, et al. Symptomatic response to varying levels of fructooligosaccharides consumed occasionally or regularly. *Eur J Clin Nutr.* 1995;49:501–507.

19. van den Heuvel EG, Schaafsma G, Muys T, et al. Nondigestible oligosaccharides do not interfere with calcium and nonheme-iron absorption in young, healthy men. *Am J Clin Nutr.* 1998;67:445–451.

20. Ohta A, Motohashi Y, Sakai K, et al. Dietary fructooligosaccharides increase calcium absorption and levels of mucosal calbindin-D9k in the large intestine of gastrectomized rats. *Scand J Gastroenterol.* 1998;33:1062–1068.

21. Morohashi T, Sano T, Ohta A, et al. True calcium absorption in the intestine is enhanced by fructooligosaccharide feeding in rats. *J Nutr.* 1998;128:1815–1818.

22. Ohta A, Motohashi Y, Ohtsuki M, et al. Dietary fructooligosaccharides change the concentration of calbindin-D9k differently in the mucosa of the small and large intestine of rats. *J Nutr.* 1998;128:934–939.

Gamma-Linolenic Acid (GLA)

Gamma-linolenic acid (GLA) is an essential omega-6 fatty acid found naturally in evening primrose oil (*Oenothera biennis*, 8 percent to 10 percent GLA), borage oil (*Borago officinalis*, 23 percent to 26 percent GLA) and black currant oil (*Ribes nigrum*, 15 percent to 20 percent GLA). In addition to GLA, the remaining fatty acid content of these plant oils is primarily linoleic acid (LA) and a small amount of alpha-linolenic acid (omega-3) and other fatty acids. In the body, GLA is synthesized from LA by the rate-limiting enzyme delta-6 desaturase. GLA can then be elongated into dihomo-GLA (DGLA). DGLA can be directed into 3 pathways: (1) conversion into 1-series (anti-inflammatory) prostaglandin (PGE_1); (2) conversion into 15-(S)-hydroxy-8, 11, 13-eicosatrienoic acid (15-HETrE), which inhibits the biosynthesis of pro-inflammatory arachidonic acid (AA) metabolites; or (3) conversion into AA by delta-5 desaturase. However, due to the limited activity of delta-5 desaturase, only a small fraction of DGLA is converted to AA. It is estimated that only 5 percent to 10 percent of the daily intake of LA is converted into GLA and its metabolites (1, 2).

A defect in delta-6 desaturase interferes with the conversion of LA to GLA. In animal studies and some human studies, many factors have been associated with impaired GLA formation: aging; diabetes; excessive alcohol intake; deficiencies of zinc, vitamin B_6, magnesium, biotin, and calcium; elevated stress hormone levels; high cholesterol levels; and viral infections (2). Atopic dermatitis, premenstrual syndrome, rheumatoid arthritis, cancer, and cardiovascular diseases have indirectly been associated with a reduced ability to convert LA to GLA. Because supplementation with GLA oils bypasses the rate-limiting enzyme (delta-6 desaturase) that converts LA to GLA, researchers have investigated the role of evening primrose, borage, and black currant oils in various diseases (1, 2).

Media and Marketing Claims	Efficacy
Reduces symptoms of PMS	↔
Eliminates pain associated with rheumatoid arthritis	↔
Clears up acne and allergic skin reactions	↔
Improves diabetic nephropathy	NR
Improves symptoms of heart disease	NR
Reduces risk of breast cancer	NR
Prevents hair loss	NR

G

Advisory

- Potential side-effects include belching, bloating, and nausea
- Doses up to 2.8 g/day appear to be safe

Drug/Supplement Interactions

- Evening primrose oil may lower seizure threshold when used with tricyclic antidepressants and anticonvulsant medications
- Borage seed should not be taken with hepatotoxic drugs
- Could potentially increase bleeding time; should be monitored by a physician if individual is taking anticoagulant drugs or supplements and should be avoided prior to surgery

KEY POINTS

- Evidence is conflicting concerning the effect of GLA supplementation on mastalgia and other symptoms of PMS. According to one reviewer, many of the clinical trials, especially those in PMS, resulted in a very large placebo response, making it difficult to show any true response (2).

- The research on the potential benefits of GLA supplements in rheumatoid arthritis is also conflicting. Some of these studies have been criticized for large number of dropouts and for failing to control concomitant use of medications. In addition, studies shorter than one year offer limited information regarding the efficacy of pharmacologic agents in the treatment of rheumatoid arthritis (3). Furthermore, the results from GLA studies may be confounded by the use of olive oil as the placebo, because one author reported that it is conceivable that olive oil itself may be beneficial to patients with rheumatoid arthritis (4). One study reported that the reduction in EPA associated with supplementation may actually have adverse clinical effects in rheumatoid arthritis because EPA is a precursor to anti-inflammatory prostaglandins (5).

- Evidence from a meta-analysis suggests that GLA from evening primrose oil may benefit patients with atopic dermatitis; however, other studies show no benefit. There is no evidence at this time indicating that GLA supplements clear acne blemishes.

- Animal and preliminary human studies are suggestive of a benefit of GLA-rich oils for patients with diabetic neuropathy. Additional, long-term controlled trials are needed.

- Overall, there is insufficient human research to draw definite conclusions about the role of GLA oils in heart disease. Preliminary evidence from animal and a few human studies suggest that GLA-rich oil may reduce blood pressure. GLA oils do not appear to affect triglyceride levels and their effect on LDL cholesterol is inconsistent. The effects of GLA supplements on reducing morbidity and/or mortality from heart disease are not known.

- There is preliminary data from one pilot study that GLA supplements may enhance the action of the breast cancer drug tamoxifen. More research is needed to clarify the potential role of GLA in treating cancer.

- Despite claims that GLA oils prevent hair loss, there is currently no evidence from controlled trials in humans demonstrating this effect. This claim may have been falsely extrapolated from a study of diabetic mice (not discussed here) that reported less alopecia and dry skin in mice supplemented with GLA compared to a placebo. Clearly, much more research is needed to determine whether GLA affects hair loss.

- Although the role of GLA in human health has been proposed in several literature reviews (1, 2), additional controlled research on the efficacy, safety, dose, and duration of treatment with GLA oils in humans is needed before specific recommendations can be made.

FOOD SOURCES

No significant typical food sources. Human breast milk contains approximately 100 mg to 400 mg GLA plus DGLA/L (2).

DOSAGE INFORMATION/BIOAVAILABILITY

Evening primrose, borage, and black currant oils are available in softgels or as a liquid oil. Dosages of GLA range from 45 mg to 300 mg per softgel, with a total suggested daily intake ranging from 500 mg to 3,000 mg (10 to 15 large capsules/softgels) taken with food. Almost all the studies of evening primrose oil have used SP116, an extract selected for consistency of composition and incorporated into commercial products (2).

Normal human endogenous production of GLA is approximately 250 mg/day to 1,000 mg/day (2). Acute administration of 280 mg GLA from 3 g evening primrose oil (SP116) resulted in a significant increase in plasma GLA concentrations in healthy volunteers that reached maximum levels in 2.7 hours to 4.4 hours. There was no significant effect on DGLA and AA levels (6). In a study of rats supplemented with GLA oils, there was a significant dose-related increase of GLA and DGLA in liver, erythrocyte, and aorta phospholipids after six weeks (7).

RELEVANT RESEARCH

GLA and PMS, Mastalgia, and Menopause

- Some researchers have suggested that symptoms of PMS may be associated with defective metabolism of omega-6 fatty acids. In a cross-sectional observational study, 250 patients with PMS, cyclic mastalgia, and noncyclic mastalgia had serum samples analyzed for fatty acid content. LA levels were normal for all patients with symptoms; however, DGLA and AA levels were significantly lower in subjects with mastalgia compared to controls. Subjects with PMS had significantly lower AA than controls. Subjects with noncyclic mastalgia had significantly lower docosahexaenoic acid levels compared to controls. The authors concluded that these results suggest a defect in the conversion of linoleic acid to other omega-6 fatty acids in this population (8). Another study reported significantly reduced DGLA and AA levels in women with cyclic mastalgia (n = 36), and significantly reduced AA in noncyclic mastalgia patients (n = 6), but no differences in plasma fatty acids in subjects with breast cysts (n = 200) when compared to blood samples from normal controls (9).

- In a systematic review of seven placebo-controlled trials testing evening primrose oil in the treatment of PMS, the authors noted that the two best controlled studies failed to show beneficial effects, although the trials were small. Only five of seven trials clearly indicated randomization. The authors had intended to complete a meta-analysis; however, inconsistent scoring and response criteria made statistical pooling inappropriate. They concluded that based on current evidence, evening primrose oil does not appear to be effective in the management of premenstrual syndrome (10).

- In a double-blind, placebo-controlled, crossover study, 38 women with PMS were randomized to receive 360 mg GLA from evening primrose oil or a placebo daily for three menstrual cycles each. There were no significant differences in PMS symptoms (psychological, fluid retention, breast) between evening primrose oil and placebo, though both groups reported improvement in subjective symptoms. The authors concluded that the improvement reported by these women with moderate PMS was solely a placebo effect (11).

- In a double-blind, placebo-controlled study, 200 women with breast cysts were randomized to receive 270 mg GLA from evening primrose oil or a placebo daily for one year. Cysts were categorized by initial electrolyte composition, and follow-up continued for one year after therapy. Recurrent cyst formation was slightly lower, but this change did not reach statistical significance in the evening primrose group compared to the placebo (12).

- In a double-blind, placebo-controlled study, 56 menopausal women suffering from hot flushes at least three times daily were randomized to receive 500 mg evening primrose oil (approximately 45 mg GLA) with 10 mg natural vitamin E or a placebo daily for six months. During the first month, no treatment was administered until baseline data were collected. Only 18 women in the treatment group and 17 women in the placebo group completed the trial. (The authors did not explain the reason for the high dropout rate.) Both groups had reductions in the mean number of hot flushes, with a greater significant overall improvement in the placebo group. The only significant improvement in the evening primrose group over the placebo group was a reduction in the maximum number of self-reported nighttime flushes. The authors concluded: "Based on the data from this small pilot study and on the lack of a hypothetical rationale for using GLA, we cannot support the use of evening primrose oil in the treatment of menopausal hot flushes" (13).

GLA and Rheumatoid Arthritis

- In a double-blind, placebo-controlled trial, 34 subjects (average age 55 y) with rheumatoid arthritis and active synovitis were randomized to receive 10.5 g black currant oil in 15 capsules (providing approximately 2,000 mg GLA) or a placebo daily for 24 weeks. Patients were maintained on a stable dose of NSAIDs and corticosteroids one month before the study and were instructed to maintain their pre-entry doses during the study. There were no significant differences in medication use between groups. Clinical assessment of disease activity (physician and patients' global assessment, pain self-assessment on a visual analogue scale, number of tender joints and joints with swelling, joint tenderness score, duration of morning stiffness, ability to do vocational activities, and grip strength) was completed every six weeks. Twenty patients dropped out of the study mainly because of the large size and number of capsules that had to be taken to achieve the target dose (14 patients in the GLA group and 13 patients in the placebo group completed the study). At 24 weeks, subjects taking black currant oil had significantly reduced signs and symptoms of disease activity compared to the baseline. Subjects receiving placebo showed no change in disease activity. However, overall clinical responses (defined as a significant change in four measures) were no better in the treatment group than in the placebo group (14). The high dropout rate (20/34) makes the results of this study difficult to evaluate.

- In a double-blind, placebo-controlled study, 37 patients with rheumatoid arthritis and active synovitis were randomized to receive 1,400 mg GLA in borage seed oil or a placebo (cottonseed oil) daily for 24 weeks. Physicians' and patients' global assessments of disease activity, joint tenderness, joint swelling, duration of morning stiffness, grip strength, and ability to do daily activities were completed before and after the study. GLA significantly reduced signs and symptoms of disease activity compared to the placebo group, which showed no change or worsening of disease. Overall clinical response (significant change in four measures) was better in the GLA group. The authors concluded that further trials of GLA oils in rheumatoid arthritis are warranted (15).

- In a double-blind, placebo-controlled study, 40 patients with rheumatoid arthritis with gastrointestinal lesions associated with NSAID use were randomized to receive 540 mg GLA from 6 g evening primrose oil plus 120 mg vitamin E or a placebo (6 g olive oil) daily for six months. Patients were assessed at the baseline and every three months for pain on a visual analogue scale, analgesic use, blood samples, and the Ritchie articular index. NSAID use did not stop during the study, but three subjects in each group reduced their dosages. Evening primrose oil was associated with a statistically significant reduction in morning stiffness at three and six months. Olive oil was associated with a significant reduction in pain and articular index at six months. There were no changes in blood parameters of inflammation. The authors concluded: "While gamma-linolenic acid may produce mild improvement in rheumatoid arthritis, olive oil may itself have unrecognized benefits" (4). Alternatively, it is possible that a placebo effect was operating.

- In a double-blind, placebo-controlled study, 49 patients with rheumatoid arthritis were randomized to receive one of three treatments daily for 12 months: (1) 540 mg GLA from evening primrose oil, (2) 240 mg eicosapentaenoic acid (EPA) plus 450 mg GLA, or (3) a placebo. At the end of the study, all subjects were given a placebo for an additional three months. There was a statistically significant subjective improvement of symptoms in subjects receiving GLA and EPA plus GLA compared to the placebo group at 12 months. GLA and EPA plus GLA were also associated with a statistically significant decrease in NSAID use. After three months of placebo, those who received active treatment relapsed. The authors concluded evening primrose oil alone or in combination with fish oil produced a subjective improvement that allowed some patients to reduce or stop treatment with NSAIDs (16).

- In a double-blind, comparative study, 20 patients with rheumatoid arthritis were randomized to receive 20 mL evening primrose oil containing 9 percent GLA or olive oil for 12 weeks. Subjects abstained from nonsteroidal anti-inflammatory drugs during the trial. Fatty acid and apolipoprotein samples were taken after overnight fasting before treatment and after 6 and 12 weeks of the study. After 12 weeks, evening primrose oil significantly increased LA, GLA, and DGLA in serum fatty acids, whereas olive oil had no effect. Evening primrose oil resulted in a small, but significant increase in AA at six weeks compared to the baseline. Evening primrose oil also significantly reduced eicosapentaenoic acid (EPA) after 6 weeks, and by an even greater amount after 12 weeks. Olive oil also significantly reduced EPA after 12 weeks. There was no effect on total cholesterol or triglycerides by either treatment; however, olive oil raised HDL cholesterol and apolipoprotein A-I concentrations slightly. The authors concluded that the decrease in serum EPA and the increase in AA concentrations induced by evening primrose oil may have adverse effects in patients with rheumatoid arthritis in light of the roles of these fatty acids as precursors of eicosanoids (EPA is a precursor to anti-inflammatory eicosanoids and AA is a precursor to inflammatory eicosanoids) (5).

- Diets enriched with 15 percent fat from borage seed oil suppressed inflammation as measured by lysosomal enzyme activity, prostaglandin E_2, leukotriene B_4 in rats with acute injury and in rats with induced arthritis compared to diets enriched with 15 percent safflower oil (17).

GLA and Skin Disorders

- In a double-blind, placebo-controlled, multicenter trial, 160 patients with atopic eczema of moderate severity were randomized to receive 500 mg borage oil (naturally contains 23 percent GLA) or a placebo daily for 24 weeks. Use of a topical cream was permitted as a rescue medication, with amount used until response being defined as the primary endpoint, and clinical improvement as a secondary efficacy criterion. Although several clinical symptoms improved compared to placebo, the overall response to borage oil was not significant. However, when a subgroup was excluded (subjects who failed to show increased erythrocyte DGLA levels, took < 70 percent of the capsules, or used the rescue cream in excess), there were statistically significant improvements observed in favor of borage oil (18).

- In a double-blind, placebo-controlled trial, 39 patients with chronic hand dermatitis were randomized to receive 600 mg GLA from evening primrose oil or a placebo daily for 16 weeks, and observation continued for another 8 weeks. Patients were assessed monthly for clinical changes using a visual analogue scale. Plasma and red blood cell lipograms, and skin biopsies were taken before therapy, after 16 weeks and at week 24. Tissue was used for histological evaluation, electromicroscopic assessment and epidermal lipid analysis. Both groups improved in clinical parameters, with no statistical difference between the groups. There was no change in the lipid composition of plasma red cells or epidermis. Ultrastructurally, skin specimens showed no change during the study (19).

- A meta-analysis of nine controlled trials (four parallel, five crossover design) of evening primrose oil (standardized extract SP116) to treat atopic dermatitis reported a statistically significant improvement over baseline in patient and physician symptom scores of inflammation, dryness, scaliness, pruritus, and overall skin involvement compared to the placebo in the parallel studies. Similar results were seen in analysis of the crossover trials; however, the difference between evening primrose oil and the placebo in the physicians' global scores did not reach statistical significance. However, there was a statistically significant improvement in pruritus compared to the placebo in the crossover studies. There was also a positive association between clinical improvement and plasma levels of DGLA and AA (20).

- In a double-blind, placebo-controlled study, 58 children with atopic dermatitis requiring topical steroids were randomized to receive 40 mg GLA from 500 mg evening primrose oil or a placebo daily for 16 weeks. (Twenty-two of the subjects also had asthma). Peak expiratory flow was measured and disease activity was assessed monthly. Subjects taking evening primrose oil had a significant increase in plasma concentrations of DGLA and AA compared to the placebo. Both groups had a significant improvement in eczema symptoms, but there were no differences between the placebo and treatment groups. There was also no therapeutic effect on asthma symptoms (21).

- In a double-blind, placebo-controlled study, 37 patients with chronic stable plaque psoriasis were randomized to receive a combination of 107 mg marine oil plus 430 mg evening primrose oil plus 10 mg vitamin E (12 capsules) or a placebo for 24 weeks. All subjects received placebo capsules for the run-in period for four weeks. Subjects were assessed every four weeks during the study. There was no significant improvement in erythema, scaling, transepidermal water loss, or psoriasis plaque thickness for treatment or control groups. Additionally, there were no differences in the overall clinical severity of psoriasis or in patient assessment of itch, redness, anxiety, and depression (22).

GLA and Diabetes

- In a double-blind, placebo-controlled, multicenter trial, 111 patients with mild diabetic neuropathy were randomized to receive 480 mg GLA from 12 evening primrose capsules or a placebo daily for one year. Neurophysiological responses to hot and cold thresholds, sensation, tendon reflexes, and muscle strength were assessed by standard tests in upper and lower limbs at 3, 6, and 12 months. For all 16 parameters measured, the change during one year in response to GLA was more favorable than the change with the placebo, and for 13 parameters this difference was significant. Specifically, GLA supplementation significantly improved 8 of 10 neurophysiological parameters and 5 of 6 neurological assessments. Gender, age, and type of diabetes did not affect the results, although treatment with GLA was more effective among persons with relatively well-controlled diabetes than among people having poorly controlled diabetes as defined by HbA_{1c} (23).

- Several studies supplementing diabetic animals with GLA-rich oils have demonstrated improvement in nerve blood flow and nerve (24–26).

GLA and Cardiovascular Disease

- In a double-blind, placebo-controlled trial, 27 men with borderline hypertension were randomized to receive 6 g black currant oil or a placebo (safflower oil) for eight weeks. Weekly blood pressure readings were recorded and blood pressure and heart reactivity were measured before and at the end of the study during a mental arithmetic test. There was a significant decrease in diastolic blood pressure in subjects taking black currant oil compared to those in the placebo group (27).

- In a placebo-controlled crossover (not randomized) study, 19 hypercholesterolemic patients (9 with elevated triglycerides) were given 3.6 mg evening primrose oil (providing 324 mg GLA) for eight weeks and a placebo (safflower oil) for eight weeks. Diets were not controlled. During treatment, levels of DGLA in plasma and red blood cell levels increased. In subjects without hypertriglyceridemia, evening primrose oil treatment resulted in a significant decrease in LDL cholesterol and plasma apolipoprotein B compared with the baseline and placebo levels (28).

- In a double-blind, placebo controlled, crossover study, 27 subjects with hypertriglyceridemia were randomized to receive either 4 g evening primrose oil (n = 13) or marine oil (n = 14) for eight weeks and a placebo (olive oil) for eight weeks. Evening primrose oil increased GLA and DGLA in plasma lipids and platelet phospholipids; however, no effect was seen on platelet function, triglycerides, or levels of total, HDL, or LDL cholesterol. In contrast, fish oil significantly reduced triglycerides in all lipoprotein fractions with a slight increase in HDL and LDL cholesterol (29).

- Evening primrose oil reduced platelet hyperaggregability in rabbits fed atherogenic diets compared to rabbits on atherogenic diets not supplemented with evening primrose oil (30).

- Rats with spontaneous hypertension that were fed diets containing evening primrose, black currant, borage, or fungal oils for seven weeks had significant reductions in blood pressure. (31).

GLA and Cancer

- In a pilot study (not randomized or blinded) of 38 elderly breast cancer patients, those receiving 2.8 g/day of GLA with tamoxifen were compared to matched controls who took tamoxifen alone. Tumor biopsies were taken to assess changes in estrogen receptor and bcl-2 expression during treatment. GLA plus tamoxifen achieved a significantly faster clinical response than tamoxifen alone by six weeks. There were significant reductions in estrogen receptor expression in both treatments, but a greater reduction was observed in GLA-supplemented subjects (32). The lack of randomization and blinding weaken the results of this trial.

SAFETY

- Long-term human trials have shown that up to 2,800 mg GLA/day is apparently well tolerated (1). It has been estimated that doses less than 100 mg GLA/kg/day are unlikely to be toxic (2).

- Borage seed contains low concentrations of unsaturated pyrrolizidine alkaloids that may cause hepatotoxic effects (33). Manufacturers state that these alkaloids are removed by washing before packaging. One review article advised against taking borage with other hepatotoxic drugs (anabolic steroids, phenothiazines, ketoconazole) (33).

- Little is known about herb-drug interactions. According to a recent review, evening primrose oil and borage seed oil may lower the seizure threshold, thus interfering with anticonvulsant medications. Neither oil should be used concomitantly with other drugs known to lower the seizure threshold (tricyclic antidepressants and phenothiazines) (33).

- Some reports of nausea, soft stools, belching, and bloating have been associated with GLA (1).

- Toxicity studies in dogs, mice, rats and rabbits providing 400 mg to 800 mg GLA from evening primrose oil/kg/day for up to two years showed no toxic or carcinogenic effects compared to corn oil (34, 35).

REFERENCES

1. Fan YY, Chapkin RS. Importance of dietary gamma-linolenic acid in human health and nutrition. *J Nutr*. 1998;128:1411–1414.
2. Horrobin DF. Nutritional and medical importance of gamma-linolenic acid. *Prog Lipid Res*. 1992;31:163–194.
3. Joe LA, Hart LL. Evening primrose oil in rheumatoid arthritis. *Ann Pharmacother*. 1993;27:1475–1477.
4. Brzeski M, Madhok R, Capell HA. Evening primrose oil in patients with rheumatoid arthritis and side-effects of nonsteroidal anti-inflammatory drugs. *Br J Rheumatol*. 1991;30:370–372.
5. Jantti J, Nikkari T, Solakivi T, et al. Evening primrose oil in rheumatoid arthritis: changes in serum lipids and fatty acids. *Ann Rheum Dis*. 1989;48:124–127.
6. Martens-Lobenhoffer J, Meyer FP. Phamacokinetic data of gamma-linolenic acid in healthy volunteers after the administration of evening primrose oil (Epogam). *Int J Clin Pharmacol Ther*. 1998;36:363–366.
7. Quoc KP, Pascaud M. Effects of dietary gamma-linolenic acid on the tissue phospholipid fatty acid composition and the synthesis of eicosanoids in rats. *Ann Nutr Metab*. 1996;40:99–108.
8. Horrobin DF, Manku MS, Brush M, et al. Abnormalities in plasma essential fatty acid levels in women with premenstrual syndrome and with nonmalignant breast disease. *J Nutr Med*. 1991;2:259–264.
9. Gateley CA, Maddox PR, Pritchard GA, et al. Plasma fatty acid profiles in benign breast disorders. *Br J Surg*. 1992;79:407–409.
10. Budeiri D, Li Wan Po A, Dornan JC. Is evening primrose oil of value in the treatment of premenstrual syndrome? *Control Clin Trials*. 1996;17:60–68.
11. Khoo SK, Munro C, Battistutta D. Evening primrose oil and treatment of premenstrual syndrome. *Med J Aust*. 1990;153:189–192.
12. Mansel RE, Harrison BJ, Melhuish J, et al. A randomized trial of dietary intervention with essential fatty acids in patients with categorized cysts. *Ann N Y Acad Sci*. 1990;586:288–294.
13. Chenoy R, Hussain S, Tayob Y, et al. Effect of oral gamolenic acid from evening primrose oil on menopausal flushing. *BMJ*. 1994;308:501–503.
14. Leventhal LJ, Boyce EG, Zurier RB. Treatment of rheumatoid arthritis with black currant seed oil. *Br J Rheumatol*. 1994;33:847–852.
15. Leventhal LJ, Boyce EG, Zurier RB. Treatment of rheumatoid arthritis with gamma-linolenic acid. *Ann Intern Med*. 1993;119:867–873.
16. Belch JJ, Ansell D, Madhok R, et al. Effects of altering dietary essential fatty acids on requirements for nonsteroidal anti-inflammatory drugs in patients with rheumatoid arthritis: a double blind placebo controlled study. *Ann Rheum Dis*. 1988;47:96–104.

17. Tate G, Mandell BF, Laposata M, et al. Suppression of acute and chronic inflammation by dietary gamma linolenic acid. *J Rheumatol.* 1989;16:729–734.
18. Henz BM, Jablonska S, Van De Kerkhof, PC, et al. Double-blind, multi-center analysis of the efficacy of borage oil in patients with atopic eczema. *Br J Dermatol.* 1999;140:685–688.
19. Whitaker DK, Cilliers J, de Beer C. Evening primrose oil (Epogam) in the treatment of chronic hand dermatitis: disappointing therapeutic results. *Dermatology.* 1996; 193:115–120.
20. Morse PF, Horrobin DF, Manku MS, et al. Meta-analysis of placebo-controlled studies of the efficacy of Epogam in the treatment of atopic eczema. Relationship between plasma essential fatty acid changes and clinical response. *Br J Dermatol.* 1989;121:75–90.
21. Hederos CA, Berg A. Epogam evening primrose oil treatment in atopic dermatitis and asthma. *Arch Dis Child.* 1996;75:494–497.
22. Oliwiecki S, Burton JL. Evening primrose oil and marine oil in the treatment of psoriasis. *Clin Exp Dermatol.* 1994;19:127–129.
23. Keen H, Payan J, Allawi J, et al. Treatment of diabetic neuropathy with gamma-linolenic acid. The Gamma Linolenic Acid Multicenter Trial Group. *Diabetes Care.* 1993;16:8–15.
24. Horrobin DF. Essential fatty acids in the management of impaired nerve function in diabetes. *Diabetes.* 1997;46(suppl 2):S90–S93.
25. Julu PO. Latency of neuroactivity and optimum period of treatment with evening primrose oil in diabetic rats. *J Lipid Mediat Cell Signal.* 1996;13:99–113.
26. Cameron NE, Cotter MA, Robertson S. Essential fatty acid diet supplementation. Effects on peripheral nerve and skeletal muscle function and capillarization in streptozocin-induced diabetic rats. *Diabetes.* 1991;40:532–539.
27. Deferne JL, Leeds AR. Resting blood pressure and cardiovascular reactivity to mental arithmetic in mild hypertensive males supplemented with black currant seed oil. *J Hum Hypertens.* 1996;10:531–537.
28. Ishikawa T, Fujiyama Y, Igarashi O, et al. Effects of gammalinolenic acid on plasma lipoproteins and apolipoproteins. *Atherosclerosis.* 1989;75:95–104.
29. Boberg M, Vessby B, Selinus I. Effects of dietary supplementation with n-6 and n-3 long-chain polyunsaturated fatty acids on serum lipoproteins and platelet function in hyper-triglyceridaemic patients. *Acta Med Scand.* 1986;220;153–160.
30. De La Cruz JP, Martin-Romero M, Carmona JA, et al. Effect of evening primrose oil on platelet aggregation in rabbits fed an atherogenic diet. *Thromb Res.* 1997;87:141–149.
31. Engler MM. Comparative study of diets enriched with evening primrose, black currant, borage, or fungal oils on blood pressure and pressor responses in spontaneously hypertensive rats. *Prostaglandins Leukot Essent Fatty Acids.* 1993;49:809–814.
32. Kenny FS, Pinder SE, Ellis IO, et al. Gamma linolenic acid with tamoxifen as primary therapy in breast cancer. *Int J Cancer.* 2000;85:643–648.
33. Miller LG. Herbal medicinals. Selected clinical considerations focusing on known or potential drug-herb interactions. *Arch Intern Med.* 1998;158:2200–2211.
34. Everett DJ, Greenough RJ, Perry CJ, et al. Chronic toxicity studies of Efamol evening primrose oil in rats and dogs. *Med Sci Res.* 1988;16:863–864.

35. Everett DJ, Perry CJ, Bayliss P. Carcinogenicity studies of Efamol evening primrose oil in rats and mice. *Med Sci Res.* 1988;16:865–866.

Gamma-Oryzanol (Phytosterols)

Gamma-oryzanol is a lipid fraction derived from rice bran oil. Oryzanol was first isolated from rice bran oil in the 1950s. A number of lipid fractions were isolated from the oil. The third (gamma) fraction isolated was oryzanol (2). It is made up of a mixture of ferulic acid esters and plant sterols (1). Similar in structure to cholesterol, the phytosterols and triterpenes that compose oryzanol include campesterol, stigmasterol, β-sitosterol, cycloartanol, and cycloartenol (2). Because phytosterols are poorly absorbed, it has been suggested that they may reduce blood cholesterol by inhibiting intestinal cholesterol absorption. In contrast, the ferulic acid portion of gamma-oryzanol is easily absorbed into the body's tissues. Ferulic acid has also demonstrated antioxidant properties *in vitro* (3–8).

Media and Marketing Claims	Efficacy
Lowers cholesterol	NR
Anabolic agent—converted into testosterone and growth hormone for bulking up	↓
Reduces oxidative stress during exercise	NR

Advisory

No reported serious adverse effects

Drug/Supplement Interactions

No reported adverse interactions

KEY POINTS

- Preliminary evidence from uncontrolled human trials and animal studies suggest that gamma-oryzanol has a potential beneficial effect on serum lipids. However, well-controlled clinical trials of gamma-oryzanol or ferulic acid supplements in humans are required before recommendations can be made.

- There is no evidence that gamma-oryzanol builds muscle by acting as an anabolic agent. In fact, one review suggested that it has the opposite effect (2). However, because absorption of phytosterols is limited, it is unlikely to have a detrimental effect on body mass.

- Although gamma-oryzanol has demonstrated antioxidant potential *in vitro* (3–8), there is no research specifically testing whether gamma-oryzanol supplements reduce oxidative stress *in vivo* caused by exercise in humans.

G

FOOD SOURCES

Gamma-oryzanol is found in rice bran oil, which is commercially available in Japan for use in salad oils and frying. The crude rice bran oil contains approximately 1.56 percent oryzanol. Of the 180 mg of plant sterols found in the typical American diet, about 4 percent is gamma-oryzanol (2). One cup of brown rice provides 18 mg, whereas white rice provides 4 mg gamma-oryzanol (2). The ferulic acid portion of gamma-oryzanol is naturally found in the bran of cereals, and in fruits and vegetables. Ferulic acid is also a metabolite of caffeic acid found in coffee (1).

DOSAGE INFORMATION/BIOAVAILABILITY

Gamma-oryzanol supplements are sold in capsules or tablets in doses ranging from 100 mg to 500 mg. Ferulic acid and rice bran oil concentrate capsules are also available as separate supplements. Phytosterols are poorly absorbed, with less than 5 percent taken up by the intestinal tract after ingestion (2).

RELEVANT RESEARCH

Gamma-Oryzanol and Cholesterol

- In an uncontrolled study, 20 chronic schizophrenic patients with dyslipidemia were given 300 mg gamma-oryzanol divided into three doses for 16 weeks. There were statistically significant decreases in total cholesterol (from 204 mg/dL to 176 mg/dL) and LDL cholesterol (from 124 mg/dL to 101 mg/dL), but not HDL levels. Apolipoprotein B decreased (from 116 mg/dL to 101 mg/dL) significantly and apolipoprotein A-II levels (from 31.7 mg/dL to 34.7 mg/dL) increased significantly (9). The results of this study should be viewed with caution because the design was not double-blinded or placebo-controlled, nor was dietary intake controlled.

- In an uncontrolled study, 80 patients with hyperlipidemia were given 300 mg gamma-oryzanol daily for six months. In type IIa and IIb hypercholesterolemic subjects, plasma cholesterol fell by 12 percent and 13 percent, respectively in the first month. The drop was significant only after three months. Plasma triglycerides significantly decreased in all subjects after three months. There was an insignificant trend for HDL cholesterol to increase (10). The results of this study should be viewed with caution because the design was not double-blinded or placebo-controlled.

- Several animal studies have shown a hypolipidemic effect of feeding gamma-oryzanol (0.5 percent to 1.0 percent of the diet) to rats, mice, and hamsters (1, 11–13). However, in one study using rats, 100 mg/kg gamma oryzanol and cycloartenol ferulic acid ester daily for 6 or 12 days did not prevent hyperlipidemia induced by high cholesterol feedings. When the treatment was given intravenously, there was a significant inhibition in serum total cholesterol (14).

Gamma-Oryzanol and Muscle Mass

- In a double-blind, placebo-controlled study, 22 weight-trained men were supplemented with 500 mg gamma-oryzanol or a placebo for nine weeks. Strength tests were taken before the study, and after four and nine weeks of a resistance exercise program. There were no significant differences between groups in one-repetition maximum muscular strength (bench press and squat) and vertical jump power. There were also no differences in testosterone, cortisol, estradiol, growth hormone, insulin, beta-endorphin, calcium, magnesium, albumin, or blood lipids. No differences between groups existed in resting cardiovascular variables. The authors concluded: "These data suggest that nine weeks of 500 mg/day of gamma-oryzanol supplementation do not influence performance or related physiological parameters in moderately weight-trained males" (15).

- One review article cites several animal studies that are suggestive of an antianabolic or catabolic effect of gamma-oryzanol. Specifically, intravenous or subcutaneous injections of phytosterols have been shown to suppress luteinizing hormone release, reduce growth hormone synthesis and release, and increase release of catecholamines, dopamine, and norepinephrine in the brain. Although it was not directly tested, the authors suggested that this hormone profile may actually reduce testosterone production (2).

SAFETY

- A study of mice fed 0 mg, 200 mg, 600 mg, or 2,000 mg gamma-oryzanol/kg body weight/day for 78 weeks showed no adverse events on general condition, body weight, food consumption, mortality, organ weight, or hematology. There were no differences in tumor incidence (16).

- There are no long-term studies on the safety of gamma-oryzanol supplementation in humans.

REFERENCES

1. de Deckere EA, Korver O. Minor constituents of rice bran oil as functional foods. *Nutr Rev.* 1996;54(11 pt 2):S120–S126.
2. Wheeler KB, Garleb KA. Gamma-oryzanol-plant sterol supplementation: metabolic, endocrine, and physiologic effects. *Int J Sport Nutr.* 1991;1:170–177.
3. Graf E. Antioxidant potential of ferulic acid. *Free Radic Biol Med.* 1992;13:435–448.
4. Garica-Conesa MT, Plumb GW, Waldron KW, et al. Ferulic acid dehydrodimers from wheat bran: isolation, purification, and antioxidant properties of 8-O-4-diferulic acid. *Redox Rep.* 1997;3:319–323.
5. Kim SJ, Han D, Moon KD, et al. Measurement of superoxide dismutase-like activity of natural antioxidants. *Biosci Biotechnol Biochem.* 1995;59:822–826.
6. Ohta T, Nakano T, Egashira Y, et al. Antioxidant activity of ferulic acid beta-glucuronide in the LDL oxidation system. *Biosci Biotechnol Biochem.* 1997;61:1942–1943.

7. Bourne LC, Rice-Evans CA. The effect of the phenolic antioxidant ferulic acid on the oxidation of low density lipoprotein depends on the pro-oxidant used. *Free Radic Res.* 1997;27:337–344.

8. Castelluccio C, Bolwell GP, Gerrish C, et al. Differential distribution of ferulic acid to the major plasma constituents in relation to its potential as an antioxidant. *Biochem J.* 1996;316(pt 2):691–694.

9. Sasaki J, Takada Y, Handa K, et al. Effects of gamma-oryzanol on serum lipids and apolipoproteins in dyslipidemic schizophrenics receiving major tranquilizers. *Clin Ther.* 1990;12:263–268.

10. Yoshino G, Kazumi T, Amano M, et al. Effects of gamma-oryzanol and probucol on hyperlipidemia. *Curr Ther Res.* 1989;45:975–982.

11. Rong N, Ausman LM, Nicolosi RJ. Oryzanol decreases cholesterol absorption and aortic fatty streaks in hamsters. *Lipids.* 1997;32:303–309.

12. Rukmini C, Raghuram TC. Nutritional and biochemical aspects of the hypolipidemic action of rice bran oil: a review. *J Am Coll Nutr.* 1991;10:593–601.

13. Seetharamaiah GS, Chandrasekhara N. Studies on hypocholesterolemic activity of rice bran oil. *Atherosclerosis.* 1989;78:219–223.

14. Sugano M, Tsuji E. Rice bran oil and cholesterol metabolism. *J Nutr.* 1997;127:521S–524S.

15. Fry AC, Bonner E, Lewis DL, et al. The effects of gamma-oryzanol supplementation during resistance exercise training. *Int J Sport Nutr.* 1997;7:318–329.

16. Tamagawa M, Otaki Y, Takahashi T, et al. Carcinogenicity study of gamma-oryzanol in B6C3F1 mice. *Food Chem Toxicol.* 1992;30:49–56.

Garlic

Garlic (*Allium sativum*), one of the top ten-selling herbal supplements in the United States, has been cultivated for medicinal and culinary purposes for 5,000 years. In Germany, garlic supplements are approved as a nonprescription medicine to lower blood cholesterol and reduce other cardiovascular risk factors. Of recent interest are the sulfur-containing compounds (S-allyl cysteine [SAC], S-allyl mercaptocysteine [SAMC], allicin, alliin, and diallyl polysulfides) that are considered to be the primary active agents in garlic. Other active components such as ajoene (produced from the combination of allicin and diallyl disulfide) also have been examined. Numerous studies have focused on the effect of garlic on hyperlipidemia, hypertension, platelet aggregability, cancer, and bacterial and fungal diseases (1–3).

Media and Marketing Claims	Efficacy
Lowers cholesterol	↑?
Controls blood pressure	↑?
Improves circulation	↑?
Reduces risk of cancer	↑?
Antibiotic, antifungal, antibacterial, antiparasitic, antiviral properties	↔

Advisory

- May cause gastrointestinal discomfort in some people
- Raw or enteric coated garlic may irritate intestinal lining; contraindicated in individuals having gastrointestinal diseases
- Should be avoided at least seven days prior to surgery due to potential increased bleeding

Drug/Supplement Interactions

- May increase bleeding when taken with other blood-thinning drugs or supplements (eg, coumadin, warfarin, ginger, ginkgo, vitamin E, flaxseed, bromelain, dong quai, fish oil, aspirin); should be monitored by a physician
- May decrease the concentration of the HIV drug saquinavir (Fortovase)

KEY POINTS

G

- Limited meta-analyses have suggested that garlic supplements reduce cholesterol and blood pressure compared to a placebo. However, the authors of the meta-analyses criticized a number of the studies included in the analysis for methodological limitations. For example, comparing the various garlic formulations (fresh, dried, powdered, oil, aged) and dosages is difficult. Additionally, blinding is difficult because of the characteristic smell in even "odor-free" preparations. Additional well-controlled, larger clinical trials are needed before garlic supplements are considered adjunctive treatment for cardiovascular disease

- One meta-analysis reported that standardized dried garlic powder supplements resulted in a mild blood pressure reduction. The authors of the meta-analysis concluded: "There is insufficient evidence at present to recommend garlic as an effective antihypertensive agent for routine clinical use. However, there is equally no evidence to suggest it is harmful, and the currently available data strongly support the likelihood of dried garlic powder therapy being beneficial for the lowering of lipid levels, and possibly against mild hypertension, at least in the short term" (4). Additional well-controlled trials are needed to verify the results of these studies.

- There is evidence that garlic (aged extract and dried powder) may reduce platelet aggregation and improve microcirculation in subjects with arterial disease. There is also preliminary evidence from studies with very small numbers of subjects suggesting that garlic enhances microcirculation in healthy individuals. More research is needed with larger sample sizes.

- Epidemiological studies are conflicting regarding the cancer-protective effects of garlic. Some observational studies show that raw or cooked garlic may reduce cancer risk, with the strongest evidence for stomach and colorectal cancers. Although animal and *in vitro* studies demonstrate anticarcinogenic effects, large-scale intervention studies are needed to determine the effectiveness of garlic supplements against cancer in human subjects.

- Garlic has been used worldwide for centuries as both a topical and oral antibacterial, antifungal, and antiviral agent. *In vitro* studies have demonstrated these properties, whereas one preliminary study of 12 subjects reported that high levels of raw garlic (10 cloves) had no effect on treatment of *Helicobacter pylori* infection (5). Controlled human studies testing the effectiveness of garlic supplements in treating the common cold, flu, or herpes virus are needed.

- The amount of garlic (equivalent to one to two raw cloves) used in most studies can be easily consumed in the diet. However, cooking garlic may destroy some of its active compounds.

FOOD SOURCES

Garlic cloves and powder (1 raw clove ≈ 3 grams—most studies used the equivalent of 2 g to 5 g raw garlic) (6). Crushing raw garlic and then allowing it to sit for 10 minutes helps retain some of the biologically active compounds that are normally destroyed when heated (7).

DOSAGE INFORMATION/BIOAVAILABILITY

Garlic powder, oil, and garlic aged in aqueous-alcoholic extract are available in capsules or enteric-coated pills. Garlic is also sold in "deodorized," "odor-free," or "odor-controlled" preparations. Most studies have used 400 mg to 1,200 mg dried powder equivalent to about 2 g to 5 g fresh garlic (one to two cloves) or 1 g to 7.2 g aged garlic extract. Some garlic manufacturers state that their supplements are standardized to 1.3 percent or 10 mg allicin or have "allicin potential." There has been some controversy regarding whether allicin must be present for supplements to be biologically active. Numerous sulfur-containing compounds, as well as some nonsulfur compounds, appear to contribute to the potential beneficial effects of garlic. Although some suggest that allicin activity may be important for cholesterol-lowering, it may not be important for anticarcinogenic properties. However, since its discovery in 1944, allicin has been known to be a highly unstable compound formed by crushing the bulb, which quickly decomposes and is transformed into other sulfur compounds (8–10). Allicin does not appear to be absorbed by the gastrointestinal tract, and has been shown to break down rapidly when administered intravenously (9, 11). In contrast, SAC was found to be rapidly absorbed and distributed in the plasma, liver, and kidney in rats, mice, and dogs (12).

RELEVANT RESEARCH

Garlic's Effect on Cholesterol Control and Atherogenesis

- A meta-analysis of 13 randomized, double-blind, placebo-controlled trials of subjects with hypercholesterolemia (n = 796 subjects) found that garlic significantly reduced total cholesterol levels from baseline compared to placebo. Six diet-controlled trials with the highest scores for methodologic quality revealed a nonsignificant difference between garlic and placebo groups (13).

- A meta-analysis of 16 trials (n = 952 subjects) compared the pooled mean difference in the change of total serum cholesterol, triglycerides, and HDL cholesterol among subjects treated with garlic therapy (powder, fresh, oil, or aged extract) and those treated with a placebo or another agent in trials lasting a minimum of four weeks. The analysis revealed a statistically significant 12 percent average reduction in total cholesterol (–0.77 mmol/L) with garlic therapy (dried powder, fresh, oil, aged extract) beyond the levels achieved with placebo. In the dried garlic powders, there were no significant differences in the size of reduction across the dose range of 600 mg to 900 mg (estimated to be equivalent to 1.8 g to 2.7 g fresh garlic) daily. Dried garlic powders also significantly reduced triglyceride levels (–0.3 mmol/L) compared to the placebo. Despite these positive results, the authors acknowledged that many of the trials had methodological shortcomings (failure to provide information on randomization or use an intention-to-treat analysis. Two trials had an open-design (not controlled) and two trials were single-blind (14).

- Another meta-analysis selected 5 of 28 garlic trials (4 trials double-blind, all placebo-controlled or parallel-group design; n = 365 subjects having elevated cholesterol) and found a significant 9 percent reduction in cholesterol following ingestion of garlic (garlic powder and liquid aged garlic extract). None of the studies monitored or controlled dietary intake. Twenty-three studies were excluded from the analysis for not providing adequate data, lacking randomization, and/or lacking proper controls. The dosages used in the studies, 600 mg to 1,000 mg, were estimated to be equivalent to one-half to one fresh clove/day (15).

- In a double-blind, placebo-controlled trial, 46 mildly to moderately hypercholesterolemic patients who had failed or were not compliant with drug therapy were randomized to receive enteric-coated garlic powder capsules (9.6 mg allicin-releasing potential) or a placebo daily for 12 weeks. All subjects were given dietary counseling to lower fat intake. Garlic supplementation was associated with a significant reduction in total cholesterol and LDL cholesterol. The placebo group had a nonsignficant increase in levels of triglycerides and LDL cholesterol. Interestingly, HDL cholesterol was significantly increased in the placebo group, but not in the garlic group (16).

- In a double-blind, placebo-controlled study, 50 patients with hypercholesterolemia were randomized to receive 900 mg garlic powder divided into three doses or a placebo daily for 12 weeks. The authors noted that the amount of powder used was equivalent to 2.7 g or approximately one clove of fresh garlic/day. There were no significant changes in levels of total cholesterol, triglycerides, LDL cholesterol, or HDL cholesterol with either treatment or between groups (17).

- In a double-blind, placebo-controlled trial, 25 patients with moderate hypercholesterolemia were randomized to receive 10 mg steam-distilled garlic oil divided into two doses or a placebo daily for 12 weeks. Garlic oil had no effect on serum lipoproteins, cholesterol absorption, or cholesterol synthesis (18). However, this study has been criticized for using steam-distilled garlic oil, which is not is not thought to be as active as other garlic preparations and for choosing a brand of garlic oil that was not readily dissolved or absorbed (19).

G

- In a double-blind, placebo-controlled trial, 115 subjects with elevated cholesterol were randomly assigned to receive 900 mg/day of dried garlic powder or a placebo for six months. Compared to the placebo, garlic had no significant effect on cholesterol (total, LDL, HDL), triglycerides, lipoproteins, or apolipoprotein A1 or B. This study was in contrast to the authors' 1994 meta-analysis (14), which showed that garlic was effective in lowering total cholesterol. The authors suggested that this difference may be because of publication bias, overestimation of treatment effects in trials with inadequate masking of treatment allocation, or a type 2 error. They concluded that "meta-analyses should be interpreted critically and with particular caution if the constituent trials are small" (20).

- In a double-blind, placebo-controlled, crossover study, 41 moderately hypercholesterolemic men were given in random order 7.2 g aged garlic extract or a placebo daily for six months before switching treatments for four additional months. All subjects were advised to follow a Step I cholesterol-reducing diet during the study. Vital signs, body weight, blood chemistry, and liver function tests were monitored throughout the study. Aged garlic extract resulted in a statistically significant 6.1 percent to 7.0 percent reduction in serum total cholesterol compared to the placebo phase and baseline evaluation. LDL cholesterol was decreased 4.6 percent compared to the placebo. In addition, the garlic extract produced a significant 5.5 percent decrease is systolic blood pressure compared to placebo and baseline. There were no significant changes in HDL cholesterol, triglycerides, or diastolic blood pressure (21).

- Other animal and *in vitro* studies have reported that aged garlic extract suppressed the development of atherosclerosis in rabbits fed high-cholesterol diets (22), inhibited oxidation of LDL cholesterol (23), protected against oxidation of vascular endothelial cells (24), and enhanced glutathione and superoxide dismutase levels in vascular endothelial cells (25).

- *See* Fish Oil for studies testing garlic and fish oil combinations in hyperlipidemic subjects.

Garlic's Effect on Blood Pressure and Cardiac Elasticity

- In a meta-analysis, eight randomized, controlled trials testing the effect of garlic on blood pressure (n = 415 subjects) lasting at least four weeks were assessed. Only three of eight studies included subjects with hypertension and all studies used the same dried garlic powder preparation in doses ranging from 600 mg to 900 mg daily (equivalent to 1.8 g to 2.7 g fresh garlic). Three of seven trials that were placebo-controlled reported a statistically significant reduction in systolic blood pressure with garlic. The overall pooled mean difference in systolic blood pressure (7.7 mm Hg) was greater in subjects taking garlic than those treated with placebo. For diastolic blood pressure, four of seven trials reported significant reductions with garlic therapy compared to the placebo. The pooled mean difference between garlic and placebo was 5.0 mm Hg for this measure. The authors concluded that garlic powder preparations were safe and may be of some benefit in subjects with mild hypertension, but that "there is still insufficient evidence to recommend it as routine clinical therapy for the treatment of hypertensive subjects" (4).

■ In a cross-sectional, observational study, 101 healthy, normotensive adults who were taking > 300 mg/day standardized garlic powder for two or more years were paired with 101 age- and sex-matched controls. Blood pressure, heart rate, and plasma lipids were similar between groups. Measures of aortic stiffness (pulse wave velocity and pressure-standardized elastic vascular resistance) were lower in the garlic group (26).

Garlic and Platelet Function

■ Fifteen subjects selected from the larger sample of 41 moderately hypercholesterolemic men (double-blind, placebo-controlled, crossover study) were examined for the effects of garlic on platelet adhesion (21). Blood samples from 10 of the subjects were available for analysis. Subjects supplemented with 7.2 g aged garlic extract daily showed a significant reduction of epinephrine- and collagen-induced platelet aggregation *ex vivo*, but no inhibition of adenosine diphosphate-induced aggregation. Platelet adhesion to fibrinogen decreased by 30 percent and a decrease in *ex vivo* lipoprotein oxidation occurred during garlic supplementation compared to the placebo period. The authors concluded: "AGE [aged garlic extract] administration can produce an inhibition of some of the platelet functions important for initiating thromboembolic events in the arterial circulation" (27).

■ In a double-blind, placebo-controlled study, 80 patients with peripheral arterial occlusive disease stage II were randomized to receive 800 mg garlic powder or a placebo for 12 weeks. The use of other therapeutic drugs was not permitted. Garlic intake resulted in a significant increase (+31 m) in walking distance when compared to the placebo group. The effect appeared at the fifth week of the study. There was a significant decrease in diastolic blood pressure, spontaneous thrombocyte aggregation, plasma viscosity, and blood cholesterol levels with garlic therapy. The authors concluded: "Garlic may be an appropriate agent especially for the long-term treatment of incipient intermittent claudication" (28).

■ In a double-blind, placebo-controlled study, 60 subjects with cerebrovascular risk factors including increased platelet aggregation were randomized to receive 800 mg enteric-coated powdered garlic or a placebo for four weeks. Garlic ingestion led to a significant inhibition of the increased ratio of circulating platelet aggregates and of spontaneous platelet aggregation. There were no significant changes in the placebo group. After a four-week washout phase, the ratio of circulating platelet aggregates and spontaneous platelet aggregation increased to initial values (run-in phase prior to garlic supplementation). The authors concluded: "Since garlic is well tolerated it would be worthwhile testing it in a controlled clinical trial for usefulness in preventing disease manifestations associated with platelet aggregation" (29).

■ In a double-blind, placebo-controlled study, 14 healthy subjects were randomly assigned to receive 85 mg garlic extract capsules (equivalent to 15 g raw garlic) or a placebo daily for six days. The effects of the same garlic preparation on platelet aggregation *in vitro* were also tested. Garlic supplements had no effect on platelet aggregation as tested by adenosine diphosphate, platelet-activating factor, and collagen. When tested *in vitro*, aggregation decreased with increasing amounts of garlic extract. However, the authors noted that concentrations *in vitro* were higher than attainable *in vivo* because of gastrointestinal pain associated with higher doses of garlic in this trial (30).

- In a double-blind, placebo-controlled, crossover study, 10 healthy subjects were randomized to receive a dose of 900 mg garlic powder/day or a placebo in random order with a two-week washout period between phases. The garlic or a placebo was administered after one hour of rest in a laboratory setting. No food or drink was permitted during the observation. Hemodynamic parameters (blood pressure and heart rate) and microcirculatory parameters (erythrocyte velocity in skin capillaries in the margin of the nail fold, capillary blood flow calculated by the diameter, and mean erythrocyte velocity) were measured before and after administration of the garlic or a placebo. Five hours after garlic administration, there was a 55 percent significant increase in mean erythrocyte velocity in the arterial capillary branch and a 45 percent increase in capillary blood flow compared to the baseline. During placebo administration, erythrocyte velocity and capillary blood flow did not change. Blood pressure and heart rate were not affected with either treatment (31).

Garlic and Cancer

- The epidemiological studies on garlic consumption and cancer risk are conflicting. Stomach cancer risk was 13 times lower for Chinese subjects consuming 20 g garlic/day than for those who ate less than 1 g/day. In the Iowa Women's Health Study, a reduced colon cancer risk was seen in women who ate garlic more than once a week (32). However, the Netherlands large-scale, prospective cohort study reported that self-reported intake of garlic supplements was not associated with a reduced risk of breast (33), colon (34), or lung cancer (35).

- A review of epidemiological studies reported that garlic (not supplemental) consumption is most strongly associated with a reduction in stomach and colorectal cancers, but that garlic pills do not appear to reduce cancer risk at any site. However, the researchers noted limitations of observational studies and emphasized the need for intervention trials (36).

- One review article cited several animal and *in vitro* studies showing a protective effect of garlic on breast, uterine, esophageal, skin, colon, stomach, bladder, prostate, and lung cancers' cell lines. The author noted that the benefits of garlic were not limited to a specific species, tissue, or carcinogen. Overall, S-allyl cysteine (SAC), a water-soluble compound, was effective in reducing the risk of chemically induced tumors in experimental animals but had no effect on established tumors. In contrast, oil-soluble compounds such as diallyl disulfide were effective in reducing the proliferation of neoplasms (32).

Garlic and Infection

- In a prospective, crossover study, 12 *Helicobacter pylori*-infected adults received test meals three times, consisting of beef, tortillas, and salad with one of the following: (1) 10 sliced, raw garlic cloves; (2) 6 sliced, fresh jalapeno peppers; (3) Pepto-Bismol (always administered last because of its ability to inhibit *H. pylori*; (4) no added drug.

At least two days elapsed between administration of each test. Urea breath-testing to evaluate the effectiveness of anti-*H. pylori* therapy was done before the first meal, the evening meal, and the following morning. Neither garlic nor jalapeno peppers had any *in vivo* effect on *H. pylori* infection (5).

- In an *in vitro* study, garlic extract exerted a dose-dependent antiviral effect against human cytomegalovirus (37).

- Another *in vitro* study garlic extract demonstrated virucidal activity against herpes simplex virus types 1 and 2, parainfluenza virus type 3, vaccinia virus, vesicular stomatitis virus, and human rhinovirus type 2 (38).

- The growth of *Candida albicans* yeast cells was inhibited by the presence of garlic extract in an *in vitro* study. The author hypothesized that anticandidal properties may be because of oxidization of thiol groups in garlic extract that inactivate enzymes and slow microbial growth (39).

SAFETY

- Garlic supplements in most studies are relatively well-tolerated with the only reported side-effects being mild gastrointestinal discomfort at high doses. One harmless side-effect is the presence of undesirable body odor even in some odor-free varieties. However, garlic applied topically has been associated with dermatitis and burns (40).

- Different garlic preparations have different effects on intestinal mucosa. One animal study reported that dried raw garlic powder caused significant damage to gut mucosa, dried boiled garlic powder caused reddening of the mucosa, and aged garlic extract had no deleterious effects (41).

- The safety of enteric-coated garlic products (designed to pass through the stomach and deposit garlic compounds in intestine) is questionable. In one study, enteric-coated garlic supplements caused a loss of epithelial cells at the top of crypts in the ileum and reddening of the gut mucosa (41).

- Toxicity studies of aged garlic extract reported no growth retardation, stomach injuries, changes in red blood cell counts, or morphological abnormalities in rats supplemented with 5 mL/kg aged garlic extract for 3 to 21 days, whereas the same amount of raw garlic juice decreased total serum protein and albumin and caused stomach ulceration (42). Rats given 2,000 mg/kg aged garlic extract five times per week for six months displayed no toxicity of tissues, organs, or cells (43). There was also no evidence of mutagenicity with aged garlic (44).

- An increase in bleeding time was reported in 50 young, healthy subjects supplemented with 10 g of raw garlic daily for two months (approximately three cloves) (45).

- Some researchers have cautioned that preoperative patients should discontinue garlic supplements or dietary use of garlic seven days prior to surgery. Data from *in vitro* and *in vivo* studies indicate that the effects of garlic on platelet function "is undesirable in the surgical patient, especially if taking other antiplatelet agents" (46, 47).

- Due to the effect of garlic on clotting time, patients taking aspirin or other blood thinning medications or supplements should only use garlic supplements after consulting with their physician (46).

- In a small study of 10 healthy subjects, garlic supplements decreased the concentration of the HIV drug saquinavir (Fortovase). It may be advisable for patients taking HIV medications to avoid garlic supplements (48).

REFERENCES

1. Blumenthal M, ed. *The Complete German Commission E Monographs Therapeutic Guide to Herbal Medicines.* Austin, Tex: American Botanical Council; 1998.
2. Abdullah TH, Kandil O, Elkadi A, et al. Garlic revisited: therapeutic for the major diseases of our time? *J Natl Med Assoc.* 1988;80:439–445.
3. Birt DF, Shull JD, Yaktine AL. Chemoprevention of Cancer. In: Shils ME, Olson JA, Shike M, Ross AC, eds. *Modern Nutrition in Health and Disease.* 9th ed. Baltimore, Md: Williams & Wilkins; 1999:1263–1295.
4. Silagy CA, Neil HA. A meta-analysis of the effect of garlic on blood pressure. *J Hypertens.* 1994;12:463–468.
5. Graham DY, Anderson SY, Lang T. Garlic or jalapeno peppers for treatment of Helicobacter pylori infection. *Am J Gastroenterol.* 1999;94:1200–1202.
6. Pennington JAT, ed. *Bowes & Church's Food Values of Portions Commonly Used.* 17th ed. Philadelphia, Pa: Lippincott; 1998.
7. Song K, Milner J. The influence of heating on the anticancer properties of garlic. *J Nutr.* 2001;131:1054S–1057S.
8. Cavallito CJ, Bailey JH. Allicin, the antibacterial principle of *Allium sativum.* Isolation, physical properties, and antibacterial action. *J Am Chem Soc.* 1944;66:1950–1951.
9. Egan-Schwind C, Eckard R, Kemper FH. Metabolism of garlic constituents in the isolated perfused rat liver. *Planta Med.* 1992;58:301–305.
10. Lawson LD, Ransom DK, Hughes BG. Inhibition of whole blood platelet-aggregation by compounds in garlic clove extracts and commercial garlic products. *Thromb Res.* 1992;65:141–156.
11. Freeman F, Kodera Y. Garlic chemistry: stability of s-(2-propenyl)-2-propene-1-sulfinothioate (allicin) in blood, solvents, and simulated physiological fluids. *J Agric Food Chem.* 1995;43:2332–2338.
12. Nagae S, Ushijima M, Hatono S, et al. Pharmacokinetics of the garlic compound S-allylcysteine. *Planta Med.* 1994;60:214–217.
13. Stevinson C, Pittler MH, Ernst E. Garlic for treating hypercholesterolemia: a meta-analysis of randomized clinical trials. *Ann Int Med.* 2000;133:420–429.
14. Silagy C, Neil A. Garlic as a lipid lowering agent—a meta-analysis. *J R Coll Physicians Lond.* 1994;28:39–45.
15. Warshafsky S, Kamer RS, Sivak SL. Effect of garlic on total serum cholesterol: a meta-analysis. *Ann Intern Med.* 1993;119(7 pt 1):599–605.
16. Kannar D, Wattanapenpaiboon N, Savige GS, et al. Hypocholesterolemic effect of an enteric-coated garlic supplement. *J Am Coll Nutr.* 2001;20:225–231.

17. Isaachsohn JL, Moser M, Stein EA, et al. Garlic powder and plasma lipids and lipoproteins: a multicenter, randomized, placebo-controlled trial. *Arch Intern Med.* 1998;158:1189–1194.

18. Berthold HK, Sudhop T, von Bergmann K. Effect of a garlic oil preparation on serum lipoproteins and cholesterol metabolism: a randomized controlled trial. *JAMA.* 1998;279:1900–1902.

19. Lawson LD. Effect of garlic on serum lipids. *JAMA.* 1998;280:1568.

20. Neil HA, Silagy CA, Lancaster T, et al. Garlic powder in the treatment of moderate hyperlipidaemia: a controlled trial and meta-analysis. *J R Coll Physicians Lond.* 1996;30:329–334.

21. Steiner M, Khan AH, Holbert D, et al. A double-blind crossover study in moderately hypercholesterolemic men that compared the effect of aged garlic extract and placebo administration on blood lipids. *Am J Clin Nutr.* 1996;64:866–870.

22. Efendy JL, Simmons DL, Campbell GR, et al. The effect of aged garlic extract, "Kyolic," on the development of experimental atherosclerosis. *Atherosclerosis.* 1997;132:37–42.

23. Ide N, Lau BHS. Garlic compounds inhibit low density lipoprotein (LDL) oxidation and protect endothelial cells from oxidized LDL-induced injury. *FASEB J.* 1997;11:A122.

24. Yamasaki T, Lin L, Lau BHS. Garlic compounds protect vascular endothelial cells from hydrogen peroxide-induced injury. *Phytother* Res. 1994;8:408–412.

25. Geng Z, Lau BHS. Aged garlic extract modulates glutathione redox cycle and superoxide dismutase activity in vascular endothelial cells. *Phytother Res.* 1997;11:54–56.

26. Breithaupt-Grogler K, Ling M, Boudoulas H, et al. Protective effect of chronic garlic intake on elastic properties of aorta in the elderly. *Circulation.* 1997;96:2649–2655.

27. Steiner M, Lin RS. Changes in platelet function and susceptibility of lipoproteins to oxidation associated with administration of aged garlic extract. *J Cardiovasc Pharmacol.* 1998;31:904–905.

28. Kiesewetter H, Jung F, Jung EM, et al. Effects of garlic coated tablets in peripheral arterial occlusive disease. *Clin Investig.* 1993;71:383–386.

29. Kiesewetter H, Jung F, Jung EM, et al. Effect of garlic on platelet aggregation in patients with increased risk of juvenile ischemic attack. *Eur J Clin Pharmacol.* 1993;45:333–336.

30. Morris J, Burke V, Mori TA, et al. Effects of garlic extract on platelet aggregation: a randomized placebo-controlled double-blind study. *Clin Exp Pharmacol Physiol.* 1995;22:414–417.

31. Jung F, Jung EM, Mrowietz C, et al. Influence of garlic powder on cutaneous microcirculation. A randomised, placebo-controlled, double-blind, cross-over study in apparently healthy subjects. *Br J Clin Pract Suppl.* 1990;69:30–35.

32. Milner JA. Garlic: its anticarcinogenic and antitumorgenic properties. *Nutr Rev.* 1996;54(11 pt 2):S82–S86.

33. Dorant E, van den Brandt PA, Goldbohm RA. Allium vegetable consumption, garlic supplement intake, and female breast carcinoma incidence. *Breast Cancer Res Treat.* 1995;33:163–170.

34. Dorant E, van den Brandt PA, Goldbohm RA. A prospective cohort study on the relationship between onion and leek consumption, garlic supplement use and the risk of colorectal carcinoma in The Netherlands. *Carcinogenesis.* 1996;17:477–484.

G

35. Dorant E, van den Brandt PA, Goldbohm RA. A prospective cohort study on allium vegetable consumption, garlic supplement use, and the risk of lung carcinoma in The Netherlands. *Cancer Res.* 1994;54:6148–6153.

36. Fleischauer AT, Arab L. Garlic and cancer: a critical review of the epidemiologic literature. *J Nutr.*2001;131:1032S–1040S.

37. Guo NL, Lu DP, Woods GL, et al. Demonstration of the antiviral activity of garlic extract against human cytomegalovirus in vitro. *Chin Med J (Engl).* 1993;106:93–96.

38. Weber ND, Andersen DO, North JA, et al. *In vitro* virucidal effects of *Allium sativum* (garlic) extract and compounds. *Planta Med.* 1992;58:417–423.

39. Ghannoum MA. Studies on the anticandidal mode of action of *Allium sativum* (garlic). *J Gen Microbiol.* 1988;134(pt 11):2917–2924.

40. Farrell Am, Straughton RC. Garlic burns mimicking herpes zoster. *Lancet.* 1996;347:1195.

41. Hoshino T, Kashimoto N, Kasuga S. Effects of garlic preparations on the gastrointestinal mucosa. *J Nutr.* 2001;131:1109S–1113S.

42. Nakagawa S, Masamoto K, Sumiyoshi H, et al. Effect of raw and extracted-aged garlic juice on growth of young rats and their organs after peroral administration [in Japanese]. *J Toxicol Sci.* 1980;5:91–112.

43. Sumiyoshi H, Kanezawa A, Masamoto K, et al. Chronic toxicity test of garlic extract in rats [in Japanese]. *J Toxicol Sci.* 1984;9:61–75.

44. Yoshida S, Hirao Y, Nakagawa S. Mutagenicity and cytoxicity tests of garlic [in Japanese]. *J Toxicol Sci.* 1984;9:77–86.

45. Gadkari JV, Joshi VD. Effect of ingestion of raw garlic on serum cholesterol level, clotting time, and fibrinolytic activity in normal subjects. *J Postgrad Med.* 1991;37:128–131.

46. Petry JJ. Surgically significant nutritional supplements. *Plast Reconstr Surg.* 1996;97:233–240.

47. Ang-Lee MK, Moss J, Yuan CS. Herbal medicines and perioperative care. *JAMA.* 2001;286:208–216.

48. Piscitelli SC, Burstein AH, Welden N. The effect of garlic supplements on the pharmacokinetics of saquinavir. *Clin Infect Dis.* 2002;34:234–238.

Ginkgo biloba

The leaves of the ginkgo tree have been used in China for centuries. It is one of the most frequently prescribed herbs for cognitive disorders in Germany and is one of the top-selling herbs in the United States (1). *Ginkgo biloba* leaves contain flavonoids, sesquiterpenes, and diterpenes (ginkgolides) that have been identified as possible active ingredients. The flavonoids are thought to act as free-radical scavengers and the ginkgolides may be platelet-activating factor (PAF) antagonists that reduce clotting time (2). Many studies, though not all well-controlled, have been conducted in Europe using a standardized extract of *Ginkgo biloba* (EGb 761).

Media and Marketing Claims	Efficacy
Enhances memory (in Alzheimer's disease patients)	↔
Improves memory and concentration (in healthy individuals)	NR
Improves circulation (in patients having intermittent claudication)	↑?
Strong antioxidant (*in vitro*)	↑

Advisory

Should be avoided at least 36 hours prior to surgery due to potential increased bleeding

Drug/Supplement Interactions

May increase bleeding when taken with other blood thinning drugs or supplements (coumadin, warfarin, garlic, ginger, vitamin E, flaxseed, bromelain, dong quai, fish oil, aspirin); should be monitored by a physician

G

KEY POINTS

- Several studies suggest that ginkgo may slow the progression of dementia, particularly in Alzheimer's disease. However, the positive effect of ginkgo appears to be small. Further, not all studies reported improvements. A physician should be involved in deciding whether to supplement with ginkgo for dementia. New research in healthy individuals suggests that ginkgo supplementation may enhance some aspects of memory. More research is needed to clarify ginkgo's effect on cognitive function in healthy people.

- Preliminary evidence suggests that ginkgo improves walking time and reduces pain in patients with peripheral vascular disease, although blood flow to legs is not improved.

- Preliminary animal and *ex vivo* studies have demonstrated the antioxidant properties of ginkgo on brain neurons.

FOOD SOURCES

None

DOSAGE INFORMATION/BIOAVAILABILITY

Ginkgo biloba is available in tincture, infusions, capsule, or tablet form. The majority of research used a 50:1 concentrated leaf extract standardized to 24 percent ginkgo flavonoid glycosides and 6 percent terpenes (EGb 761). Manufacturers recommend taking 40 mg to 80 mg extract three times daily.

RELEVANT RESEARCH

Ginkgo's Effect on Alzheimer's Disease and Dementia

- Researchers summarized the effects of ginkgo on cognitive function in Alzheimer's patients in a meta-analysis of randomized, placebo-controlled, double-blind design. Of 50 articles reviewed, most did not meet inclusion criteria primarily because of a lack of clear diagnosis. Of the four studies selected (total subjects = 212, lasting three to six months, 120 mg to 230 mg ginkgo), there was a significant effect in favor of ginkgo that translated into a modest 3 percent difference in the Alzheimer Disease Assessment Scale-cognitive subtest (3).

- In a double-blind, placebo-controlled, multicenter trial, 214 subjects with mild to moderate dementia (either Alzheimer's dementia or vascular-related dementia) were randomized to receive a placebo or *Ginkgo biloba* EGb 761 (160 mg or 240 mg) for 12 weeks. After 12 weeks, the initial ginkgo users were randomized again to either continued treatment or to a placebo for another 12 weeks. Outcome measures included neuropsychological testing, clinical assessment, self-perceived health and memory status, and self-reported level of daily life activities. An intention-to-treat analysis showed no effect on each of the outcome measures for subjects taking ginkgo compared to the placebo after 12 or 24 weeks. After 12 and 24 weeks, the combined ginkgo dose groups performed slightly, but significantly, better on self-reported activities of daily life. However, they performed slightly worse in regard to self-perceived health. No beneficial effects of the higher ginkgo dose were observed. Additionally, no subgroups appeared to benefit from ginkgo treatment. No negative side-effects were reported (4).

- In a double-blind, placebo-controlled, multicenter trial, 309 patients older than 45 years with Alzheimer's disease or multi-infarct dementia were randomized to receive 120 mg *Ginkgo biloba* extract tablets (EGb 761) or a placebo daily for 52 weeks. Only 202 subjects completed the study (main reasons for dropout were noncompliance of subjects, caregiver request, and ineffective intervention). At weeks 12, 24, and 52, cognitive impairment, daily living and social behavior, and changes in psychopathology were assessed by the Alzheimer's Disease Assessment Scale (ADAS-Cog), Geriatric Evaluation by Relative's Rating Instrument (GERRI), and the Clinical Global Impression of Change (CGIC), respectively. Regarding cognitive function (ADAS-cog), the placebo group became significantly worse, whereas no significant change was observed in the ginkgo group. Regarding GERRI, a mild improvement was observed for ginkgo subjects, while the placebo group worsened, resulting in a significant difference between groups. There were no differences between groups on CGIC or reported side-effects (not specified). The authors concluded that ginkgo was safe and capable of stabilizing, and in some cases improving, cognitive performance and social function of demented patients for six months to one year (5).

- In a double-blind, placebo controlled study, 216 patients with mild to moderate Alzheimer's disease or multi-infarct dementia were randomized to receive 240 mg *Ginkgo biloba* extract (EGb 761) or a placebo for 24 weeks after a four-week run-in period. Only 156 patients completed the trial. Psychopathological changes, attention and memory, and activities of daily life were variables measured by CGIC, Syndrom-Kurztest (SKT), and Nurnberger Alters-Beobachtungsskala, respectively. Clinical efficacy was defined as a response in at least two of the three variables. A significant clinical response was seen in 28 percent of the ginkgo group compared to 10 percent for the placebo. When patients were analyzed by diagnosis, a greater benefit of ginkgo was seen for Alzheimer's patients than multi-infarct dementia patients (6).

- In a double-blind, placebo-controlled study, 20 outpatients aged 50 y to 80 y with mild to moderate dementia of the Alzheimer's type were randomized to receive 240 mg *Ginkgo biloba* extract (EGb 761) or a placebo for three months. The SKT, ADAS-cog, CGIC psychometric tests and electroencephalograms (EEG) were evaluated at the start and at monthly intervals during the study. Regarding attention and memory (SKT), the ginkgo-treated group had a poorer baseline than the placebo group but experienced a significant improvement after treatment compared to the placebo group, whose scores worsened. There were no significant differences between groups on ADAS-cog, CGIC and EEG findings, although there were insignificant trends of improvement on these parameters (7).

Ginkgo for Memory and Concentration in Healthy People

- In a double-blind, placebo-controlled crossover study, 20 healthy young subjects received one of four treatments in random order: (1) 120 mg ginkgo; (2) 230 mg ginkgo; (3) 360 mg ginkgo; (4) a placebo for one acute dose. Cognitive performance was assessed using the Cognitive Drug Research (CDR) computerized assessment immediately prior to dosing and 1, 2.5, 4, and 6 hours after. The CDR has four primary cognitive factors described as speed of attention, accuracy of attention, speed of memory, and quality of memory. The 240-mg and 360-mg doses of ginkgo significantly improved the speed of attention factor at 2.5 hours through six hours compared to placebo. However, not all performance measures were positive, some indicated that ginkgo had a negative effect on performance (8).

- In a double-blind, placebo-controlled study, 256 healthy, middle-aged subjects were randomized to receive a placebo or a combination of ginkgo and panax ginseng in two dosing regimens (60 mg ginkgo + 100 mg ginseng or 120 mg ginkgo + 200 mg ginseng) for 14 weeks. At baseline and at week s 4, 8, 12 and 14, subjects performed a series of tests of attention and memory from the CDR computerized assessment system prior to morning dosing and again at one, three and six hours later. Subjects also completed questionnaires about mood, quality of life, and sleep quality. The gingko/ginseng mixture significantly improved results on an Index of Memory Quality. However, the design of the study does not identify whether the ginkgo, the ginseng, or the combination of both herbs is responsible for the improvement in memory (9).

- In a double-blind, placebo-controlled study, 48 cognitively healthy subjects (ages 55 y to 86 y) were randomized to receive 180 mg ginkgo extract EGb 761 or a placebo daily for six weeks. Cognitive function was evaluated by a series of neuropsychological tests at baseline and at six weeks. Ginkgo treatment was associated with significant improvement on a task assessing speed of processing abilities (eg, Stroop Color and Word Test color-naming task) compared to use of a placebo. There was a trend favoring improved performances in the ginkgo group in three of the four remaining tasks that involved a timed speed of processing component, but this did not reach statistical significance. In contrast, no improvements were observed with ginkgo in relation to any of the objective memory measures. The subjects' self-assessment of memory significantly improved with use of ginkgo compared to the placebo (10).

- In a double-blind, placebo-controlled study, 31 patients older than 50 y with mild to moderate memory impairment were randomized to receive 120 mg *Gingko biloba* extract (EGb 761) divided into three doses or a placebo daily for six months. Assessments were taken at weeks 0, 12, and 24 using a range of psychometric tests. Gingko had a beneficial effect on cognitive function as demonstrated by statistically significant improvement on the Digit Copying subtest of the Kendrick battery at weeks 12 and 24, and a statistically significant superior effect on the median response speed on a classification task than the placebo at week 24. However, subjects taking ginkgo performed worse over time on the digit recall task compared to the placebo group. The authors hypothesized that the opposing results in the digit recall task may have reflected a change in strategy employed by the patients (11).

- In a double-blind, placebo-controlled, crossover study, eight healthy, female subjects were randomized to receive 120 mg, 240 mg, or 600 mg *Ginkgo biloba* extract and a placebo in random order. Two weeks prior to the test, all subjects underwent training on psychological test procedures. One hour following treatment, subjects completed several psychological tests, subjective ratings of drug effects, and a Sternberg memory scanning test. A reduction in reaction time on the memory scanning test was observed only with the 600-mg dose. There were no significant effects of ginkgo on the other parameters measured (12).

- A systematic review of 40 European trials testing ginkgo extract to improve cerebral insufficiency (characterized by symptoms of concentration and memory difficulties, confusion, fatigue, depression, and anxiety) found that only 8 of the trials were well-controlled. The authors noted that all 40 trials reported positive results and suggested there may have been a publication bias (13).

Ginkgo and Peripheral Vascular Disease

- A meta-analysis of eight randomized, placebo-controlled, double-blinded trials was performed to evaluate the efficacy of ginkgo extract for intermittent claudication. There was a significant difference in the increase in pain-free walking distance in favor of ginkgo (+33 m). The authors concluded that ginkgo "is superior to placebo in the symptomatic treatment of intermittent claudication. However, the overall treatment effect is modest and of uncertain clinical relevance" (14).

- In a double-blind, placebo-controlled, multicenter trial, 111 patients with peripheral occlusive arterial disease (average age = 61 y) were randomized to receive 120 mg *Ginkgo biloba* extract (EGb 761) or a placebo for 24 weeks. The distance of pain-free walking on a treadmill was measured after weeks 0, 8, 16, and 24. Pain-free walking and maximal walking distance were significantly greater in the ginkgo subjects. Doppler studies measuring blood flow were unchanged in both groups. Subjective assessment showed an amelioration of symptoms in both groups (15).

- In a placebo-controlled trial, 37 patients with stage 2 peripheral vascular disease were randomized to receive *Ginkgo biloba* extract (EGb 761) or a placebo daily for six months. Ginkgo-treated subjects had a significant improvement in walking distance compared to the placebo group, which improved insignificantly. Doppler studies did not show any improvement in the perfusion of the ischemic leg (16).

Ginkgo and Antioxidant Properties in the Brain

- Treatment of rats with *Ginkgo biloba* extract one hour before ischemia caused by occlusion of the carotid artery (followed by reperfusion) produced a significant decrease in mitochondrial brain lipid peroxide content compared to control. Ginkgo administration attenuated the decrease in superoxide dismutase after ischemia. The authors concluded: "*Ginkgo biloba* extract could protect the brain against possible ischemic injury induced by free-radical production" (17).

- An *ex vivo* study found that pretreatment of neurons from rats with *Gingko biloba* extract (10 µg/mL) attenuated the death of neurons undergoing oxidative stress from hydrogen peroxide. This effect was less pronounced when the extract was administered immediately or 60 minutes after the start of oxidative injury (18).

- Another *ex vivo* study found *Gingko biloba* extract (EGb 761) inhibited apoptosis in rat neuronal cells caused by hydrogen peroxide. Apoptosis (cell death characterized by shrinkage and DNA fragmentation) is thought to play a central role in the pathogenesis of neurodegenerative diseases. The authors hypothesized that the protective effect of ginkgo was because of the direct scavenging of hydroxyl radicals and to the indirect inhibition of lipid peroxidation (19).

SAFETY

- There are no controlled studies testing the safety of ginkgo supplementation in humans for longer than one year.

- Very seldom mild gastrointestinal upset, headache, or allergic skin rash have been reported (1).

- Because the ginkgolides act as inhibitors of platelet-activating factor, supplementation could affect clotting time. Patients taking anticoagulant medications, aspirin, or vitamin E should discuss ginkgo supplementation with their physician prior to using it (20).

- Surgical patients should discontinue use of ginkgo at least 36 hours before surgery due to potential increase risk of bleeding (20).

- A case report of subdural hematoma was associated with long-term use of *Ginkgo biloba* supplements (21).

REFERENCES

1. Blumenthal M, ed. *The Complete German Commission E Monographs Therapeutic Guide to Herbal Medicines.* Austin, Tex: American Botanical Council; 1998.

2. Smith PF, Maclennan K, Darlington CL. The neuroprotective properties of the *Ginkgo biloba* leaf: a review of the possible relationship to platelet-activating factor (PAF). *J Ethnopharmacol.* 1996;50:131–139.

3. Oken BS, Storzbach DM, Kaye JA. The efficacy of *Ginkgo biloba* on cognitive function in Alzheimer disease. *Arch Neurol.* 1998;55:1409–1415.

4. van Dongen, Martien CJ, van Rossum E, et al. The efficacy of ginkgo for elderly people with dementia and age-associated memory impairment: new results of a randomized clinical trial. *J Am Ger Soc.* 2000;48:1183–1194.

5. Le Bars PL, Katz MM, Berman N, et al. A placebo-controlled, double-blind, randomized trial of an extract of *Ginkgo biloba* for dementia. *JAMA.* 1997;278:1327–1332.

6. Kanowski S, Herrmann WM, Stephan K, et al. Proof of efficacy of the *Ginkgo biloba* special extract EGb 761 in outpatients suffering from mild to moderate primary degenerative dementia of the Alzheimer type or multi-infarct dementia. *Pharmacopsychiatry.* 1996;29:47–56.

7. Maurer K, Ihl R, Dierks T, et al. Clinical efficacy of *Ginkgo biloba* special extract EGB 761 in dementia of the Alzheimer type. *J Psychiatr Res.* 1997;31:645–655.

8. Kennedy DO, Scholey AB, Wesnes KA. The dose-dependent cognitive effects of acute administration of ginkgo biloba to healthy young volunteers. *Psychopharmacology (Berl).* 2000;151:416–423.

9. Wesnes KA, Ward T, McGinty A, et al. The memory enhancing effects of *Ginkgo biloba*/Panax ginseng combination in healthy middle-aged volunteers. *Psychopharmacology (Berl).* 2000;152:353–361.

10. Mix JA, Crews WD. An examination of *Ginkgo biloba* extract EGb 761 on the neuropsychological functioning of cognitively intact older adults. *J Altern Complement Med.* 2000;6:219–229.

11. Rai GS, Shovlin C, Wesnes KA. A double-blind, placebo-controlled study of *Ginkgo biloba* extract ("tanakan") in elderly outpatients with mild to moderate memory impairment. *Curr Med Res Opin.* 1991;12:350–355.

12. Subhan Z, Hindmarch I. The psychopharmacological effects of *Ginkgo biloba* extract in normal healthy volunteers. *Int J Clin Pharmacol Res.* 1984;4:89–93.

13. Kleijnen J, Knipschild P. *Ginkgo biloba* for cerebral insufficiency. *Br J Clin Pharmacol.* 1992;34:352–358.

14. Pittler MH, Ernst E. *Ginkgo biloba* extract for the treatment of intermittent claudication: a meta-analysis of randomized trials. *Am J Med.* 2000;108:276–281.

15. Peters H, Kieser M, Holscher U. Demonstration of the efficacy of *Ginkgo biloba* special extract EGb 761 on intermittent claudication—a placebo-controlled, double-blind multicenter trial. *Vasa.* 1998;27:106–110.

16. Thomson GJ, Vohra RK, Carr MH, et al. A clinical trial of *Ginkgo biloba* extract in patients with intermittent claudication. *Int Angiol.* 1990;9:75–78.

G

17. Seif-El-Nasr M, El-Fattah AA. Lipid peroxide, phospholipids, glutathione levels and superoxide dismutase activity in rat brain after ischemia: effect of *Ginkgo biloba* extract. *Pharmacol Res.* 1995;32:273–278.

18. Oyama Y, Chikahisa L, Ueha T, et al. *Ginkgo biloba* extract protects brain neurons against oxidative stress induced by hydrogen peroxide. *Brain Res.* 1996;712:349–352.

19. Ni Y, Zhao B, Hou J, et al. Preventive effect of *Ginkgo biloba* extract on apoptosis in rat cerebellar neuronal cells induced by hydroxyl radicals. *Neurosci Lett.* 1996;214:115–118.

20. Ang-Lee, Moss J, Yuan CS. Herbal medicines and perioperative care. *JAMA.* 2001;286:208–216.

21. Rowin J, Lewis SL Spontaneous bilateral subdural hematomas associated with chronic *Ginkgo biloba* ingestion. *Neurology.*1996; 46:1775–1776.

Ginseng

Ginseng is the collective term used to describe several species of plants belonging to the genus *Panax*. Asian ginsengs (*Panax ginseng* C.A. Meyer and *Panax japonicus* C.A. Meyer) have been used medicinally for more than 2,000 years in China, Japan, and Korea. American ginseng (*Panax quinquefolius L*) grows in North America and is largely exported to the Orient. Siberian/Russian ginseng (*Eleuthrococcus senticosus*) is not considered a true "ginseng" because it is not in the genus *Panax*. (Although Siberian ginseng [*E senticosus*] is not related botanically to Asian or American ginseng, it is included here because it is often promoted with *Panax ginseng* products.)

The bioactive compounds in the *Panax* plant are believed to be the saponins (or ginsenosides) found in the roots. Several ginsenosides have been identified and are labeled ginsenoside R_x, (where x is a, b_1, b_2, c, d, e, f, g_1, g_2, g_3, h_1, h_2, or o). Eleutherosides that are believed to be the active agents in Siberian ginseng, have different chemical structures than do ginsenosides. Ginseng plants contain varying levels of several different saponins that appear to exert opposing pharmacological effects. It has been proposed that this natural variation may explain the conflicting studies reported in the literature. Other reasons for differing results may be related to time of harvest, lack of standardization of bioactive compounds, variability in dosage, administration, and type of ginseng used (1, 2, 3).

Media and Marketing Claims	Efficacy
Improves exercise performance	↓
Energy and mood booster	NR
Heart tonic	↔
Aphrodisiac	NR
Adaptogen—helps normalize imbalances in different disease states	NR
Helps control blood sugar in diabetes	NR

G

Advisory

- Some studies have shown a potential hypoglycemic effect; diabetics should have their blood glucose levels monitored
- Should be discontinued at least seven days prior to surgery due to potential increased bleeding

Drug/Supplement Interactions

- May interfere with phenelzine (MOA inhibitor), corticosteroids, digoxin, diabetes medications, and estrogen therapy
- May increase bleeding when taken with other blood-thinning drugs or supplements (coumadin, warfarin, garlic, ginger, ginkgo, vitamin E, flaxseed, bromelain, dong quai, fish oil, aspirin); should be monitored by a physician
- Use with caffeine may stimulate hypertension

KEY POINTS

- Although hundreds of ginseng studies have been conducted in Asia, most of the research has not been translated into English and thus is difficult to review. Furthermore, confusion is exacerbated by the difference in Eastern compared to Western interpretations of the effects of ginseng. For instance, Eastern traditional medicine practitioners would suggest that the actions of opposing ginsenosides "adapt" to meet the patient's individual mental or physical state. Western practitioners would assume that the differing actions of the ginsenosides neutralize each other (4). The results from the research are insufficient to support or refute either argument.

- Controlled studies do not support ginseng use to enhance exercise performance and reduce fatigue in humans. There are several studies that purportedly show an ergogenic benefit, but they have been criticized for lacking sufficient controls and blinding (1, 2).

- Although animal trials suggest some benefit in boosting energy, there is little comparable research in humans.

- Preliminary studies have demonstrated varying effects of the different ginsenosides on cardiovascular function. Ginseng has exerted both a lowering and raising effect on blood pressure. In *in vitro* and animal studies, ginseng inhibited platelet aggregation, decreased lipid peroxidation, and reduced experimentally induced free-radical damage. More controlled clinical trials are needed in humans.

- Scientists have suggested a hypothesis for the possible aphrodisiac effect of ginseng involving the production of nitric oxide, which may enhance penile blood flow. However, sufficient data to support this hypothesis are lacking.

- Animal data and a few small studies of patients with diabetes suggest that ginseng may exert a hypoglycemic effect; however, much more controlled clinical research is needed to verify this effect.

- Epidemiological evidence suggests a possible lower risk of cancer associated with ginseng consumption in Korea. Ginseng has also exhibited potential anticancer effects in animal and *in vitro* studies.

- Because of the complex chemical composition of the ginseng root and lack of controlled studies, it is not surprising that there is inconclusive evidence in any of the areas of research. Variations in harvest time/maturity of plant roots, different methods of preparation, lack of standardized preparation, and varying dosages and administrations of ginseng have made drawing conclusions about the efficacy of this herb very difficult. Animal studies have also been criticized for using very high doses to achieve short-term effects ("forced pharmacology") and for administering intravenous as opposed to oral ginseng (4). Overall, there have been few placebo-controlled, double-blind, clinical studies using ginseng preparations with known ginsenoside contents. As noted by one recent review, such studies are essential if there is to be a general acceptance of ginseng by Western medicine (3).

FOOD SOURCES

Fresh ginseng root is available at health food stores and Asian markets.

DOSAGE INFORMATION/BIOAVAILABILITY

Ginseng (Asian, American, or Siberian/Russian) is available in capsules, tablets, tinctures, powders and teas. Products usually provide 100 mg to 400 mg of dried extract equivalent to 0.5 g to 2.0 g of ginseng root. Ginseng roots are air-dried, producing "white ginseng," or steam treated, yielding "red ginseng." Although products claim to be standardized with 4 percent to 7 percent ginsenosides, a survey of 50 commercial ginseng products sold in 11 countries found the ginsenoside concentrations varied greatly, with some products containing no ginseng compounds at all (5). Several studies have used G115, a *Panax ginseng* CA Meyer *(P ginseng)* extract standardized to contain 13 ginsenosides at a level of 4 percent. Animal studies have shown a rapid absorption of ginsenoside Rg_1 following an oral dose (6).

The American Botanical Council's Ginseng Evaluation Program (GEP) reported the results of a seven-year study that examined 500 commercial ginseng product for content and consistency. One component of the program was an encoded blinded study of 13 Asian ginseng products for lot-to-lot consistency assessed by: 1) frequency of acceptable R_{b1}/R_{g1} value; 2) percentage of lots (within a product) that met claim for total ginsenoside content; and 3) percent relative standard deviation of total ginsenoside content. Overall, most products were reasonably consistent. However, GEP found that the term "standardized" on labels was frequently inappropriate, confusing, or misleading (7).

RELEVANT RESEARCH

Ginseng and Exercise Performance

- In a double-blind, placebo-controlled study, 28 nonathlete subjects were randomized to receive 200 mg *P ginseng* (7 percent standardized ginsenosides) or a placebo daily for three weeks. Before and at the end of the study period, subjects completed a maximal exercise test on a cycle ergometer. There were no significant effects of ginseng administration on exercise time, workload, VO_{2max}, heart rate, plasma lactate, or hematocrit at peak, or rate of perceived exertion at 150 watts, 200 watts, or peak. The authors concluded: "This study does not support an ergogenic effect on peak aerobic exercise performance following a three-week supplementation period in healthy, young adults with moderate exercise capacities and unrestricted diets" (8).

- In a double-blind, placebo-controlled trial, 36 young, healthy men (not athletes) were randomized to receive 200 mg or 400 mg of a standardized ginseng extract capsules (G115) or a placebo daily for eight weeks. This dosage was equivalent to 1 g to 2 g *P ginseng* root. Thirty-one subjects completed the study. Submaximal and maximal aerobic exercise parameters were measured before and after the trial. Ginseng had no effect on oxygen consumption, respiratory exchange ratio, minute ventilation, blood lactic acid, heart rate, and rate of perceived exertion (9).

- In a double-blind, placebo-controlled, crossover study, eight subjects of various fitness levels received in random order ginseng (8 mg/kg/day or 16 mg/kg/day *P quinquefolius* standardized extract—560 mg or 1,120 mg for a person weighing 70 kg) or a placebo for seven days each separated by a one week washout period between treatments. The ginseng preparation was prepared by the researchers and was further tested for the presence of three ginsenosides: R_{b1}, R_c, and R_e. Subjects performed three bouts of exhaustive exercise on a cycle ergometer prior to supplementation (control trial), after ginseng administration, and after the placebo. There were no differences in time to exhaustion, blood lactate, free fatty acids, VO_2, ventilation, and perceived exertion. The authors concluded: "The data indicate that with one week of pretreatment there is no ergogenic effect of ingesting the ginseng saponin extract" (10).

- In a double-blind, placebo-controlled, crossover study, 50 male gym teachers received in random order capsules containing an unspecified amount of *P ginseng* extract (G115) in combination with dimethylamino-ethanol bitartrate (choline complex), vitamins, and minerals, or a placebo daily for six weeks each, separated by a one-week washout period. The ginseng-choline complex significantly enhanced total workload and maximal oxygen uptake during maximal exercise tests compared to the placebo. The ginseng-choline complex also resulted in statistically significant lower oxygen consumption, plasma lactate levels, ventilation, CO_2 production and heart rates during exercise. The effects of the ginseng-choline supplement were more pronounced in subjects with lower VO_{2max} capacities (11). In this study, the potential effects of ginseng could not be separated from those of other ingredients in the combined supplement regimen.

- In a double blind, placebo-controlled study, 20 elite distance runners were randomly assigned in matched pairs (matched by gender, body weight, and 10-K race pace) to receive 60 drops (3.4 mL) of *E senticosus L* (Siberian ginseng) extract containing eleutherosides B and E or a placebo daily for six weeks. Every two weeks, and two weeks after the study's end, subjects completed a 10-minute treadmill run at their 10 km pace and a maximal treadmill test. Siberian ginseng had no effect on time to exhaustion, heart rate, VO$_{2max}$, rate of perceived exertion, respiratory exchange ratio, or serum lactate (12).

- In a double blind, placebo-controlled, crossover, pilot study, 9 highly trained men were given in random order 1.2 g *E senticosus* (Siberian ginseng) or placebo for seven days prior to 120 minute cycle followed by a simulated 10 km time cycle trial. Diet was controlled during each seven day period. Oxygen consumption, respiratory exchange ratio, and heart rate were recorded every 30 minutes, and rate of perceived exertion, plasma lactate and glucose were recorded every 20 minutes during the steady state cycling. There were no differences between either treatment at any point during the steady state or timed cycle trials (13)

- According to a comprehensive review, although some studies have suggested that ginseng or its active components may prolong survival to physical or chemical stress in animals, there is lack of compelling evidence demonstrating the ability of ginseng to consistently enhance physical performance in humans (1, 2).

Ginseng for Mood and Cognitive Function

- In a double-blind, placebo-controlled study, 83 healthy male and female adults (mean age = 27 y) were randomized to receive one of three treatments for eight weeks: (1) a placebo; (2) 200 mg *P ginseng* (G115); or (3) 400 mg *P ginseng* (G115). Prior to intervention and after 56 to 60 days of supplementing, subjects' positive and negative affect was assessed by the 20-item Positive Affect Negative Affect Scale (PANAS) and total mood disturbance was measured by the 65-item Profile of Mood States Inventory (POMS). Ginseng had no effect on psychological well-being (affect or mood) at either dose compared to the placebo (14).

- In a double-blind, placebo-controlled (not randomized) trial, 60 geriatric patients received a commercial product containing 40 mg *P ginseng* extract (G115) and vitamins and minerals or a placebo daily for eight weeks. Length of stay in the hospital, activities of daily living, cognitive function (measured using the Mini-Mental State Examination, Kendrick Object Learning test, and the Trail Making test) and symptoms of depression and anxiety were assessed. Forty-nine subjects finished the study (25 in the placebo group, 24 in the ginseng group). Reasons for dropping out included: lack of motivation; difficulty swallowing the capsules; and clinical events unrelated to treatment (one hip fracture and one death in the placebo group). There were no differences between groups, except the placebo group had a significant improvement on one cognitive function test (Kendrick Object Learning Test). The authors concluded there was no identifiable benefit of the ginseng complex as adjuvant to treatment and rehabilitation of geriatric patients (15). The potential effects of ginseng could not be separated from those of other ingredients in the combined supplement regimen. In addition, the lack of randomization weaken the findings of this study.

- Rats orally administered *P ginseng* root (20 mg/kg and 50 mg/kg) for five days showed improvement in anxiolytic activity compared to a placebo when tested against several paradigms of experimental anxiety (16).

- Animal studies have shown ginseng to enhance learning and memory in passive avoidance tests (2).

- See *Ginkgo biloba* for study of a ginkgo and ginseng combination use.

Ginseng and Cardiovascular Disease

- *In vitro* and animal studies suggest that ginseng inhibits platelet aggregation, decreases lipid peroxidation during ischemia, and protects against experimentally-induced free radical injury (17). Researchers have suggested that ginseng may be cardioprotective by stimulating endothelial production of nitric oxide (NO), an antioxidant and vasodilator (3, 17).

- Ginsenosides have exhibited both vasoconstriction and vasodilation effects in *ex vivo* studies using blood vessels taken from dogs, rabbits, and humans (18).

Ginseng and Sexual Function

- Traditional Chinese medicine has long used ginseng as an aphrodisiac. It has been hypothesized that ginseng may act as an aphrodisiac by enhancing nitric oxide (NO) production, which plays a potential role in stimulating penile erection (3, 17).

- In an *in vitro* study, NO release by endothelial cells of rabbit corpus cavernosum (penile tissue) was enhanced by the addition of ginsenosides (19).

- In a placebo-controlled (not blinded) study, 90 patients with erectile dysfunction not because of organic causes were randomly assigned to one of three groups for three months: (1) 300 mg *P ginseng*/day; (2) trazodone (antidepressant)/day; or (3) placebo. Changes in frequency of intercourse, premature ejaculation, and morning erections after treatment were not changed in any group. However, improvements in early detumescence, penile rigidity and girth, libido, and patient satisfaction were greater in the ginseng group compared to the placebo or trazodone-treated groups. None of the treatments resulted in complete remission of erectile dysfunction (20). The lack of blinding in this study may have introduced bias.

Ginseng and Diabetes

- In a placebo-controlled, pilot (not blinded) study, 10 type 2 diabetic patients were randomly administered 0 (placebo), or 3, 6, or 9 g ground American ginseng root in capsules at 120, 80, 40, and 0 minutes before a 25 g oral glucose challenge. Blood glucose was measured before ingestion of treatments and at 0, 15, 30, 45, 60, and 90 minutes from the start of the challenge. Compared with use of a placebo, either the 3-g, 6-g, or 9-g doses of ginseng significantly reduced postprandial glycemia at 30, 45, and 120 minutes. There was no difference in response between the 3-g, 6-g, or 9-g doses (21). The lack of blinding in this study may have introduced bias.

- In a randomized, crossover design study, 12 healthy subjects received 16 treatments: a placebo, or 1 g, 2 g, or 3 g American ginseng at 30, 20, 10, or 0 minutes before a 25-g oral glucose challenge. Blood was collected at 0, 15, 30, 45, 60, and 90 minutes after the start of the challenge. Compared to use of the placebo, glycemia was significantly lower during the last 45 minutes of the test with 1 g, 2 g, or 3 g of ginseng. There were no differences among results for the doses. Glycemia in the last hour of the test was significantly lower when ginseng was given 40 minutes before the challenge, but not when given sooner. The authors concluded that ginseng reduces postprandial glycemia in healthy subjects in a time-dependent, but not dose dependent, manner (22).

- In a double-blind, placebo-controlled study, 36 newly diagnosed patients with type 2 diabetes were treated with 100 mg or 200 mg ginseng extract daily (species and percent ginsenosides were not identified) or a placebo for eight weeks. Subjective tests of mood, vigor, memory, sleep, physical activity, and well-being were self-rated on linear analog scales. Psychophysical performance was evaluated by time to complete a numbered diagram. Fasting blood glucose, serum lipids, glycosylated hemoglobin, serum aminoterminalpropetide (PIIINP), and fasting serum immunoreactive insulin (IRI) and C-peptide were also measured. Subjects were given individual and group-based instruction on diabetes management including diet and glucose monitoring. Ginseng therapy resulted in a significant reduction in fasting blood glucose, elevation in mood, and improvement of psychophysical performance, but had no effect on memory, sleep, serum lipids, or IRI. The 200-mg dose resulted in a significant improvement in glycosylated hemoglobin and PIIINP and increased physical activity. The authors speculated that ginseng elevated subjects' mood, which may have improved self-care and physical activity, and thus led to improved glucose balance (23).

- Korean and American ginsenosides and Siberian eleuthorosides were found to exert a hypoglycemic effect in mice with experimentally induced hyperglycemia (24–26).

Ginseng and Cancer

- A case-control study of 905 pairs of case and control subjects matched by age, sex, and date of admission to the Korea Cancer Center Hospital reported a statistically significant decrease in cancer cases with increasing frequency of *P. ginseng.*CA. Meyer intake. Ginseng extract and powder appeared to be associated with a lower risk of cancer than did fresh sliced ginseng, ginseng juice, or tea (27). A second case-control study of 1,987 pairs of subjects reported similar results. On the site of cancer, the odds ratios were 0.47 for cancer of the lip, oral cavity, and pharynx; 0.20 for esophageal cancer; 0.36 for stomach cancer; 0.42 for colorectal cancer; 0.48 for liver cancer; 0.22 for pancreatic cancer; 0.18 for laryngeal cancer; 0.55 for lung cancer; and 0.15 for ovarian cancer. In cancers of the female breast, uterine cervix, urinary bladder, and thyroid gland, however, there was no association with ginseng intake (28). It is important to note that recall data of ginseng intake were used, rather than plasma levels of ginsenosides.

- According to one review, a five-year prospective cohort study of 4,587 Korean subjects more than 40 years old reported a significant decreased risk of cancer incidence in ginseng consumers (relative risk of 0.48) compared to nonconsumers. The risk was lowered as the frequency of ginseng intake increased, demonstrating a significant dose-responsive effect (29).

- The same review summarized animal and *in vitro* research on ginseng and cancer. The author noted that ginsenosides have demonstrated *in vitro* antimutagenic activity, inhibition of tumor cell lines in mice and humans, and immunmodulating activity. Other constituents of ginseng (polysaccharides, polyacetylenes) have also exhibited potential cancer-protective effects (29).

SAFETY

- No serious adverse effects have been reported in the research among subjects consuming ginseng for short periods of time. Reports of hypertension, nervousness, sleeplessness, acne, edema, headache, and diarrhea have been associated with ingestion of > 3 g ginseng root/day (equivalent to approximately 600 mg ginseng extract) (30).

- According to the German Commission E monographs, Siberian ginseng root, but not *Panax* ginseng root, is contraindicated for those with hypertension (31). Ginseng should be taken up to three months and a repeated course is feasible.

- No treatment-related changes in body weight, hematology, or clinical chemistry were observed in dogs orally administered 15 mg ginseng extract (G115)/kg for 90 days (32).

- There are limited data on potential drug-herb or herb-herb interactions with ginseng. One review concluded: "Ginseng may cause headache, tremulousness, and manic episodes in patients treated with phenelzine sulfate [antidepressant, MAO Inhibitor] . . . Ginseng should also not be used with estrogens or corticosteroids because of possible additive effects. . . . Ginseng may interfere with digoxin pharmacodynamically or with digoxin monitoring. . . . Ginseng may affect blood glucose levels and should not be used in patients with diabetes mellitus" (33).

- Use of Siberian ginseng was associated with elevated digoxin levels in a 74-year-old man using digoxin therapy. Levels returned to the therapeutic range after ginseng was discontinued (34).

- Ginseng has been reported to have mild hormonal effects similar to those of estrogen. Cases of both postmenopausal bleeding and amenorrhea have been documented with ginseng use (35).

- One review article summarized research suggesting that ginseng blocks the analgesic effects of opioids (morphine) and inhibits the tolerance to and dependence on opioids and psychostimulants (36).

- Ginsenosides may inhibit platelet aggregation and increase bleeding time; therefore, one review suggested that ginseng use be discontinued at least seven days prior to surgery (37).

- Although ginseng may slow coagulation, in one case report, ginseng was associated with the opposite effect: it decreased the efficacy of warfarin (38).

- An *in vitro* study examined the effects of ginsenosides (Rb_1, Rb_2, Rc, Rd, Re, Rf, and Rg_1) and eleutherosides (B and E) on P450 enzyme pathway. The authors of the experiments concluded that the ginsendosides and eleutherosides tested are *not* likely to inhibit the metabolism of coadministered medications in which the primary route of elimination is via cytochrome P450 (eg, anti-HIV drugs, oral contraceptives, or transplant drug therapies) (39).

- One woman developed cerebral arteritis after ingesting a large quantity of ethanol-extracted ginseng (prepared from 60 slices of ginseng root stewed with 400 mL rice wine) (40).

REFERENCES

1. Bahrke MS, Morgan WR. Evaluation of the ergogenic properties of ginseng. *Sports Med.* 1994;18:229–248.
2. Bahrke MS, Morgan WR. Evaluation of the ergogenic properties of ginseng: an update. *Sports Med.* 2000;29:113–133.
3. Gillis CN. *Panax ginseng* pharmacology: a nitric oxide link? *Biochem Pharmacol.* 1997;54:1–8.
4. Sonnenborn U, Proppert Y. Ginseng (Panax ginseng CA Meyer). *Br J Phytother.* 1991;2:3–14.
5. Cui J, Garle M, Eneroth P, et al. What do commercial ginseng preparations contain? *Lancet.* 1994;344:134.
6. Odani T, Tanizawa H, Takino Y. Studies on the absorption, distribution, excretion and metabolism of ginseng saponins: the absorption, distribution, and excretion of ginsenoside R_{g1} in the rat. *Chem Pharm Bull (Tokyo).* 1983;31:292–298.
7. Hall T, Lu ZZ, Yat PN, et al. Evaluation of consistency of standardized Asian ginseng products in the ginseng evaluation program. *HerbalGram.* 2001;52:31–45.
8. Allen JD, McLung J, Nelson AG, et al. Ginseng supplementation does not enhance healthy young adults' peak aerobic exercise performance. *J Am Coll Nutr.* 1998;17:462–466.
9. Engels HJ, Wirth JC. No ergogenic effects of ginseng (*Panax ginseng* CA Meyer) during graded maximal aerobic exercise. *J Am Dietet Assoc.* 1997;97:1110–1115.
10. Morris AC, Jacobs I, McLellan TM, et al. No ergogenic effect of ginseng ingestion. *Int J Sport Nutr.* 1996;6:263–271.
11. Pieralisi G, Ripari P, Vecchiet L. Effects of a standardized ginseng extract combined with dimethylaminoethanol bitartrate, vitamins, minerals, and trace elements on physical performance during exercise. *Clin Ther.* 1991;13:373–382.
12. Dowling EA, Redondo DR, Branch JD, et al. Effect of *Eleutherococcus senticosus* on submaximal and maximal exercise performance. *Med Sci Sports Exerc.* 1996;28:482–489.
13. Eschbach LF, Webster MJ, Boyd JC, et al. The effect of Siberian ginseng (*Eleutherococcus senticosus*) on substrate utilization and performance. *Int J Sport Nutr Exerc Metab.* 2000;10:444–451.
14. Cardinal BJ, Engels HJ. Ginseng does not enhance psychological well-being in healthy, young adults: results of a double-blind, placebo-controlled randomized clinical trial. *J Am Diet Assoc.* 2001;101:655–660.
15. Thommessen B, Laake K. No identifiable effect of ginseng (Gericomplex) as an adjuvant in the treatment of geriatric patients. *Aging (Milano).* 1996;8:417–420.
16. Bhattacharya SK, Mitra SK. Anxiolytic activity of *Panax ginseng* roots: an experimental study. *J Ethnopharmacol.* 1991;34:87–92.

G

17. Chen X. Cardiovascular protection by ginsenosides and their nitric oxide releasing action. *Clin Exp Pharmacol Physiol.* 1996;23:728–732.

18. Chen X, Gillis CN, Moalli R. Vascular effects of ginsenosides in vitro. *Br J Pharmacol.* 1984;82:485–491.

19. Chen X, Lee TJ. Ginsenosides-induced nitric oxide-mediated relaxation of the rabbit corpus cavernosum. *Br J Pharmacol.* 1995;115:15–18.

20. Choi HK, Seong DH, Rha KH. Clinical efficacy of Korean red ginseng for erectile dysfunction. *Int J Impot Res.* 1995;7:181–186.

21. Vuksan V, Stavro MP, Sievenpiper JL, et al. Similar postprandial glycemic reductions with escalation of dose and administration time of American ginseng in type 2 diabetes. *Diabetes Care.* 2000;23:1221–1226.

22. Vuksan V, Sievenpiper JL, Wong J, et al. American ginseng (*Panax quinquefolius L*) attenuates postprandial glycemia in a time-dependent but not dose-dependent manner in healthy individuals. *Am J Clin Nutr.* 2001;73:753–758.

23. Sotaniemi EA, Haapakoski E, Rautio A. Ginseng therapy in non-insulin-dependent diabetic patients. *Diabetes Care.* 1995;18:1373–1375.

24. Konno C, Sugiyama K, Kano M, et al. Isolation and hypoglycemic activity of Panaxans A, B, C, D, and E, glycans of *Panax ginseng* roots. *Planta Med.* 1984;50:434–436.

25. Hikino H, Takahashi M, Otake K, et al. Isolation and hypoglycemic activity of eleutherans A, B, C, D, E, F, and G: glycans of *Eleutherococcus senticosus* roots. *J Nat Prod.* 1986;49:293–297.

26. Oshima Y, Sato K, Hikino H. Isolation and hypoglycemic activity of quinquefolans A, B, and C, glycans of *Panax quinquefolium* roots. *J Nat Prod.* 1987;50:188–190.

27. Yun TK, Choi SY. A case-control study of ginseng intake and cancer. *Int J Epidemiol.* 1990;19:871–876.

28. Yun TK, Choi SY. Preventive effect of ginseng intake against various human cancers: a case control study on 1,987 pairs. *Cancer Epidemiol Biomarkers Prev.* 1995;4:401–408.

29. Yun TK. Experimental and epidemiological evidence of the cancer-preventive effects of *Panax ginseng* CA Meyer. *Nutr Rev.* 1996;54(11 pt 2):S71–S81.

30. Siegel RK. Ginseng abuse syndrome: problems with the panacea. *JAMA.* 1979;241:1614–1615.

31. Blumenthal M, ed. *The Complete German Commission E Monographs Therapeutic Guide to Herbal Medicines.* Austin, Tex: American Botanical Council; 1998.

32. Hess FG, Parent RA, Stevens KR, et al. Effect of subchronic feeding of ginseng extract G115 in beagle dogs. *Food Chem Toxicol.* 1983;21:95–97.

33. Miller LG. Herbal medicinals: selected clinical considerations focusing on known or potential drug-herb interactions. *Arch Intern Med.* 1998;158:2200–2211.

34. McRae S. Elevated serum digoxin levels in patient taking digoxin and Siberian ginseng. *CMAJ.* 1996;155:293–295.

35. Greenspan EM. Ginseng and vaginal bleeding. *JAMA.* 1983;249:2018.

36. Takahashi M, Tokuyama S. Pharmacological and physiological effects of ginseng on actions induced by opioids and psychostimulants. *Methods Find Exp Clin Pharmacol.* 1998;20:77–84.

G

37. Ang-Lee, Moss J, Yuan CS. Herbal medicines and perioperative care. *JAMA.* 2001;286:208–216.

38. Janetzky K, Morreale AP. Probable interaction between warfarin and ginseng. *Am J Health Syst Pharm.* 1997;54:692–693.

39. Henderson GL, Harkey MR, Gershwin ME, et al. Effects of ginseng components on c-DNA-expressed cytochrome P450 enzyme catalytic activity. *Life Sci.* 1999;65:209–214.

40. Ryu SJ, Chien YY. Ginseng-associated cerebral arteritis. *Neurology.* 1995;45:829–830.

Glucosamine

Glucosamine is an amino-monosaccharide that is synthesized in the body from glucose and glutamine by chrondrocytes (cells that form cartilage). It functions as a building block in substances found in articular cartilage (1). Glucosamine supplements have gained popularity as an alternative to non-steroidal anti-inflammatory drugs (NSAIDS) for arthritis relief. NSAIDs, while effective in decreasing pain and inflammation, have been associated with serious adverse effects including gastrointestinal complications and cartilage degeneration (2, 3). In contrast, glucosamine is thought to have a good safety record and may have potential chondroprotective effects (4).

Some researchers suggest that supplying exogenous glucosamine provides the extra raw materials needed to keep the joint healthy. Glucosamine appears to stimulate the production of molecules that provide strength and elasticity to the joint. Specifically, in vitro and animal studies report that glucosamine sulfate enhances production of collagen, glycosaminoglycans (GAGs), and proteoglycans in the joint matrix. Collagen is a thick protein that physically connects cartilage to tissue for tensile strength. GAGs are large polysaccharides that include chrondroitin sulfate, keratan sulfate, and hyaluronic acid. Proteoglycans are made up of chains of GAGs arranged on a protein core. They function by attracting water to produce an elastic layer, thereby cushioning and protecting cartilage from mechanical stress (1, 5).

Media and Marketing Claims	Efficacy
Relieves osteoarthritis pain	↑?
Improves joint structure	NR
Heals tendons and ligaments damaged from sports injuries	NR
Improves symptoms of tendonitis and bursitis	NR

Advisory

- No reported serious adverse effects in short-term studies
- Controversial effect of glucosamine on blood glucose control; to be safe, diabetics should have glucose levels monitored

Drug/Supplement Interactions

No reported adverse interactions

KEY POINTS

- Preliminary evidence suggests that glucosamine may improve symptoms of osteoarthritic patients compared to a placebo, or at least as effectively as NSAIDs. A meta-analysis suggested that glucosamine and chondroitin combinations provided significant pain relief. However, some of these studies have been criticized for poor methodology, and not all of them are suggestive of a benefit. A large, long-term, controlled multicenter trial of glucosamine plus chondroitin is currently being conducted in the United States to further determine the efficacy, dosage, and safety of these supplements in treating osteoarthritis.

- One controlled study using radiological evidence suggests that glucosamine may have a structure-modifying effect on osteoarthritis by slowing knee joint degeneration. Further studies are needed to confirm these results.

- Although glucosamine is part of the structure that makes up tendons, ligaments, and cartilage, there is currently little or no evidence demonstrating that supplementation repairs damaged tendons and ligaments from sports-related injuries.

- Likewise, there is currently no published controlled research investigating the effects of glucosamine on tendonitis or bursitis.

FOOD SOURCES

None

DOSAGE INFORMATION/BIOAVAILABILITY

Glucosamine is available in tablets, capsules, or powders as glucosamine sulfate, glucosamine hydrochloride, or N-acetyl-D-glucosamine (NAG). Glucosamine supplements are derived from the exoskeleton of the crustacean chitin. It is often combined with chondroitin sulfate (see Chondroitin). Manufacturer's labels suggest taking 1,500 mg glucosamine/day divided into three doses. In one human study, 90 percent of orally ingested glucosamine sulfate was absorbed and diffused into bone and articular cartilage (6). Another study supplemented human subjects with 1 g polymeric (sustained-release) NAG or nonpolymeric NAG and found that both forms are absorbed and raise serum glucosamine levels (7).

RELEVANT STUDIES

Glucosamine Sulfate (GS) and Osteoarthritis

- In a double-blind, placebo-controlled study, 212 Belgium patients with knee osteoarthritis were randomized to receive 1,500 mg glucosamine sulfate or a placebo daily for three years. Disease progression was assessed by x-raying knee joint-space width at baseline and after one and three years. Subjects assigned to placebo had significant progressive joint-space narrowing. In contrast, there were no significant losses in joint-space in subjects taking glucosamine. Symptoms worsened in patients taking placebos compared to an improvement in symptoms in glucosamine-treated subjects. Treatment was well tolerated with no differences in safety or early withdrawal between the groups. The authors concluded that glucosamine may have a positive structure-modifying effect on osteoarthritis of the knee (8).

- In a double-blind, placebo-controlled study, 98 male patients (age range 34 y to 81 y, mean age = 63 y) being treated for osteoarthritis pain of the knee were randomized to receive 1,500 mg glucosamine sulfate or placebo daily for two months. Pain intensity both at rest and while walking was assessed by a visual analog scale at baseline, and after 30 days and 60 days. There were no differences in pain between groups at baseline or at any point of the study. The authors noted that their study was in contrast to most other studies investigating glucosamine. They suggested that the lack of benefit could be due to the fact that their subjects tended to be older, heavier, and had more severe arthritis than other trials (9).

- In a double-blind, placebo-controlled trial, 49 subjects with temporomandibular joint (TMJ) osteoarthritis were randomized to receive 1,500 mg glucosamine sulfate or ibuprofen (1,200 mg) daily for 90 days. TMJ pain and function, pain-free, and voluntary maximum mouth opening, Brief Pain Inventory questionnaire and masticatory muscle tenderness were assessed after a one-week washout period and at day 90. Additionally, acetaminophen (500 mg) for breakthrough pain was evaluated every 30 days to day 120. Within-group analysis reported significant improvements in all variables in both treatment groups, with no differences in acetaminophen use. There were no significant differences in positive clinical responses between the groups. However, between days 90 and 120 (after discontinuation of treatment), the glucosamine group had a significantly greater reduction in TMJ pain during function and effect of pain with daily activities and a decrease in acetaminophen use when compared to subjects who had taken ibuprofen. The authors suggested that glucosamine appears to have a carryover effect (10).

- In a double-blind, parallel study, 200 hospitalized patients with clinically documented knee osteoarthritis were randomized to receive 1,200 mg GS divided into three doses or 1,200 mg ibuprofen divided into three doses for four weeks. Only occasional use of NSAIDs (type, dose, and amount not specified) as a rescue therapy were permitted. Patients were not permitted to exercise or apply heat or cold therapy to the knees during the trial. The treatments were equally effective as assessed by improvement on Lesquesne's Index (which assesses functional status and quality of life), although there was an insignificant trend for the ibuprofen group to respond sooner. The ibuprofen group had significantly more adverse effects, such as gastrointestinal discomfort, than did the glucosamine group (35 percent versus 6 percent). The authors did not report information on NSAID use (11).

- In a double-blind, parallel, group trial, 40 patients with osteoarthritis in the knee (ages 48 y to 66 y) were given 1,500 mg GS or 1,200 mg ibuprofen daily for two months. Articular pain was scored on a 0 to 3 rating before treatment and at weeks 1, 2, 4, and 8. Presence of swelling, body weight, and hematological data were also recorded. Pain scores decreased faster during the first two weeks with ibuprofen treatment. However, the reduction in pain in patients on GS continued throughout the trial and pain was significantly lower with glucosamine as compared to ibuprofen by week 8. There were no differences in swelling or any other parameters measured between the two groups (12).

- In a double-blind, placebo-controlled trial, 20 patients (ages 45 y to 73 y) with osteoarthritis were randomized to receive three doses of 250 mg GS or a placebo daily for six to eight weeks. No analgesics or NSAIDs were permitted during the study. There was a significant alleviation of symptoms (articular pain, joint tenderness, restricted movement) in GS-supplemented subjects compared to the placebo group. In addition, symptoms were relieved earlier with GS compared to placebo. GS supplements did not alter hematologic parameters, erythrocyte sedimentation rate, urinalysis and X-rays (13).

Glucosamine Hydrochloride (HCL) and Chondroitin Combinations in Arthritis

- A meta-analysis was performed examining 15 trials of glucosamine and chondroitin preparations. Studies were selected if they were double-blinded, controlled, randomized and lasted for four or more weeks' duration. In addition, studies were only included if subjects had knee or hip osteoarthritis. The pooled results suggested that glucosamine and chondroitin significantly improved osteoarthritis symptoms with moderate (glucosamine) to large effects (chondroitin). The researchers noted that the benefits might be exaggerated due to issues of quality and publication bias. Specifically, important demographic details including age, sex, radiological stage of arthritis, duration of disease, and use of analgesics and NSAIDs were not provided in many of the studies (14).

- In a double-blind, placebo-controlled study, 93 patients with knee osteoarthritis were randomized to receive a placebo or 2,000 mg glucosamine HCL plus 1,600 mg sodium chondroitin sulfate for six months. The treatment group had a significantly greater improvement in scores on the Lesquesne's Index compared to placebo. There was also a significant drop in pain medication used in the treatment group compared to the placebo (15).

- In a double-blind, placebo-controlled study, 118 subjects with knee osteoarthritis were randomized to receive 1,500 glucosamine HCL plus 1,200 sodium chondroitin sulfate plus 228 mg manganese ascorbate or a placebo daily for eight weeks. Two weeks before the study, subjects were examined and instructed to take only prescribed acetaminophen for pain. At baseline, patients were examined and prescribed acetaminophen and given either glucosamine or placebo. At week 4, the prescriptions for acetaminophen were renewed. At weeks 4 and 8, patients returned diaries and unused medications, and were examined. The Western Ontario and McMaster University Osteoarthritis Index (WOMAC) questionnaire was given before, at baseline and the end of the study. Ninety-eight subjects completed the study, dropout was due to scheduling conflicts, violating study protocol, etc. The primary endpoint (difference in WOMAC pain score from baseline to week 8) was not significant in either group. However, during weeks 5 through 8, there was a significant improvement in the knee exam and in the response to daily diary pain question ("How much pain do you have today compared to yesterday?") in the glucosamine group. However, there was no difference between responses to "Are you better than at the start of the trial?" (40 percent of the placebo and 49 percent of glucosamine subjects answered yes). The authors concluded that although the primary endpoint was not met, sufficient positive trends in favor of glucosamine suggest the need for larger trials (16).

- In a double-blind, placebo-controlled, crossover study, 34 Navy SEALs and divers with degenerative joint disease of the knee or back (average age = 43 y) were given in random order 1,500 glucosamine HCL plus 1,200 sodium chondroitin sulfate plus 228 mg manganese ascorbate or a placebo for eight weeks each. Patients were not permitted NSAIDs but were allowed acetaminophen for pain during the study. Subjects were assessed at the baseline and at week 7 to 8 for each treatment period. A summary disease score incorporated results of pain and functional questionnaires, physical examination scores, and running times (time to run 100 yards and to run up and down a tower with 80 stairs, touching every stair). Glucosamine plus chondroitin supplementation was associated with a significant improvement in the overall summary disease score compared to the placebo. Specifically, significant improvements were seen in the patients' assessment of treatment result and the visual analogue score (VAS) for pain. However, trends in physical examination scores, acetaminophen use, disability scores of Lesquesne and Roland, patient assessment of handicap, and physician assessment of severity were not different between treatments. There was also no change in running times or range of motion. When the knee data were separated from back data, the improvements in summary disease scores, patients self-assessment, and VAS for pain were mainly attributable to improvements in knee symptoms. None of the trends for low back pain reached significance. Treatment had no adverse effects on vital signs, occult blood testing, and hematologic parameters. The authors concluded that the combination of glucosamine and chondroitin relieved symptoms of knee osteoarthritis, but that a larger data set is needed to determine the value of this therapy for spinal degenerative joint disease (17).

- In September of 1999, the National Institutes of Health (NIH) allocated money for the first U.S. double-blind, placebo-controlled, randomized, multicenter trial of more than 1,000 patients with osteoarthritis of the knee. This study is currently in process and consists of four arms: (1) use of glucosamine alone; (2) chondroitin sulfate alone; (3) glucosamine plus chondroitin together; and (4) a placebo. The subjects will be evaluated at monthly intervals for 16 weeks. Medical evaluations and x-rays will be used to verify diagnoses. The primary outcome will be measured as improvement in pain, with improvement in function as the secondary outcome. The final report is expected in 2005.

- There are several studies (published as abstracts) showing improvements (reduction in lameness, increased flexion, preservation of joint capsule) in degenerative joint disease in dogs and horses supplemented with glucosamine HCL and sodium chondroitin sulfate (18–21).

SAFETY

- A three year study of glucosamine sulfate reported no serious adverse effects (8).

- There were no reported serious adverse effects with glucosamine in the cited studies.

- Some researchers have suggested that there may be a potential for adverse effects of glucosamine on glucose metabolism in diabetics (1, 22, 23). A three-year trial reported no changes in glycemic homeostasis (8). Short-term glucosamine infusions appeared to have no effect on insulin sensitivity in healthy subjects (22, 23). Further research is needed to determine the effects of glucosamine in people with diabetes.

- Because glucosamine is a derivative of shellfish, a potential exists for a reaction to occur in those allergic to shellfish. However, there are no reported cases of allergies to glucosamine supplements.

REFERENCES

1. Barclay TS, Tsourounis C, McCart GM. Glucosamine. *Ann Pharmacother.* 1998;32:574–579.
2. Gabriel SE, Jaakkimainen L, Bombardier C. Risk for serious gastrointestinal complications related to use of nonsteroidal anti-inflammatory drugs: a meta-analysis. *Ann Intern Med.* 1991;115:787–796.
3. Palmoski MJ, Brandt KD. Effects of some nonsteroidal anti-inflammatory drugs on proteoglycan metabolism and organization in canine articular cartilage. *Arthritis Rheum.* 1980;23:1010–1020.
4. de los Reyes GC, Koda RT, Lien EJ. Glucosamine and chondroitin sulfates in the treatment of osteoarthritis: a survey. *Prog Drug Res.* 2000;55:81–103.
5. da Camara CC, Dowless GV. Glucosamine sulfate for osteoarthritis. *Ann Pharmacother.* 1998;32:580–587.
6. Setnikar I, Palumbo R, Canali S, et al. Pharmacokinetics of glucosamine in man. *Arzneimittelforschung.* 1993;43:1109–1113.
7. Talent JM, Garcy RW. Pilot study of oral polymeric N-acetyl-D-glucosamine as a potential treatment for patients with osteoarthritis. *Clin Ther.* 1996;18:1184–1190.
8. Reginster JY, Deroisy R, Rovai LC, et al. Long-term effects of glucosamine sulfate on osteoarthritis progression: a randomized, placebo-controlled clinical trial. *Lancet.* 2001;357:247–248.
9. Rindone JP, Hiller D, Collacott E, et al. Randomized, controlled trial of glucosamine for treating osteoarthritis of the knee. *West J Med.* 2000. 172:91–94.
10. Thie NM, Prasad NG, Major PW. Evaluation of glucosamine sulfate compared to ibuprofen for the treatment of temporomandibular joint osteoarthritis: a randomized double-blind controlled 3 month clinical trial. *J Rheumatol.* 2001;28:1347–1355.
11. Muller-Fabbender H, Bach G, Haase W, et al. Glucosamine sulfate compared to ibuprofen in osteoarthritis of the knee. *Osteoarthritis Cartilage.* 1994;2:61–69.
12. Lopes Vaz A. Double-blind clinical evaluation of the relative efficacy of ibuprofen and glucosamine sulfate in the management of osteoarthrosis of the knee in out-patients. *Curr Med Res Opin.* 1982;8:145–149.

13. Pujalte JM, Llavore EP, Ylescupidez FR. Double-blind clinical evaluation of oral glucosamine sulfate in the basic treatment of osteoarthrosis. *Curr Med Res Opin.* 1980;7:110–114.

14. McAlindon TE, LaValley MP, Gulin JP, et al. Gluocosamine and chondroitin for treatment of osteoarthritis: a systematic quality assessment and meta-analysis. *JAMA.* 2000;283:1469–1475.

15. Das AK, Eitel J, Hammad T. Efficacy of a combination of FCHG49 glucosamine hydrochloride, TRH122 low molecular weight sodium chondroitin sulfate and manganese in the treatment of osteoarthritis of the knee. *Osteoarthritis Cartilage.* 2000;8:343–350.

16. Houpt JB, McMillan R, Wein C, et al. Effect of glucosamine hydrochloride in the treatment of pain of osteoarthritis of the knee. *J Rheumatol.* 1999;26:2423–2430.

17. Leffler CT, Philippi AF, Leffler SG, et al. Glucosamine, chondroitin, and manganese ascorbate for degenerative joint disease of the knee or low back: a randomized, double-blind, placebo-controlled pilot study. *Mil Med.* 1999;164:85–91.

18. Hanson RR, Smalley LR, Huff GK, et al. Oral treatment with a glucosamine-chondroitin sulfate compound for degenerative joint disease in horses: 25 cases. *Equine Pract.* 1997;19:16–21.

19. Canapp SO, McLaughlin RM, Hoskinson JJ, et al. Scintigraphic evaluation of glucosamine HCL and chondroitin sulfate as treatments for acute synovitis in dogs. In: Abstracts of ACVS Veterinary Symposium Small Animal Proceedings; October 8–11, 1998; Chicago, Ill.

20. Hulse DS, Hart D, Slatter M, et al. The effect of cosequin in cranial cruciate deficient and reconstructed stifle joints in dogs. In: Abstracts of Veterinary Orthopedic Society, 25th Annual Conference; February 21–28, 1998.

21. McNamara PS, Barr SC, Idouraine A, et al. Effects of an oral chondroprotective agent (Cosequin) of cartilage metabolism and canine serum. In: Abstracts of Proceedings of the 24th Annual Conference of Veterinary Orthopedic Society; March 1–8, 1997; Big Sky, Mont.

22. Monauni T, Zenti MG, Cretti A, et al. Effects of glucosamine infusion on insulin secretion and insulin action in humans. *Diabetes.* 2000;49:926–935.

23. Pouwels MJ, Jacobs JR, Span PN, et al. Short-term glucosamine infusion does not affect insulin sensitivity in humans. *J Clin Endocrinol Metab.* 2001;86:2099–2103.

Glutamine

Glutamine, a nonessential amino acid, is the most abundant free amino acid in skeletal muscle and plasma. It is a fuel source for the gut mucosal cells, lymphocytes, macrophages, endothelial cells, and renal tubular cells. Body stores of glutamine decrease during trauma, infection, surgery, acidosis, and physical stress. Increased gluconeogenesis and hepatic, gut, and renal uptake of glutamine during catabolic states may account for the depletion of plasma glutamine. Because the demands for muscle glutamine exceed the supply during stress, many researchers consider glutamine to be conditionally essential (1, 2, 3).

Glutamine has considerable scientific evidence of efficacy for certain disease states in the acute care setting when administered by a qualified health professional. For more details about glutamine supplementation on catabolic states, cancer, intestinal function, organ transplants, and burn injuries, see reference 3. This section will only review nonacute care marketing claims for glutamine.

Media and Marketing Claims	Efficacy
Keeps the immune system strong and prevents infection during heavy exercise training	↔

Advisory

No reported serious adverse effects

Drug/Supplement Interactions

No reported adverse interactions

KEY POINTS

- Research suggests that strenuous exercise is associated with reduced plasma glutamine levels and impaired immune function.

- The limited research on the role of glutamine supplements on immunity after intensive activity yielded inconsistent results and used only small numbers of subjects, and thus is difficult to interpret. Laboratory studies have not shown improvements in immune parameters with glutamine ingestion, whereas field studies suggest glutamine supplementation after endurance exercise may reduce the incidence of self-reported infection. More controlled research is needed to determine the efficacy, dosage, and timing before recommendations can be made (4).

- One strategy to maintain plasma glutamine levels may be to consume carbohydrates between repeated exercise bouts. Carbohydrates not only may attenuate glutamine levels from dropping, but there is a large body of research (not discussed here) demonstrating that carbohydrate ingestion also enhances exercise performance by replenishing glycogen stores (5).

FOOD SOURCES

Glutamine is a nonessential amino acid found predominantly in protein-rich foods. It is also synthesized in the body from glutamic acid.

DOSAGE INFORMATION/BIOAVAILABILITY

Glutamine is available in capsules, pills, and sports beverages in the form of L-glutamine. It is also found in protein powder supplements. Products provide anywhere from 0.5 g to 20 g glutamine per serving. Plasma glutamine increases approximately two hours after eating meals, especially ones having protein-rich foods (6).

RELEVANT RESEARCH

Plasma Glutamine Levels and Immunity During Exercise Training

- Research suggests that there is a transient decrease in plasma glutamine following acute exercise and from chronic overtraining (7, 8).

- Athletes with overtraining syndrome (OTS) have been reported to have low plasma glutamine levels. In one study, 40 athletes diagnosed with OTS had significantly lower plasma glutamine levels than did a group of controls (9). In another study, 10 male athletes with OTS also had significantly lower plasma glutamine levels compared to sedentary controls. No other hematological or immunological parameter differed among subjects (10).

- Decreased plasma glutamine levels and an impairment in the number and activity of CD4+ T cells were observed in untrained subjects after an eight-week anaerobic exercise program (11).

- Serum glutamine levels declined and natural killer and lymphokine activated killer cell activities were suppressed in triathletes after a half-ironman race (12).

Glutamine Supplementation and Immunity During Exercise

- In placebo-controlled, crossover study, eight male subjects performed three bouts of ergometer cycle exercise lasting 60, 45, and 30 minutes at 75 percent VO_{2max} separated by two hours. Each subject randomly underwent two trials separated by 30 days: (1) 9 equal doses of 100 mg glutamine/kg body weight 30 minutes before, at the end, and 30 minutes after exercise session; or (2) a placebo. The authors chose this dosage regimen based on pilot studies showing that this regimen maintained plasma glutamine levels. During placebo administration, subjects had lowered plasma glutamine levels compared to the glutamine phase. Circulating lymphocytes, phytohemagglutinin-stimulated lymphocyte proliferative response, and lymphokine-activated killer (LAK)-cell activity declined two hours after each bout of exercise in both groups. However, glutamine supplementation had no effect on these immune responses to exercise (13).

- Data were summarized from eight double-blind, placebo-controlled studies of a total of 151 athletes (middle-distance, marathon, and ultramarathon runners and elite rowers) who were supplemented with a placebo or 5 g glutamine dissolved in 330 mL water immediately after and two hours after a marathon, ultramarathon or intensive rowing (total glutamine = 10 g). The incidence of infection was assessed in each subject by questionnaire for seven days after exercise. The number of athletes reporting no infection was significantly higher in the glutamine-supplemented subjects (81 percent) compared to the placebo (49 percent). The authors concluded that glutamine supplementation after prolonged exercise might restore glutamine to physiological levels, thus making glutamine more available to immune cells (14).

G

- In a randomized, placebo-controlled study, 18 athletes were given 5 g glutamine in solution or a placebo 15 minutes and 1 hour after running a marathon (total glutamine intake = 10 g). Blood samples were taken 30 minutes prior to the race, and 15 minutes, 1 hour, and 16 hours postrace. A third group of 12 runners who received no treatment (controls) also had blood samples drawn. In all groups, plasma glutamine was decreased immediately after and 1 hour after the marathon and returned to pre-exercise levels by 16 hours post-race. Glutamine had no effect on T-lymphocytes, which were reduced to below pre-exercise levels in all groups (15).

Glutamine and Glycogen Stores

- Eighteen subjects were randomly assigned to receive an infusion of glutamine, alanine plus glycine, or saline 30 minutes after completing glycogen-depleting exercise (90 minutes cycling at 70 percent to 140 percent maximal oxygen capacity). Muscle glutamine increased 16 percent during glutamine infusion while it decreased or remained unchanged during alanine plus glycine and saline infusions, respectively. Two hours after exercise, there was a significant increase in muscle glycogen in the glutamine-infused group compared to the other two groups (16). Exercise performance was not determined.

- Seven male distance runners with depleted glycogen stores performed a 60-minute treadmill run after a 14-hour fast or after a high‑carbohydrate meal. Plasma glutamine did not change in response to exercise when runners fasted, but increased when fed. The authors stressed the importance of dietary carbohydrate intake between repeated bouts of exercise to lessen the decrease in plasma glutamine (17).

SAFETY

- In the cited studies, glutamine was well-tolerated. However, there are no long-term studies testing the safety of high-dose glutamine supplementation.

REFERENCES

1. Lacey JM, Wilmore DW. Is glutamine a conditionally essential amino acid? *Nutr Rev.* 1990;48:297–309.
2. Walsh NP, Blannin AK, Robson PJ, et al. Glutamine, exercise and immune function. Links and possible mechanisms. *Sports Med.* 1998;26:177–191.
3. Abcouwer SF, Souba WW. Glutamine and arginine. In: Shils ME, Olson JA, Shike M, Ross AC, eds. *Modern Nutrition in Health and Disease.* 9th ed. Baltimore, Md: Williams & Wilkins; 1999:559–569.
4. Shephard RJ, Shek PN. Heavy exercise, nutrition, and immune function: is there a connection? *Int J Sports Med.* 1995;16:491–497.
5. Coleman EJ. Carbohydrate—the Master Fuel. In: Berning JR, Steen SN, eds. *Nutrition for Sport and Exercise.* 2nd ed. Gaithersburg, Md: Aspen Publishers; 1998:21–44.

6. Castell LM, Liu CT, Newsholme EA. Diurnal variation of plasma glutamine in normal and fasting humans. *Proc Nutr Soc.* 1995;54:118A.

7. Rowbottom DG, Keast D, Morton AR. The emerging role of glutamine as an indicator of exercise stress and overtraining. *Sports Med.* 1996;21:80–97.

8. Keast D, Arstein D, Harper W, et al. Depression of plasma glutamine concentration after exercise stress and its possible influence on the immune system. *Med J Aust.* 1995;162:15–18.

9. Parry-Billings M, Budgett R, Koutedakis Y, et al. Plasma amino acid concentrations in the overtraining syndrome: possible effects on the immune system. *Med Sci Sports Exerc.* 1992;24:1353–1358.

10. Rowbottom DG, Keast D, Goodman C, et al. The haematological, biochemical, and immunological profile of athletes suffering from the overtraining syndrome. *Eur J Appl Physiol.* 1995;70:502–509.

11. Hack V, Weiss C, Friedmann B, et al. Decreased plasma glutamine level and CD4+ T cell numbers in response to 8 wk of anaerobic training. *Am J Physiol.* 1997;272(5 pt 1):E788–E795.

12. Rohde T, MacLean DA, Hartkopp A, et al. The immune system and serum glutamine during a triathlon. *Eur J Appl Physiol.* 1996;74:428–434.

13. Rohde T, MacLean DA, Pedersen BK. Effect of glutamine supplementation on changes in the immune system induced by repeated exercise. *Med Sci Sports Exerc.* 1998;30:856–862.

14. Castell LM, Newsholme EA. The effects of oral glutamine supplementation on athletes after prolonged exhaustive exercise. *Nutrition.* 1997;13:738–742.

15. Castell LM, Poortmans JR, Leclercq R, et al. Some aspects of the acute phase response after a marathon race, and the effects of glutamine supplementation. *Eur J Appl Physiol.* 1997;75:47–53.

16. Varnier M, Leese GP, Thompson J, et al. Stimulatory effect of glutamine on glycogen accumulation in human skeletal muscle. *Am J Physiol.* 1995;269(2 pt 1):E309–E315.

17. Zanker CL, Swaine IL, Castell LM, et al. Responses of plasma glutamine, free tryptophan, and branched-chain amino acids to prolonged exercise after a regime designed to reduce muscle glycogen. *Eur J Appl Physiol.* 1997;75:543–548.

Glycerol

Glycerol, a three-carbon molecule, makes up the structural core of triglycerides and phospholipids. It is produced endogenously and is present in the body as a component of stored fat and as free glycerol in body fluids. Through gluconeogenesis, glycerol can be converted into glucose in the liver. Intravenous or oral administration of glycerol increases blood osmolarity, resulting in fluid retention in the body with the exception of the brain and eyes. Because glycerol does not penetrate these areas, it has been prescribed to decrease intracranial pressure in serious clinical conditions such as stroke, Reye's syndrome, meningitis, and encephalitis and to lower intraocular pressure in glaucoma. Sports scientists are investigating glycerol loading prior to exercise as a possible way to maintain hydration and thus enhance exercise performance (1–3).

Media and Marketing Claims	Efficacy
Improves hydration status and enhances exercise	↑?
Improves exercise in hot and humid conditions	NR

Advisory

- May cause headache, nausea, or blurred vision
- Causes fluid retention; not for use by patients with edema, congestive heart failure, renal disease, hypertension

Drug/Supplement Interactions

No reported adverse interactions

KEY POINTS

- There is preliminary evidence that glycerol ingestion results in a state of hyperhydration for exercise lasting less than two hours. However, the limited research and small numbers of subjects used in varying states of physical fitness is conflicting regarding the efficacy of glycerol in enhancing physical performance or improving thermoregulation. Until more studies are completed determining the efficacy, dosage, and timing of glycerol ingestion, the claim that glycerol "enhances sport performance" is unsupported.

- It is important to warn individuals deciding to use glycerol products that the supplement may produce headache and blurred vision, which could interfere with athletic performance.

- Because of the potential for serious adverse effects, individuals with compromised health status (ie, congestive heart failure, diabetes, hypertension, renal disease) should avoid ingesting glycerol.

FOOD SOURCES

Glycerol or glycerine is a food additive in processed foods, medications, and skin products. Glycerol yields 4.32 calories/g when oxidized to carbon and water (2).

DOSAGE INFORMATION/BIOAVAILABILITY

Glycerol is available in drugstores as glycerin or glycerine in oral and topical formulations. It is also sold as glycerate in individual packets and is in some sports beverages. Glycerol products marketed to athletes recommend taking about approximately 1 g glycerate/kg to be mixed with a large volume of water (≈1.5 L). For a person weighing 70 kg, manufacturers recommend different doses ranging from 60 mL to 177 mL glycerate (2 oz to 6 oz) consumed with water (1). Researchers have used varying doses of glycerol and water generally 1 hour to 1.5 hours before exercise. Glycerol is easily absorbed with plasma levels peaking at approximately 60 minutes to 90 minutes after ingestion (2).

RELEVANT RESEARCH

Glycerol and Hydration

- In a double-blind, placebo-controlled study, 11 nonexercising male subjects participated in two separate acute trials of hyperhydration and a third control trial without hydration. Subjects drank: (1) water plus 1.5 g glycerol per liter of the subject's measured total body water (TBW), or (2) plain water matched for taste and color. Change in TBW was calculated by subtracting urine volumes from the volume of liquid ingested. Total ingested volume was equal to 37 mL/L TBW (average volume was 1,765 mL). Three hours after ingestion, glycerol intake resulted in significantly greater fluid retention (500 mL) than water intake alone (60 percent water retention with glycerol vs 32 percent water). Both glycerol and water increased blood and plasma volumes, but there were no differences between the groups. There were no differences in heart rate, diastolic blood pressure, mean arterial blood pressure, and pulse pressure between groups. However, systolic blood pressure was significantly higher during the final 60 minutes in glycerol-treated subjects compared to subjects receiving the placebo (114 mm Hg vs 109 mm Hg) (3).

- In a double-blind, placebo-controlled, crossover study, seven subjects were randomly assigned to ingest a large volume of fluid (39.2 or 51.1 mL/kg/day) with glycerol (2.9 g/kg/day to 3.1 g/kg/day) and without glycerol in experiments lasting 32 or 49 hours. Subjects reported to the lab four times per day for meals, blood draws, and urine collection. Mean glycerol intake was 235 g/24 hours (equivalent to 940 kcal). In both trials, glycerol ingestion resulted in a significant reduction in urine volume compared to placebo. Water retention with glycerol (fluid intake less urine volume) was approximately 700 mL. During glycerol ingestion, mean serum glycerol values rose after four hours; however, there were no significant changes observed in plasma osmolality, hemotocrit, or hemoglobin. The authors noted that the osmolality data was difficult to explain, as they had expected it to increase with glycerol ingestion. They concluded that it is possible to hyperhydrate for extended periods of time, thereby reducing the amount of fluid intake needed before or during bouts of negative fluid balance situations such as during strenuous exercise (4).

- In a double-blind, crossover study, eight competitive cyclists were given either a glycerol solution (1 g/kg body mass) in a diluted carbohydrate drink or a placebo (carbohydrate drink alone) prior to completing a 60-minute cycle ergometer trial(30 minutes fixed workload phase and 30 minutes variable workload phase). The total fluid intake in each trial was 22 mL/kg body mass. Glycerol intake expanded body water by approximately 600 mL over the placebo. Glycerol also significantly increased performance by

G

5 percent compared to the placebo. There were no differences in rectal temperature, sweat rate, or cardiac frequency between treatment phases (5).

Glycerol and Thermoregulation

- In a double-blind, controlled, crossover study, eight heat-acclimated male subjects were hydrated in five separate trials in random order prior to 120 minutes of treadmill exercise in the heat (35ringC): (1) euhydration (determined by plasma osmolality), (2) glycerol hyperhydration (1.2 g glycerol/kg lean body mass [LBM]) with water replacement equivalent to sweat loss, (3) glycerol hyperhydration with no water replacement, (4) hyperhydration with water replacement equivalent to sweat loss, and (5) hyperhydration with no water replacement. Hyperhydration was achieved by drinking 3.9 mL/kg LBM of either a glycerol solution (containing 1.2 g glycerol/kg LBM) or plain water, followed by drinking a large volume of water (25.2 mL/kg LBM). The total volume of fluid consumed during a 30-minute period was 29.1 mL/kg. Glycerol hyperhydration with or without water replacement had no effect on body temperature, whole body sweating rate, sweating threshold temperature, sweating sensitivity, or heart rate compared to water hyperhydration or euhydration. The authors concluded that neither water nor glycerol hyperhydration provide a thermoregulatory advantage over maintaining euhydration during exercise-heat stress (6).

- In a controlled trial, six untrained subjects were administered three different hydration protocols in randomized order on three separate days: (1) glycerol (1 g/kg body weight) plus a large volume of water (21.4 mL/kg), (2) large volume of water (21.4 mL/kg), or (3) limited fluid (3.3 mL/kg). Two and a half hours after fluid intake, subjects performed 90 minutes of treadmill exercise at 60 percent VO_{2max} in a hot, dry environment (42ringC). Urine volume prior to exercise was significantly decreased with glycerol ingestion. Glycerol ingestion resulted in a significantly lower rectal temperature and significantly elevated sweat rate during exercise compared to trials with water alone. The authors concluded: "These data support the hypothesis that glycerol-induced hyperhydration reduces the thermal burden of moderate exercise in the heat" (7).

Glycerol and Exercise Performance

- In a double-blind, placebo-controlled, crossover study, 11 trained subjects were randomly assigned to drink a glycerol solution (1.2 g/kg glycerol in 26 mL/kg water) or water (placebo) over a 90-minute period prior to exercise on a cycle ergometer (74 percent VO_{2max}). A second study was completed using the same pre-exercise regimen with the addition of a carbohydrate replacement drink (5 percent glucose) given to seven subjects during exercise. In both studies, glycerol intake resulted in significantly reduced heart rate and prolonged endurance time. Body temperature (rectal) was not affected by glycerol (8).

- In a placebo-controlled trial, nine subjects completed four trials of cycling for 90 minutes at 50 percent VO_{2max} while consuming one of four solutions (total = 650 mL) every 15 minutes: 10 percent glycerol drink, 6 percent carbohydrate (CHO) drink, CHO drink plus 4 percent glycerol, and water (placebo). Glycerol ingestion attenuated the decrease in plasma volume associated with water intake alone. Heart rate, esophageal temperature, sweat rate, ratings of perceived exertion, cortisol, and aldosterone levels measurements were taken. There were no substantial cardiovascular, metabolic, hormonal, or thermoregulatory advantages associated with glycerol ingestion (9).

SAFETY

- According to a recent review article, several studies have shown no adverse side-effects with glycerol ingestion, whereas other studies have reported adverse effects in 10 percent to 25 percent of the subjects (1). Reported side-effects include nausea, headache, and blurred vision, attributed to fluid drawn away from the cranial and ocular regions. Symptoms appear to intensify as the dose increases (8).

- Hyperglycemia in diabetic patients has also been reported with intravenous glycerol (2).

- In one small study, glycerol ingestion raised systolic blood pressure but had no effect on diastolic pressure (3).

- Because glycerol appears to cause fluid retention, it should be avoided by patients with edema, congestive heart failure, renal disease, hypertension, and other conditions that may be exacerbated by retaining excess fluid.

REFERENCES

1. Wagner DR. Hyperhydrating with glycerol: implications for athletic performance. *J Am Diet Assoc.* 1999;99:207–212.
2. Frank MS, Nahata MC, Hilty MD. Glycerol: a review of its pharmacology, pharmacokinetics, adverse reactions, and clinical use. *Pharmacotherapy.* 1981;1:147–160.
3. Freund BJ, Montain SJ, Young AJ, et al. Glycerol hyperhydration: hormonal, renal, and vascular fluid responses. *J Appl Physiol.* 1995;79:2069–2077.
4. Koenigsberg PS, Martin KK, Hlava HR, et al. Sustained hyperhydration with glycerol ingestion. *Life Sci.* 1995;57:645–653.
5. Hitchins S, Martin DT, Burke L, et al. Glycerol hyperhydration improves cycle time trial performance in hot humid conditions. *Eur J Appl Physiol Occup Physiol.* 1999;80:494–501.
6. Latzka WA, Sawka MN, Montain SJ, et al. Hyperhydration: thermoregulatory effects during compensable exercise-heat stress. *J Appl Physiol.* 1997;83:860–866.
7. Lyons TP, Riedesel ML, Meuli LE, et al. Effects of glycerol-induced hyperhydration prior to exercise in the heat on sweating and core temperature. *Med Sci Sports Exerc.* 1990;22:477–483.
8. Montner P, Stark DM, Riedesel ML, et al. Pre-exercise glycerol hydration improves cycling endurance time. *Int J Sports Med.* 1996;17:27–33.
9. Murray R, Eddy DE, Paul GL, et al. Physiological response to glycerol ingestion during exercise. *J Appl Physiol.* 1991;71:144–149.

Goldenseal (Hydrastis canadensis)

Originally used orally and topically by Native Americans to treat a variety of conditions such as dyspepsia, diarrhea, whooping cough, mouth sores, anorexia, eye infections, and fever, goldenseal was one of the top ten-selling herbs in the United States in 1997 (1, 2). The active constituents in goldenseal are believed to be isoquinoline alkaloids. Berberine (2 percent to 3 percent) and hydrastine (2 percent to 4 percent) have been identified as the major alkaloids. Although there is a lack of pharmacological and clinical research on goldenseal, several studies have been conducted on the isolated alkaloid berberine (1). Other herbs that contain berberis alkaloids include barberry (*Berberis vulgaris*), Oregon grape (*Mahonia aquifolium*), barberry bush (*Berberis aristata*) and the Chinese herb goldthread (*Coptis chinensis*). Extracts from berberine containing plants have been used in antidiarrheal medications in Ayurvedic medicine in India and in traditional medicine in China (3).

Media and Marketing Claims	Efficacy
Herbal antibiotic; reduces mucous and soothes sore throat	NR
Protects against traveler's diarrhea	NR
Helps symptoms associated with menstrual difficulties	NR
Masks drug use in urine tests	NR

Advisory

- Lack of scientific data in humans to evaluate safety
- Berberine (an isolated component of goldenseal) in doses of 200 mg to 1,200 mg is not associated with any adverse effects

Drug/Supplement Interactions

No reported adverse interactions

KEY POINTS

- Marketing claims about goldenseal cannot be supported at this time because of a lack of clinical research. A component of goldenseal, berberine, appears to have antibiotic and antiparasitic actions *in vitro* and in animal studies. However, there is conflicting evidence on the efficacy of berberine sulfate on enterotoxin-induced secretory diarrhea in infected humans.

- Although some proponents have used anecdotal evidence and historical use to suggest that goldenseal reduces mucous production, soothes sore throats, alleviates dyspepsia, and stimulates menstrual flow, clinical trials are lacking to verify these claims.

- There is no evidence that goldenseal masks drug use in urine tests. Some products claiming to "detoxify" the urine also suggest drinking massive quantities of fluid before urine testing, which would act as a dilutant and decrease drug detection.

FOOD SOURCES

None

DOSAGE INFORMATION/BIOAVAILABILITY

The dried roots and rhizome of the goldenseal plant are available in capsules, tinctures, and teas, often combined with echinacea. Dosages range from 500 mg to 2,000 mg of the dried extract, 1 mL liquid extract, or 2 mL to 4 mL tincture. It is often recommended for short-term use to help treat infections and promote healing. Some goldenseal products are standardized to contain 5 percent hydrastine. There are no recent studies on the absorption and bioavailability of goldenseal. In a study completed 30 years ago, berberine was found to be poorly absorbed across the human small intestine (4).

RELEVANT RESEARCH

Goldenseal/Berberine and Antibiotic Activity

- No studies have tested the effects of goldenseal on infection. However, studies supplementing with berberine (an alkaloid in goldenseal) are reported here.

- In an *in vitro* study, berberine sulfate blocked the adherence of *Streptococci pyogenes* to host cells by releasing adhesin lipoteichoic acid from the streptococcal cell surface and by preventing the formation of or dissolving lipoteichoic acid-fibronectin complexes. Berberine inhibited streptococci growth but did not have bactericidal actions. The author speculated that berberine may be useful in treating infections such as tonsillitis and respiratory, urinary, and skin infections as caused by group A *Streptococci* because berberine both inhibits adhesion and growth of this organism (5).

- An *in vitro* study found berberine sulfate inhibited the growth of the parasites *Giardia lamblia, Trichomonas vaginalis,* and *Entamoeba histolytica* (6). Another *in vitro* study showed berberine had antiparasitic activity against *Leishmania donavani* (7).

- In an *in vitro* study, berberine sulfate had no effect on bacterial growth or the synthesis of major outer membrane proteins of the *Escherichia coli* enterotoxin. However, berberine sulfate did block adhesion of bacteria to host cells. The authors hypothesized that the anti-infectious activity of berberine in *E coli*-induced urinary tract infections could interfere with the adhesion of uropathogenic organisms to the urinary tract, but this has not been tested in humans (8).

Goldenseal/Berberine and Infectious Diarrhea

- No studies have tested goldenseal in digestive disorders. However, studies supplementing with berberine (an alkaloid in goldenseal) are reported here.

- In a parallel trial, 165 subjects from Bangladesh with acute diarrhea caused by enterotoxigenic *E coli* and *Vibrio cholerae* were randomized to receive 400 mg berberine sulfate, 1,200 mg berberine sulfate plus tetracycline in a single oral dose or no treatment (control). Patients with *E coli* infections who received berberine had significantly lower mean stool volumes than controls during three consecutive eight-hour periods after treatment. After 24 hours, significantly more subjects treated with berberine stopped having diarrhea compared to controls (42 percent vs 20 percent). In patients with cholera who received 400 mg berberine, stool volume significantly decreased during the second eight-hour period after treatment compared to controls, but not during the first or third period. Among cholera patients, there were no differences in stool output between patients receiving berberine and tetracycline compared to controls (9).

- In a double-blind, placebo-controlled trial, 400 subjects with acute watery diarrhea were randomized to receive 400 mg berberine, 2,000 mg tetracycline, a combination of the two, or a placebo divided into four doses per day. Of 185 patients with cholera, those given tetracycline or tetracycline plus berberine had reduced volume and frequency of diarrhea stools, duration of diarrhea, and volumes and frequency of required oral rehydration. Berberine alone had no effect. Of the 215 patients with non-cholera diarrhea, neither berberine nor tetracycline had any benefit compared to the placebo (3).

- Berberine has been shown to inhibit the intestinal secretory response to enterotoxins (*V cholerae* and *E coli*) in animal and *ex vivo* studies (10–13). These effects were apparent when administered before or after enterotoxin binding and when berberine was given either intraluminally or parentally (9).

Goldenseal and Masking of Urinary Drug Tests

- It is a popular myth that ingestion of goldenseal prior to urinary drug testing can mask the detection of illicit drug use. Early urine tests relied on thin-layer chromatography, in which goldenseal may have interfered with the detection of morphine. However, goldenseal would have no effect in current urine analysis techniques (immunoassays and gas chromatography-mass spectrometry) (14).

- There are no studies testing the effect of goldenseal on urinary drug test results.

SAFETY

- Because there is a dearth of research on goldenseal, data on safety and toxicity are not known. Berberine has been used acutely in studies with no serious adverse effects reported in doses ranging from 200 to 1,200 mg.

- Berberine resulted in a significant decrease in mean bilirubin serum protein binding in rats, due to a persistent elevation of serum concentrations of unbound and total bilirubin. The author of this study cautioned against the use of berberine-containing herbs by pregnant women and jaundiced infants (15). (Note: Because of the lack of safety data for most botanicals, pregnant women and infants should not use *any* herbal supplement without physician approval.)

REFERENCES

1. Blumenthal M, ed. *The Complete German Commission E Monographs Therapeutic Guide to Herbal Medicines.* Austin, Tex: American Botanical Council; 1998.

2. Foster S. *Botanical Series No. 309—Goldenseal.* Austin, Tex: American Botanical Council; 1996.

3. Khin-Maung-U, Myo-Khin, Nyunt-Nyuny-Wai, et al. Clinical trial of berberine in acute watery diarrhea. *Br Med J (Clin Res Ed).* 1985;291:1601–1605.

4. Bhide MB, Chavan SR, Duttak NK. Absorption, distribution, and excretion of berberine. *Indian J Med Res.* 1969;57:2128–2131.

5. Sun D, Courtney HS, Beachey EH. Berberine sulfate blocks adherence of *Streptococcus pyogenes* to epithelial cells, fibronectin, and hexadecane. *Antimicrob Agents Chemother.* 1988;32:1370–1374.

6. Kaneda Y, Torii M, Tanaka T, et al. *In vitro* effects of berberine sulfate on the growth and structure of *Entamoeba histolytica, Giardia lamblia,* and *Trichomonas vaginalis. Ann Trop Med Parasitol.* 1991;85:417–425.

7. Ghosh AK, Bhattacharyya FK, Ghosh DK. *Leishmania donovani*: amastigote inhibition and mode of action of berberine. *Exp Parasitol.* 1985;60:404–413.

8. Sun D, Abraham SN, Beachey EH. Influence of berberine sulfate on synthesis and expression of Pap fimbrial adhesion in uropathogenic *Escherichia coli. Antimicrob Agents Chemother.* 1988;32:1274–1277.

9. Rabbani GH, Butler T, Knight J, et al. Randomized controlled trial of berberine sulfate therapy for diarrhea due to enterotoxigenic *Escherichia coli* and *Vibrio cholerae. J Infect Dis.* 1987;155:979–984.

10. Sack RB, Froehlich JL. Berberine inhibits intestinal secretory response of *Vibrio cholerae* and *Escherichia coli* enterotoxins. *Infect Immun.* 1982;35:471–475.

11. Zhu B, Ahrens FA. Effect of berberine on intestinal secretion mediated by *Escherichia coli* heat-stable enterotoxin in jejunum of pigs. *Am J Vet Res.* 1982;43:1594–1598.

12. Zhu B, Ahrens F. Antisecretory effects of berberine with morphine, clonidine, L-phenylephrine, yohimbine, or neostigmine in pig jejunum. *Eur J Pharmacol.* 1983;96:11–19.

13. Tai YH, Feser JF, Marnane WG, et al. Antisecretory effects of berberine in rat ileum. *Am J Physiol.* 1981;241:G253—G258.

14. Morgan JP. Urine tests for drug use: are they reliable? *HerbalGram.* 1988;32:46–51, 70.

15. Chan E. Displacement of bilirubin from albumin by berberine. *Biol Neonate.* 1993;63:201–208.

Green Tea Extract

Tea (*Camellia sinensis*) is one of the most popular beverages in the world. Of the total tea manufactured worldwide from *Camellia sinensis*, 78 percent is black, 20 percent is green, and 2 percent is oolong tea. Green tea is an integral part of Japanese and Chinese cultures and is consumed at an average of three cups per day. Although green, oolong, and black teas are made from the same species of tea plant, they each have different chemical compositions. The fresh tea leaf contains flavonoids, a large group of polyphenolic compounds with antioxidant properties. The polyphenols found in green tea, known as catechins, make up 30 percent to 50 percent of the dry tea leaf weight. Green tea is produced by steaming and drying the tea leaves, which preserves the polyphenol content. During black tea production, natural fermentation occurs, causing complexation of most of the polyphenols, with the retention of the antioxidant properties. Oolong tea is semifermented and is intermediate in polyphenol composition between green and black teas (1–3).

One cup of green tea provides approximately 100 mg to 200 mg polyphenols, which include epigallocatechin gallate (EGCG), epicatechin (EC), and epicatechin gallate (ECG). EGCG is present in the highest concentrations and is thought to be the most biologically active ingredient in green tea. Green tea also contains caffeine (3 percent to 5 percent dry weight), minerals (6 percent to 8 percent), and free amino acids (4 percent) (1–3). Regular varieties contain caffeine (approximately 10 mg to 50 mg caffeine/cup), but green tea is also available decaffeinated.

Green tea extract is the primary focus here because currently there are no black tea supplements on the market.

Media and Marketing Claims	Efficacy
Strong antioxidant (*in vitro*)	↑
Strong antioxidant (*in vivo*)	↑?
Reduces risk of cancer	↑?
Protects the heart	NR
Fights viruses and bacteria	NR

Advisory

Contains caffeine—use caution if caffeine-sensitive

Drug/Supplement Interactions

- Green tea extract may interfere with iron absorption
- Not to be used with any medications that have negative interactions with caffeine

KEY POINTS

- The polyphenols in green tea have demonstrated antioxidant capacities *in vitro* and *in vivo*.

- Although much more research is needed, there is evidence from *in vitro*, animal, and epidemiological studies suggesting that green tea has anticarcinogenic activity. The first controlled, clinical trial of oral green tea supplements in cancer patients was conducted to determine the maximum tolerated dose and toxicity, but now future studies are needed to provide efficacy data.

- Controlled clinical trials in humans drinking green tea or supplementing green tea extract (equivalent to 16 cups of tea) have not shown a lipid-lowering effect or a consistent protective effect on markers of oxidative stress. Additional clinical research is needed to delineate the role of green tea in cardiovascular disease.

- There is preliminary evidence from *in vitro* studies suggesting that green tea extract inhibits bacterial growth and that polyphenols from green and black tea inhibit the influenza virus. Further research is needed to verify the significance of green tea extract or beverage intake in the prevention or treatment of infections in humans.

- Although there is a large body of research on green tea beverage consumption, the research on concentrated supplements is in its infancy. For this reason and because of the potential health benefits of tea, drinking green and black tea can be part of a healthful diet. More information on the safety and efficacy of green tea supplements is needed before recommendations regarding their use can be made.

FOOD SOURCES

Infusions made from green tea leaves

DOSAGE INFORMATION/BIOAVAILABILITY

Green tea extract is sold in capsules providing 100 mg to 600 mg green tea standardized to 50 percent catechins (polyphenols). Consumption of 1.5 g and 3.0 g of green tea solids dissolved in 500 mL water resulted in a maximum plasma concentration of tea catechins within 1.4 hours to 2.4 hours (4). The half-life of EGCG (5.0 hours to 5.5 hours) was greater than EGC or EC (2.5 hours to 3.4 hours) (4).

RELEVANT RESEARCH

Green Tea and Antioxidant Activity

- Several *in vitro* studies have demonstrated antioxidant properties of green tea (3, 5–8).

- In a study by the US Department of Agriculture, a serving of green or black tea brewed for five minutes in 5 oz of boiling water had more antioxidant activity (as measured by the Oxygen Radical Absorbance Capacity-ORAC assay) than individual servings of commonly consumed fruits and vegetables (8).

- Green tea consumption in smokers decreased oxidative DNA damage (8-OHdG in white blood cells and urine), lipid peroxidation (malondialdehyde in urine), and free radical generation (2,3-DHBA in urine). In nonsmokers, there was also a decrease in overall oxidative stress (9).

- In a double-blind, placebo-controlled study, 20 healthy nonsmoking female subjects (ages 23 y to 50 y) were randomized to receive 3 g green tea extract (equivalent to 10 cups of tea) or a placebo daily for four weeks. The background diet was rich in linoleic acid and contained 27 percent fat, 14 percent protein, and 59 percent carbohydrate. Fasting blood samples and five 24-hour urine specimens were collected before and at the end of the study. Same samples were taken from 10 control subjects. Green tea extract significantly decreased plasma malondialdehyde concentration (marker of lipid peroxidation) compared to the placebo. There was no effect of green tea on serum lipids, indicators of antioxidant status, urinary 8-isoprostaglandin F2 alpha (marker of oxidative stress), 2, 3 dinorthromboxane B_2, nitric oxide metabolites, or coagulation indicators. The authors concluded that green tea extract resulted in a small but significant reduction of lipid peroxidation, but did not have specific effects on other markers related to cardiovascular diseases (10).

Green Tea and Cancer

- Several animal studies have demonstrated anticarcinogenic activity of tea polyphenols in carcinogen-induced tumors in stomach, duodenum, colon, pancreas, mammary glands, liver, lung, skin, and prostate cancer (3, 11–15). *In vitro* studies have shown green tea polyphenols to increase activity of antioxidant and detoxifying enzymes, block nitrosamines, suppress tumor growth by inhibition of tumor necrosis factor-α release, modulate DNA replication and repair, and inhibit estrogen receptor interaction in mammary cancer (2, 3, 16, 17).

- A review article summarized 31 epidemiological studies of reported green tea consumption and cancer risk. Of 5 studies reporting on colon cancer, 3 reported an inverse relationship, 1 reported an insignificant inverse trend and 1 found a positive relationship with green tea intake. For rectal cancer, 1 of 4 studies reported an inverse relationship, but increased risks were apparent in 2 studies. Both studies on urinary bladder cancer reported an inverse association. Of the 10 studies on stomach cancer, 6 suggested an inverse and 3 reported a positive relationship. Two of 3 studies report an inverse relationship of green tea and pancreatic cancer. Although studies examining esophageal cancer had mixed results, there was a consistent positive association between cancer risk and temperature of tea (defined as very hot or scalding hot). Of the total studies in the review, 17 demonstrated reduced risk, 7 reported increased risk, 3 showed no association, and 5 reported an increased risk of cancer with scalding hot temperature (17).

- In a retrospective study, 472 Japanese patients with stages I, II, and III breast cancer were evaluated for green tea consumption prior to clinical cancer diagnosis. Increased green tea intake was significantly correlated with decreased numbers of axillary lymph node metastases among premenopausal but not postmenopausal patients with stage I and II cancer. Green tea was also associated with increased expression of progesterone receptors and estrogen receptors among postmenopausal subjects. Increased consumption of green tea was associated with a significant decrease in recurrence of stage I and II breast cancer after seven years. Specifically, the recurrence rate was 16.7 percent among those consuming ≥ 5 cups, and 24.3 percent among those consuming ≤ 4 cups/day. No improvement in prognosis was seen in stage III patients (18).

- The effects of green tea and coffee among Korean cigarette smokers were examined in 52 healthy male subjects (ages 20 y to 52 y). Blood specimens were obtained from non-smokers (group 1), smokers (group 2), smokers consuming green tea (group 3), and smokers drinking coffee (group 4). Daily intake of green tea and coffee was 2 to 3 cups/day for six months in groups 3 and 4. The mean number of smoking years (> 10 cigarettes/day) ranged from 13 years to 14 years. The frequencies of sister chromatid exchange—SCE (biomarker of mutagenesis) in mitogen-stimulated peripheral lymphocytes were determined. SCE rates were significantly elevated in smokers vs nonsmokers; however, the frequency of SCE in smokers who consumed green tea was comparable to that of nonsmokers. In contrast, coffee did not exhibit a significant inhibitory effect on smoking-induced SCE (19).

- The first phase I trial of oral green tea extract in cancer patients investigated the safety and pharmacology of the extract. Forty-nine patients (ages 27 y to 77 y) with incurable malignancy, not on chemotherapy or radiotherapy, and with a life expectancy of at least 16 weeks were given green tea extract capsules in varying doses after meals one or three times daily for four weeks up to a maximum of six months, depending on tolerance. Doses ranged from 0.5 to 5.05 g/m^2 once daily and dose levels of 1.0 to 2.2 g/m^2 three times daily were also explored. Lung, head, and neck cancers were the most frequent diagnoses among the subjects. Mild to moderate toxicities were seen at most dose levels and were reversed after discontinuing green tea extract. Dose-limiting toxicities were deemed related to caffeine and included neurologic (agitation, dizziness, insomnia, tremors) and gastrointestinal (bloating, dyspepsia, flatulence, nausea, vomiting) side-effects. Maximum tolerated doses were found to be 4.2 g/m^2 once daily or 1.0 g/m^2 three times daily. After eight weeks, an accumulation of caffeine related to dosage was seen in plasma, whereas epigallocatechin gallate levels did not accumulate in plasma. The authors recommended that future studies use a dose of 1.0 g/m^2 (about 7 to 8 Japanese cups [120 mL per cup] of green tea three times daily), because this amount appeared to be well tolerated with minimal side-effects. The researchers concluded that the doses they investigated are safe for at least six months in cancer patients (20).

Tea and Cardiovascular Disease

- Epidemiological studies suggest that tea consumption (green or black) is associated with decreased risk of cardiovascular disease and stroke (21, 22).

- In a single-blind, placebo-controlled, *ex vivo* study, 64 healthy smokers were randomized to drink 6 cups black tea, green tea, or water per day, or a supplement of 3.6 g green tea polyphenols/day (equivalent to 18 cups green tea) for four weeks. Subjects were instructed by a dietitian to maintain normal eating habits and avoid red wine. Blood samples were taken at the baseline and at the end of the study. Compared to the control, there were no significant different effects shown by green tea or black tea consumption on plasma cholesterol, triglycerides, HDL and LDL cholesterol, plasma vitamins C and E, beta-carotene, and uric acid. There were also no differences found in parameters of LDL oxidation *ex vivo*. Intake of green tea polyphenol supplements had no significant effect on any of the parameters measured except a decrease in plasma vitamin E concentrations compared to controls (23).

- In a parallel comparison trial, 48 subjects were randomized to drink six cups black tea, green tea, or water (control) daily for four weeks. Blood samples were taken at the baseline and at the end of the study. Neither green nor black tea affected serum lipid concentrations, resistance of LDL to oxidation *ex vivo*, or markers of oxidative damage *in vivo*. However, green tea slightly increased total antioxidant activity of plasma. The *in vitro* experiment showed a decrease in LDL oxidation only after incubation with very high concentrations of green or black tea, higher than achievable *in vivo*. The authors concluded: "Future research should focus on mechanisms by which tea flavonoids may reduce the risk of cardiovascular disease other than by increasing the intrinsic antioxidant status of LDL" (24).

- In a cross-sectional study, 371 subjects from five regions in Japan were evaluated for green tea intake and lipid levels. Mean serum concentrations of total cholesterol, triglycerides, and HDL cholesterol were compared to three levels of daily green tea intake (4 cups). After researchers adjusted for dietary and nondietary factors, green tea was not associated with lipid levels (25).

- In a cross-sectional study, 1,371 Japanese men (aged more than 40 y) were evaluated for green tea consumption and associated lipid levels and liver function. Increased consumption of green tea was significantly associated with decreased serum total cholesterol and triglyceride levels. There was also a significant association of green tea with increases in HDL cholesterol levels together with a decreased proportion of LDL and VLDL cholesterol, which resulted in a lowered atherogenic index (26).

- In an *in vitro* study, green tea extract inhibited peroxidation in LDL cholesterol catalyzed by copper with malondialdehyde as a parameter of antioxidant activity. The polyphenol component showed the strongest antioxidant effect, followed by theanine. Caffeine had a limited effect (27).

Tea's Antibacterial and Antiviral Properties

- In an *in vitro* study, extracts of green tea, black tea, or coffee inhibited the growth of various bacteria causing diarrhea (*Vibrio cholerae, Salmonella typhimurium, and Salmonella typhi*) (28).

- In an *in vitro* study, four kinds of Japanese green tea extract demonstrated antibacterial and bactericidal actions against 24 bacterial strains isolated from subjects' infected root canals (29).

- In an *in vitro* study, tea polyphenols inhibited the absorption of the influenza virus A and B to canine kidney cells and blocked the infectiousness of the influenza virus (30).

SAFETY

- One study examining toxicity and pharmacological effects of green tea extract in cancer patients reported no serious adverse effects with doses of 1 g/m^2 (three times daily) to 4.2 g/m^2 (once daily) for six months. The $1 \text{ g/m}2$ dose corresponds to about seven to eight Japanese cups of tea three times daily. Side-effects (gastrointestinal and neurological) were determined to be caffeine-related (20).

- Green tea as a beverage has been consumed safely in China for more than 4,000 years (3).

- Green tea supplements contain caffeine. Individuals sensitive to caffeine should use caution.

- In one study, green tea extract added to foods reduced dietary nonheme iron absorption in young women (31).

REFERENCES

1. Graham HN. Green tea composition, consumption, and polyphenol chemistry. *Prev Med.* 1992;21:334–350.
2. Fujiki H, Suganuma M, Okabe S, et al. Japanese green tea as a cancer preventive in humans. *Nutr Rev.* 1996;54(11 pt 2):S67—S70.
3. Kuroda Y, Hara Y. Antimutagenic and anticarcinogenic activity of tea polyphenols. *Mutat Res.* 1999;436:69–97.
4. Yang CS, Chen L, Lee MJ, et al. Blood and urine levels of tea catechins after ingestion of different amounts of green tea by human volunteers. *Cancer Epidemiol Biomarkers Prev.* 1998;7:351–354.
5. Wei H, Zhang X, Zhao JF, et al. Scavenging of hydrogen peroxide and inhibition of ultraviolet light-induced oxidative DNA damage by aqueous extracts from green and black teas. *Free Radic Biol Med.* 1999;26:1427–1435.
6. Grinberg LN, Newmark H, Kitrossky N, et al. Protective effects of tea polyphenols against oxidative damage to red blood cells. *Biochem Pharmacol.* 1997;54:973–978.
7. Lin AM, Chyi BY, Wu LY, et al. The antioxidative property of green tea against iron-induced oxidative stress in rat brain. *Chin J Physiol.* 1998;41:189–194.
8. Prior RL, Cao G. Antioxidant capacity and polyphenolic components of teas: implications for altering *in vivo* antioxidant status. *Proc Soc Exp Biol Med.* 1999;220:255–261.
9. Klaunig JE, Xu Y, Han C, et al. The effect of tea consumption on oxidative stress in smokers and nonsmokers. *Proc Soc Exp Biol Med.* 1999;220:249–254.
10. Freese R, Basu S, Hietanen E, et al. Green tea extract decreases plasma malondialdehyde concentration but does not affect other indicators of oxidative stress, nitric oxide production, or hemostatic factors during a high linoleic acid diet in healthy females. *Eur J Nutr.* 1999;38:149–157.
11. Fujiki H, Suganuma M, Okabe S, et al. Cancer inhibition by green tea. *Mutat Res.* 1998;402:307–310.
12. Hibasami H, Komiya T, Achiwa Y, et al. Induction of apoptosis in human stomach cancer cells by green tea catechins. *Oncol Rep.* 1998;5:527–529.
13. Yang CS, Yang GY, Landau JM, et al. Tea and tea polyphenols inhibit cell hyperproliferation, lung tumorigenesis, and tumor progression. *Exp Lung Res.* 1998;24:629–639.
14. Wang ZY, Huang MT, Ferraro T, et al. Inhibitory effect of green tea in the drinking water on tumorigenesis by ultraviolet light and 12-o-tetradecanoylphorbol-13-acetate in the skin of SKH-1 mice. *Cancer Res.* 1992;52:1162–1170.
15. Paschka AG, Butler R, Young CY. Induction of apoptosis in prostate cancer cell lines by the green tea component (-)-epigallocatechin-3-gallate. *Cancer Lett.* 1998;130:1–7.
16. Fujiki H, Suganuma M, Okabe S, et al. Mechanistic findings of green tea as cancer preventive for humans. *Proc Soc Exp Biol Med.* 1999;220:225–228.

G

17. Bushman JL. Green tea and cancer in humans: a review of the literature. *Nutr Cancer.* 1998;31:151–159.

18. Nakachi K, Suemasu K, Suga K, et al. Influence of drinking green tea on breast cancer malignancy among Japanese patients. *Jpn J Cancer Res.* 1998;89:254–261.

19. Lee IP, Kim YH, Kang MH, et al. Chemopreventive effect of green tea (*Camellia sinensis*) against cigarette smoke-induced mutations (SCE) in humans. *J Cell Biochem Suppl.* 1997;27:68–75.

20. Pisters KM, Newman RA, Coldman B, et al. Phase I trial of oral green tea extract in adult patients with solid tumors. *J Clin Oncol.* 2001;19:1830–1838.

21. Hertog MG, Feskens EJ, Hollman PC, et al. Dietary antioxidant flavonoids and risk of coronary heart disease: the Zutphen Elderly Study. *Lancet.* 1993;342:1007–1011.

22. Keli SO, Hertog MG, Feskens EJ, et al. Dietary flavonoids, antioxidant vitamins, and incidence of stroke: the Zutphen Study. *Arch Intern Med.* 1996;156:637–642.

23. Princen HM, van Duyvenvoorde W, Buytenhek R, et al. No effect of consumption of green and black tea on plasma lipid and antioxidant levels and on LDL oxidation in smokers. *Arterioscler Thromb Vasc Biol.* 1998;18:833–841.

24. van het Hof KH, de Boer HS, Wiseman SA, et al. Consumption of green or black tea does not increase resistance of low-density lipoprotein to oxidation in humans. *Am J Clin Nutr.* 1997;66:1125–1132.

25. Tsubono Y, Tsugane S. Green tea intake in relation to serum lipid levels in middle-aged Japanese men and women. *Ann Epidemiol.* 1997;7:280–284.

26. Imai K, Nakachi K. Cross sectional study of effects of drinking green tea on cardiovascular and liver disease. *BMJ.* 1995;310:693–696.

27. Yokozawa T, Dong E. Influence of green tea and its three major components upon low-density lipoprotein oxidation. *Exp Toxicol Pathol.* 1997;49:329–335.

28. Shetty M, Subbannayya K, Shivananda PG. Antibacterial activity of tea (*Camellia sinensis*) and coffee (Coffee arabica) with special reference to *Salmonella typhimurium. J Commun Dis.* 1994;26:147–150.

29. Horiba N, Maekawa Y, Ito M, et al. A pilot study of Japanese green tea as a medicament: antibacterial and bactericidal effects. *J Endod.* 1991;17:122–124.

30. Nakayama M, Suzuki K, Toda M, et al. Inhibition of the infectivity of influenza virus by tea polyphenols. *Antiviral Res.* 1993;21:289–299.

31. Samman S, Sandstrom B, Toft MB, et al. Green tea or rosemary extract added to foods reduces nonheme-iron absorption. *Am J Clin Nutr.* 2001;73:607–612.

5-Hydroxy-Tryptophan (5-HTP)

5-Hydroxy-tryptophan, or 5-HTP,[1] is derived from the seed of the African plant *Griffonia simplica*. 5-HTP is a metabolite of the essential amino acid L-tryptophan, and both are pre-

---

[1] 5-HTP supplements should not be confused with L-tryptophan supplements; the latter are currently banned in the U.S. due to safety issues.

cursors to the neurotransmitter serotonin in the body. Serotonin regulates several processes in the body, including sleep, emotions, pain sensitivity, and addictive cravings. If there is a sufficient supply of L-tryptophan and its metabolite 5-HTP in the body, serotonin will be produced. Scientists believe that low levels or insufficient activity of serotonin and/or norepinephrine may cause depression. In addition, low levels of serotonin may also be involved in sleep disorders, obesity, excessive appetite, low pain sensitivity, and anxiety. In theory, therapeutic use of 5-HTP would result in bypassing the step where L-tryptophan converts into 5-HTP by the enzyme tryptophan hydroxylase. The chemical make-up of 5-HTP allows it to cross the blood-brain barrier, whereas L-tryptophan requires a transport molecule to enter the central nervous system. Thus, it is theorized that supplementing 5-HTP would initiate a more immediate and abundant conversion of 5-HTP into the neurotransmitter serotonin (1, 2).

Media and Marketing Claims	Efficacy
Reduces depression	↑?
Reduces carbohydrate cravings and aids weight loss	NR
Reduces pain	NR
Alleviates stress	NR

Advisory

- Some 5-HTP supplements have been reported to be contaminated with impurities that my cause illness.
- Case report of eosinophilia-myalgia syndrome occurring in a family taking 5-HTP
- May cause gastrointestinal symptoms, including nausea and stomach pain, with initial use

Drug/Supplement Interactions

Should not be combined with triclyclic antidepressants, monoamine oxidase inhibitors (MAOI), serotonin reuptake inhibitors (ie, Prozac, Zoloft, Paxil)

KEY POINTS

- Theoretically, 5-HTP, a precursor to serotonin, might have a variety of beneficial effects because a lack of serotonin appears to be involved in mood disorders, sleep, pain sensitivity, addiction, and satiety.

- Preliminary, small trials of 5-HTP in depressive subjects suggest an antidepressant effect. However, many of the studies have been criticized for having small sample sizes, lack of placebo use or blinding, short duration, or unclear diagnosis of depression. More evidence is needed from long-term, large-scale, controlled trials to determine efficacy. Severely depressed individuals should be under the care of a mental health professional, and should not self-supplement using 5-HTP without physician approval.

- Small, poorly controlled trials report that 5-HTP supplementation reduces appetite, lowers carbohydrate cravings, and stimulates weight loss. It is significant that 5-HTP also causes mild nausea, which could also have contributed to the reported loss of appetite and weight. Well-controlled research in larger numbers of subjects is needed to validate the claim that 5-HTP is an effective tool for weight reduction.

- Controlled studies are needed to determine whether 5-HTP reduces the perception of pain. One unblinded study reported a reduction in pain in fibromyalgia patients, but this needs to be confirmed in a well-designed, double-blind study.

- Evidence is lacking to support the use of 5-HTP for stress reduction.

FOOD SOURCES

None

DOSAGE INFORMATION/BIOAVAILABILITY

5-HTP is available in capsules and tablets in amounts ranging from 50 mg to 100 mg. Studies have used a range of doses from 100 mg to 1,200 mg/day. Some manufacturers suggest taking 100 mg per day on an empty stomach (2). However, because 5-HTP may cause mild nausea in some patients, some researchers recommend taking it with food.

5-HTP appears to be well absorbed, with approximately 70 percent reaching the bloodstream (2). Absorption is not affected by ingesting it with other amino acids (2). 5-HTP has been associated with increases in the cerebrospinal fluid levels of 5-hydroxyindolacetic acid, the primary metabolite of serotonin, suggesting that 5-HTP stimulates serotonin release (1).

RELEVANT RESEARCH

5-HTP and Depression

- A number of uncontrolled and controlled studies of 5-HTP for depression were published in the 1970s and early 1980s. In a review of seven controlled studies with a combined total of 78 subjects, 5-HTP was found to be effective in five of these trials (1).

- In a double-blind, comparative, multicenter study in Switzerland, 63 patients with severe depression were randomized to receive 300 mg 5-HTP or 150 mg fluvoxamine with meals daily for six weeks. No other antidepressant medications were permitted during the study. Subjects were assessed with the Hamilton Rating Scale for Depression (HRSD), Clinical Global Impression (CGI) scale, and their own self-assessment. There were no significant differences in the level of depression between groups. Both treatment groups showed significant improvements in depressive symptoms as assessed by the HRSD, CGI, and self-assessment. However, there were no significant differences in improvement between the two groups. 5-HTP-treated subjects had lesser degrees of severity of adverse events (mostly mild gastrointestinal disturbance, nausea) than fluvoxamine. Ingestion of 5-HTP had no effect on liver enzymes and other routine laboratory tests (3).

- In a double-blind, placebo-controlled study, 26 subjects hospitalized for depression were randomized to receive 300 mg L-5-HTP or placebo daily for 28 days. All subjects also received 50 mg/day chlorimipramine (antidepressant). Depressive symptoms were evaluated weekly by the HRSD and at baseline and study end by the CGI scale and Zung's Depression Status Inventory (ZDSI). All subjects improved on the HRDS, with the L-5-HTP group showing significantly greater improvement. ZDSI scores were also significantly improved with the L-5-HTP group. No statistical analysis was performed on CGI evaluation (no explanation given). The authors concluded that more improvement in the overall clinical picture and symptoms was obtained with 5-HTP plus chlorimipramine than with chlorimipramine plus placebo. The parameters that improved more than others were mood, insomnia, work and activities, agitation, anxiety, general and gastrointestinal somatic disturbances, and hypochondriasis. Tolerability was good in both groups (4).

5-HTP and Appetite

- In a double-blind, placebo-controlled study, 28 obese patients were randomized to receive either 900 mg 5-HTP (300 mg 30 minutes before each meal) or placebo daily for 12 weeks. Subjects were prescribed a 1,200 calorie diet during weeks 6 to 12. Subjects were evaluated every two weeks for weight, feeding behavior, energy intake (assessed by three-day diet records). To investigate the effect on appetite, patients were asked to report the presence of symptoms such as meat aversion, taste and smell alteration, nausea/vomiting, and early satiety. Patient compliance to 5-HTP was confirmed by urinary excretion of the 5-HTP metabolite (5-hydroxy-indoleacetic acid). Eight subjects dropped out of the study (three in the 5-HTP group, five in the control group) for reasons unrelated to treatment. 5-HTP subjects had a significant reduction in weight throughout the study (approximately 5 percent of the basal body weight). There were no significant changes in body weight with the placebo group. Mean total energy intake was significantly lowered in the 5-HTP subjects, but not in the placebo group. Subjects receiving 5-HTP showed a significant 50 percent reduction of their intake of carbohydrates during both six-week phases of the study, but there was no change in carbohydrate intake in the placebo group. Subject reports of satiety were significantly greater with 5-HTP administered than with the placebo. Episodic nausea was reported by 80 percent of 5-HTP subjects during the first six weeks, and then reduced to 20 percent of subjects for the remaining six weeks. There were no other differences in symptoms between the two groups (5).

- In a pilot study, 14 overweight, hyperphagic women (aged 24 y to 51 y) were randomized to receive a placebo or 300 mg 5-HTP 30 minutes before each meal (900 mg total) for 12 weeks. During the first 6 weeks, subjects were not given dietary instruction. During the last 6 weeks, subjects were prescribed a 1,200-calorie diet. Every two weeks, subjects were assessed for body weight, diet diary, self evaluation of appetite and satiety, and anorexia (measured by a questionnaire). The prevalence of anorexia was higher in the 5-HTP group than in the placebo group during both periods of observation (no statistical analysis reported). Early satiety was responsible for the reduced food intake in most 5-HTP subjects. However, in the first seven weeks, nausea was present in 70 percent of the 5-HTP subjects. Interestingly, this side effect could have also been responsible for the loss of appetite. This study was not blinded and lacked statistical analysis; thus, the results should be viewed with caution (6).

5-HTP and Fibromyalgia

- In a placebo-controlled study, 200 subjects diagnosed with fibromyalgia and who experienced migraines were randomized to one of four groups for one year: (1) 400 mg 5-HTP/day; (2) tricyclic antidepressants; (3) monoamine oxidase inhibitors (MAOIs); and (4) 5-HTP plus MAOIs. After an initial washout of one month, all subjects were given placebo for one month before beginning the 12 months of treatment. Pain levels were recorded in a daily diary and on a visual analogue scale (VAS) during the washout, the initial placebo phase, and during the main study. At the end of 12 months, all groups showed significant improvement over the placebo, with the combination of 5-HTP plus MAOIs being the most effective. The effect of treatment on migraine was not evaluated. This study was not blinded, and therefore the results should be reviewed with caution (7).

SAFETY

- 5-HTP may cause gastrointestinal symptoms (nausea, heartburn); users may need to start with lower doses and gradually increase them for better tolerability.

- In 1989, the supplement L-tryptophan was banned due to an outbreak of eosinophilia-myalgia syndrome (EMS) in more than 1,500 people, resulting in 30 deaths. EMS, a serious systemic illness that results in elevated white blood cells and severe muscle pain, was believed to be caused by consuming contaminated L-tryptophan produced by a fermentation process by one manufacturer in Japan. There is some concern about the purity of 5-HTP, because EMS-like symptoms have been reported with its use (8, 9).

- There is one confirmed case of EMS-related syndrome in a mother and her children after taking 5-HTP (8).

- One study analyzed eight commercially available synthetically and naturally derived 5-HTP supplements and found contamination by an impurity known as "peak X" in all supplements tested. Peak X is similar to impurities found in the banned L-tryptophan supplements (9).

- In theory, 5-HTP should not be combined with other serotonin-enhancing drugs to avoid serotonin syndrome, which can cause agitation, confusion, blood pressure fluctuations, and diaphoresis. However, this effect has not been reported in the literature.

REFERENCES

1. Meyers S. Use of neurotransmitter precursors for treatment of depression. *Altern Med Rev.* 2000;5:64–71.

2. Birdsall, TC. 5-hydroxytryptophan: a clinically effective serotonin precursor. *Altern Med Rev.*1998;3:271–280.
3. Poldinger W, Calanchini B, Schwarz W. A functional-dimensional approach to depression: serotonin deficiency as a target syndrome in a comparison of 5-hydroxytryptophan and fluvoxamine. *Psychopathology.* 1991;24:53–81.
4. Nardini M, De Stefano R, Iannuccelli M, et al. Treatment of depression with L-5-hydroxytryptophan combined with chlorimipramine, a double-blind study. *Int J Clin Pharmacol Res.* 1983;3:239–250.
5. Cangiano C, Ceci F, Cascino A, et al. Eating behavior and adherence to dietary prescriptions in obese adult subjects treated with 5-hydroxytryptophan. *Am J Clin Nutr.* 1992;56:863–867.
6. Cangiano C, Ceci F, Cairella M, et al. Effects of 5-hydroxytryptophan on eating behavior and adherence to dietary prescriptions in obese adult subjects. *Adv Exp Med Biol.* 1991;294:591–593.
7. Nicolodi M, Sicuteri F. Fibromyalgia and migraine, two faces of the same mechanism: Serotonin as the common clue for pathogenesis and therapy. *Adv Exp Med Biol.* 1996;398:373–379.
8. Michelson D, Page SW, Casey R, et al. An Eosinophilia-Myalgia Syndrome related disorder associated with exposure to L-5-Hydroxytryptophan. *J Rheumatol.* 1994;21:2261–2265.
9. Klarskov K, Johnson KL, Benson LM, et al. Eosinophilia-myalgia syndrome case-associated contaminants in commercially available 5-hydroxytryptophan. *Adv Exp Biol.* 1999;58:461–468.

β-Hydroxy-Methylbutyrate (HMB)

β-Hydroxy β-Methylbutyrate (HMB) is a metabolite of the branched-chain amino acid leucine. Approximately 5 percent to 10 percent of the leucine in the body is metabolized into HMB. HMB is believed to be converted into HMB-CoA in muscle, mammary tissue and certain immune cells to synthesize cholesterol necessary to maintain cell function. Humans endogenously produce an estimated 0.2 g to 0.4 g HMB/day in the liver and muscle depending on individual dietary leucine intake. Studies showing that HMB increases lean tissue mass and enhances the immune system in farm animals prompted the addition of HMB to animal feed. Because of the positive results from animal studies researchers began to test the effects of HMB supplements on lean body mass in humans (1–4).

Media and Marketing Claims	Efficacy
Increases muscle strength	↔
Increases lean body mass and reduces body fat	↑?
Decreases muscle breakdown after exercise	↔

Advisory

No reported serious adverse effects in short-term studies

Drug/Supplement Interactions

No reported adverse interactions

KEY POINTS

- Preliminary evidence from some studies suggests that 3 g HMB/day may increase strength and lean body mass in male, female, and elderly exercisers. However, not all trials reported strength gains or improvements in body composition with HMB supplementation.
- There is preliminary evidence that HMB may reduce markers of muscle damage from exercise. However, whether this effect actually enhances exercise performance remains to be tested.

FOOD SOURCES

Food	HMB (mg/Serving) *
Catfish (3 oz)	0.204–1.505
Squash (½ c)	0.267
Avocado (1 c)	0.165
Cauliflower (1 c)	0.110
Asparagus (1 c)	0.108
Cheese (1.5 oz)	0.055
Grapefruit (½)	0.026

Source: Data from Zhang Z, Coates C, Rathmacher J (5)
*Serving sizes calculated from values from Reference 5.

Ingesting food sources of the amino acid leucine (animal products, soybeans and other legumes) enhances endogenous HMB production.

HMB is found in most foods in low amounts, but is 4 to 10 times higher in alfalfa leaves (in animal feed), poultry by-products, and certain vegetables (5).

DOSAGE INFORMATION/BIOAVAILABILITY

HMB is sold as calcium-HMB in tablets, capsules and in some nutrition bars with suggested doses ranging from 1 g to 3 g/day. Each tablet provides 0.3 g to 0.5 g, so it is often necessary to take six to nine tablets or capsules to reach the recommended dosage. HMB is often sold in products containing creatine-monohydrate, glutamine, carnitine, DHEA, and/or N-acetyl cysteine (NAC).

RELEVANT RESEARCH

HMB and Strength, Body Composition, and Muscle Damage

- In a double-blind, placebo-controlled study, 37 untrained males were matched based on their body weights and assigned to one of three groups: 0 mg, 38 mg, or 76 mg HMB/kg body weight daily for eight weeks. These doses corresponded to about 0 g (placebo), 3 g, and 6 g HMB per day, respectively. Subjects performed resistance training three times per week at 80 percent of the maximum amount of weight they could lift at one time (one repetition maximum, RM). No differences were observed in 1 RM strength among the groups during the study. The 38 mg/kg dose had a greater increase in peak isometric torque than the placebo or the 76 mg/kg group. The 76 mg/kg group had a greater increase in peak isokinetic torque than the other groups. The placebo group had significantly higher plasma creatine phosphokinase activity (measure of muscle damage) than both HMB groups at 48 hours after the initial training bout. No differences were noted in body fat between the three groups. However, the 38 mg/kg group exhibited a greater increase in fat-free mass (6).

- In an unblinded study, healthy subjects on controlled diets were randomly assigned to one of two experiments. In study 1, (n = 41) untrained male subjects ages 19 y to 22 y were randomly assigned to one of three levels of HMB powder (0 g, 1.5 g, or 3.0 g HMB/day) and two protein levels (117 g or 175 g/day). All subjects weight trained 1.5 hours, three times per week for three weeks. In study 2, 32 trained male subjects took 0 g HMB/day or 3 g HMB/day and weight trained for two to three hours, six days a week for seven weeks. In study 1, HMB significantly decreased the weight trained-induced rise in muscle proteolysis as measured by urine 3-methylhistidine during the first two weeks. Also, a significant increase in the amount of weight lifted was seen in HMB-supplemented subjects during each successive week compared to unsupplemented subjects. In study 2, fat-free mass assessed by total body electrical conductance (TOBEC) was statistically significantly increased in HMB subjects at two and four to six weeks, but not at the end of the study. The authors concluded, "1.5 or 3 g HMB/day can partly prevent exercise-induced proteolysis and/or muscle damage and result in larger gains in muscle function associated with resistance training" (7). The results of this study have limited application because neither researchers nor subjects were blinded, which could have introduced bias.

- In a double-blind, placebo-controlled study, 36 women and 39 men (ages 20 y to 40 y) were randomized to receive 3 g HMB or a placebo daily in two gender cohorts. All subjects trained three times per week for four weeks. There were no significant differences in strength gains based on prior training status or gender with HMB supplementation. Combined male and female HMB groups had a significant greater increase in upper body strength (bench press) than the placebo group. There was also a trend toward a greater increase in fat-free weight with HMB groups compared to the placebo, but this difference did not reach statistical significance (8).

- In a double-blind, placebo-controlled study, 31 older adults (average age = 70 y) engaging in weight training two days per week and walking three days per week were ran-

H

domly assigned to receive 3 g HMB/day or a placebo for eight weeks. Skinfold tests (SF) and computerized tomography (CT) measured fat and lean body mass. When total body mass was measured by SF, HMB-supplemented subjects tended toward increased fat-free mass gain, but this did not reach statistical significance. HMB supplementation was significantly associated with an increase in percentage of body fat loss determined by SF and CT scan compared to the placebo group. There were no significant differences between groups on upper- and lower-body strength (assessed using five different exercises and summing the one repetition maximum for each lift) (9).

- In a double-blind, placebo-controlled study, 40 experienced resistance-trained athletes were matched and randomly assigned to receive a powdered carbohydrate-protein supplement with 0 g, 3 g, or 6 g HMB for 28 days. Blood and urine samples, dual x-ray absoptiometry determined body composition, and isotonic bench press and leg press one RM were measured at baseline and at day 28. HMB significantly increased blood and urine HMB concentrations. However, there were no differences between groups on general markers of body anabolic or catabolic status, muscle and liver enzyme efflux, fat-free mass, fat mass, percent body fat, or measures of strength (10).

HMB and Endurance Exercise

- In a small, double-blinded, crossover design study, eight male competitive cyclists took three different supplements (3 g HMB, 3 g leucine, or a placebo) for two weeks at a time with two-week washout periods between each one. Before and following each trial, subjects completed a maximal oxygen peak test (VO_2) on a cycle ergometer. Blood samples were taken during the last 20 seconds of each stage and immediately following exercise to determine maximal lactate levels. HMB supplementation resulted in a statistically significant increase in VO_2 peak and time to reach VO_2 peak compared to leucine and placebo trials. There was no effect on maximal lactate concentration, but lactate threshold (a predictor of exercise performance) was significantly increased with HMB and leucine compared to the placebo. There were no changes in plasma fatty acids or the respiratory exchange ratio, though HMB was associated with higher blood glucose levels. The authors suggested that HMB may alter cellular and/or mitochondrial proteins resulting in an increase in oxidative potential and/or blood buffer capacity. They stressed the need for further research in endurance athletes to determine whether the increases in lactate threshold due to HMB actually influence performance (11).

- In a double-blind, placebo-controlled study, 13 male and female subjects (ages 20 y to 50 y) were paired according to run performance and randomized to receive 3 g HMB/day or a placebo for six weeks. At the end of six weeks, subjects ran a 20-k race. Creatine kinase (CK) and lactate dehydrogenase (LDH) were measured to assess muscle damage at the start of the study, before and after the race, and one to four days after the race. Plasma CK and LDH levels were elevated in all subjects postrace; however, on days 2 and 3 post-race, HMB supplemented subjects had significantly lower CK and LDH levels. There were no changes in the percentage of fat free mass between groups. The authors concluded that HMB may help prevent exercise-induced muscle damage (12).

SAFETY

- To date, there are no long-term studies (> 8 weeks) using HMB supplements (3 g/day).

- One review article summarized the safety data of 3 g HMB daily supplemented in nine human studies lasting three to eight weeks duration. HMB did not negatively affect any markers of organ and tissue function or emotional state in any of the studies. In addition, adverse events assessed by a weekly questionnaire did not reveal any safety issue. The only notable changes were positive and included decreases in total cholesterol, LDL cholesterol, and systolic blood pressure (13).

- Doses up to 76 mg/kg (about 5.5 g for a person weighing 79 kg) for eight weeks had no adverse effects on liver enzymes, lipid profiles, renal function, or the immune system in 37 untrained collegiate males (14).

REFERENCES

1. Nissen S, Abumrad NN. Nutritional role of the leucine metabolite β-hydroxy β-methyl-butyrate (HMB). *J Nutr Biochem.* 1997;8:300–311.
2. Nissen S, Fuller JC, Sell J, et al. The effect of β-hydroxy β-methylbutyrate on growth, mortality, and carcass qualities of broiler chickens. *Poult Sci.* 1994;73:137–155.
3. Nissen S, Faidley TD, Zimmerman R, et al. Colostrol milk fat percentage and pig performances are enhanced by feeding the leucine metabolite β-hydroxy β-methylbutyrate to sows. *J Anim Sci.* 1994;72:2332–2337.
4. Van Koeving MT, Dolezal HG, Gill DR, et al. Effects of β-hydroxy β-methylbutyrate on performance and carcass quality of feedlot steers. *J Anim Sci.* 1994;72:1927–1935.
5. Zhang Z, Coates C, Rathmacher J. Occurrence of β-hydroxy β-methyl butyrate in foods and feeds. *FASEB J.* 8:A464.
6. Gallagher PM, Carrithers JA, Godard MP, et al. Beta-hydroxy-beta-methylbutyrate ingestion, Part I: effects on strength and fat free mass. *Med Sci Sports Exerc.* 2000;32:2109–2115.
7. Nissen S, Sharp R, Ray M, et al. Effect of leucine metabolite β-hydroxy β-methylbutyrate on muscle metabolism during resistance-exercise training. *J Appl Physiol.* 1996;81:2095–2104.
8. Panton L, Rathmacher JA, Baier S, et al. Nutritional supplementation of the lecuine metabolite beta-hydroxy-beta-methylbutyrate (HMB) during resistance training. *Nutrition.* 2000;16:734–739.
9. Vukovich MD, Stubbs NB, Bohlken RM, et al. Body composition in 70-year-old adults responds to dietary β-hydroxy β-methylbutyrate (HMB) similarly to that of young adults. *J Nutr.* 2001;131:2049–2052.
10. Kreider RB, Ferreira M, Wilson M, et al. Effects of calcium β-hydroxy β-methylbutyrate (HMB) supplementation during resistance-training on markers of catabolism, body composition and strength. *Int J Sports Med.* 1999;20:503–509.
11. Vukovich MD, Dreifort GD.. Effect of β-hydroxy β-methylbutyrate (HMB) on the onset of blood lactate accumulation and VO_2 peak in endurance trained cyclists. *J Strength Cond.* 2001;15:491–497.

H

12. Knitter A, Panton L, Rathmacher JA, et al. Effects of β-hydroxy β-methylbutyrate on muscle damage after a prolonged run. *J Appl Physiol.* 2000;89: 1340–1344.

13. Nissen S, Sharp L, Panton L, et al. β-hydroxy β-methylbutyrate (HMB) supplementation in humans is safe and may decrease cardiovascular risk factors. *J Nutr.* 2000; 130: 1937–1945.

14. Gallagher PM, Carrithers JA, Godard MP, et al. Beta-hydroxy-beta methylbutyrate ingestion, part II: effects on hematology, hepatic and renal function. *Med Sci Sports Exerc.* 2000;32:2116–2119.

Hydroxycitric Acid (Garcinia cambogia)

Hydroxycitric acid (HCA) is a compound derived from the fruit of a plant called *Garcinia cambogia* (also called Malabar tamarind) found in Southeast Asia. HCA was first isolated in the late 1800s and was discovered to be a potent competitive inhibitor of the enzyme ATP-citrate-lyase in the 1960s. This enzyme converts citrate, a product of the Krebs cycle produced from carbohydrate breakdown, into acetyl coenzyme A. Acetyl coenzyme A is a substrate for fatty acid and cholesterol synthesis. Because of this biological action of HCA, some scientists theorized that HCA may inhibit fat synthesis (1, 2).

Media and Marketing Claims	Efficacy
Reduces body weight and body fat	↓
Reduces appetite	↓

Advisory

- No reported serious adverse effects
- No long-term studies to evaluate safety

Drug/Supplement Interactions

No reported adverse interactions

KEY POINTS

Preliminary controlled trials testing the active ingredient in *Garcinia cambogia*, hydroxycitric acid, do not support its use as a weight loss aid. Although some research has reported beneficial effects on body composition, these trials have been criticized for poor design, and for using the herb in combination with other ingredients. Further controlled, clinical research is needed to build on the present studies and determine the safety and efficacy of the compound.

FOOD SOURCES

Not an ingredient or component of food in Western cultures. In India, the dried fruit and rinds of the fruit are used in cooking.

DOSAGE INFORMATION/BIOAVAILABILITY

Garcinia cambogia extract is sold in tablets, capsules, and powders standardized to about 50 percent HCA. Manufacturers recommend taking from 250 mg to 1,500 mg HCA per day (500 mg to 3,000 mg *Garcinia cambogia*) 30 minutes to 60 minutes prior to eating. Some suggest that a high-fiber diet may inhibit absorption of HCA (2, 3). Excessive levels of calcium (used to stabilize HCA) and low solubility in water are also factors that may reduce bioavailability of HCA and that exist in some commercial HCA extracts (3, 4).

RELEVANT RESEARCH

- In a double-blind, placebo-controlled, crossover study, 11 overweight male subjects were randomized to one of three treatments for two weeks each separated by four-week washout periods. Subjects consumed three self-selected meals (with no restrictions on type or amount of food) and four iso-energetic snacks daily with either no supplementation (placebo), 500 mg HCA, or 500 mg HCA plus 3 mg medium-chain triglycerides. Each intervention ended with a 36-hour stay in a respiration chamber. There was a significant loss in body weight in all groups, but this did not differ among groups. In addition, 24-hour energy expenditure, fat oxidation, and satiety did not differ among groups. The authors did note that the subjects were in a state of moderate negative energy balance, as evident by weight loss of > 1 kg, and that this action may explain why HCA was not effective in reducing appetite and inhibiting fat synthesis (because the conversion of citrate into acetyl coenzyme A only occurs when energy intake exceeds requirements) (5).

- In a double-blind, placebo-controlled study, 89 overweight female subjects (weighing 10 lb to 20 lb over their ideal body weight) were randomized to receive 400 mg HCA three times per day or a placebo for 12 weeks. Treatment was administered 30 minutes to 60 minutes prior to meals for a total dose of 1,200 mg/day. Subjects were counseled to adhere to a 1,200-calorie-exchange, 30-percent-fat diet. Weight and body composition were assessed at baseline and every other week for the 12 weeks. Food intake and appetite variables were assessed at baseline and monthly. Both groups experienced significant loss of weight, although mean weight loss with HCA (↓3.7 kg) was significantly greater than with the placebo (↓ 2.4 kg). The reduction in fat mass was not significant. No significant effects were observed on appetite indices (hunger ratings, mean ratings of desire to eat, fullness or sensation of thirst, stomach growling, headache, or irritability). Further, the appetite indices were not associated with energy intake or body weight change within the active treatment subjects (6).

H

- In a double-blind, placebo-controlled study, 135 overweight, healthy subjects (ages 18 y to 65 y) were randomized to receive 1,500 mg HCA or a placebo daily for 12 weeks. HCA was administered approximately 30 minutes prior to meals. Both groups were prescribed a high-fiber, low-calorie diet plan (20 percent fat, 50 percent carbohydrate, 30 percent protein) and asked to maintain a stable physical activity level. Diet compliance was not quantitatively monitored during the study. Body weight was measured biweekly, and fat mass was measured at baseline and at study's end using four methods (dual-energy x-ray absorptiometry [DXA] scanner, skinfold thickness, underwater weighing, and bioimpedance analysis). Eighty-four subjects completed the trial (42 subjects in each group). The number of dropouts was not related to adverse events. Patients in both groups lost significant amounts of weight at the end of the trial; however, there was no difference between groups in estimated percentage of body fat mass loss. Blood or tissue levels of hydroxycitric acid were not measured in this study (1).

- The authors of the above study also reviewed seven earlier HCA trials (five abstracts, two peer-reviewed controlled trials, and one open trial reported in an industrial publication). Five of the seven studies reported significant effects of HCA alone or in combination with other ingredients on weight and fat loss. However, the studies noted several limitations, including coadministration of HCA with other potentially active ingredients (chromium, chitosan, carnitine, caffeine) in five of the studies and use of inaccurate body composition method, and failure to publish study results in peer-reviewed journals (1).

- In a double-blind, placebo-controlled, crossover study, 10 sedentary male subjects (ages 22 y to 38 y, body mass index 22.4 kg/m^2 to 37.6 kg/m^2) were given in random order 3,000 mg HCA or a placebo for three days each. The objective of the study was to determine the effect of HCA on marker substrates of altered metabolism and the effect on the respiratory quotient (RQ) and energy expenditure in humans following an overnight fast and during a bout of exercise. The effects of treatment on metabolic parameters with or without moderate exercise (30 minutes at 40 percent maximal aerobic fitness (VO$_{2max}$) and 15 minutes at 60 percent VO$_{2\,max}$) was investigated during four laboratory visits. Energy expenditure measured by indirect calorimetry and RQ were measured for 150 minutes following an overnight fast. Blood levels of glucose, insulin, glucagons, lactate and beta-hydroxybutyrate (marker of increased fat oxidation) were assessed. HCA treatment did not lower RQ or affect energy expenditure during rest or during exercise compared with placebo treatment. The blood levels measured were not significantly different between treatment groups under fasting conditions. The authors concluded that the results do not support the hypothesis that HCA alters the short-term rate of fat oxidation in the fasting state during rest or exercise while subjects maintain a typical Western diet (approximately 30 percent to 35 percent total calories as fat) (7).

- In one animal study, both lean and obese young rats were fed HCA for 39 days. In the lean rats, HCA decreased body weight, food intake, body fat percentage, and fat cell size. In the obese rat, food intake and body weight were reduced, but the percent of body fat was not affected. Obese rats maintained a fat cell size equivalent to their obese controls. Obese rats had a reduction in fat cell number during treatment; however, posttreatment fat cell numbers increased (8).

SAFETY

- No long-term studies have evaluated the safety of HCA supplements in humans.
- Twelve weeks of supplementing 1,500 mg HCA to overweight subjects appeared to be safe, with no reports of serious adverse effects (1, 6).

REFERENCES

1. Heymsfield SB, Allison DB, Vasselli JR, et al. *Garcinia cambogia* (hydroxycitric acid) as a potential antiobesity agent. *JAMA.* 1998; 280:1596–1600.
2. Badmaev V, Majeed M, Conte AA, et al. *Garcinia cambogia* for weight loss [letter]. *JAMA.* 1999;282:233.
3. Schaller JL. *Garcinia cambogia* for weight loss [letter]. *JAMA.* 1999; 282:234.
4. Firenzuoli F. *Garcinia cambogia* for weight loss [letter]. *JAMA.* 1999; 282: 234.
5. Kovacs EMR, Westerterp-Plantenga MS, Saris WHM. The effects of 2-week ingestion of (-)-hydroxycitrate and (-)-hydroxycitrate combined with medium-chain triglycerides on satiety, fat oxidation, energy expenditure and body weight. *Int J Obesity.* 2001;25:1087–1094.
6. Mattes RD, Bormann L. Effects of (-)-hydroxycitric acid on appetitive variables. *Physiol Behav.* 2000;71:87–94.
7. Kriketos AD, Thompson HR, Greene H, et al. (-)-Hydroxycitric acid does not affect energy expenditure and substrate oxidation in adult males in a post-absorptive state. *Int J Obes Relat Metab Disord.* 1999;23:867–873.
8. Greenwood MR, Cleary MP, Gruen R, et al. Effect of (-)-hydroxycitrate on development of obesity in the Zucker obese rat. *Am J Physiol.* 1981;240:E72—E78.

Isoleucine

See Branched-Chain Amino Acids (BCAAs).

Kava (*Piper methysticum*)

Kava (also known as kava-kava) is a perennial plant native to the Pacific Islands. For centuries, kava roots have been ground into a bitter-tasting drink for ceremonial occasions in the South Pacific. The kava beverage, a psychoactive drink, is valued for its minor tranquilizing and relaxant effects. Kava pyrones (also referred to as kava lactones), the active components of the kava plant, are generally considered to be responsible for its sedative qualities.

The mechanism of action on the central nervous system is not known. *In vitro* studies have found that certain pyrones block norepinephrine uptake. Recent studies have suggested that kava has monoamine (MAO) uptake inhibition properties. Research is conflicting regarding the capacity of kava to bind to the gamma-aminobutyric acid (GABA)-receptors in the brain (prescription sedatives bind to these receptors) (1–4).

Media and Marketing Claims	Efficacy
Promotes sleep and relaxation	↑?
Sleep and relaxation aid	NR

Advisory

- Concern with liver toxicity; associated with 25 cases of serious liver damage in Europe. Patients with liver disease or Parkinson's disease should absolutely not use kava. More information is needed on safe use by healthy individuals.
- May affect motor reflexes; users should exercise caution when driving/operating heavy machinery
- Not to be used for more than three months without medical advice

Drug/Supplement Interactions

- Potential additive, sedative affects when combined with alcohol, antianxiety medications (benzodiazepines), barbiturates, and other psychopharmalogical agents
- May decrease effectiveness of drugs used in Parkinson's disease (levodopa)

KEY POINTS

- The FDA released a letter to health professionals seeking information on liver injury and kava products in December 2001 after approximately 25 reports of hepatic toxicity associated with the use of kava were reported in Germany and Switzerland. To date, there have been no reported cases in the United States. Whether these cases were due to contamination of the product has not been resolved. More information about the safety of kava is needed before it can be used without concern.
- There is preliminary evidence that kava may play a role in reducing anxiety in nonpsychotic anxiety disorders. However, more research is needed before specific recommendations can be made.
- Although various books discussing kava suggest that the herb induces a deep, restful sleep and relieves insomnia and nervousness (1), controlled clinical trials are lacking to substantiate these effects. However, if kava does indeed reduce anxiety as suggested in controlled trials, this could theoretically improve sleep. Well-designed trials are needed to determine the role of kava in healthy and sleep-disordered subjects.

FOOD SOURCES

Kava beverage (consumed in the South Pacific, prepared by infusing dried kava powder in cold water for several minutes)

DOSAGE INFORMATION/BIOAVAILABILITY

Kava is sold in liquid or powdered herbal extract preparations. Some products are standardized to contain 30 percent kava pyrones/lactones (equivalent to 60 mg to 120 mg kava pyrones). Most of the research on anxiety used a standardized kava extract, WS 1490. WS 1490 is standardized to contain 70 percent kava pyrones (providing about 210 mg kava pyrones per 300 mg daily dose). Kava can also be taken as a tea. Some products suggest taking kava on an empty stomach to maximize purported sedative effects.

RELEVANT RESEARCH

Kava and Anxiety

- A meta-analysis of three double-blind, placebo-controlled, randomized German trials (total subjects = 198) of kava extract for the treatment of anxiety reported a significant reduction in the total score on the Hamilton Rating Scale for Anxiety in favor of kava extract. The studies used a standardized extract of kava (WS 1490) providing 300 mg (210 mg kavalactones) per day. Of seven trials initially selected, all reported the superiority of kava extract over a placebo, suggestive of a publication bias. Four studies were excluded from the analysis because they did not have sufficient data for statistical pooling. Few adverse effects were reported, but they included restlessness, drowsiness, tremor, and headache. The authors concluded that their findings warrant further and more rigorous research on the risk-benefit relation of kava (5).

- In a double-blind, placebo-controlled multicenter study, 101 German outpatients with anxiety disorders clinically documented by DSM-III-R were randomized to receive a standardized kava extract (WS 1490) providing 210 mg kavalactones or a placebo for 25 weeks. The total Hamilton Anxiety Scale (HAMA) score showed a pronounced decrease in both groups; however, patients taking kava scored significantly better from week 8 until the end of the study. Kava was also found to be significantly more effective than placebo on HAMA subscores somatic and psychic anxiety, Clinical Global Impression, Self-Report Symptom Inventory-90 Items revised, and the Adjective Mood Scale. The authors noted that WS 1490 had none of the tolerance problems typically associated with tricyclics and benzodiazepines (6).

- In a double-blind, placebo-controlled study, 58 patients with anxiety disorders were randomized to receive 100 kava extract WS 1490 three times/day or a placebo preparation for four weeks. Patients taking kava had a significant reduction in anxiety as measured by the Hamilton Anxiety Scale. The magnitude of anxiety reduction in the kava group increased during the course of the study (p < 0.02 at week 8; p < 0.001 at weeks 16 to 24) (7).

K

- In Germany, double-blind, placebo-controlled studies of kava extract have demonstrated anxiety reduction activity in patients with anxiety disorders (7, 8). These studies were not available for review in English.

Kava and Memory

- In a double-blind, placebo-controlled, crossover study, 12 healthy young male subjects were given 200 mg kava extract WS 1490 three times/day for five days, the antianxiety medication oxazepam (placebo for days 1 to 3, 15 mg the day before testing, and 75 mg on the morning of the experiment), or a placebo for five days. Each treatment was separated by 12-day washout periods. Subjects were asked to identify within a list of visually presented words those that were shown for the first time and those that were repeated. During oxezepam treatment, there was a significant slowing of reaction time and a reduction in the number of correct responses. During kava ingestion there was an insignificant trend toward increased recognition rate compared to the placebo (9).

SAFETY

- The FDA released a letter seeking information on liver injury and kava products in December 2001. Twenty-five cases of serious liver toxicity were associated with kava products in Germany and Switzerland. However, there have been no reports of injury in the United States. It is not known whether these cases were due to a contamination of products or a particular component found in kava. More information is needed to demonstrate the safety of this herb (10).

- A 50-year-old man developed acute hepatitis and required liver transplantation after taking kava extract (210 kavalactones to 280 kavalactones/day) for two months. The authors of the case report noted that heavy kava intake has been associated with increased levels of gamma-glutamyltransferase, suggesting potential hepatotoxicity (11).

- The German Commission E reports that kava use should be discontinued if side-effects such as discoloration of skin, hair, and nails, enlargement of pupils, or disturbance of ocularmotor equilibrium develop. The Commission E also states that kava is contraindicated in pregnancy, nursing, and endogenous depression. It should not be combined with alcohol, barbiturates, and psychopharmacological agents because of possible potentiation of sedative effects (12).

- Kava should not be taken for longer than three months without medical advice (12).

- Due to its sedative properties, kava could adversely affect motor reflexes and judgment for driving and/or operating heavy machinery (12).

- An interaction between kava and the antianxiety medication Xanax (a benzodiazepine) produced a lethargic and disoriented state in a 54-year-old man. The authors suggested that kava may have an additive sedating effect to benzodiazepines since they may act on the same receptor and areas of the central nervous system (13). Additionally, if transitioning from antianxiety drugs to kava, must be under medical supervision due to potential adverse effects.

- The mechanism of action of kava is not fully understood. Recent *in vitro* studies reported MAO-inhibitor qualities of kava pyrones (3, 4). If kava does act as an MAO inhibitor, foods containing large amounts of tyramine (cheese, red wine, smoked or pickled foods, beer, yogurt) should be avoided. To date, however, there are no reports of kava-induced hypertensive reactions that can occur when MAO inhibitors are combined with tyramine.

- In Australia, heavy kava beverage consumption (300 g to 400 g/week) has been associated with scaly rash, malnutrition, abnormal liver function tests, and dyskinesia (14, 15).

- Cases of kava extract-associated dermopathy have been reported. Two to three weeks of kava use was associated with papules and plaques on the face, arms, back, and chest (16, 17).

- Tremors, muscle spasms, or abnormal movements can be brought about by kava that may decrease the effectiveness of anti-Parkinson's medications. This would apply also to the movement problems caused by antipsychotic medications (18).

K

REFERENCES

1. Singh YN. Kava: an overview. *J Ethnopharmacol.* 1992;37:13–45.
2. Anonymous. *Piper methysticum* (kava kava). *Altern Med Rev.* 1998;3:458–460.
3. Uebelhack R, Franke L, Schewe HJ. Inhibition of platelet MAO-B by kava pyrone-enriched extract from *Piper methysticum* Forster (kava kava). *Pharmacopsychiatry.* 1998;31:187–192.
4. Seitz U, Schule A, Gleitz J. [3H]-monoamine uptake inhibition properties of kava pyrones. *Planta Med.* 1997;63:548–549.
5. Pittler MH, Ernst E. Efficacy of kava extract for treating anxiety: systematic review and meta-analysis. *J Clin Psychopharmacol.* 2000;20:84–89.
6. Volz HP, Kieser M. Kava-kava extract WS 1490 versus placebo in anxiety disorders—a randomized placebo-controlled 25-week outpatient trial. *Pharmacopsychiatry.* 1997;30:1–5.
7. Kinzler E, Kromer J, Lehmann E. Effect of a special kava extract in patients with anxiety-tension and excitation states of nonpsychotic genesis. Double blind study with placebos over 4 weeks [in German]. *Arzneimittelforschung.* 1991;41:584–588.
8. Warnecke G. Neurovegetative dystonia in the female climateric. Studies on the clinical efficacy and tolerance of kava extract WS 1490. [In German.] *Fortschr Med.* 1991;109:120–122.
9. Munte TF, Heinze HJ, Matzke M, et al. Effects of oxazepam and an extract of kava roots (*Piper methysticum*) on event-related potentials in a word recognition task. *Neuropsychobiology.* 1993;27:46–53.

10. Letter to Health Care Professionals about FDA seeking information on liver injury and kava products. U.S. Food and Drug Administration. Available at: *www.cfsan.fda.gov/~dms/ds-ltr27.html.* Accessed July 7, 2002.

11. Escher M, Desmeules J, Giostra E, et al. Hepatitis associated with kava, an herbal remedy for anxiety. *BMJ.* 2001;322:139.

12. Blumenthal M, ed. *The Complete German Commission E Monographs Therapeutic Guide to Herbal Medicines.* 1st ed. Boston, Mass: Integrative Medicine Communications; 1998.

13. Almeida JC, Grimsley EW. Coma from the health food store: Interaction between kava and alprazolam. *Ann Intern Med.* 1996;125:940–941.

14. Mathews JD, Riley MD, Fejo L, et al. Effects of the heavy usage of kava on physical health: summary of a pilot survey in an Aboriginal community. *Med J Aust.* 1988;148:548–555.

15. Spillane PK, Fisher DA, Currie BJ. Neurological manifestations of kava intoxication. *Med J Aust.* 1997;167:172–173.

16. Jappe U, Franke I, Reinhold D, et al. Sebotropic drug reaction resulting from kava-kava extract therapy: a new entity? *J Am Acad Dermatol.* 1998;38:104–106.

17. Schmidt P, Boehncke WH. Delayed-type hypersensitivity reaction to kava-kava extract. *Contact Dermatitis.* 2000;42:363–364.

18. Herbs and Drugs Can Make a Bad Mix. *Tufts University Health & Nutrition Letter.* July 1999.

α-Lipoic Acid

See Alpha-Lipoic Acid.

Lactobacillus Acidophilus

See Acidophilus.

Lecithin/Choline

Lecithin, also known as phosphatidylcholine, is a phospholipid that is approximately 13 percent choline by weight and is found in the cell membranes and lipoproteins of plants and animals. Choline, an amine, is a precursor of the phospholipids lecithin and sphingomyelin, and the neurotransmitter acetylcholine. As part of these compounds, choline is involved in memory storage, muscle control, cell membrane signaling, and many other functions.

Because it can be synthesized in the body if excess methionine is present, choline is an essential nutrient only when demand for it exceeds the endogenous production. Although a normal diet provides sufficient choline to maintain healthy organ function, some populations are at risk for deficiency, including infants, pregnant or lactating women, patients with cirrhosis, and patients fed with total parenteral nutrition (TPN) (1). Several studies have reported that choline deficiency associated with long-term TPN administration results in hepatic steatosis (2–4). In healthy humans, diets deficient in choline have resulted in reduced plasma choline concentrations and the development of liver dysfunction (5). Because steatosis and liver dysfunction can be reversed in these conditions following lecithin or choline supplementation, choline is now generally recognized as a "conditionally" essential nutrient for normal liver function (6, 7).

Media and Marketing Claims	Efficacy
Improves exercise endurance	↓
Improves dementia in Alzheimer's patients	↓
Improves memory, thinking ability, and muscle control	NR
Reduces liver degeneration	NR

Advisory

- Regarded as safe at doses below the Tolerable Upper Intake Level (UL): 3.5 g choline/day for adults > 19 y
- Side-effects associated with high doses (> 20 g choline) include gastrointestinal symptoms, fishy body odor, urinary incontinence, and diarrhea

Drug/Supplement Interactions

No reported adverse interactions

L

KEY POINTS

- Research suggests that choline is a conditionally essential nutrient. Deficiency is not a concern for most people because choline and lecithin are available in a wide variety of foods. The National Academy of Sciences states that "Although an AI is set for choline, there are few data to assess whether a dietary supply is needed at all stages of the life cycle and it may be that the choline requirement can be met by endogenous synthesis during some of these stages" (7).

- Study results are conflicting about whether choline levels decline during exercise. However, the limited research in small numbers of subjects shows that lecithin/choline supplements do not appear to improve exercise performance.

- In general, choline/lecithin supplements have not been shown to improve symptoms of Alzheimer's disease. Limited studies in bipolar disorder subjects do not provide sufficient evidence to warrant lecithin supplementation for bipolar disorder.

- Controlled trials are needed to assess the claim that supplemental lecithin/choline improves memory and thinking in healthy subjects.

- Although rare, choline deficiency has been associated with hepatic steatosis during long-term TPN administration, which is corrected by choline supplementation. However, there is currently no evidence that additional choline/lecithin intake from supplements can prevent or treat liver degeneration in individuals without deficiency.

FOOD SOURCES

The estimated average intake in the typical American diet is 700 mg to 1,000 mg choline/day. However, depending on food choices, it is possible to take in more than 2,000 mg choline in one day (4). Rich sources of choline are egg yolks, spinach, organ meats, nuts, and wheat germ. Choline is available in food as lecithin and free choline. Lecithin is used as an emulsifier in processed foods such as mayonnaise, ice cream, and salad dressings.

Food	Free Choline (mg)	Lecithin (mg)	Total Choline (mg)
Egg (1 large)	0.2	2,009	282.3
Beef steak (3.5 oz)	0.8	466	68.8
Peanut butter (2 tbsp)	13.0	97	26.1
Cauliflower (½ c)	6.8	107	22.2
Coffee (6 oz)	18.6	2	19.3
Orange (1)	2.9	53	10.4
Lecithin powder (1 tbsp/7.5 g)	—	1,725	250

Source: Data from Canty DJ, Zeisel SH (6)

DOSAGE INFORMATION/BIOAVAILABILITY

In 1998, the National Academy of Sciences Food and Nutrition Board set the Adequate Intake (AI) for choline as 425 mg for adult females and 550 mg for adult males. The AI for pregnancy is 450 mg/day. No RDA was set due to a lack of data or uncertainty in the data (7). Choline, in the form of choline chloride, choline bitartrate, or lecithin, is available as tablets, capsules, powders, and in some sport beverages. Much of the commercial lecithin sold is a mixture of phospholipids and may contain less than 50 percent actual lecithin (8). Some manufacturers supply 90 percent to 98 percent lecithin powder derived from soybeans. Manufacturers recommend a variety of doses ranging from 1 g to 20 g of lecithin (about 1 to 10 tablespoons of powder).

Dietary choline is absorbed in the small intestine, some of which is metabolized by gut bacteria. Lecithin is broken down by phospholipases and is absorbed into the lymph as chylomicrons via the thoracic duct, and the remaining free choline enters the portal circulation (1, 7).

RELEVANT RESEARCH

Choline and Exercise

- Plasma choline concentrations were reduced by approximately 40 percent in trained runners following a 26-km race. The authors hypothesized that the reductions in plasma choline associated with strenuous exercise may reduce acetylcholine release and could thereby affect endurance or performance (9).

- In a placebo-controlled, pilot study (not blinded), 12 male and female marathon runners were randomized to receive 2.2 g lecithin (1.1 g choline) or a placebo beginning one day prior to a marathon. Fasting, pre- and postmarathon plasma and five-hour urine collection were taken. Runners were asked to estimate finish time based on recent performance and training. Performance enhancement was measured by comparing the actual vs predicted finish times, noting whether there were significant differences. All subjects completed the marathon. Plasma free choline decreased significantly in the placebo group and increased significantly in the lecithin group. No changes in plasma phospholipid-bound choline were noted in either group. Actual finish time to predicted finish time ratios did not differ between groups, suggesting that lecithin did not enhance performance. The authors noted that a much larger, controlled study is needed to confirm these results (10).

- In a placebo-controlled, randomized, crossover (not blinded) study of 10 elite triathletes, an acute dose of 0.2 g lecithin/kg one hour before exercise prevented a decrease in plasma choline after two hours of cycling. During placebo administration, plasma choline concentrations dropped an average of 16.9 percent. The effect of reduced choline levels and exercise performance was not tested (11).

- In a double-blind, crossover design study, 20 cyclists rode either at 150 percent power output or 70 percent output to exhaustion one hour after drinking a beverage with or without choline bitartrate (2.43 g). Neither group depleted serum choline during exercise with or without choline and there were no differences in fatigue times and work performance between groups. The authors concluded: "Trained cyclists do not deplete choline during supramaximal brief or prolonged submaximal exercise, nor do they benefit from choline supplementation to delay fatigue under these conditions (12).

Choline and Neurological Disorders

- In the 1970s and 1980s, several small studies tested the use of choline or lecithin in Alzheimer's patients. The theory was that by increasing plasma acetylcholine levels through choline supplementation, dementia symptoms would subside. Alzheimer's disease is believed to be associated with a defect in the enzyme choline acetyl transferase and production of the neurotransmitter acetylcholine by this enzyme is enhanced when more choline is available to the brain. Although occasionally some patients with Alzheimer's did respond to choline or lecithin treatment (13), the overall findings of the research are not suggestive of a benefit with choline or lecithin supplements (4, 6).

- A systematic review of 11 randomized trials of lecithin in patients with Alheimer's disease (265 subjects) and Parkinsonian dementia (21 subjects) concluded that lecithin had no benefit (14).

- A small, double-blind, placebo-controlled trial of six patients with bipolar disorder reported that 10 mg lecithin three times a day dissolved in ice cream had a therapeutic effect on symptoms of mania (hallucinations, delusions, incoherent speech) in five patients compared to the placebo phase (15). However, the dose used was so small ($\approx$ 4 mg choline), it is unlikely that such a quantity could ameliorate manic symptoms.

SAFETY

- Regarded as safe in doses below the Tolerable Upper Intake Level (UL) of 3.5 g choline per day for adults 19 years and older (7).

- Safety of choline is not well-studied. Side-effects associated with high oral doses of choline (20 g) include gastrointestinal symptoms, urinary incontinence, and diarrhea.

- Excess choline (> 20 g) may cause a fishy odor because of breakdown of trimethylamine in the intestine (8).

- A depression of dopamine receptors and a disturbance of neurotransmitter balance may be a concern when taking chronically high doses of choline (8).

REFERENCES

1. Zeisel SH. Choline and phosphytidylcholine. In: Shils ME, Olson JA, Shike M, Ross AC, eds. *Modern Nutrition in Health and Disease.* 9th ed. Philadelphia, Pa: Lea & Febiger; 1999:513–523.
2. Buchman AL, Dubin M, Jenden D, et al. Lecithin increases plasma free choline and decreases hepatic steatosis in long-term total parenteral nutrition patients. *Gastroenterology.* 1992;102:1363–1370.
3. Buchman AL, Dubin MD, Moukarzel AA, et al. Choline deficiency: a cause of hepatic steatosis during parenteral nutrition that can be reversed with intravenous choline supplementation. *Hepatology.* 1995;22:1399–1403.
4. Shronts EP. Essential nature of choline with implications for total parenteral nutrition. *J Am Diet Assoc.* 1997;97:639–646, 649.
5. Zeisel SH. Choline: an important nutrient in brain development, liver function, and carcinogenesis. *J Am Coll Nutr.* 1992;11:473–481.
6. Canty DJ, Zeisel SH. Lecithin and choline in human health and disease. *Nutr Rev.* 1994;52:327–339.
7. Institute of Medicine, Food and Nutrition Board. *Dietary Reference Intakes for Thiamin, Riboflavin, Niacin, Vitamin B-6, Folate, Vitamin B-12, Panthothenic Acid, Biotin, and Choline.* Washington, DC: National Academy Press; 1998.
8. Linder MC. Nutrition and metabolism of vitamins. In: Linder MC, ed. *Nutritional Biochemistry and Metabolism with Clinical Applications.* 2nd ed. Norwalk, Conn: Appleton & Lange; 1991:127.
9. Conlay LA, Saboujian LA, Wurtman RJ. Exercise and neuromodulators: choline and acetylcholine in marathon runners. *Int J Sports Med.* 1992;13:S141—S142.
10. Buchman AL, Awal M, Jenden D, et al. The effect of lecithin supplementation on plasma choline concentrations during a marathon. *J Am Coll Nutr.* 2000;19:768–770.
11. Von Allworden HN, Horn S, Kahl J, et al. The influence of lecithin on plasma choline concentrations in triathletes and adolescent runners during exercise. *Eur J Appl Physiol.* 1993;67:87–91.
12. Spector SA, Jackman MR, Sabounjian LA, et al. Effect of choline supplementation on fatigue in trained cyclists. *Med Sci Sports Exerc.* 1995;27:668–673.

13. Little A, Levy R, Chuaqui KP, et al. A double-blind, placebo-controlled trial of high dose lecithin in Alzheimer's disease. *J Neurol Neurosurg Psychiatry.* 1985;48:736–742.

14. Higgins JP, Flicker L. Lecithin for dementia and cognitive impairment. *Cochrane Database Syst Rev.* 2000;2:CD001015.

15. Cohen BM, Lipinski JF, Altesman RI. Lecithin in the treatment of mania: double-blind, placebo-controlled trials. *Am J Psychiatry.* 1982;139:1162–1164.

Leucine

See Branched-Chain Amino Acids (BCAAs).

Lysine

Lysine is an essential amino acid involved in the synthesis of cross-linking proteins (collagen and elastin) and is a precursor of carnitine. Low-lysine diets produce lower growth rates and nitrogen retention in animals and humans than diets in which the lysine/tryptophan ratio is 5 or higher. (Proteins are considered to have a high biological value if they have approximately five to eight times as much lysine as tryptophan by weight.) Of all the essential amino acids, lysine is one of the most strongly conserved by the body. Lysine is usually the limiting amino acid in diets based on grains (1).

Media and Marketing Claims	Efficacy
Stops growth of the herpes virus	↔
Enhances calcium absorption	NR
Reduces chest pain	NR

Advisory

Doses of 3g/day regarded as safe

Drug/Supplement Interactions

Competes with the amino acid arginine for absorption

KEY POINTS

- Research is conflicting on the role of lysine in treating herpes simplex infection. Dietary protein intake and lysine:arginine ratios were not controlled in any of the studies, although subjects were instructed to avoid arginine-rich foods. The amount supplemented in these studies was comparable to an amount that can be obtained from the diet (see food sources). Although more research is needed on the potential role of lysine against herpes infection, these patients can be encouraged to increase consumption of lysine-rich foods within the context of an overall healthful diet.

L

- Preliminary animal studies and one human trial suggest that lysine enhances calcium absorption and retention. Controlled clinical trials are needed to more clearly determine the potential role of supplemental lysine in the treatment or prevention of osteoporosis.

- Evidence from case studies is not sufficient to support the claim that lysine reduces angina. Controlled clinical trials are needed to verify this claim.

FOOD SOURCES

Lysine is found in animal proteins and in potatoes and legumes (lentils, soybeans, lima bean). Wheat flour, maize, rice, oats, and peanuts are low in lysine. Lysine is easily damaged during the processing of foods and animal feeds (2). Dietary lysine intakes are highly variable and can be as low as 2 g/day if protein intake is 50 g/day, and as high as 8 g to 9 g/day on a diet high in calories and animal protein (1). Estimated dietary lysine requirements for adults are 12 mg/kg/day (3).

Food	Lysine (mg/Serving)
Beef, ground (3.5 oz)	1,892
Salmon, Atlantic (3 oz)	1,727
Tofu, firm (½ c)	1,309
Beans, black (1 c)	1,064
Milk, nonfat (1 c)	818
Peanuts (½ c)	621
Cheese, mozzarella (1 oz)	559
Egg (1)	452
Spinach, boiled (½ c)	164
Corn, boiled (½ c)	116
Bread, whole wheat (1 slice)	85

Source: Data from Pennington, JAT (4)

DOSAGE INFORMATION/BIOAVAILABILITY

Lysine is sold as free form L-lysine hydrochloride usually in 500-mg tablets or capsules. It is also sold in combination with other amino acids supplements. Studies have shown that free lysine hydrochloride added to food or in supplements is absorbed at a similar rate as amino acids from dietary proteins (1).

RELEVANT RESEARCH

Lysine and Herpes Simplex Virus

- Researchers have hypothesized that lysine may treat the herpes simplex virus because its growth appears to be inhibited by high intracellular concentrations of lysine and low levels of arginine (5, 6).

- In a double-blind, placebo-controlled, multicenter study, 52 subjects with genital and oral-facial herpes simplex infection were randomized to receive 1,000 mg of lysine as lysine monohydrochloride divided into three doses or a placebo daily for six months. Subjects were instructed to avoid foods containing large amounts of arginine, but this was not monitored. There was a significant decrease in the average number of infections, decrease in symptoms, and decrease in severity and healing time with lysine. Specifically, subjects treated with lysine had 2.4 fewer herpes outbreaks and 2.3 fewer days of infection compared to the placebo (7).

- In a double-blind, placebo-controlled, crossover study, 26 subjects with a history of recurring genital herpes lesions received in random order 1,000 mg lysine or a placebo daily for six months each. For one year prior to the study, subjects recorded the frequency of herpetic lesions. All subjects were instructed to avoid foods high in arginine content, but this was not monitored. At the end of the first six-month period, the frequency of lesions in those subjects given lysine did not differ significantly from those given the placebo (39 lesions in the lysine group vs 44 lesions in the placebo group). In contrast, subjects who began taking lysine during the second six-month test period reported significantly fewer lesions than those who had reverted to placebo (12 lesions in the lysine group vs 31 in the placebo group). The authors speculated that a placebo effect may have occurred during the first six-month period. Low serum lysine concentrations were associated with a significant increase in lesion frequency, and high concentrations were associated with a significant decrease in lesion frequency. The serum lysine to arginine ratio showed no correlation with lesion occurrence. The authors concluded: "Prophylactic lysine may be useful in managing selected cases of recurrent herpes simplex labialis *if* serum lysine levels can be maintained at adequate concentrations" (8).

- In a double-blind, placebo-controlled study, 21 patients with a history of severe frequently occurring herpes simplex infection were randomized to receive 1,200 mg lysine as lysine hydrochloride divided into three doses or a placebo for four to five months. Patients were evaluated at baseline, at three months, and at the end of the study. Subjects were instructed to avoid arginine-rich foods and to keep a diary of symptoms. There were no changes in episode frequency, duration, or severity of episodes between groups (9).

- In a double-blind, placebo-controlled, crossover study, 41 patients with recurrent herpes simplex infections were randomized to receive one of four treatments for 48 weeks: (1) 1248 mg lysine as lysine monohydrochloride for 24 weeks, followed by a placebo for 24 weeks; (2) reverse of group 1; (3) 624 mg lysine for 24 weeks followed by a placebo; or (4) reverse of group 3. Subjects were instructed to avoid arginine-rich foods and increase lysine foods, but this was not monitored. Patients were assessed at the baseline, 12, 24, 36, and 48 weeks. In the high-dose lysine group, there was a significant decrease in herpes outbreaks compared to the placebo phase. There were no significant changes in the lower dose lysine group. There were also no differences in self-reported healing times among groups (10).

L

Lysine and Calcium Metabolism/Bone Health

- In a comparative study, 30 women aged 33 y to 65 y (15 healthy, 15 having osteoporosis) were given an acute oral load of calcium chloride (3 g elemental calcium) administered either with or without 400 mg lysine. Both the lysine and control groups experienced an increase in plasma total calcium. A progressive increase in urinary calcium excretion was observed after calcium alone but not in the calcium plus lysine-treated healthy subjects. In a second study, 45 osteoporotic postmenopausal women were randomized to receive one of three treatments: (1) 800 mg lysine, (2) 800 mg valine, or (3) 800 mg tryptophan. Lysine, but not valine or tryptophan, significantly increased intestinal absorption of calcium as measured by fractional absorption of calcium by stable isotope administration. The authors concluded: "Our results suggest that L-lysine can both enhance intestinal calcium absorption and improve the renal conservation of the absorbed calcium. The combined effects may contribute to a positive calcium balance, thus suggesting a potential usefulness of L-lysine supplements for both preventative and therapeutic interventions in osteoporosis" (11).
- Lysine supplementation in animals has been shown to increase calcium absorption (11).

Lysine and Angina

- Three case studies of patients with coronary heart disease supplemented with 2 g to 6 g lysine/day reported a reduction in angina and an increase in exercise capacity (12–14). These findings should be viewed with caution because they are case reports and thus lack proper controls.

SAFETY

- L-lysine supplements in daily doses up to 3 g lysine (3.75 g lysine monohydrate), divided among meals, would not elevate the proportion of lysine in the dietary protein beyond that in meat and would be safe for chronic use (1). However, chronic administration of higher doses is not warranted until their clinical value and safety have been established by appropriate clinical studies (1).
- Lysine and arginine are antagonistic because they share a common transport system in the blood. Excess lysine intake may interfere with arginine metabolism (1).
- Diets high in lysine (4 percent to 5 percent) or with a high lysine:arginine ratio were reported to have a hypercholesterolemic effect in animal studies (15–17).
- To date, there have been no reported cases of acute toxicity with lysine supplementation (1).

REFERENCES

1. Flodin NW. The metabolic roles, pharmacology, and toxicology of lysine. *J Am Coll Nutr.* 1997;16:7–21.

2. Ostrowski HT. Analysis for availability of amino acid supplements in foods and feeds: biochemical and nutritional implications. *Adv Exp Med Biol.* 1978;105:497–547.

3. Matthews DE. Proteins and amino acids. In: Shils ME, Olson JA, Shike M, Ross AC, eds. *Modern Nutrition in Health and Disease.* 9th ed. Philadelphia, PA: Lea & Febiger; 1999:11–48.

4. Pennington JAT. *Bowes and Church's Food Values of Portions Commonly Used.* 17th ed. Philadelphia, Pa: Lippincott-Raven Publishers; 1998.

5. Tankersley RW Jr. Amino acid requirements of herpes simplex virus in human cells. *J Bacteriol.* 1964;87:609–613.

6. Griffith RD, DeLong DC, Nelson JD. Relation of arginine-lysine to herpes simplex growth in tissue culture. *Chemotherapy.* 1981;27:209–213.

7. Griffith RS, Walsh DE, Myrmel KH, et al. Success of L-lysine therapy in frequently recurrent herpes simplex infection. Treatment and prophylaxis. *Dermatologica.* 1987;175:183–190.

8. Thein DJ, Hurt WC. Lysine as a prophylactic agent in the treatment of recurrent herpes simplex labialis. *Oral Surg Oral Med Oral Pathol.* 1984;58:659–666.

9. DiGiovanna JJ, Blank H. Failure of lysine in frequently recurrent herpes simplex infection. Treatment and prophylaxis. *Arch Dermatol.* 1984;120:48–51.

10. McCune MA, Perry HO, Muller SA, et al. Treatment of recurrent herpes simplex infections with L-lysine monohydrochloride. *Cutis.* 1984;34:366–373.

11. Civitelli R, Villareal DT, Agnusdei D, et al. Dietary L-lysine and calcium metabolism in humans. *Nutrition.* 1992;8:400–405.

12. McBeath M, Pauling L. A case history: lysine/ascorbate-related amelioration of angina pectoris. *J Orthomolec Med.* 1993;8:77–78.

13. Pauling L. Third case report on lysine-ascorbate-related amelioration of angina pectoris. *J Orthomolec Med.* 1993;8:137–138.

14. Pauling L. Case report: lysine/ascorbate-related amelioration of angina pectoris. *J Orthomolec Med.* 1991;6:144–146.

15. Kurowska EM, Carroll KK. Hypercholesterolemic responses in rabbits to selected groups of dietary essential amino acids. *J Nutr.* 1994;124:364–370.

16. Sanchez A, Rubano DA, Shavlik GW, et al. Cholesterolemic effects of the lysine/arginine ratio in rabbits after initial early growth. *Arch Latinoam Nutr.* 1988;38:229–238.

17. Leszcynski DE, Kummerow FA. Excess dietary lysine induces hypercholesterolemia in chickens. *Experientia.* 1982;38:266–267.

M

Ma Huang *(Ephedra sinica)*

Ma huang, the dried stem of the three ephedra species (*Ephedra sinica, Ephedra equisetina, Ephedra intermedia*), has been a part of Chinese medicine for 5,000 years. The herb has traditionally been used for a number of conditions including colds, flu, fever, chills, headache, edema, asthma, wheezing, and lack of perspiration. The alkaloids of ma huang, ephedrine and pseudoephedrine, are found in many over-the-counter cold and asthma medications (synthetic form) and dietary supplements (botanical form). Ephedra alkaloids are powerful central nervous system (CNS) stimulants. Ephedrine, a sympathomimetic agent, causes vasoconstriction and cardiac stimulation. Pseudoephedrine enhances bronchodilation and decreases symptoms of nasal congestion.

There is considerable controversy surrounding the safety and regulation of this herb. Serious side-effects including rapid heart beat, hypertension, arteriole constriction, and even death led to the FDA's 1996 warning to avoid ma huang/ephedrine-containing dietary supplements. Because dietary supplements containing ephedrine alkaloids can pose serious health risks, the FDA proposed labeling requirements in June 1997 that would require: (1) warning labels to state: "Taking more than the recommended serving may result in heart attacks, seizures, or death"; (2) products to be limited to 8 mg of ephedrine or related alkaloid per serving, with a maximum daily dosage of 24 mg; (3) supplement use to be limited to no more than seven days; (4) to not combine products with other herbal stimulants (kola nut, guarana) and caffeine with ephedrine. However, in August 1999, a report by the U.S. General Accounting Office (GAO) concluded that although the FDA was justified in addressing the safety of ephedra supplements given the number of adverse events, additional evidence was needed to support the proposed limits on dosage and duration. In March 2000, FDA conceded that its original proposal should be reassessed in light of the GAO's recommendations. The agency also released a new set of 140 reported adverse events for public comment and asked independent reviewers to assess the validity of these events. At press time, FDA has not officially published any new guidelines on ephedra products. The FDA website (*http://vm.cfsan.fda.gov/~dms/ds-ephed.html*) lists up-to-date information on regulations (1, 2, 3).

Media and Marketing Claims	Efficacy
Speeds metabolism for weight loss (Danger!)	↑?
Improves asthma symptoms	↑?
Nasal decongestant	↑?
Herbal ecstasy—euphoric feelings and enhanced sexual sensations	NR

Advisory

- Associated with serious adverse effects, including heart attack, hypertension, stroke, insomnia, tremors, death
- Individuals with hypertension, cardiovascular disease, thyroid disease, diabetes, neurological disorders, and men experiencing difficulty urinating due to an enlarged prostate should not use ma huang/ephedra products
- Individuals should not supplement without medical supervision

Drug/Supplement Interactions

- Excessive CNS and cardiovascular stimulation may occur when ma huang is combined with MAO inhibitors, medications containing pseudoephedrine or ephedrine, or large sources of caffeine, such as weight-loss remedies or caffeine-containing analgesics
- Ma huang/ephedra should not be combined with any medications used to treat heart disease, hypertension, depression, Parkinson's disease, asthma, diabetes

- Potential excessive CNS stimulation when combined with other stimulant herbs such as kola nut and guarana

KEY POINTS

- Ma huang/ephedra is a "natural" product with drug-like actions. Unfortunately, the alkaloid content of ma huang is variable. This makes self-medicating potentially dangerous, especially if products contain unusually high amounts of ephedrine or if taken in excess. Stricter regulations and warning labels have been proposed as a way to help avert potential health risks associated with these products. Some manufacturers are already voluntarily including warnings on their labels to prevent misuse by unwary supplement users. The regulation of ephedra products remains a controversial topic that has sparked heated debates among the public, the dietary supplement industry, FDA, health professionals, researchers, and politicians.

- Studies have found that ephedrine plus caffeine increases weight loss and reduces body fat in healthy, obese subjects. In clinical trials, herbal preparations of ephedra with kola nut or guarana have been associated with palpitations, increased heart rate, transient rises in blood pressure, insomnia, irritability, and chest pain. Many experts feel that the risks associated with self-supplementing with ephedra products far outweigh the weight loss benefits.

- Although ephedra alkaloids appear to be effective bronchodilators and nasal decongestants, there is currently greater consistency in FDA-approved over-the-counter or prescription drugs that contain approved levels of pseudoephedrine and ephedrine (4). Until extracts of ma huang (providing standardized concentrations of ephedra or pseudoephedrine) can be guaranteed to be properly formulated, dosed, and labeled, ma huang/ephedra supplements are not recommended for use in asthma or bronchial congestion.

- Ephedrine is similar in chemical structure to the illegal drug methamphetamine or "ecstasy," which produces a feeling of increased energy and euphoria. Some manufacturers have used this fact to falsely claim that ma huang produces the same effects "naturally." Although ma huang may seem to increase energy because of its stimulatory effect on the CNS, there is no evidence that it produces a "high" similar to that from amphetamines. In March 2000, FDA stated that "street drugs" containing ephedra and marketed as dietary supplements are not legal because they are considered unapproved and misbranded drugs.

FOOD SOURCES

None

DOSAGE INFORMATION/ BIOAVAILABILITY

Ma huang *(E sinica)* contains up to 3.3 percent ephedra alkaloids. Currently, ma huang is sold in tablets, capsules, tinctures, and teas in doses ranging from 5 mg to 75 mg ephedrine alkaloids. This is compared to asthma medications that contain 24 mg ephedrine hydrochloride and cold medications that contain 60 mg to 120 mg pseudoephedrine hydrochloride. Supplements are prepared from either the powdered stems and aerial portions of the herb or from dried herbal extracts. The powdered stems and aerial portions typically contain lower levels of ephedra alkaloids than the dried extracts, which contain much higher alkaloid concentrations (5). It is of note that traditional use of ma huang as documented in the Chinese literature was to prepare the extract using the whole herb over a longer period of time than other herbs in the prescription (5). Furthermore, it was only to be extracted once (not twice), and this whole process differs from the standard commercial formulation of ephedra supplements (6).

An analysis of nine commercial ma huang products showed varying levels of alkaloids ranging from 0.3 mg to 56 mg, with one product having no detectable ephedrine-type alkaloids (7). A separate analysis of 20 ephedra products reported variability in ephedra alkaloid contents (ephedrine content ranged from 1.1 mg to 15.3 mg per dose) (8). In addition, there were significant lot-to-lot variations in alkaloid content in four samples, and half of the products had discrepancies between label claims for ephedra alkaloid content and actual content (in excess of 20 percent). Ma huang supplements formulated as extracts (found in most dietary supplements) are more rapidly absorbed than those formulated from the ground stem and aerial portions. The mean values of the rate of absorption and maximum plasma levels was 0.49 hours to 3.9 hours for the powdered herb and 1.36 hours to 2.8 hours for the extract formulations (5, 8, 9).

RELEVANT RESEARCH

Ephedra (Ma Huang) vs Ephedrine

- A randomized, crossover study of 10 subjects investigated the pharmacokinetics of ephedrine from three commercially available ma huang products compared to a 25-mg ephedrine hydrochloride capsule. Pharmacokinetic parameters for botanical ephedrine were found to be similar to the synthetic form. The authors concluded: "The increased incidence of ma huang toxicity does not stem from differences in the absorption of botanical ephedrine compared with synthetic ephedrine; rather it results from accidental overdose often prompted by exaggerated off-label claims and a belief that 'natural' medicinal agents are inherently safe" (10).

Ephedrine (Synthetic) and Weight Loss

- In a double-blind, placebo-controlled study, 67 overweight men and women (ages 25 y to 55 y) were randomized to receive ma huang and gurana (72 mg ephedrine alkaloids plus 240 mg caffeine/Metabolife 356) or a placebo daily for eight weeks. Subjects were excluded if they had diabetes; thyroid, kidney, liver, or heart diseases; cancer; anemia; hypertension; or use of medication other than contraceptives, hormone replacement therapy, or specific allergy preparations. Subjects were encouraged to limit dietary fat content to 30 percent of calories and exercise moderately. Baseline evaluation included medical and nutrition history, exam, blood and urine studies, and electrocardiogram (ECG) and body composition measurements. Twenty-four subjects in each group completed the study. The ma huang/guarana group had significant greater loss of weight, body fat, and waist and hip circumferences compared to the placebo. The herbs were also associated with significant reductions in serum triglyceride levels. There were no differences between groups in systolic or diastolic blood pressure; however, when the rise over baseline was compared for all subjects at each time point, mean systolic pressure was significantly greater at week 6 in the ephedra/gurana group. In addition, heart rate (beats/minute) was significantly higher with the ephedra/guarana combination throughout the study. There was a slight, but significant, rise in fasting blood glucose level that did not exceed normal ranges with the ephedra/guarana supplementation compared to the placebo. No abnormalities were observed with ECG in either group at baseline or week 8. Eight of the ma huang/guarana-treated subjects (23 percent) and zero from the placebo group withdrew from the study because of adverse side-effects. These subjects withdrew in the first two weeks because of elevated blood pressure, palpitations, extreme irritability, and chest pain. Subjects that remained in the study reported a higher rate of side-effects than in the placebo group, but no serious or lasting negative effects. The authors noted that the physiological responses observed with ephedra/guarana (heart rate, transient elevation in glucose and blood pressure) are more pronounced in patients using the prescription drug sibutramine approved by FDA for obesity. The authors concluded that critical questions regarding risk/benefit must be determined. In particular, the researchers asked whether the risk/benefit ratio should be greater for an over-the-counter remedy that can be purchased by medically unsupervised individuals compared to a prescription drug that is used only under physician supervision. (11)

M

- In a double-blind, placebo-controlled study, 30 healthy, overweight subjects were randomized to receive Xenadrine (40 mg ephedrine alkaloids, 10 mg synephrine, 400 mg caffeine, 30 mg salicin) or a placebo divided into two doses daily for eight weeks. All subjects were instructed by a dietitian to follow a National Cholesterol Education Step One diet and performed cross-training exercise three times per week under the guidance of an exercise physiologist. Subjects taking the ephedrine combination supplement lost a significant amount of weight compared to the placebo group (—3.14 kg vs. —2.05 kg). The experimental group experienced a 16 percent decrease in body fat compared to a 1 percent increase for the placebo group, which was significant. There were no significant changes in blood pressure, serial electrocardiograms, pulse, serum chemistries, or caloric intake (12).

- In a double-blind, placebo-controlled trial (published as an abstract), 167 weight-stable men and women (mean BMI = 31.4) were randomized to receive ma huang plus koala nut (90 mg ephedrine/day + 192 mg caffeine/day) or a placebo daily for six months. Forty-six subjects in the herbal group and 38 subjects in the placebo group completed the study. The ephedra/caffeine combination significantly lowered body weight, percent body fat, and BMI. Blood pressure was transiently increased and heart rate was persistently significantly increased, but no cardiac arrhythmias were observed. Self-reported symptoms of dry mouth, heartburn, insomnia, and diarrhea were significantly greater in the ephedra/koala nut group, but there were no differences in reported chest pain, palpitations, irritability, nausea, and constipation (13). The full paper of this study was not available for review.

- According to a review published in 1995, prior to the FDA's warnings about ephedra, several studies suggest that ephedrine coadministered with methylxanthines (caffeine) enhances fat loss. Ephedrine plus caffeine is thought to act by centrally suppressing appetite and peripherally stimulating fat oxidation. The authors noted one trial in which ephedrine plus caffeine was as effective as dexfenfluramine. The authors concluded that more research is needed to identify combinations of sympathomimetics and methylxanthines with improved efficiency and safety. They also stated that long-term trials and studies in males are lacking (14).

- In a double-blind, placebo controlled study, 180 obese patients on a low-calorie diet were treated daily with either ephedrine/caffeine combination (60 mg/600 mg), ephedrine (60 mg), caffeine (600 mg) or a placebo divided into three doses for six months. Withdrawals from the trial (39 subjects dropped out) were equally distributed among the four treatments. Mean weight loss was statistically significantly greater with the combination treatment (–16.6 kg) compared to placebo (–13.2 kg) from months 2 to 6. Weight loss using ephedrine alone or caffeine alone was similar to that of the placebo group. Patients receiving ephedrine, caffeine, or the combination experienced tremors, insomnia, and dizziness, which subsided after two months. Blood pressure fell in all four groups (15).

SAFETY

- The FDA had compiled numerous reports of "adverse events" for ma huang including heart attack, stroke, tremors, insomnia, and death in individuals otherwise in good health after using ma huang/ephedrine products (1).

- Independent researchers were asked by FDA to review 140 reports of adverse events related to ephedra alkaloids reported between June 1997 and March 1999. Each event was assessed and categorized into definitely, probably or possibly related to supplements containing ephedra. Of the 43 events categorized as "definitely or probably" related to ephedra use (31 percent of the total), 3 cases resulted in death, 7 cases resulted in permanent impairment, 4 cases required ongoing medical treatment, and 29 cases had full recoveries. Most of these adverse events were related to cardiovascular symptoms, with hypertension as the single most frequent negative event, followed by palpitations, tachycardia, or both, stroke, and seizures (16).

- Ma huang was assessed for cytotoxicity under different conditions *in vitro*. The summarized results were: (1) cytotoxicity was not entirely related to ephedrine alkaloid content, suggesting the presence of other toxins in the herb; (2) grinding the herb increased the cytotoxicty; (3) ma huang extracts had a very high toxicity on neuronal cells compared to other cell lines; and (4) toxicity was reduced by boiling the whole herb for two hours (6).

- Case reports of ischemic and hemorrhagic stroke have been associated with ephedrine use (17).

- In one case, a healthy college student died from necrosis of the heart muscle after six months of taking a daily sports drink containing 25 mg to 50 mg ephedrine (18).

- A 58-year-old woman taking ma huang for 4.5 months and omeprazole for four years developed acute hepatitis, which her physicians associated with use of the herb (19).

- Ephedrine-induced nephrolithiasis has been reported with use of ma huang extract (20).

- Individuals with hypertension, cardiovascular disease, thyroid disease, diabetes, neurological disorders, and men experiencing difficulty urinating because of an enlarged prostate should take special precautions to avoid ma huang/ephedra because it acts as a heart and CNS system stimulant (1, 2). To prevent potential excessive CNS and cardiovascular stimulation, ma huang/ephedrine supplements should not be combined with MAO inhibitors, medications containing pseudoephedrine or ephedrine, or other caffeine-containing weight-loss remedies (1).

- The German government's *Commission E Monographs of Herbal Medicines* states that ephedra is contraindicated in individuals with anxiety, restlessness, high blood pressure, glaucoma, cerebral insufficiency, adenoma of prostate with residual urine accumulation, pheochromocytoma, thyrotoxicosis. Side-effects of the herb are listed as: insomnia, motor restlessness, irritability, headaches, nausea, vomiting, disturbances of urination, tachycardia, and in higher doses cardiac arrhythmia, drastic increases in blood pressure, and development of dependency (21).

REFERENCES

1. Dietary supplements containing ephedrine alkaloids; proposed rule (21 CFR 111). *Fed Regist.* June 2, 1997;62(pt 2):30678–30724.
2. Blumenthal M, King P. Ma huang: a review of the botany, chemistry, medicinal uses, safety concerns, and legal status of ephedra and its alkaloids. *HerbalGram.* 1995;34:22.
3. United States General Accounting Office. Dietary Supplements: Uncertainties in analyses underlying FDA's proposed rule on ephedrine alkaloids. GAO publication no. GAO/HEHS/GGD-99–90 July 1999.
4. Blanc PD, Kuschner WG, Katz PP, et al. Use of herbal products, coffee or black tea, and over-the-counter medications as self-treatments among adults with asthma. *J Allergy Clin Immunol.* 1997;100:789–791.
5. Gurley BJ, Gardner SF, Hubbard MA. Content versus label claims in ephedra-containing dietary supplements. *Am J Health-Syst Pharm.* 2000;57:963–969.
6. Lee MK, Cheng BW, Che CT, et al. Cytotoxicity assessment of ma-huang (ephedra) under different conditions of preparation. *Toxicol Sci.* 2000;56:424–430.
7. Betz JM, Gay ML, Mossaba MM, et al. Chiral gas chromatographic determination of ephedrine-type alkaloids in dietary supplements containing ma huang. *J AOAC Int.* 1997;80:303–315.
8. Gurley B. Extract versus herb: effect of formulation on the absorption on rate of botanical ephedrine from dietary supplements containing Ephedra (ma huang). *Thera Drug Monit.* 2000;22:497.

9. White LM, Gardner SF, Gurley BJ, et al. Pharmacokinetics and cardiovascular effects of ma-huang (*Ephedra sinica*) in normotensive adults. *J Clin Pharmacol.* 1997;37:116–122.

10. Gurley BJ, Gardner SF, White LM, et al. Ephedrine pharmacokinetics after ingestion of nutritional supplements containing *Ephedra sinica* (ma huang). *Ther Drug Monit.* 1998;20:439–445.

11. Boozer CN, Nasser JA, Heymsfield SB, et al. An herbal supplement containing ma huang-guarana for weight loss: a randomized, double-blind, trial. *Int J Obes Relat Metab Disord.* 2001;25:316–324.

12. Kalman DS, Colker CM, Shi Q, et al. Effects of a weight-loss aid in healthy overweight adults: double-blind, placebo-controlled clinical trial. *Curr Ther Res.* 2000;61:199–205.

13. Boozer CN, Daly PA, Blanchard D, et al. Herbal ephedra/caffeine for weight loss: a 6-month trial. *FASEB J.* 2001;15:A403.

14. Astrup A, Breum L, Toubro S. Pharmacological and clinical studies of ephedrine and other thermogenic agonists. *Obes Res.* 1995;3:537S—540S.

15. Astrup A, Breum L, Toubro S, et al. The effect and safety of an ephedrine/caffeine compound compared to ephedrine, caffeine, and placebo in obese subjects on an energy restricted diet. A double blind trial. *Int J Obes Relat Metab Disord.* 1992;16:269–277.

16. Haller CA, Benowitz NL. Adverse cardiovascular and central nervous system events associated with dietary supplements containing ephedra alkaloids. *N Engl J Med.* 2000;343:1833–1888.

17. Bruno A, Nolte KB, Chapin J. Stroke associated with ephedrine use. *Neurology.* 1993;43:1313–1316.

18. Theoharides TC. Sudden death of a healthy college student related to ephedrine toxicity from a ma-huang-containing drink. *J Clin Psychopharmacol.* 1997;17:437–439.

19. Borum ML. Fulminant exacerbation of autoimmune hepatitis after the use of ma huang. *Am J Gastroenterol.* 2001;96:1654–1655.

20. Powell T, Hsu FF, Turk J, et al. Ma huang strikes again: ephedrine nephrolithiasis. *Am J Kidney Dis.* 1998;32:153–159.

21. Blumenthal M, ed. *The Complete German Commission E Monographs Therapeutic Guide to Herbal Medicines.* Austin, TX: American Botanical Council; 1998.

Magnesium

The second most abundant intracellular cation in the body, magnesium is involved in more than 300 enzymatic reactions. It interacts closely with other electrolytes (calcium, potassium), plays a role in neuromuscular activity, excitation, and contraction, and is involved in bone function. Magnesium also stabilizes the structure of adenosine triphosphate (ATP) in ATP-dependent enzyme reactions. The body contains a total of 20 g to 28 g magnesium, with 60 percent in bone, 27 percent in muscle, 1 percent in extracellular fluid, and the remainder in soft tissue and other fluids. Hypomagnesemia may result from renal dysfunction, endocrine disorders, malabsorption syndromes, use of loop diuretics or digitalis, chronic alcoholism, diabetes mellitus, and excessive diarrhea. A deficiency is associated with cardiac and neuromuscular changes including muscle weakness, spasms, tetany, convulsions, hypokalemia, hypocalcemia, and arrhythmias (1).

Media and Marketing Claims	Efficacy
Supports a healthy heart	↔
Lowers blood pressure	↔
Improves diabetes because diabetics are often deficient in magnesium	?↑
Alleviates migraine headaches	↔
Improves symptoms of PMS	↔
Enhances exercise performance	↓

Advisory

- Considered safe in supplemental doses below the Tolerable Upper Intake Level (UL): 350 mg/day
- Hypermagnesemia can occur with supplement use in individuals with kidney disease

Drug/Supplement Interactions

Magnesium supplements used with magnesium-containing drugs (antacids, cathartics) may supply high doses of magnesium and may be associated with diarrhea and dehydration/electrolyte imbalances

KEY POINTS

M

- Magnesium is necessary for the proper functioning of muscle, including the heart muscle. A deficiency (rare in healthy individuals) results in negative effects on cardiac and neuromuscular functions. There is preliminary evidence that magnesium supplements may be beneficial for individuals with mitral valve prolapse. Larger, controlled clinical trials are needed to substantiate the potential role of magnesium supplements in various heart conditions. If dietary intake is not adequate, patients with cardiovascular diseases should be encouraged to consume magnesium-rich foods and take a magnesium supplement providing no more than the UL.

- The role of magnesium supplements in reducing blood pressure has not been confirmed. Epidemiological studies have suggested an inverse relationship between dietary magnesium and blood pressure. The data from clinical trials is conflicting and the reduction in blood pressure, if any, appears to be small. Loop and thiazide diuretics, used in the treatment of hypertension, can induce magnesium depletion that can be corrected by increasing intake of magnesium-rich foods and/or by taking a magnesium supplement providing no more than the UL provided that renal function is normal.

- Patients with diabetes are at risk for poor magnesium status. However, magnesium supplements generally have not improved glycemic control in type 1 or 2 diabetics. This may be because these studies have not been able to fully restore subjects' intracellular magnesium status. This has been difficult to evaluate because of methodological problems in assessment, the study length, or magnesium dose. Longer studies are needed to determine the effect of supplements on the morbidity and mortality of patients with diabetes. This population should be encouraged to increase dietary magnesium and/or take a supplement if necessary only if there is no sign of renal insufficiency. A physician should be consulted to make recommendations regarding magnesium supplementation in patients at risk for renal insufficiency.

- The research in support on the efficacy of magnesium in migraine headaches is conflicting and requires further study.

- Preliminary research suggests that magnesium supplements may reduce mild premenstrual symptoms. In one study, only symptoms of fluid retention were affected, whereas in another, only symptoms related to mood were improved. More research is needed in this population.

- Although athletes competing in weight-controlled sports may not be meeting the RDA for magnesium, research from well-controlled studies generally does not support an ergogenic benefit of magnesium supplements. Athletes should be advised to consume an adequate amount of magnesium from a varied, balanced eating plan.

FOOD SOURCES

Good sources of magnesium are whole grains, dark green leafy vegetables, nuts, legumes, and fish.

Food	Magnesium (mg)
Spinach, (½ c)	78
Beans, black (½ c)	60
Potato, baked, with skin	55
Peanuts (1 oz)	50
Sea bass (3 oz)	45
Rice, brown (½ c)	42
Squash, butternut (½ c)	30
Milk, nonfat (1 c)	28
Chicken breast, skinless (half)	25

Source: Data from Pennington JAT (2)

DOSAGE INFORMATION/BIOAVAILABILITY

Under the recent Dietary Reference Intakes (DRIs), the revised RDA for magnesium is 400 mg for males aged 19 y to 30 y, 310 mg for females aged 19 y to 30 y, 420 for males ≥ 31 y, and 320 for females ≥ 31 y (3). Magnesium is sold in single preparations, in combination with calcium, or in multivitamin mineral supplements providing 10 mg to 500 mg in the form of magnesium citrate, aspartate, acetate, glycinate, hydroxide, lactate, carbonate, chloride, pidolate, or oxide. In one study, magnesium citrate was found to be more soluble and bioavailable than magnesium oxide supplements (4). Because magnesium oxide and hydroxide are not soluble, they are often used as an osmotic laxative (1). Absorption of dietary magnesium varies from 14 percent to 70 percent depending on the dosage (fractional absorption is inversely related to intake). The kidneys regulate magnesium excretion and conserve the mineral when intake is low (1). Diets high in saturated fats, sugar, caffeine, and alcohol may increase magnesium needs (5).

RELEVANT RESEARCH

Magnesium Status and Intake

- Magnesium status is difficult to assess because plasma levels represent only 1 percent of total body magnesium and are not reflective of intracellular stores. A variety of diagnostic tests are used to assess magnesium nutriture, but none of them are flawless. Blood mononuclear cell magnesium concentrations are thought to be more reliable than serum levels. Likewise, ionized magnesium (IMg^{2+}) is considered a better indicator of magnesium status than total serum concentrations. Urinary levels of magnesium increase with supplementation but do not provide a quantitative measure of magnesium status (1).

- Magnesium depletion is common among patients in intensive care (1). In one study, approximately 50 percent of critically ill patients presented with magnesium depletion that was related to a higher morbidity and mortality than magnesium-replete patients (6).

- Risk factors associated with poor magnesium status include: uncontrolled diabetes mellitus, cardiovascular disease, alcohol ingestion, severe diarrhea and steatorrhea, and the use of renal magnesium-wasting drugs (ie, loop diuretics such as furosemide) (1).

Magnesium and Cardiovascular Disease

- In a prospective, observational study (Atherosclerosis Risk in Communities—ARIC), 13,922 subjects from four US communities free of coronary heart disease (CHD) were followed for four to seven years. After adjusting for sociodemographics, waist:hip ratio, smoking, alcohol, exercise, diuretics, fibrinogen, cholesterol levels, and hormone replacement therapy, the relative risk of developing CHD was statistically significantly correlated to low serum magnesium levels in women, but not men (the relative risk from the highest to lowest quartile of serum magnesium in women was 1.00, 0.92, 0.48, and 0.44). However, the adjusted relative risk of developing CHD was not statistically correlated with dietary magnesium intake in women or men (7). Results from the same ARIC population were reported in an earlier analysis of 15,248 subjects. Mean serum magnesium was significantly lower in subjects with prevalent cardiovascular disease, hypertension, and diabetes. Dietary magnesium was inversely associated with serum insulin, HDL cholesterol, and systolic and diastolic blood pressure (8).

- The serum magnesium levels in 141 subjects with mitral valve prolapse syndrome (MVP) aged 16 y to 57 y were compared with 40 healthy controls aged 19 y to 49 y living in the same area. There was a significant difference in the incidence of low magnesium levels between MVP subjects and controls (60 percent vs 5 percent). MVP patients (n = 70) with low serum magnesium were entered into a double-blind, crossover study and were supplemented in random order with magnesium or a placebo daily for five weeks each (week 1 = 497 mg [21 mmol] magnesium as magnesium carbonate; weeks 2 to 5 = 330 mg [14 mmol] magnesium). Serum magnesium increased significantly with magnesium supplementation (0.63 ± 0.11 mmol/L to 0.73 ± 0.08 mmol/L), but not with the placebo. Symptoms of MVP, intensity of anxiety (assessed by Spielberger's psychological questionnaire), and daily catecholamine excretion were determined. After five weeks of magnesium therapy, the mean number of symptoms per patient decreased significantly compared to the baseline. Specifically, there was a significant reduction in weakness, chest pain, dyspnea, palpitations, and anxiety after magnesium supplementation. The number of symptoms during magnesium supplementation decreased after five weeks (from 10.4 symptoms ± 2.1 to 5.6 ± 2.5). The placebo had no statistically significant effect on mean number of symptoms (8.5 symptoms ± 3.7 at the baseline to 8.9 ± 2.9 at five weeks). Mean daily excretion of catecholamines (norepinephrine and epinephrine) decreased significantly with magnesium but not with placebo. The authors hypothesized that the reduction in symptoms could have been caused by an antiadrenergic effect of magnesium (9).

- One review article reported research indicating that magnesium-deficient diets cause arterial and myocardial lesions in animal models. The author cautioned that treatment of cardiovascular disease (with digitalis or diuretics) may exacerbate an underlying magnesium deficit that could cause cardiac arrhythmias (10).

Magnesium and Blood Pressure

- More than 12 controlled trials have investigated the effects of magnesium supplements in patients with hypertension. Most of these trials have produced inconsistent results (11).

- In a double-blind, placebo-controlled, randomized study, 300 women from the Nurses Health Study II with normal blood pressure whose reported intake of magnesium, potassium, and calcium were between the 10th and 15th percentile, received daily supplements of 336 mg (14 mmol) magnesium as magnesium lactate, or 1,200 mg calcium, or 40 mmol potassium, all three supplements together, or a placebo for 16 weeks. The mean reductions in systolic and diastolic blood pressures between treatment and placebo groups were statistically significant for the potassium-supplemented group (↓2.0 mm Hg systolic, ↓1.7 mm Hg diastolic), but not for the calcium- or magnesium-supplemented groups. The combination supplement did not enhance the blood pressure-lowering effect of potassium supplements alone (11).

- In a double-blind, placebo-controlled trial, 698 healthy subjects with high-normal diastolic blood pressure (80 mm Hg to 89 mm Hg) were randomized to receive one of three treatments daily for six months: (1) 360 mg magnesium as magnesium diglycine, (2) 1,000 mg calcium, or (3) placebo. Overall analysis revealed no significant changes in blood pressure at three or six months among groups. Analyses stratified by baseline intakes of calcium, magnesium, sodium, or initial blood pressures also showed no effect with supplementation (12).

- In a double-blind, placebo-controlled trial, 14 subjects with mild to moderate hypertension were randomized to receive 360 mg (15 mmol) magnesium as magnesium pidolate or a placebo daily for six months. There were no significant differences between groups in blood pressure at rest, during sympathetic stimulation induced by cold, isometric exercise, or during the tilt test (13).

Magnesium and Diabetes

- Hypomagnesemia occurs in an estimated 30 percent of patients with type 2 diabetes, especially those not under good metabolic control (1, 14–16).

- In a double-blind, placebo-controlled trial, 128 Brazilian patients with type 2 diabetes treated by diet or diet with oral medication were randomized to receive one of three treatments daily for 30 days: (1) 497 mg (20.7 mmol) magnesium as magnesium oxide, (2) 994 mg (41.4 mmol) magnesium, or (3) a placebo. Magnesium levels in plasma, mononuclear cell, and urine were assessed. Fasting blood glucose, HbA_{1c}, and fructosamine were taken as measures of glycemic control. At the baseline, 48 percent had low plasma magnesium and 31 percent had low intramononuclear cell magnesium levels. Intracellular magnesium was significantly lower than in healthy controls (n = 62 blood donors). Lower-dose magnesium supplementation did not affect plasma or intracellular levels of magnesium, nor did it improve glycemic control. With the higher dose of magnesium, there was an insignificant trend toward increasing plasma, intracellular, and urine magnesium and a significant fall in fructosamine. There were no correlations between plasma and intracellular magnesium, or between magnesium concentrations and glycemic control (17).

- In a placebo-controlled (not blinded) study, 50 moderately controlled, type 2 diabetics requiring insulin were randomized to receive 360 mg (15 mmol) magnesium as magnesium aspartate-hydrochloride or a placebo daily for three months. Glycemic control, blood pressure, and plasma lipids were measured before and after three months. Plasma magnesium concentrations and urinary magnesium excretion were higher after supplementation compared to the placebo, but there was no effect on erythrocyte magnesium. There were no significant differences in glycemic control (glucose, HbA_{1c}), lipids, or blood pressure between groups (18). The results of this study should be viewed with caution because of the lack of blinding, which may have introduced bias.

- In an open, pilot study, 11 patients with type 1 diabetes with stable metabolic parameters and persistently low values of erythrocyte magnesium were given 450 mg magnesium (as magnesium carbonate plus oxide) for 10 weeks following an intravenous magnesium loading test. During intravenous loading, plasma ionized magnesium decreased and erythrocyte magnesium increased significantly together with an increased storage of urinary magnesium demonstrated by a classical retention test. However, supplementation did not result in normalization of magnesium parameters. There were no significant changes in glycosylated hemoglobin A_{1c}, total cholesterol, HDL cholesterol, or triglycerides. The authors concluded that in states of chronic magnesium depletion such as insulin-dependent diabetes mellitus it is difficult to replete

M

and maintain the magnesium body stores. They suggested that long-term studies in a large group of patients are necessary (19).

Magnesium and Migraine Headaches

- According to one review, 50 percent of patients have lowered levels of ionized magnesium during an acute migraine attack. The author further discussed the potential role of magnesium in the pathogenesis of migraines, noting that magnesium concentration affects serotonin receptors, nitric oxide synthesis and release, and other migraine-related receptors and neurotransmitters (20).

- In a double-blind, placebo-controlled, prospective multicenter study, 69 patients experiencing two to six migraine attacks per month without aura, and a history of migraine for at least two years, were randomized to receive 480 mg (20 mmol) magnesium or a placebo divided into two doses daily for 12 weeks. All patients were followed at the baseline for four weeks before the start of the study. There were no differences between groups in the number of migraine days or migraine attacks. Final assessments of efficacy by doctor and patients showed no benefit of magnesium supplementation. The trial was discontinued because interim analysis revealed a lack of response to treatment. Forty-five percent of patients receiving magnesium experienced mild adverse effects (soft stool, diarrhea) compared to 23 percent in the placebo group (21).

- In a double-blind, placebo-controlled, multicenter study, 81 subjects with a mean migraine attack frequency of 3.6 per month were randomized to receive 576 mg (24 mmol) magnesium (as trimagnesium dicitrate) daily or a placebo for 12 weeks. All patients were followed at the baseline for four weeks prior to treatment. At weeks 9 to 12, self-reported attack frequency was significantly reduced by 41.6 percent in the magnesium group compared to a 15.8 percent reduction in the placebo group. The number of days with migraine and the drug consumption for symptomatic treatment per patient also decreased significantly in the magnesium group. Intensity of attacks and drug consumption per attack tended to decrease with magnesium, but was not statistically significant. Diarrhea and gastric irritation occurred in 4 percent to 18 percent of the treatment group (22).

- In a case-control (not blinded, not placebo-controlled) study at an outpatient headache clinic, a consecutive sample of 40 patients presenting with moderate or severe headache of any type (16 migraine headaches without aura, 9 cluster headaches, 4 tension headaches, 11 chronic migrainous headaches) were given an acute bolus of 1 g intravenous magnesium sulfate. These subjects were compared to a group of 60 healthy controls (not age- or sex-matched). Total serum magnesium, serum ionized magnesium (IMg^{2+}), and ionized calcium were measured. Eighty percent of the patients experienced complete elimination of pain within 15 minutes of magnesium infusion, which was statistically significant. Patients demonstrating no return of headache or associated symptoms within 24 hours of magnesium infusion had the lowest initial basal levels of IMg^{2+}. Nonresponders had significantly elevated total magnesium levels compared to responders. The authors concluded that measurement of serum IMg^{2+} levels may have a practical application in many types of headache patients and that low serum and brain tissue ionized magnesium levels may precipitate headache symptoms in susceptible patients (23). However, it is important to note that a placebo-control was lacking which would have strengthened the findings.

Magnesium and Premenstrual Syndrome (PMS)

- Blood magnesium measures across the menstrual cycle were studied in 26 women with confirmed PMS and 19 female controls of the same age. Lower magnesium concentrations (in erythrocyte and mononuclear blood cells but not plasma) in PMS patients at each sampling time were statistically lower than controls. However, the lower magnesium concentrations were not confined to the luteal phase when PMS symptoms typically occur. Additionally, magnesium measures did not correlate with severity of mood symptoms (24). Another study of 105 women with PMS reported that erythrocyte magnesium concentration, but not plasma magnesium, was significantly lower than that of a normal population (25).

- In a double-blind, placebo-controlled, crossover study, 38 women were randomized to receive 200 mg magnesium as magnesium oxide or a placebo daily for two menstrual cycles each. Subjects kept a daily record of symptoms grouped into six categories (anxiety, craving, depression, hydration, other, and total overall symptoms). In the first menstrual cycle, there was no difference among treatment results. In the second month there was a significant reduction of symptoms of "hydration" (weight gain, swelling of upper extremities, breast tenderness, abdominal bloating) with magnesium supplementation compared with placebo (26).

- In a double-blind, placebo-controlled study, 32 women with confirmed PMS were randomized to receive 360 mg magnesium (as magnesium pyrrolidone carboxylic acid) or a placebo divided into three doses/day from the 15th day of the menstrual cycle to the onset of menstrual flow for two cycles. Subjects had completed baseline recording of PMS symptoms for two months prior to supplementation. Blood samples were taken at the baseline, premenstrually, and in the second and fourth months of treatment. The Menstrual Distress Questionnaire score of the cluster "pain" was significantly reduced in the second month in both the treatment and placebo groups; however, only the magnesium group had a significant effect on both the total Menstrual Distress Questionnaire score and the cluster "negative affect." In the second month, the magnesium group had a statistically significant increase in magnesium in lymphocytes and polymorphonuclear cells, but no change in plasma and erythrocyte concentrations. In contrast, the placebo group had no significant changes in the magnesium levels in any of the cellular compartments (27).

- In a double-blind, placebo-controlled, crossover study, 44 women (average age = 32 y) were given in random order one of four treatments for one menstrual cycle: (1) 200 mg magnesium (oxide); (2) 50 mg vitamin B_6; (3) magnesium plus B_6; or (4) a placebo. During the study, each subject recorded daily symptoms on a five-point scale in a menstrual diary of 30 symptoms that were grouped into categories (anxiety, craving, depression, hydration, other). Urinary magnesium output was not affected by treatment, suggesting poor absorption of the magnesium. There were no overall differences

M

in symptoms between the treatments, however, a modest significant reduction in premenstrual anxiety-related symptoms was associated with the magnesium plus B_6 combination (28).

Magnesium and Exercise Performance

- Several studies have reported that athletes competing in weight-controlled sports often do not consume recommended dietary magnesium intakes because of food restriction practices (29).

- In a meta-analysis, researchers examined 12 studies of magnesium supplementation for exercise and reported that most evidence is not suggestive of a benefit of supplementation on performance (strength, anaerobic, aerobic). When only peak treadmill speed during a VO_{2max} test was examined, the evidence is equivocal. They noted several limitations with the studies making it difficult to analyze including varying exercise modes and intensities; variable training statuses and ages of subjects; subject selection favoring males; varying doses (116 mg to 500 mg/day); lack of magnesium status assessment; and lack of dietary magnesium intake controlled (30).

- In a double-blind, placebo-controlled study, 20 athletes with low-normal serum magnesium levels were randomized to receive 500 mg magnesium as magnesium oxide or a placebo daily for three weeks. Supplementation did not increase the magnesium concentration in serum or any cellular compartment studied. Serum magnesium only correlated with red cell magnesium and mononuclear leukocyte magnesium correlated with nuclear magnetic resonance-measured muscle cell magnesium concentration. There was no effect of magnesium on exercise performance by submaximal and maximal ergometer measurements, neuromuscular activity, or muscle-related symptoms. The authors concluded: "Magnesium supplementation in athletes with low-normal serum magnesium did not improve performance and failed to increase the body's magnesium stores. Serum magnesium appears to be a poor indicator for magnesium in skeletal muscle or most other cellular compartments, but the concentration of magnesium in mononuclear leukocytes might be used as an indicator of skeletal muscle magnesium when magnetic resonance is not available" (31).

- In a small, double-blind, placebo-controlled study, 20 marathon runners were assigned to receive 365 mg magnesium daily or a placebo for four weeks before and six weeks after a marathon race. Subjects were pair-matched by performance on a treadmill test. Magnesium supplementation did not increase muscle or serum magnesium concentrations. There were no differences between groups on the extent of muscle damage or the rate of recovery of muscle function. There were also no significant differences in age, mass, height, peak treadmill running velocity, and marathon racing times between groups. Serum and muscle magnesium did not differ between groups, although serum magnesium levels fell in all subjects after the marathon. The authors concluded that runners who have adequate magnesium status would not experience a benefit from supplementation (32).

- In a double-blind, placebo-controlled study, 26 untrained subjects received a magnesium supplement (magnesium oxide) equivalent to 8 mg/kg body weight/day (560 mg magnesium for a 70-kg man) or a placebo during seven weeks of a weight training program. Body composition and strength (pre- and postquadriceps torque measurements) were assessed before and after the study. Both groups gained strength; however, the magnesium group had a statistically significant increase in absolute quadriceps torque, relative torque adjusted for body weight, and relative torque adjusted for lean body mass compared to the control (33). This study has been criticized for not assessing magnesium status and because the placebo group had an average magnesium intake less than the RDA (34).

SAFETY

- The tolerable upper intake level (UL) for magnesium from supplements/pharmacological agents is set at 350 mg/day in addition to magnesium intake from food and water (3).

- Magnesium supplements are considered relatively nontoxic since for healthy individuals with normal kidney function because they are capable of eliminating excessive amounts. However, soft stools and osmotic diarrhea have been reported by some subjects supplemented with more than 500 mg elemental magnesium daily, which could result in dehydration and neurological symptoms (1).

- Hypermagnesemia can occur in renal-insufficient patients who chronically ingest magnesium-containing drugs (antacids or cathartics). The toxic effects of elevated serum magnesium can result in hypotension, nausea, decreased mental status, alterations in cardiac function, paralysis, central nervous system disorders, and death (1).

M

REFERENCES

1. Shils ME. Magnesium. In: Shils ME, Olson JA, Shike M, Ross AC, eds. *Modern Nutrition in Health and Disease.* 9th ed. Philadelphia, Pa: Lea & Febiger; 1999:169–192.
2. Pennington JA. *Bowes and Church's Food Values of Portions Commonly Used.* 17th ed. Philadelphia, Pa: Lippincott-Raven Publishers; 1998.
3. Institute of Medicine, Food and Nutrition Board. *Dietary Reference Intakes for Calcium, Phosphorus, Magnesium, Vitamin D, and Fluoride.* Washington, DC: National Academy Press; 1997.
4. Lindberg JS, Zobitz MM, Poindexter JR, et al. Magnesium bioavailability from magnesium citrate and magnesium oxide. *J Am Coll Nutr.* 1990;9:48–55.
5. Schaafsma G. Bioavailability of calcium and magnesium. *Eur J Clin Nutr.* 1997;51:S13–S16.
6. Olerich MA, Rude RK. Should we supplement magnesium in critically ill patients? *New Horiz.* 1994;2:186–192.
7. Liao F, Folsom AR, Brancati FL. Is low magnesium concentration a risk factor for coronary heart disease? The Atherosclerosis Risk in Communities (ARIC) Study. *Am Heart J.* 1998;136:480–490.

8. Ma J, Folsom AR, Melnick SL, et al. Associations of serum and dietary magnesium with cardiovascular disease, hypertension, diabetes, insulin, and carotid arterial wall thickness: the ARIC study. Atherosclerosis Risk in Communities Study. *J Clin Epidemiol.* 1995;48:927–940.

9. Lichodziejewska B, Klos J, Rezler J, et al. Clinical symptoms of mitral valve prolapse are related to hypomagnesemia and attenuated by magnesium supplementation. *Am J Cardiol.* 1997;15:768–772.

10. Seelig M. Cardiovascular consequences of magnesium deficiency and loss: pathogenesis, prevalence and manifestations—magnesium and chloride loss in refractory potassium repletion. *Am J Cardiol.* 1989;63:4G–21G.

11. Sacks FM, Willet WC, Smith A, et al. Effect on blood pressure of potassium, calcium, and magnesium in women with low habitual intake. *Hypertension.* 1998;31:131–138.

12. Yamamoto ME, Applegate WB, Klag MJ, et al. Lack of blood pressure effect with calcium and magnesium supplementation in adults with high-normal blood pressure. Reports from phase I of the Trials of Hypertension Prevention (TOHP). Trials of Hypertension Prevention (TOHP) Collaborative Research Group. *Ann Epidemiol.* 1995;5:96–107.

13. Ferrara LA, Iannuzzi R, Castaldo A, et al. Long-term magnesium supplementation in essential hypertension. *Cardiology.* 1992;81:25–33.

14. Resnick L, Altura BT, Gupta R, et al. Intracellular and extracellular magnesium depletion in type 2 (non-insulin-dependent) diabetes mellitus. *Diabetologia.* 1993;36:767–770.

15. Crook M, Couchman S, Tutt P, et al. Erythrocyte, plasma total, ultrafiltrable and platelet magnesium in type 2 (non-insulin-dependent) diabetes mellitus. *Diabetes Res.* 1994;27:73–79.

16. Vanroelen L, Gaal L, Van Rooy P, et al. Serum and erythrocyte magnesium level in type I and type II diabetes. *Acta Diabetol.* 1985;22:185–190.

17. Lima M, Cruz T, Pousada JC, et al. The effect of magnesium supplementation in increasing doses on the control of type 2 diabetes. *Diabetes Care.* 1998;21:682–686.

18. DeValk HW, Verkaaik R, van Rijn HJ, et al. Oral magnesium supplementation in insulin-requiring Type 2 diabetic patients. *Diabet Med.* 1998;15:503–507.

19. De Leeuw I, Engelen W, Vertommen J, et al. Effect of intensive IV + oral magnesium supplementation on circulating ion levels, lipid parameters, and metabolic control in Mg-depleted insulin-dependent diabetic patients (IDDM). *Magnes Res.* 1997;10:135–141.

20. Mauskop A, Altura BM. Role of magnesium in the pathogenesis and treatment of migraines. *Clin Neurosci.* 1998;5:24–27.

21. Pfaffenrath V, Wessely P, Meyer C, et al. Magnesium in the prophylaxis of migraine—a double-blind placebo-controlled study. *Cephalalgia.* 1996;16:436–440.

22. Peikert A, Wilimzig C, Kohne-Volland R. Prophylaxis of migraine with oral magnesium: results from a prospective, multi-center, placebo-controlled and double-blind randomized study. *Cephalalgia.* 1996;16:257–263.

23. Mauskop A, Altura BT, Cracco RQ, et al. Intravenous magnesium sulfate rapidly alleviates headaches of various types. *Headache.* 1996;36:154–160.

24. Rosenstein DL, Elin RJ, Hosseini JM, et al. Magnesium measures across the menstrual cycle in premenstrual syndrome. *Biol Psychiatry.* 1994;35:557–561.

25. Sherwood RA, Rocks BF, Stewart A, et al. Magnesium and the premenstrual syndrome. *Ann Clin Biochem.* 1986;23:667–670.

26. Walker AF, De Souza MC, Vickers MF, et al. Magnesium supplementation alleviates premenstrual symptoms of fluid retention. *J Women's Health.* 1998;7:1157–1165.

27. Facchinetti F, Borella P, Sances G, et al. Oral magnesium successfully relieves premenstrual mood changes. *Obstet Gynecol.* 1991;78:177–181.

28. De Souza MC, Walker AF, Robinson PA, et al. A synergistic effect of a daily supplement for one month of 200 mg magnesium plus 50 mg vitamin B$_6$ for the relief of anxiety-related premenstrual symptoms: a randomized, double-blind, crossover study. J Womens Health *Gend Based Med.* 2000;9:131–139.

29. Haymes EM, Clarkson PM. Minerals and trace minerals. In: Berning JR, Nelson S, eds. *Nutrition for Sport and Exercise.* 2nd ed. Gaithersburg, Md: Aspen Publishers Inc; 1998:91–92.

30. Newhouse IJ, Finstad EW. The effects of magnesium supplementation on exercise performance. *Clin J Sport Med.* 2000;10:195–200.

31. Weller E, Bachert P, Meinck HM, et al. Lack of effect of oral Mg-supplementation on Mg in serum, blood cells, and calf muscle. *Med Sci Sports Exerc.* 1998;30:1584–1591.

32. Terblanche S, Noakes TD, Dennis SC, et al. Failure of magnesium supplementation to influence marathon running performance or recovery in magnesium-replete subjects. *Int J Sport Nutr.* 1992;2:154–164.

33. Brilla LR, Haley TF. Effect of magnesium supplementation on strength training in humans. *J Am Coll Nutr.* 1992;11:326–329.

34. Clarkson PM, Haymes EM. Exercise and mineral status of athletes: calcium, magnesium, phosphorus, and iron. *Med Sci Sports Exerc.* 1995;27:831–843.

M

Melatonin

Synthesized from tryptophan, melatonin is the major hormone produced by the pineal gland located in the brain. Studies have shown that melatonin plays a role in regulating circadian rhythm and reducing core body temperature. Reduced melatonin secretions have been associated with aging, Alzheimer's disease, diabetes, cancer, and cardiovascular disease; however, its role in the etiology and pathophysiology of these conditions is unknown. Additionally, melatonin has been studied as a potential anticancer agent based on evidence from *in vitro* and animal research suggesting that the hormone has antiproliferative, antioxidative, and immunostimulatory mechanisms of action. Melatonin became available in 1993 as a dietary supplement marketed as a sleep-aid for insomnia and jet lag (1–4).

Media and Marketing Claims	Efficacy
Regulates sleep	↔
Reduces jet lag	↔
Reduces cancer risk through antioxidant properties	NR
Slows the aging process	NR
Increases sex drive	NR

Advisory

Not known whether long-term use inhibits endogenous melatonin production

Drug/Supplement Interactions

- Melatonin production is increased with administration of fluvoxetine/Prozac (antidepressant); the additive effect of melatonin supplementation is unknown
- Endogenous melatonin production may be reduced by beta-blockers (antihypertensive), valproic acid (anticonvulsant), corticosteroids (anti-inflammatory), fluvoxetine/Prozac (antidepressant)
- Melatonin administered with chemotherapy drugs may reduce side-effects or enhance drug efficacy; combination should only be used under the supervision of an oncologist

KEY POINTS

- Studies of melatonin supplements and sleep have yielded contradictory results. Much of the research suggests that melatonin hastens sleep onset, though this has not been consistent across all studies. One review article attributes contradictory results to study design differences with varying times of melatonin administration, dosage levels, types of subjects (normal vs insomniacs) and subjective vs objective measures of improvement. The authors concluded: "There is not yet a convincing body of evidence using generally accepted measures that melatonin administration improves sleep in insomniacs with noncircadian sleep disturbance" (5).

- Until large-scale, clinical trials testing the safety, efficacy, drug interactions, and effects on disease states are completed, supplementation with melatonin cannot be recommended with certainty. Individuals with sleep disorders or jet lag should instead consider maximizing nighttime endogenous melatonin production by avoiding alcohol and caffeine, which lower melatonin levels, increasing exposure to light during the day, avoiding sleeping late and taking naps longer than 30 minutes, and sleeping in a cool, dark environment.

- There is some evidence from preliminary controlled studies that high doses of melatonin administered in addition to chemotherapy may reduce some, but not all, chemotherapy-induced side-effects and increase one-year survival time. Several other open studies (not discussed here) also reported some benefit with melatonin. More definitive research is needed before any recommendations can be made regarding melatonin administration and cancer. The decision to supplement with melatonin should be made under the supervision of a patient's oncologist.

- Evidence from controlled clinical trails is lacking to support the claim that melatonin slows the aging process.

- Although the pineal gland secretes higher levels of melatonin during sexual maturation than during adulthood (6), there is currently no evidence from controlled clinical trials that melatonin supplements enhance sexual function or drive.

FOOD SOURCES

A minimal amount of melatonin is found in food, although more extensive studies are needed to define the levels of melatonin in a wider variety of food products (7). Melatonin is produced by plants, with the highest known amounts found in rice, barley, sweet corn, and oats (8). According to one report, in order to ingest 3 mg melatonin, one would have to eat 120 bananas or 30 bowls of rice (9). Unknown variables such as absorption from the gut and processing by the liver make it difficult to calculate how much a melatonin-containing food would have to be consumed to affect mood/sleep at the current time (7).

DOSAGE INFORMATION/BIOAVAILABILITY

Melatonin is sold capsules and tablets with manufacturer's recommending doses ranging from 3 mg to 5 mg (studies have used doses ranging from 0.1 mg to 2,000 mg). Some researchers have raised concerns about the safety, purity, and potency of melatonin sold in health food stores and pharmacies (2). Melatonin is absorbed rapidly and has a half-life in plasma of about 45 minutes (3). Labels suggest taking melatonin supplements a few hours before sleep time. Although the research is not conclusive, timing of administration varies depending on whether melatonin is used to advance the body clock (as in eastward travel), to treat delayed sleep phase syndrome, or to treat elderly or insomniac patients. Sach, Lewy, and Hughes describe melatonin administration as developed by the Sleep and Mood Disorders Laboratory at Oregon Health Sciences University (3).

RELEVANT STUDIES

Melatonin and Sleep

- In a double-blind, placebo-controlled, crossover study, 22 patients with delayed sleep phase syndrome received in random order placebo or 5 mg melatonin daily for four weeks, with a one week washout period between treatments. Subjects could take the treatment between 7 pm and 9 pm, and were restricted to a sleep period from 12 am to 8 am. Two consecutive overnight polysomnographic recordings were performed at baseline and after each four-week period. Sleep onset latency was significantly reduced during melatonin treatment compared to baseline and placebo. Melatonin did not alter total sleep time or subjective measures of sleepiness, fatigue, and alertness compared to baseline and placebo, but there was a significant reduction in total sleep time during placebo treatment. No adverse effects were noted (10).

- In a double-blind, placebo-controlled, crossover design study, 14 insomniac patients aged 55 y to 80 y (diagnosis verified by interview and polysomnogram) took 0.5 mg/day of melatonin in four treatment conditions: (1) an immediate release dose 30 minutes before bedtime, (2) a controlled-release dose 30 minutes before bedtime, (3) an immediate-release dose four hours after bedtime, and (4) a placebo. Each trial lasted for two weeks with two-week washout periods. Polysomnographic monitoring was

M

recorded on in subjects' homes on day 11 and 12. Subjects wore wrist actigraphs (records changes in movement/activity) 24 hours/day for each day of the study. All melatonin trials resulted in a significant shortened sleep latency compared to the placebo. However, melatonin did not sustain sleep or improve total sleep time, efficiency, or wake time after sleep onset. Furthermore, melatonin did not improve subjective self-reports of sleep quality. Subjects with lower melatonin levels did not preferentially respond to melatonin supplements. The authors concluded that their study "does not provide strong support for the melatonin replacement treatment strategy for age-related sleep-maintenance insomnia" (11).

- In a double-blind, placebo-controlled, crossover design study, 12 elderly patients with insomnia were randomly assigned to receive 2 mg controlled-release melatonin daily for three weeks each with a one-week washout period. In all subjects the excretion of the major melatonin metabolite (6-sulphatoxymelatonin) during the night was lower than normal or delayed in comparison to noninsomniac seniors. Sleep quality was measured by wrist actigraphy. There was a significant improvement in sleep efficiency and a significantly shorter wake time after sleep onset with melatonin compared to the placebo. Although there were no differences in total sleep time, the authors concluded that controlled-release melatonin replacement therapy appeared to improve sleep quality in a small group of elderly patients" (12).

- In a double-blind, placebo-controlled, crossover design study, eight male subjects (aged 14 y to 61 y) with delayed sleep phase syndrome were randomized to receive a placebo or 5 mg/day melatonin taken five hours before sleep onset for four weeks each with a one-week washout period between treatments. Differences between treatment were based on within-subject differences in changes of sleep log timings and alertness self-rating scores and the subject's overall assessment. In all subjects, sleep onset time and wake time were significantly earlier after melatonin supplementation. However, average total sleep time was less with melatonin than placebo. The authors concluded that melatonin may act as a "phase-setter" for sleep-wake cycles in patients with delayed sleep phase syndrome (13).

- In a double-blind, placebo-controlled study, 34 elderly subjects with insomnia who were taking benzodiazepines to induce sleep were randomized to receive 2 mg controlled-release melatonin or a placebo nightly for six weeks. Subjects were encouraged to reduce their benzodiazepine dosage by 50 percent during week 2, by 75 percent during weeks 3 and 4, and eliminate it by weeks 5 and 6. In a second single-blind phase of the study, melatonin was administered for six weeks to all subjects and encouraged to discontinue benzodiazepine therapy. Drug intake and subjective sleep quality scores were reported daily. By the end of the first phase, 14 of 18 subjects taking melatonin but only 4 of 16 placebo subjects were able to discontinue benzodiazepine therapy, and the difference between groups was significant. In addition, sleep quality scores were significantly higher in the melatonin group. Six additional subjects in the placebo group eliminated benzodiapine therapy during the open phase. Follow-up six months later revealed that of the 24 subjects in the melatonin group who discontinued the sleep drug, 19 maintained good sleep quality (14).

Melatonin for Jet Lag and Night Shift Work

- In double-blind, placebo-controlled study, 257 Norwegian physicians who had visited New York for five days were randomized to receive one of four regimens: (1) a placebo; (2) 5.0 mg melatonin at bedtime; (3) 0.5 mg melatonin at bedtime; or (4) 0.5 mg taken on a shifting schedule. Jet lag ratings were made on the day of travel from New York back to Oslo (six hours eastward) and for the next six days in Norway. Main outcome measures were scores on the Columbia Jet Lag Scale (identifies prominent daytime symptoms of jet lag). In all groups, there was a marked increase in total jet lag score on the first day home, followed by improvement during the next five days. However, there were no differences in jet lag, sleep onset, time of awakening, hours slept, or hours napping among any of the groups (15).

- In a double-blind, placebo-controlled study, 137 subjects flying from Switzerland to the United States and back (six to nine time zones) received randomly one of four treatments on the eastbound flight back to Switzerland and at bedtime on four consecutive nights after the flight: (1) 5 mg melatonin; (2) 10 mg zolpidem (hypnotic); (3) a combination of the two; or (4) a placebo. Alleviation of jet lag was assessed by daily sleep logs, symptoms questionnaires, and the Profile of Mood States (POMS). On the last day of treatment, all subjects completed Visual Analog Scales (VAS) on overall jet lag ratings and treatment effectiveness. At baseline and during the days postflight, motor activity was measured by wrist-worn ambulatory monitors.in a subgroup of subjects (n = 49). Only 79 percent of the subjects took the medication between 5 pm and 9 pm as instructed; 21 percent ingested the treatment later. All active treatments were associated with a significant reduction in jet lag severity, with zolpidem rated as the most effective (it significantly improved subjective sleep quality on night flights, reduced overall jet lag feelings, and alleviated sleep disturbances and confusion associated with jet lag). However, zolpidem and the combination of melatonin/zolpidem were not tolerated as well as melatonin alone. Confusion associated with jet lag, morning sleepiness, and nausea were highest in the combination group, and this was confirmed by actigraphy, which showed a significantly reduced motor activity in the first hour after waking only in the combination group. The authors suggested that future research evaluate using one dose of zolpidem for sleep while on the aircraft, and melatonin for the following days after the intercontinental flight (16).

- In a double-blind, placebo-controlled trial, 29 army personnel involved in rapid deployment missions and night operations in the Middle East were given 10 mg melatonin or a placebo daily five to seven days before travel and for five days after arrival, approximately 30 minutes prior to bedtime. Cognitive performance was tested before and after travel, and activity rhythms (wrist-worn activity monitors) were recorded for 13 continuous days. Melatonin advanced bedtimes and rise times and maintained sleep durations between seven and eight hours. The placebo group awoke earlier and retired to bed later (average 37 minutes later), resulting in a shorter sleep duration (five to seven hours) than melatonin-treated subjects. In the melatonin group there were significantly fewer errors than the placebo group in a dual-task vigilance test. The authors concluded "exogenous melatonin can be an effective adjunct of maintaining alertness

M

and preventing sleep loss in rapid deployment missions requiring eastward travel and nighttime duty hours" (17).

- In a double-blind, placebo-controlled trial, 52 flight crew employees were randomly assigned to three groups: early melatonin (5 mg melatonin for 3 days before arrival continuing for five days after returning home), late melatonin (placebo for three days followed by 5 mg melatonin for five days), and a placebo. All subjects began taking capsules at 7 am to 8 am Los Angeles time two days prior to their departure from home to New Zealand (NZ) (corresponding to 2 am to 3 am NZ time). Subjects then took one capsule on the return flight at 12 pm NZ time and continued taking one capsule between 10 pm to 12 pm for five days after arrival in New Zealand. (Researchers did not indicate why the large window of time from 10 pm to 12 pm was chosen). For six days after arrival home, subjects completed daily questionnaires measuring subjective impressions of fatigue, jet lag, activity, and sleepiness. Subjects in the late melatonin group reported less jet lag and sleep disturbance than did the placebo group. However, subjects in the early melatonin group reported a worse recovery of energy and alertness than did the placebo group. The authors concluded that timing of the melatonin dose appeared to affect the subjective effects of jet lag (18).

- In a small double-blind, placebo-controlled study, 17 subjects flew from London to San Francisco, where they stayed for two weeks before returning. Subjects were given 5 mg melatonin or a placebo at 6 pm local time, three days before returning home to London. On their return flight home, subjects continued taking melatonin at 2 pm to 4 pm for four more days. On day 7 of melatonin administration, after returning home, subjects were asked to rate their jet lag. Subjects taking melatonin reported significantly less severe jet lag than subjects taking a placebo (19).

- In a double-blind, placebo-controlled, crossover study, 18 emergency physicians working between two and five consecutive night shifts were given 10 mg sublingual melatonin or a placebo each morning after night shifts. Although there were trends toward improvement, melatonin intake did not have a significant effect on self-reported day sleep and night alertness (20).

- In a similar double-blind, placebo-controlled, crossover study, 19 emergency medicine residents who worked at least two night shifts per week received in random order 1 mg melatonin or a placebo 30 minutes to 60 minutes prior to their daytime sleep session, for three consecutive days after each night shift. Subjects crossed over to their other treatment during their subsequent night shifts the following week. Quality of daytime sleep was assessed by wrist actigraphs (a device that measures sleep motion and correlates with sleep efficiency, total sleep time, time in bed, and sleep latency). The Profile of Mood States (POMS) and the Stanford Sleepiness Scale (SSS) were given to evaluate mood and sleepiness. There were no differences in any of the parameters measured between either treatment (21).

Melatonin and Cancer

- In a controlled trial, 80 patients with metastatic solid tumors who were in poor clinical condition (lung, breast, and gastrointestinal cancers) were randomized to receive chemotherapy alone or chemotherapy plus melatonin (20 mg/day). Melatonin resulted in a significant reduction in frequency of thrombocytopenia, malaise, and asthenia compared to controls. There was an insignificant trend toward less stomatitis and neuropathy with melatonin, but it had no effect on alopecia and vomiting. The authors concluded: "This pilot study seems to suggest that concomitant administration of the pineal hormone melatonin during chemotherapy may prevent some chemotherapy-induced side-effects, particularly myelosuppression and neuropathy" (22).

- In a controlled study, 50 patients with brain metastases caused by solid neoplasms were randomized to receive supportive care alone (steroids plus anticonvulsant drugs) or supportive care plus melatonin (20 mg/day). The survival at one year, free-from-brain-progression period and mean survival time were significantly higher in patients treated with melatonin (9/24 melatonin subjects vs 3/26 control subjects). The control subjects had a significant increase in metabolic and infective complications compared to melatonin-treated subjects (23). Another randomized controlled study providing melatonin intravenously plus chemotherapy to advanced nonsmall-cell lung cancer patients reported a significant increase in percent of one-year survival compared to chemotherapy alone (15/34 melatonin subjects vs 7/36 control subjects) (24).

- One study investigated the effect of 20 mg melatonin compared to no treatment on the disease-free survival of 30 melanoma patients surgically treated for regional node recurrence. Patients were instructed to take melatonin every day until disease recurrence. After a median follow-up of 31 months, the melatonin-treated subjects had a significantly higher percentage of disease-free survival compared to controls (10/14 melatonin subjects vs 5/16 control subjects) (25).

- In a study of 250 metastatic solid tumor patients (lung, breast, gastrointestinal, head and neck cancers), 20 mg melatonin daily plus chemotherapy reduced the frequency of thrombocytopenia, neurotoxicity, cardiotoxicity, stomatitis, and asthenia compared to chemotherapy alone (26).

- Animal and *in vitro* studies are contradictory regarding the oncostatic effect of melatonin. Some have shown an antitumor effect on breast cancer and colon cancer cells (27, 28), whereas others have shown no effect (29, 30).

SAFETY

- To date, short-term, human studies in small numbers of subjects have not reported any harmful effects of melatonin supplementation (3). However, cases of acute poisoning have not been reported partially because of problems in assessment of toxicity (31).

- The toxicity of 10 mg melatonin/day for 28 days was assessed in 40 volunteers randomly assigned to melatonin (n = 30) or placebo (n =10) in a double-blind fashion. Melatonin had no effect on complete blood count; urinalysis; sodium, potassium, and calcium levels; total protein levels; albumin; blood glucose; triglycerides; total cholesterol, HDL, LDL, and VLDL cholesterol; urea; creatinine; uric acid; liver enzymes; thyroid hormones (T3, T4, TSH); ratio of leutinizing hormone to follicle stimulating hormone; cortisol; and serum melatonin (32).

- Researchers stress that the long-term effects and the safety of melatonin supplementation have not been studied. One review article warned that metabolites formed from taking high doses of melatonin could have unknown dangerous consequences. Furthermore, high doses could induce very high melatonin concentrations and possibly desensitize melatonin receptors. Melatonin supplements could also theoretically suppress endogenous production of the compound, which could further aggravate sleep disorders (33).

- A double-blind, placebo-controlled study of nine healthy men in a sleep laboratory reported that morning administration of melatonin impaired psychomotor function for six hours. Morning supplementation of melatonin may affect alertness and reflexes, and caution should be used by users of melatonin when driving (34).

- β-blockers, specifically lipophilic β-blockers, inhibit endogenous melatonin release (35). Other drug-nutrient interactions are not known.

REFERENCES

1. Defrance R, Quera-Salva MA. Therapeutic applications of melatonin and related compounds. *Horm Res.* 1998;49:142–146.
2. Cupp MJ. Melatonin. *Am Fam Physician.* 1997;56:1421–1425.
3. Sack RL, Lewy AJ, Hughes RJ. Use of melatonin for sleep and circadian rhythm disorders. *Ann Med.* 1998;30:115–121.
4. Panzer A, Viljoen M. The validity of melatonin as an oncostatic agent. *J Pineal Res.* 1997;22:184–202.
5. Mendelson WB. Efficacy of melatonin as a hypnotic agent. *J Biol Rhythms.* 1997;12:651–656.
6. Cavallo A, Ritschel WA. Pharmacokinetics of melatonin in human sexual maturation. *J Clin Endocrinol Metab.* 1996;81:1882–1886.
7. Reiter RJ, Tan DX, Burkhardt S, et al. Melatonin in plants. *Nutr Rev.* 2001;59:286–290.
8. Hattori A, Migitaka H, Iigo M, et al. Identification of melatonin in plants and its effects on plasma melatonin levels and binding to melatonin receptors in vertebrates. *Biochem Mol Biol Int.* 1995;35:627–634.
9. Lamberg L. Melatonin potentially useful but safety, efficacy remain uncertain. *JAMA.* 1996;276:1011–1014.
10. Kayumov L, Brown G, Jindal R, et al. A randomized, double-blind, placebo-controlled crossover study of the effect of exogenous melatonin on delayed sleep phase syndrome. *Psychosom Med.* 2001;63:40–48.
11. Hughes RJ, Sack Rl, Lewy AJ. The role of melatonin and circadian phase in age-related sleep-maintenance insomnia: assessment in a clinical trial of melatonin replacement. *Sleep.* 1998;21:52–68.
12. Garfinkel D, Laudon M, Nof D, et al. Improvement of sleep quality in elderly people by controlled-release melatonin. *Lancet.* 1995;346:541–544.
13. Dahlitz M, Alvarez B, Vignau J, et al. Delayed sleep phase syndrome response to melatonin. *Lancet.* 1991;337:1121–1124.

14. Garfinkel D, Zisapel N, Wainstein J, et al. Facilitation of benzodiazepine discontinuation by melatonin: a new clinical approach. *Arch Intern Med.* 1999;159:2456–2460.

15. Spitzer RL, Terman M, Williams JB, et al. Jet lag: clinical features, validation of a new syndrome-specific scale, and lack of response to melatonin in a randomized, double-blind trial. *Am J Psychiatry.* 1999;156:1392–1396.

16. Suhner A, Schlagenhauf P, Hofer I, et al. Effectiveness and tolerability of melatonin and zolpidem for the alleviation of jet lag. *Aviat Space Environ Med.* 2001;72:638–646.

17. Comperatore CA, Lieberman HR, Kirby AW, et al. Melatonin efficacy in aviation missions requiring rapid deployment and night operations. *Aviat Space Environ Med.* 1996;67:520–524.

18. Petrie K, Dawson AG, Thompson L, et al. A double-blind trial of melatonin as a treatment for jet lag in international cabin crew. *Biol Psychiatry.* 1993;33:526–530.

19. Arent J, Aldous M, Marks V. Alleviation of jet lag by melatonin: preliminary results of controlled double blind trial. *Br Med J.* 1986;292:1170.

20. Jorgensen KM, Witting MD. Does exogenous melatonin improve day sleep or night alertness in emergency physicians working night shifts? *Ann Emerg Med.* 1998;31:699–704.

21. Jockovich M, Cosentino D, Cosentino L, et al. Effect of exogenous melatonin on mood and sleep efficiency in emergency medicine residents working night shifts. *Acad Emerg Med.* 2000;7:955–958.

22. Lissoni P, Tancini G, Barni S, et al. Treatment of cancer chemotherapy-induced toxicity with the pineal hormone melatonin. *Support Care Cancer.* 1997;5:126–129.

23. Lissoni P, Barni S, Ardizzoia A, et al. A randomized study with the pineal hormone melatonin versus supportive care alone in patients with brain metastases due to solid neoplasms. *Cancer.* 1994;73:699–701.

24. Lissoni P, Paolorossi F, Ardizzoia A, et al. A randomized study of chemotherapy with cisplatin plus etoposide versus chemoendocrine therapy with cisplatin, etoposide and the pineal hormone melatonin as a first-line treatment of advanced nonsmall cell lung cancer patients in a poor clinical state. *J Pineal Res.* 1997;23:15–19.

25. Lissoni P, Brivio F, Barni S, et al. Adjuvant therapy with the pineal hormone melatonin in patients with lymph node relapse due to malignant melanoma. *J Pineal Res.* 1996;21:239–242.

26. Lissoni P, Barni S, Mandala M, et al. Decreased toxicity and increased efficacy of cancer chemotherapy using the pineal hormone melatonin in metastatic solid tumor patients with poor clinical status. *Eur J Cancer.* 1999;35:1688–1692.

27. Lemus-Wilson A, Kelly PA, Blask DE. Melatonin blocks the stimulatory effects of prolactin on human breast cancer cell growth in culture. *Br J Cancer.* 1995;72:1435–1440.

28. Anisimov VN, Popovich IG, Zabezhinski MA. Melatonin and colon carcinogenesis: I. Inhibitory effect of melatonin on development of intestinal tumors induced by 1,2-dimethylhydrazine in rats. *Carcinogenesis.* 1997;18:1549–1553.

29. Panzer A, Lottering ML, Bianchi P, et al. Melatonin has no effect on the growth, morphology, or cell cycle of human breast cancer (MCF-7), cervical cancer (HeLa), osteosarcoma (MG-63), or lymphoblastoid (TK6) cells. *Cancer Lett.* 1998;122:17–23.

30. Papazisis KT, Kouretas D, Geromichalos GD, et al. Effects of melatonin on proliferation of cancer cell lines. *J Pineal Res.* 1998;25:211–218.

M

31. Holleman BJ, Chyka PA. Problems-assessment of acute melatonin overdose. *South Med J.* 1997;90:451–453.
32. de Lourdes M, Seabra V, Bignotto M, et al. Randomized, double-blind clinical trial, controlled with placebo, of the toxicology of chronic melatonin treatment. *J Pineal Res.* 2000;29:193–200.
33. Guardiola-Lemaitre B. Toxicology of melatonin. *J Biol Rhythms.* 1997;12:697–706.
34. Graw P, Werth E, Krauchi K, et al. Early morning melatonin administration impairs psychomotor vigilance. *Behav Brain Res.* 2001;121:167–172.
35. Nagtegaal E, Smits M, Swart W, et al. Melatonin secretion and coronary heart disease. *Lancet.* 1995;346:1299.

Methylsulfonylmethane (MSM)

Methylsulfonylmethane or MSM, is a naturally occurring sulfur-containing compound found in the body. It is an odorless, water-soluble derivative of dimethylsulfoxide (DMSO). DMSO was first used as an industrial solvent in paint thinners and antifreeze. Later, it was used in veterinary medicine and approved for human use for arthritis. DMSO is currently available in health food stores as a topical ointment for arthritis and as a prescription drug for intravesicular instillation for interstitial cystitis. Clinical trials in the 1960s and 1970s reported that topical DMSO has an analgesic effect in patients with osteoarthritis, rheumatoid arthritis, gout, and soft tissue conditions, although not all studies demonstrate benefits. In addition, some uncomfortable side-effects such as odor and garlic taste in the mouth are associated with DMSO. Because MSM is a metabolic product of DMSO and is odorless, it has been hypothesized that it might have the same beneficial effects on arthritis and other inflammatory diseases. Despite the numerous websites, *The Miracle MSM* book, and anecdotal data that support use of MSM, there is a lack of research to substantiate these claims (1, 2).

Media and Marketing Claims	Efficacy
Relieves arthritis	NR
Decreases allergy symptoms	NR
Improves asthma symptoms	NR
Treats ulcers and heartburn	NR
Reduces muscular pain	NR

Advisory

- There are no studies evaluating the safety of MSM
- Some anecdotal reports of mild gastrointestinal discomfort

Drug/Supplement Interactions

No reported adverse interactions

KEY POINTS

- Only one double-blind, placebo-controlled study has been performed in humans. This study, conducted by a researcher who holds an MSM patent, reported significant improvements in arthritis symptoms with oral supplementation. Overall, much more research is needed to determine the efficacy and safety of this supplement.

- There are no clinical trials available to evaluate MSM's effect on allergies, asthma, gastrointestinal disorders, or muscular pain.

FOOD SOURCES

Small amounts of MSM in milk, fish, grains, and fruits and vegetables (1)

DOSAGE INFORMATION/BIOAVAILABILITY

MSM is sold in capsules or tablets (often with glucosamine) with some manufacturers recommending doses ranging from 500 mg to 8,000 mg daily. MSM is also available in topical creams. MSM is produced synthetically from DMSO.

RELEVANT RESEARCH

MSM and Arthritis

- In a double-blind, placebo-controlled study, 14 subjects with osteoarthritis were given 2,250 mg MSM or placebo daily for six weeks. Pain reduction was reported in 80 percent of the MSM patients compared to 18 percent in the placebo group. Sample size was too small to perform statistical analysis. This pilot study was reported only as an abstract, and is included here because it has been cited in testimonials for MSM supplements(3).

SAFETY

- There are no studies evaluating the safety of MSM supplements. One controlled trial reported no adverse effects with 2,250 mg daily for six weeks.

- There are some anecdotal reports that MSM may cause mild gastrointestinal discomfort.

REFERENCES

1. Kolasinski SL. Dimethylsulfoxide (DMSO) and methysulfonylmethane (MSM) for the treatment of arthritis. *Alternative Medicine Alert*; 2000:115–119.
2. John H, Laudahn G. Clinical experiences with the topical application of DMSO in orthopedic diseases: evaluation of 4180 cases. *Annals N Y Acad Sci.* 1967;141:506–516.

3. Lawrence RM, Methylsulfonylmethane: a double-blind study of its use in degenerative arthritis. *Int J Anti-Aging Med.* 1998;1:50.

Minerals

See Boron, Calcium, Chromium, Magnesium, Potassium, Selenium, Vanadium (Vanadyl Sulfate), *and* Zinc.

N-Acetylcysteine (NAC)

N-acetylcysteine (NAC) is derivative of the sulfur containing amino acid cysteine. First introduced as a mucolytic drug in the 1960s, NAC has also been used successfully as an antidote for acetaminophen toxicity (1). In the body, NAC is a precursor of reduced glutathione (GSH), an endogenous antioxidant. Because NAC has demonstrated antioxidant activity *in vitro* and can be converted into the antioxidant glutathione, it has been proposed to be beneficial in treating conditions such as acute and chronic bronchitis, acute respiratory distress syndrome, HIV infection, and some cardiovascular diseases (2–5).

Media And Marketing Claims	Efficacy
Prevents and treats flu	?↑
Reduces symptoms related to HIV	?↑
Prevents free-radical damage from exercise	NR

Advisory

Mild side-effects include nausea and skin rash

Drug/Supplement Interactions

- NAC decreases toxicity of acetominophen overdose
- Intravenous NAC along with nitroglycerin has been associated with hypotension in cardiac patients

KEY POINTS

- Although NAC has been used in Europe to treat bronchitis, acute respiratory distress disease, and other lung diseases (4), there is only recent preliminary evidence that NAC may reduce symptoms related to the influenza virus in elderly subjects. Additional studies are needed to confirm this use.

- Studies in HIV-positive patients suggest that NAC can raise glutathione levels, improve parameters of immune function, and in one open trial, NAC increased survival.

Controlled clinical trials are needed in this population to further determine effects on survival.

- There is currently a lack of well-controlled clinical trials demonstrating that oral NAC supplementation in humans has a favorable effect on exercise performance by reducing oxidative damage or enhancing immunity.

FOOD SOURCES

NAC is a form of cysteine found in animal proteins (eggs, dairy, meat/poultry/fish) and soybeans (6).

Food	Cysteine (mg/Serving)*
Chicken, roasted, skinless and boneless (½ breast)	318.2
Soybeans, green, (1 c)	203.4
Beef, lean (3 oz)	190.4
Egg (1 large)	144.5
Peanut butter (2 tbsp)	116.8
Milk, whole (1 c)	73.2
Cheese, cheddar (1½ oz)	53.2

Serving sizes calculated from values from Reference 7.

DOSAGE INFORMATION/BIOAVAILABILITY

There is no RDA for NAC. NAC is sold in tablets providing doses of 200 mg to 600 mg. Most manufacturers suggest taking 1,200 mg to 2,400 mg per day with food.

RELEVANT RESEARCH

NAC and Influenza Virus and Bronchitis

- Several European studies since 1980 have reported that prophylactic treatment with NAC (600 mg/day) may reduce the duration—and in some trials, the incidence—of chronic bronchitis (8–13).

- A meta-analysis of NAC used in bronchopulmonary disease was conducted in studies from 1980 through 1995. Of 21 trials reviewed, eight double-blind, placebo-controlled studies lasting from two to six months were selected for analysis. NAC dosages varied from 400 mg (one study), 600 mg (five studies), 1,200 mg (one study), and 600 mg three times per week (one study). The primary endpoint was the incidence of acute exacerbations in seven of eight trials and clinical assessment in the other. The results showed that NAC therapy had a significant effect compared to a placebo. The authors concluded that oral NAC may prevent acute exacerbations of chronic bronchitis and thus may decrease morbidity and health care costs (14)

- In a randomized, double-blind multicenter study in Italy, 262 subjects (mainly aged > 65 years, 62 percent with nonrespiratory chronic degenerative diseases such as cardiovascular disease, arthritis, and diabetes) were randomized to receive effervescent tablets of 1,200 mg NAC divided into two doses or a placebo daily for six months. Subjects' self-reported signs and symptoms of influenza-like episodes were assessed based on the presence of two or more of the following: fever; asthenia; anorexia; headache; myalgia/arthralgia; sore throat; rhinitis; cough, and catarrh. At monthly intervals, clinicians evaluated patients' symptom diaries and performed a complete medical examination. Patients were instructed to call clinicians soon after the onset of any sign or symptom, at which time additional clinical examinations were performed as needed. The NAC-supplemented subjects experienced a statistically significant decrease in influenza-like episodes, severity of condition, and length of time confined to bed as compared to the placebo group. Additionally, local and systemic symptoms were significantly reduced in the NAC group. Although NAC supplementation did not prevent subclinical influenza infection as assessed by antibody response to the A/H_1N_1 Singapore 6/86 virus, only 25 percent of the virus-infected NAC group developed a symptomatic form vs 79 percent in the placebo group; the difference between treatments was significant (4).

NAC and HIV

- Because AIDS patients typically have decreased levels of glutathione in their lymphocytes and plasma, some researchers have suggested that NAC may benefit AIDS patients by increasing intracellular levels of glutathione, thereby potentially suppressing HIV replication (15). Although clinical studies have shown that low GSH levels are associated with poor survival in HIV-infected subjects (15), the effectiveness of NAC supplementation has not been confirmed.

- Daily NAC supplementation (3,200 mg to 8,000 mg) during an eight-week randomized, double-blind, placebo-controlled trial restored blood GSH levels in subjects with CD4 counts < 200 compared to a placebo. After this phase, the majority of subjects in both arms of the study were offered NAC for a six-month open-label phase. Survival was evaluated two years after initiation of NAC. During the two-year period NAC-supplemented subjects (n = 25) with a CD4 < 200 survived significantly longer than a comparable group of non-NAC supplemented subjects (n = 19). Despite this finding, the authors emphasized that "no conclusion can be drawn until NAC is administered in a properly controlled prospective clinical trial with survival as a primary endpoint." The authors also stated that if GSH deficiency is indeed a key determinant of survival in HIV-related disease, infected individuals should avoid drugs known to deplete GSH (eg, alcohol and acetaminophen) (15).

- In a double blind, placebo-controlled trial, 81 HIV-positive patients (low GSH, CD4 T cells < 500 micro/L, and no opportunistic infections) were randomized to receive 8,000 mg NAC in effervescent tablets dissolved in water each day for eight weeks. The trial was followed by an optional open label drug for up to 24 weeks. Blood GSH levels and T-cell GSH levels significantly increased in NAC supplemented subjects to normal levels. Baseline GSH levels in the placebo group did not change during the study. NAC was well tolerated during the eight-month study. The authors suggested that since NAC appeared to increase protection against oxidative stress and enhanced the immune system, that NAC therapy could be valuable in other conditions of GSH deficiency or oxidative stress such as rheumatoid arthritis, Parkinson's disease, hepatitis, liver cirrhosis, septic shock, and diabetes. In addition, they advised HIV-infected individuals to avoid drugs and activities that further deplete GSH such as ultraviolet light, alcohol, acetaminophen and other drugs that are toxic to GSH levels (16).

- In a double-blind, placebo-controlled trial, 40 HIV patients on antiretroviral therapy and 29 patients not on antiretroviral drugs were randomized to receive NAC (dose individually adjusted dependent on plasma glutamine levels) or a placebo daily for seven months. Immunological parameters (natural killer cell, T-cell functions and the viral load) were the main outcome measures. NAC-supplemented subjects had a significant increase in immunological functions and plasma albumin concentrations. NAC had an inconsistent effect on the viral load, which the authors noted requires further study. The authors hypothesized that the impairment of immune function in HIV-positive patients results at least partly from cysteine deficiency which can be replenished by NAC supplementation. They concluded: "Because immune reconstitution is a major goal of HIV therapy, the consistent improvement in several immunological functions in our two randomized studies on NAC strongly suggests that HIV-infected patients with or without antiretroviral therapy should receive NAC treatment" (17).

- In a double-blind, placebo-controlled trial, 45 HIV patients not on retroviral drugs were randomized to receive 400 mg NAC twice daily or a placebo for four months. Before the study, subjects had low plasma cysteine levels, high free-radical activity in neutrophils, and increased tumor necrosis factor-α (TNF). After treatment, plasma cysteine levels increased to normal and the decline of the CD4+ lymphocyte count apparent prior to the study was less severe after NAC supplementation compared to placebo. The NAC group also significantly reduced TNF-α levels. However, NAC had no effect on free-radical production by neutrophils (18).

- In a double-blind, controlled study, 238 HIV-positive patients were randomized to receive 3 g NAC or no treatment one hour before each dose of the antibiotic trimethoprim-sulfamethoxazole (TMP-SMX) twice daily. TMP-SMX was initiated as primary *Pneumocystis carinii* pneumonia prophylaxis. It was hypothesized that adverse reactions to TMP-SMX observed in HIV-positive individuals may be due to systemic glutathione deficiency that may be ameliorated by NAC supplementation. Within two months, 45 patients had to discontinue TMP-SMX because of fever, rash, or pruritis. NAC had no effect on hypersensitivity reaction to the antibiotic (19).

- One *in vitro* study tested the effects of NAC on the cytotoxicity of neutrophils and mononuclear cells from HIV-infected and healthy subjects. NAC enhanced various forms of cytotoxicity and "may be beneficial to AIDS patients whose defects in leukocyte cytotoxicity may be due to glutathione depletion." However, the authors did note

N

that at very high concentrations (far exceeding what could be achieved *in vivo*) the cytotoxic response of neutrophils was inhibited (20).

- In an *in vitro* study, NAC increased HIV-1 gene expression in macrophages. The authors note that *in vivo*, macrophages are a reservoir for HIV-1 and have been implicated in the neurological complication that affects one-third of AIDS patients. The authors conclude that "NAC treatment of AIDS patients might increase the viral burden in the brain and therefore worsen the prognosis of neurological complications" (21). However, the negative effects of NAC noted in this *in vitro* study have not been reported *in vivo*.

- An *in vitro* study tested the effects of NAC or zinc on murine bone marrow progenitor cells exposed to zidovudine (AZT). Both NAC and zinc significantly protected the cells from AZT-induced toxicity (22).

NAC and Exercise

- In a double-blind, placebo-controlled study, 14 oarsmen were randomized to receive 6 g NAC or a placebo daily for three days prior to performing a six-minute "all-out" ergometer rowing trial. NAC did not attenuate the reduction in lymphocyte proliferation and natural killer cell activity associated with intense exercise, nor did it affect levels of lymphocyte subsets (CD4+, CD8+, CD16+, CD19+ cells) as compared to the placebo (23).

- Other research has reported that NAC may reduce oxidative stress and muscle fatigue. However, one study was uncontrolled (24) and the other study was not applicable to supplementation because NAC was administered intravenously during exercise (25).

SAFETY

- NAC has been used for three decades with few side-effects (mild side-effects include nausea and skin rash). No adverse effects were reported in HIV-positive patients supplemented with 6,000 mg to 8,000 mg NAC/day for one year.

- One case of anaphylactic reaction with angioedema following oral administration of NAC (70 mg/kg every four hours) for acetaminophen poisoning was reported (26).

REFERENCES

1. Smilkstein MJ, Gary MD, Knapp MS, et al. Efficacy of oral N-acetylcysteine in the treatment of acetaminophen over-dose. *J Med.* 1988;24:1557–1562.
2. Moldeus P, Cotgreave IA, Berggren M. Lung protection by thiol-containing antioxidant: N-acetylcysteine. *Respiration.* 1986;50:S31—S42.
3. Droge W, Gross A, Hack V, et al. Role of cysteine and glutathione in HIV infection and cancer cachexia: therapeutic intervention with N-acetylcysteine. *Adv Pharmacol.* 1997;38:581–600.

4. De Flora S, Grassi C, Carati L. Attenuation of influenza-like symptomatology and improvement of cell-mediated immunity with long-term N-acetylcysteine treatment. *Eur Respir J.* 1997;10:1535–1541.

5. Flanagan RJ, Meredith TJ. Use of N-acetylcysteine in clinical toxicology. *Am J Med.* 1991;91:131S–139S.

6. Linder MC, ed. *Nutritional Biochemistry and Metabolism.* 2nd ed. Norwalk, Conn: Appleton & Lange; 1991.

7. Stipanuk MH. Homocysteine, cysteine, and taurine. In Shils ME, Olson JA, Shike M, Ross AC (eds.). Modern Nutrition in Health and Disease, 9th ed. Philadelphia, PA: Lea & Febiger; 1999:543–559.

8. Multicenter Study Group. Long-term acetylcysteine in chronic bronchitis: a double-blind, controlled study. *Eur J Respir Dis.* 1980;61:93–108.

9. Boman G, Backer U, Larsson S, et al. Oral acetylcysteine reduces exacerbation rate in chronic bronchitis: a report of a trial organized by the Swedish Society for Pulmonary Diseases. *Eur J Respir Dis.* 1983;64:404–415.

10. Rasmussen JB, Glennow G. Reduction in days of illness after long-term treatment with N-acetylcysteine controlled release tablets in patients with chronic bronchitis. *Eur J Respir Dis.* 1988;1:351–355.

11. British Thoracic Society Research Committee. Oral N-acetylcysteine and exacerbation rate in patients with chronic bronchitis and severe airways obstruction. *Thorax.* 1985;40:832–835.

12. Parr DG, Huitson A. Oral N-acetylcysteine in chronic bronchitis. *Br J Dis Chest.* 1987;81:341–348.

13. Riise BT, Larsson S, Larsson P, et al. The intrabronchial microbial flora in chronic bronchitis patients: a target for N-acetylcysteine therapy? *Eur Respir J.* 1994;7:94–101.

14. Grandjean EM, Berthet P, Ruffman R, et al. Efficacy of oral long-term N-acetylcysteine in chronic bronchopulmonary disease: a meta-analysis of published double-blind, placebo-controlled clinical trials. *Clin Ther.* 2000;22:209–221.

15. Herzenberg LA, De Rosa SC, Dubs JG, et al. Glutathione deficiency is associated with impaired survival in HIV disease. *Proc Natl Acad Sci USA.* 1997;94:1967–1972.

16. De Rosa SC, Zaretsky MD, Dubs JG, et al. N-acetylcysteine replenishes glutathione in HIV infection. *Eur J Clin Invest.* 2000;30:915–929.

17. Breitkreutz R, Pittack N, Nebe CT, et al. Improvement of immune functions in HIV infection by sulfur supplementation: two randomized trials. *J Mol Med.* 2000;78:55–62.

18. Akerlund B, Jarstrand C, Lindeke B, et al. Effect of N-acetylcysteine (NAC) treatment on HIV-1 infection: a double-blind placebo-controlled trial. *Eur J Clin Pharmacol.* 1996;50:457–461.

19. Walmsley SL, Khorasheh S, Singer J, et al. A randomized trial of N-acetylcysteine for prevention of trimethorprim-sulfamethoaxazole hypersensitivity reactions in *Pneumocystis carinii* pneumonia prophylaxis (CTN 057). Canadian HIV Trials Network 057 Study Group. *J Acquir Immune Defic Syndr Hum Retrovirol.* 1998;19:498–505.

20. Roberts RL, Aroda VR, Ank BJ. N-Acetylcysteine enhances antibody-dependent cellular cytotoxicity in neutrophils and mononuclear cells from healthy adults and human immunodeficiency virus-infected patients. *J Infect Dis.* 1995;172:1492–1502.

N

21. Nottet H, Moelans II, de Vos NM, et al. N-acetyl-L-cysteine-induced up-regulation of HIV-1 gene expression in monocyte-derived macrophages correlates with increased NF-KB DNA binding activity. *J Leukoc Biol.* 1997;61:33–39.

22. Gogu SR, Agrawal KC. The protective role of zinc and N-acetylcysteine in modulating zidovudine induced hematopoietic toxicity. *Life Sci.* 1996;59:1323–1329.

23. Nielsen HB, Secher NH, Kappel M, et al. N-acetylcysteine does not affect the lymphocyte proliferation and natural killer cell activity responses to exercise. *Am J Physiol.* 1998;275:R1227—R1231.

24. Sen CK, Rankinen T, Vaisanen S, et al. Oxidative stress after human exercise: effect of N-acetylcysteine supplementation. *J Appl Physiol.* 1994;76:2570–2577.

25. Reid MB, Stokic DS, Koch SM, et al. N-acetylcysteine inhibits muscle fatigue in humans. *J Clin Invest.* 1994;94:2468–2474.

26. Mroz LS, Benitez JG, Krenzelok EP. Angiodema with oral N-acetylcysteine. *Ann Emerg Med.* 1997;30:240–241.

Niacin

See Vitamin B$_3$ (Niacin).

Noni Juice

Noni juice is a liquid supplement made from the fruit of the noni plant (*Morinda citrifolia*) found in Polynesia, China, and India. The juice is available through local noni distributors who are part of a multilevel marketing firm. Noni juice advertisements and marketing literature feature endorsements by physicians and testimonials that the juice can heal a variety of health conditions. Noni is a relatively new supplement, only available in the United States since 1996.

Media and Marketing Claims	Efficacy
Prevents cancer	NR
Relieves arthritis pain	NR
Improves immunity, especially in autoimmune disorders	NR
Normalizes cholesterol level	NR
Regulates sleep	NR
Improves digestion	NR

Advisory

High potassium content of noni juice could cause hyperkalemia in patients with kidney disease

Drug/Supplement Interactions

No reported adverse interactions

KEY POINTS

- Preliminary experimental and animal studies suggest that a polysaccharide in the noni fruit may exert some anticancer activity. However, there is no research in humans at this time to substantiate these results. Further, the quantity of this polysaccharide needed and whether it is bioavailable when given in the form of noni juice are not known.

- There are currently no published clinical trials available to support the use of noni juice to treat or prevent any health condition.

FOOD SOURCES

None

DOSAGE INFORMATION/BIOAVAILABILITY

Noni juice is sold in bottles prepared from ripened Tahitian noni fruit. The juice is extracted from the mashed fruit and bottled for use. A typical serving is 8 ounces. Not all noni juices are pasteurized. There is no scientific data on the purported active ingredients; thus, bioavailability is not known.

RELEVANT RESEARCH

- In an animal study, a polysaccharide isolated from noni juice was found to enhance the survival of mice having Lewis lung cancer. Noni juice extract stimulated the release of tumor necrosis factor-alpha, interleukin-1beta (IL-1beta), IL-10, IL-12 p70, interferon-gamma (IFN-gamma) and nitric oxide, but had no effect on IL-2 and suppressed IL-4 release. The polysaccharide also improved survival time when combined with suboptimal doses of standard chemotherapeutic drugs (1).

- In an *in vitro* study, two isolated glycosides from the noni fruit inhibited cancer cells in the mouse epidermal JB6 cell line (2).

SAFETY

- Noni juice is a significant source of potassium similar to the amount in orange juice. There is one report of a man with renal insufficiency who presented with hyperkalemia after self-medicating with noni juice (3).

REFERENCES

1. Hirazumi A, Furusawa E. An immunomodulatory polysaccharide-rich substance from the fruit juice of Morinda citrifolia (noni) with antitumor activity. *Phytother Res.* 1999; 13:380–387.
2. Liu G, Bode A, Ma WY, et al. Two novel glycosides from the fruits of Morinda citrifolia (noni) inhibit AP-1 transactivation and cell transformation in the mouse epidermal JB6 cell line. *Cancer Res.* 2001;61:5749–5756.
3. Mueller BA, Scott MK, Sowinski KM, et al. Noni juice (*Morinda citrifolia*): a hidden potential for hyperkalemia? *Am J Kidney Dis.* 2000;35:330–332.

Pancreatin

The pancreas secretes enzymes (pancreatin) into the gastrointestinal tract to aid digestion. Pancreatin contains three classes of enzymes: (1) amylases, which hydrolyze starch molecules into sugars; (2) lipases, which hydrolyze fat molecules (insufficient lipase causes steatorrhea); and (3) proteases (chymotrypsin, trypsin, and carboxypeptidase), which digest protein into amino acids. Oral supplementation of pancreatin is an established medical treatment for such diseases as chronic pancreatitis, cystic fibrosis, and pancreatic cancer. Less frequently, pancreatic enzymes have been prescribed for celiac disease, inflammatory bowel disease, primary biliary cirrhosis, total gastrectomy, and dyspepsia (1, 2).

Media and Marketing Claims	Efficacy
Helps control digestive disorders	?↑
Supports healthy digestion and absorption	NR
Enhances the immune system	NR

Advisory

Not known whether long-term use inhibits endogenous enzyme production in healthy people

Drug/Supplement Interactions

May decrease effectiveness of diabetes medication acarbose (Precose)

KEY POINTS

- Pancreatic enzymes are effective in the treatment of documented gastrointestinal disorders if there is clinical evidence of pancreatic insufficiency (chronic pancreatitis). Pancreatic function may be impaired in nonpancreatic digestive disorders including inflammatory bowel disease, celiac disease, malabsorption conditions, hepatobiliary disease, gastrectomy, and dyspepsia. The few studies on enzyme treatment for "nonpancreatic" disorders suggest that short-term pancreatin administration does not appear to benefit subjects with dyspepsia but may have some application in young children with celiac disease. Further, controlled trials are needed to elucidate the effects and determine dosage of supplemental enzymes in subjects with these intestinal disorders.

- At the current time, there is no evidence available suggesting that the digestion process is enhanced by exogenous enzyme supplementation in healthy subjects. Controlled clinical research is needed to determine whether supplemental enzymes enhance digestion in healthy individuals and whether their long-term use is safe.

- There is little research available to evaluate the marketing claim that exogenous pancreatic enzymes improve immunity. There is preliminary evidence from *in vitro* studies that pancreatin in combination with other proteolytic enzymes is cytotoxic to tumor cells; however, no controlled clinical trials have tested this effect. (*See also* Bromelain.)

FOOD SOURCES

None (pancreatic enzymes from meat products are destroyed by cooking). Pancreatic enzymes are produced endogenously.

DOSAGE INFORMATION/BIOAVAILABILITY

Pancreatic enzymes derived from the bovine and porcine pancreas are available in tablets and capsules. The United States Pharmacopoeia (USP) has set standards for the level of activity of pancreatin. Each milligram must have a minimum of 25 USP units of amylase, 2 USP units of lipase, and 25 USP units of protease activity. One USP standard is referred to as pancreatin $1 \times$ (500 mg) which provides 12,500 USP units amylase activity, 1,000 USP units of lipase activity, and 12,500 USP units of protease activity. Many commercial products are sold as four times USP standard or pancreatin $4 \times$ USP (50,000 USP units amylase activity, 4,000 USP units lipase activity, and 50,000 USP units protease) equivalent to 2,000 mg. Pancreatin is also available as $10 \times$ USP or 5,000 mg. To prevent inactivation of enzymes by gastric acid, many preparations are enteric-coated. The activity of individual preparations depends on a variety of factors, including pH of gastrointestinal secretions, the intestinal location where the enteric-coated enzyme disintegrates (gastric acid destroys enzymes), and whether the enzyme is consumed with food (3, 4). In patients with pancreatic insufficiency, pancreatin is taken with meals to enhance effectiveness (2).

RELEVANT RESEARCH

Pancreatin and Gastrointestinal Disorders

- In a single-blind, placebo-controlled, crossover design study, 37 patients with nonulcer dyspepsia took a placebo or 30,000 mg pancreatin (units not specified) divided into three doses daily for 24 days each. All subjects underwent endoscopy prior to the study that revealed no significant clinical differences between subjects. Subjects recorded their global dyspeptic complaints on a visual analogue scale each day of the trial. There were no differences in gastrointestinal symptoms (abdominal pain, nausea, heartburn, stool abnormalities, early satiety) between treatments (5).

- In a double-blind, placebo-controlled study, 40 pediatric patients (mean age = 14.5 months) diagnosed with celiac disease were randomly assigned to receive the contents of two capsules of pancreatic enzymes with every meal (1 capsule = 5,000 IU lipase, 2,900 IU amylase, 330 IU protease) or a placebo for 60 days. On the day of diagnosis, day 30, and day 60 after beginning isocaloric gluten-free diets, a series of anthropometric measures were taken. After 30 days, subjects administered pancreatin had significantly greater weight gain, weight-for-age, weight-for-height, height Z score (observed height–mean height for sex and age ÷ standard deviation for sex and age), arm circumference, and subscapular and tricep fold measurements compared to the placebo group. After 60 days, there were no differences between groups. The authors concluded that pancreatic enzyme therapy appeared to be useful in improving anthropometric measures in young children with celiac disease in the first 30 days after diagnosis, with apparent attenuation of the benefits thereafter (6).

Pancreatin and Immunity

- A review article hypothesized the potential beneficial role of pancreatic enzymes in immune complex diseases (AIDS, rheumatoid arthritis, multiple sclerosis, Crohn's disease, ulcerative colitis). The authors suggested that enzyme supplementation removes tissue-bound immune complexes, thereby enhancing immune function (increased macrophage and NK cell activity), which may be beneficial to HIV-positive patients (7). However, no controlled clinical trials have adequately tested this hypothesis.

- *See* Bromelain for additional studies of combination enzyme supplements that include pancreatin.

SAFETY

- The effects of long-term use of exogenous enzymes by healthy subjects is unknown, including the theoretical possibility that it permanently reduces the ability of the digestive system to secrete endogenous enzymes. In one study, pancreatic enzymes acutely administered to healthy subjects reduced postprandial endogenous pancreatic secretion; however, there were no reported acute adverse effects on bile acid secretion, gastroduodenal motility, or gastrointestinal hormone release (8).

- Individuals with hypersensitivity to pork may react unfavorably to pancreatic extracts of porcine origin (3).

- Pancreatic extracts form insoluble complexes with folic acid, which may impair folate absorption (3).

- Dietary fiber may interfere with the activity of enzymes *in vitro* and *in vivo* (9). One review article stated that pancreatic enzymes should not be coingested with high-fiber meals (3).

REFERENCES

1. Gullo L. Indication for pancreatic enzyme treatment in non-pancreatic digestive diseases. *Digestion.* 1993;54(suppl):43–47.
2. Raimondo M, Dimagno EP. Nutrition in Pancreatic Disorders. In: Shils ME, Olson JA, Shike M, eds. *Modern Nutrition in Health and Disease.* 9th ed. Philadelphia, Pa: Lea & Febiger; 1999:1169–1176.
3. Lankisch PG. Enzyme treatment of exocrine pancreatic insufficiency in chronic pancreatitis. *Digestion.* 1993;54(suppl):21–29.
4. Guarner L, Rodriguez R, Guarner F, et al. Fate of oral enzymes in pancreatic insufficiency. *Gut.* 1993;34:708–709.
5. Kleveland PM, Johannessen T, Kristensen P, et al. Effect of pancreatic enzymes in non-ulcer dyspepsia. A pilot study. *Scand J Gastroenterol.* 1990;25:298–301.
6. Carroccio A, Iacono G, Montalto G, et al. Pancreatic enzyme therapy in childhood celiac disease. *Dig Dis Sci.* 1995;40:2555–2560.
7. Stauder G, Ransberger K, Steichhan P, et al. The use of hydrolytic enzymes as adjuvant therapy in AIDS/ARC/LAS patients. *Biomed Pharmacother.* 1988;42:31–34.
8. Dominguez-Munoz JE, Birckelbach U, Glasbrenner B, et al. Effect of oral pancreatic enzyme administration on digestive function in healthy subjects: comparison between two enzyme preparations. *Ailment Pharmacol Ther.* 1997;11:403–408.
9. Leng-Peschlow E. Interference of dietary fibres with gastrointestinal enzymes in vitro. *Digestion.* 1989;44:200–210.

Pantothenic Acid

Pantothenic acid (pantethine) is an essential water-soluble B vitamin. It is physiologically active as part of two coenzymes: acetyl coenzyme A (CoA) and acyl carrier protein. Pantothenic acid functions in the oxidation of fatty acids and carbohydrates for energy production and the synthesis of fatty acids, ketones, cholesterol, phospholipids, steroid hormones, and amino acids. Because pantothenic acid is widely distributed in foods, a deficiency is extremely rare. Depletion studies have shown that deficiency is associated with fatigue and depression in humans and dysfunction in adrenal cortex, nervous system, and respiratory function in animals (1).

Media and Marketing Claims	Efficacy
Lowers cholesterol	NR
Increases energy and improves sports performance	↓
Improves for rheumatoid arthritis	NR
Reduces stress	NR

Advisory

- No reported serious adverse effects
- No Tolerable Upper Intake Level (UL) has been set

P

Drug/Supplement Interactions

No reported adverse interactions

KEY POINTS

- There is a lack of well-controlled studies testing the effects of pantothenic acid in cholesterol reduction. Much more research is needed to verify the cholesterol-lowering claims, which are apparently based on poorly controlled studies.

- The limited research on pantothenic acid/pantethine does not suggest an ergogenic benefit during exercise with supplementation.

- Much more research is needed to determine the potential role of pantothenic acid supplements in treating rheumatoid arthritis.

- Although pantothenic acid has been referred to as the "antistress" vitamin by supplement marketers because of its central role in adrenal cortex function and cellular metabolism, there is currently no evidence from controlled studies to suggest that pantothenic acid reduces feelings of stress or anxiety.

FOOD SOURCES

Pantothenic is found in most plant and animal foods. Good sources are found in liver, egg yolk, fresh vegetables, legumes, yeast, and whole grains. The average American diet provides approximately 5.8 mg pantothenic acid daily. Pantothenic acid is stable at a neutral pH. It has been estimated that 15 percent to 20 percent of pantothenic acid in raw meat is destroyed by cooking and that 37 percent to 78 percent of the vitamin is lost in vegetables during processing (1).

Food	Pantothenic Acid (mg)
Mushrooms, (½ c)	1.68
Potato, baked with skin	1.12
Chicken breast (3.5 oz)	0.92
Egg (1)	0.70
Catfish (3 oz)	0.65
Lentils (½ c)	0.63
Beef, broiled, ground, lean (3.5 oz)	0.38
Rice, brown (½ c)	0.28

Source: Data from Pennington JAT (2)

DOSAGE INFORMATION/BIOAVAILABILITY

There is no RDA for pantothenic acid; however, the adequate intake (AI) is set at 5 mg/day for adult men and women (3). Pantothenic acid is available in multivitamin supplements and single preparations in doses ranging from the 5 mg to 500 mg in the form of calcium or sodium pantothenate or panthenol. Pantethine, a metabolite of pantothenic acid used in several studies, is also available in supplements. Information on pantothenic acid bioavailability in humans is limited (4). However, in one controlled study, the bioavailability of dietary pantothenate (5.8 mg/day) ranged from 40 percent to 61 percent in healthy men (5).

RELEVANT RESEARCH

Pantothenic Acid/Pantethine and Cholesterol

- In a double-blind, placebo-controlled crossover study, 29 patients (11 with type IIB hyperlipidemia, 15 with type IV, and 3 with isolated low HDL cholesterol levels) were given in random order 900 mg pantethine daily or a placebo for eight weeks each. In type IIB patients, pantethine significantly lowered plasma total and LDL cholesterol. In type IV patients, pantethine had a variable effect on LDL levels. In type IIB and type IV patients, plasma triglyceride levels were reduced when pantethine was given as the first treatment, but less so when the regime was preceded by the placebo. There was no change in HDL cholesterol in type IV or low HDL cholesterol patients (6).

- Four uncontrolled studies have tested the effect of pantethine supplements on blood lipids, but the results are unreliable because of the lack of proper controls and small sample size (7–10).

Pantothenic Acid/Pantethine and Exercise Performance

- In a double-blind, placebo-controlled study, six highly trained cyclists were randomized to receive 1.8 g of a pantethine/pantothenic acid compound plus 1 g allithiamin (an efficiently absorbed thiamin derivative) or a placebo for seven days prior to a 50-km ride on a cycle ergometer followed by a 2,000-m time trial. This protocol was completed on two separate occasions. There were no significant differences in measures of heart rate, respiratory gas exchange, ratings of perceived exertion, and blood lactate, glucose, and free fatty acids between groups. There were also no differences in time to complete the 2,000-m trial. The authors concluded that supplementation with allithiamin and pantethine does not alter exercise metabolism or exercise performance (11).

- In a double-blind, placebo-controlled study, 18 highly trained distance runners were given 1 g pantothenic acid or a placebo daily for two weeks. Subjects were instructed not to change their diets or training schedule. At the start and end of the study, each subject completed two treadmill runs to exhaustion separated by two weeks. There were no significant differences between groups in run time, pulse rate, blood cortisol, or blood glucose levels (12).

Pantothenic Acid and Arthritis

- In a double-blind, placebo-controlled trial, 94 patients with arthritis (27 with rheumatoid arthritis) were randomized to receive calcium pantothenate (titrated up from 500 mg for two days, 1,000 mg for three days, 1,500 mg for four days, and 2,000 mg for the remainder) or a placebo daily for two months. Patients were only permitted to take

P

paracetamol for pain. There were no significant reductions in either group in the duration of morning stiffness or disability. Both groups experienced significant relief of pain, although neither resulted in any reduction of paracetamol. Physician assessment did not differ between treatment groups. When rheumatoid arthritis subjects were analyzed separately, the group receiving pantothenate showed significant reductions in morning stiffness, disability, pain, but not paracetamol use. The placebo group had no changes. The authors did not speculate about why pantothenate appeared to benefit rheumatoid arthritis patients but not osteoarthritic subjects (13).

SAFETY

- High doses of calcium pantothenate are relatively nontoxic in rats, dogs, rabbits, and humans. The LD_{50} for mice was 10 g/kg body weight, which led to death from respiratory failure (1).

- The tolerable upper intake level (UL) for pantothenate has not been established.

REFERENCES

1. Plesofsky-Vig N. Pantothenic Acid. In: Shils ME, Olson JA, Shike M, Ross AC, eds. *Modern Nutrition in Health and Disease*. 9th ed. Philadelphia, Pa: Lea & Febiger; 1999:423–432.
2. Pennington JAT. *Bowes and Church's Food Values of Portions Commonly Used*. 17th ed. Philadelphia, Pa: Lippincott; 1998.
3. Institute of Medicine, Food and Nutrition Board. *Dietary Reference Intakes for Thiamin, Riboflavin, Niacin, Vitamin B-6, Folate, Vitamin B-12, Pantothenic Acid, Biotin, and Choline*. Washington, DC: National Academy Press; 1998.
4. van den Berg H. Bioavailability of pantothenic acid. *Eur J Clin Nutr*. 1997;51:S62-S63.
5. Tarr JB, Tamura T, Stokstad EL. Availability of vitamin B_6 and pantothenate in an average American diet in man. *Am J Clin Nutr*. 1981;34:1328–1337.
6. Gaddi A, Descovich GC, Noseda G, et al. Controlled evaluation of pantethine, a natural hypolipemic compound, in patients with different forms of hyperlipidemia. *Atherosclerosis*. 1984;50:73–83.
7. Coronel F, Torneo F, Torrente J, et al. Treatment of hyperlipidemia in diabetic patients on dialysis with a physiological substance. *Am J Nephrol*. 1991;11:32–36.
8. Eto M, Watanabe K, Chonan N, et al. Lowering effect of pantethine on plasma beta-thromboglobulin and lipids in diabetic mellitus. *Artery*. 1987;15:1–12.
9. Donati C, Barbi G, Cairo G, et al. Pantethine improves the lipid abnormalities of chronic hemodialysis patients: results of a multicenter trial. *Clin Nephrol*. 1986;25:70–74.
10. Bertolini S, Donati C, Elicio N, et al. Lipoprotein changes induced by pantethine in hyperlipoproteinemic patients: adults and children. *Int J Clin Pharmacol Ther Toxicol*. 1986;24:630–637.
11. Webster MJ. Physiological and performance responses to supplementation with thiamin and pantothenic acid derivatives. *Eur J Appl Physiol*. 1998;77:486–491.

12. Nice C, Reeves AG, Brinck-Johnsen T, et al. The effects of pantothenic acid on human exercise capacity. *J Sports Med Phys Fitness.* 1984;24:26–29.

13. General Practitioner Research Group. Calcium pantothenate in arthritic conditions. A report from the General Practitioner Research Group. *Practitioner.* 1980;224:208–211.

Phosphatidylserine

Phosphatidylserine (PS) is a naturally occurring phospholipid obtained from the brain cortex. PS is involved in neuronal membrane function and may influence membrane-mediated biological activities and receptor functions. It is believed to cause biochemical brain changes by acting on neurotransmitter systems (acetylcholine, norepinephrine, serotonin, dopamine) (1, 2). Because PS plays a role in the functioning of brain cells, some proponents have proposed administering oral PS to prevent or reverse age-related neurochemical deficits. Additionally, PS may also be involved in blunting corticotrophin (ACTH) and cortisol production associated with physical stress. Because elevated cortisol levels have a protein catabolic effect on skeletal muscle and have been associated with overtraining (3), proponents of PS supplementation have extrapolated applications for body builders.

Media and Marketing Claims	Efficacy
Improves age-related memory loss	?↑
Raises IQ	NR
Reduces the production of cortisol, inhibiting muscle breakdown	NR

Advisory

Potential for contamination in supplements derived from bovine cortex

Drug/Supplement Interactions

No reported adverse interactions

KEY POINTS

- Several studies suggest that phosphatidylserine (BC-PS) may improve learning and memory (recall of misplaced objects and numbers, face recognition) in older individuals with cognitive disorders.

- There is currently no evidence from controlled trials that phosphatidylserine raises IQ or improves recall of frequently misplaced objects and memory of numbers in healthy individuals with normal cognitive function.

- Limited research exists regarding the ability of BC-PS to blunt the physical stress response to exercise. More research is needed to determine whether PS is indeed beneficial to athletes.

P

FOOD SOURCES

Common foods have insignificant amounts of PS, although the total estimated daily intake is 80 mg/day (4).

DOSAGE INFORMATION/BIOAVAILABILITY

PS is sold in 100 mg to 400 mg tablets, capsules, powders, and chewing gum synthetically derived from soybean lecithin (SL-PS). Note that most studies have used PS derived from bovine cortex (BC-PS). Labels recommend taking doses ranging from 100 mg to 800 mg/day. Some products combine SL-PS with other phospholipids including lecithin and cephalin.

RELEVANT RESEARCH

PS and Cognitive Function in the Aging Population

- In a double-blind, placebo-controlled, multicenter study in Italy, 494 elderly subjects with moderate to severe cognitive impairment as determined by the Mini Mental State Examination and the Reisberg Global Deterioration scale were randomized to receive 300 mg BC-PS/day or a placebo for six months. Changes in behavior and cognitive performance were measured using the Plutchik Geriatric Rating Scale and the Buschke Selective Reminding Test at baseline, and at three and six months. Of the 494 patients enrolled, 425 (215 PS and 210 placebo-treated subjects) completed the six-month trial. Reasons for dropout included poor compliance, worsening of pre-existing conditions, and side-effects (dizziness in one PS subject and dizziness, itching, gastric distress, and psychomotor agitation in seven placebo subjects). After three and six months, PS significantly improved cognitive and behavioral parameters such as improvements in storage and retrieval during verbal learning, and a reduction in loss of motivation, initiative, interest in the environment, and socialization compared to the placebo. Clinical evaluation and laboratory tests demonstrated that PS was well-tolerated (2).

- In a double-blind, placebo-controlled study, 149 subjects with age-associated memory impairment were randomized to receive 200 mg BC-PS or a placebo for 12 weeks. Fourteen subjects did not complete the study, and these subjects were equally divided between treatments. The PS subjects improved significantly on performance tests related to learning and memory tasks of daily life such as face, name, object, and telephone number recognition and recall. Within PS supplemented subjects, those who had scored at a relatively low level before treatment were more likely to benefit from PS (5).

- In a double-blind, placebo-controlled study, 51 patients (mean age = 71 y) in the early stages of Alzheimer's disease were randomized to receive 300 mg BC-PS or a placebo daily for 12 weeks. Efficacy measures included a 12-item, clinical global improvement scale (CGI), a 25-item psychiatric rating scale completed by a study psychiatrist based on an extended interview with each patient, and the Memory Assessment Clinics Family Rating Scale. After 12 weeks, the PS group had significant improvements on 3 of the

12 CGI variables (ability to maintain concentration and two overall global items on the scale). On the psychiatric rating scale, PS-supplemented subjects significantly improved on 5 of 25 parameters related to memory impairment and ability to recall names and events compared to the placebo subjects. At 12 weeks, no differences between groups were apparent on ratings by family members. However, family members rated significant improvement with PS at weeks 6 and 9. The authors stressed that PS exerted a mild therapeutic effect, which may not be effective for middle- and late-stage Alzheimer's patients who have extensive neuronal damage (6).

- In a placebo-controlled study in Italy, 10 elderly women hospitalized for depressive disorders were given 15 days of a placebo (to obtain a complete washout from previous medications) followed by 30 days of 300 mg BC-PS/day. Changes in depression, memory, and general behavior were assessed before and after the placebo and after PS treatment using the Hamilton Rating Scale for Depression, Gottfries-Brane-Steen Rating Scale, Nurse's Observation Scale for Inpatient Evaluation, and Buschke Selective Reminding Test. Depressive symptoms were marked before treatment, did not change after the placebo, and were significantly reduced by PS treatment. PS treatment also resulted in a significant improvement in memory (recall, long-term retrieval) compared to the placebo. Biochemical blood tests did not suggest any possible mechanisms of action of PS in improving cognitive and psychological parameters (7). The results of this study should be viewed with caution because treatment was not randomized or blinded.

- Additional double-blind, placebo-controlled studies have shown that 300 mg of BC-PS improved cognitive function in patients with senile dementia, and Alzheimer's and Parkinson's disease (8–10).

PS and Physical Stress

- In a double-blind, placebo-controlled, crossover study, eight healthy men underwent three experiments with a bicycle ergometer. Just prior to exercise, within 10 minutes, each subject received intravenously 50 mg or 75 mg of intravenous PS (from bovine cortex) or placebo. Blood samples were taken 30 minutes prior to exercise and at 0, 7, 14, 21, 40, and 80 minutes after the start of exercise. The exercise protocol consisted of three bouts of 6 minutes each, using a progressive workload. There was a significant decrease in ACTH and cortisol for both the PS treatments, but not for the placebo. PS did not significantly affect plasma levels of growth hormone, prolactin, epinephrine, norepinephrine, glucose, or dopamine. The effect of PS on exercise performance was not tested (11).

- In a double-blind, placebo-controlled, crossover design study, the same exercise protocol was repeated using oral BC-PS instead of intravenous administration. Nine healthy men underwent three 10-day courses of treatment with a placebo, 200 mg BC-PS, or 400 mg BC-PS twice per day. BC-PS at 400 mg twice daily attenuated the exercise-induced ACTH and cortisol responses. The authors concluded "chronic administration of PS may counteract stress-induced activation of the hypothalamo-pituitary-adrenal axis in man" (12).

P

SAFETY

- Bovine-derived PS supplements are taken from the bovine cortex. Although there have been no adverse reports in studies using BC-PS, some researchers warned: "In terms of safety, the brain cortex is not a suitable material for food use, because some encephalopathies such as mad cow disease (bovine spongiform encephalopathy) or Kuru disease in humans are orally infectious through prior contaminated brain" (4) This concern led to the development of soybean-lecithin derived PS (SL-PS) supplements.

- To date, however, bovine-cortex derived phosphatidylserine (BC-PS) has been shown in numerous studies to be well tolerated for up to six months with no serious side-effects.

REFERENCES

1. Calderini G, Bellini F, Bonetti AC, et al. Pharmacological properties of phosphatidylserine in the aging brain. *Clin Trials J.* 1987;24:9–17.
2. Cenacchi T, Bertoldin T, Farina C, et al. Cognitive decline in the elderly: a double-blind, placebo controlled, multicenter study on efficacy of phosphatidylserine administration. *Aging (Milano).* 1993;5:123–133.
3. Urhausen A, Gabriel H, Kindermann W. Blood hormones as markers of training stress and overtraining. *Sports Med.* 1995;20:251–276.
4. Sakai M, Yamatoya H, Kudo S. Pharmacological effects of phosphatidylserine enzymatically synthesized from soybean lecithin on brain functions in rodents. *J Nutr Sci Vitaminol (Tokyo).* 1996;42:47–54.
5. Crook TH, Tinkleberg J, Yesavage J, et al. Effects of phosphatidylserine in age-associated memory impairment. *Neurology.* 1991;41:644–649.
6. Crook T, Petrie W, Wells C, et al. Effects of phosphatidylserine in Alzheimer's disease. *Psychopharmacol Bull.* 1992;28:61–66.
7. Maggioni M, Picotti GB, Bondiolotti GP, et al. Effects of phosphatidylserine therapy in geriatric patients with depressive disorders. *Acta Psychiatr Scand.* 1990;81:265–270.
8. Funfgeld EW, Baggen M, Nedwidek P, et al. Double-blind study with phosphatdiylserine (PS) in Parkinsonian patients with senile dementia of Alzheimer's type (SDAT). *Prog Clin Biol Res.* 1989;317:1235–1246.
9. Amaducci L. Phosphatidylserine in the treatment of Alzheimer's disease: results of a multicenter study. *Psychopharmacol Bull.* 1988;24:130–134.
10. Delwaide PJ, Gyselynck-Mambourg AM, Hurlet A, et al. Double-blind randomized controlled study of phophatidyserine in senile demented patients. *Acta Neurol Scand.* 1986;73:136–140.
11. Monteleone P, Beinat L, Tanzillo C, et al. Effects of phosphatidylserine on the neuroendocrine response to physical stress in humans. *Neuroendocrinology.* 1990;52:243–248.
12. Monteleone P, Maj M, Beinat L, et al. Blunting by chronic phosphatidylserine administration of the stress-induced activation of the hypothalamo-pituitary-adrenal axis in healthy men. *Eur J Clin Pharmacol.* 1992;41:385–388.

Potassium

Potassium, the most abundant intracellular cation, is one of the major minerals responsible for maintaining osmotic pressure in the intra- and extracellular environments. The steep potassium gradient from inside to outside cells, sustained by the sodium pump, creates the membrane potential and membrane charge found in every cell. Potassium is involved in the regulation of neuromuscular excitability and contraction, glycogen formation, protein synthesis, and correction of imbalances in acid-base metabolism. Excessive extracellular potassium levels (hyperkalemia) interfere with normal heart and nervous function and may be caused by acidosis and tissue damage (myocardial infarction or renal failure). Hypokalemia, although rare, may result from poor dietary intake, gastrointestinal losses due to diarrhea or laxative use, bulimia, advanced liver disease, or excessive renal losses due to diuretic therapy. Nondiuretic medications such as steroids, carbenoxolone, and digoxin, and excess natural licorice, also negatively affect potassium status (1, 2).

The role of potassium as it relates to blood pressure and high sodium diets has been investigated. Epidemiological studies have reported an inverse relationship between potassium intake and blood pressure in hypertensive patients (3).

Media and Marketing Claim	Efficacy
Lowers blood pressure	?↑

Advisory

- High dose potassium chloride prescriptions (6,000 mg to 12,000 mg KCL/day) have been associated with gastrointestinal lesions, hemorrhage, and obstruction mainly in patients with delayed intestinal transit time
- Could cause hyperkalemia in patients with kidney disease

Drug/Supplement Interactions

- Potential for hyperkalemic reaction when combined with ACE inhibitors (Capoten, Vasotec)
- Potential dangerous elevation in potassium levels when potassium supplements or salt substitutes containing potassium are combined with potassium-sparing diuretics

P

KEY POINTS

- There is suggestive evidence that potassium supplements result in small, but significant reductions in blood pressure, particularly among individuals with hypertension or those consuming diets low in potassium. However, there is also evidence from the DASH study that a diet rich in fruits, vegetables, and low-fat dairy foods, with reduced saturated and total fat (dietary potassium intake = 4,415 mg/day) is associated with substantial reductions in systolic and diastolic blood pressure.

- Diets high in sodium, processed foods, and low in fruits, vegetables, dairy, and whole grains may not provide enough potassium to meet minimum requirements. Some diuretic medications also cause potassium losses. Adjusting the diet to include more potassium-rich whole foods is preferable to over-the-counter potassium supplements. In addition, it is possible to achieve potassium intakes comparable to doses used in the blood pressure studies by increasing consumption of fruits, vegetables, low-fat dairy, and legumes (*see* Food Sources). Many potassium-rich foods are also excellent sources of many other beneficial nutrients such as fiber, phytochemicals, vitamins, and minerals that play a role in disease prevention.

- Because of potential serious adverse effects, potassium supplements should only be taken when prescribed by a physician.

FOOD SOURCES

Food	Potassium (mg)	Sodium (mg)
Figs (10)	1331	21
Beans, kidney (1 c)	713	4
Avocado (½ medium)	530	53
Molasses, blackstrap (1 tbsp)	498	11
Juice, orange (1 c)	473	2
Banana (1 medium)	451	1
Milk, nonfat (1 c)	406	126
Salmon (3 oz)	327	52
Sweet potato (½ c)	302	21
Mushrooms (½ c)	278	2
Chicken breast (½)	240	70
Sunflower seeds (1 oz)	139	1
Bread, whole wheat (1 slice)	71	148
Cheese, mozzarella (1 oz)	19	106

Note: Many processed foods are relatively high in sodium and low in potassium.
Source: Data from Pennington JAT (4)

DOSAGE INFORMATION/BIOAVAILABILITY

Potassium supplements are available in liquids, tablets, or capsules in the form of potassium gluconate, aspartate, citrate, or hydrochloride. Each dose provides no more than 99 mg per serving as mandated by the FDA because of potential dangers associated with self-dosing (*see* Safety). Potassium is also available in higher amounts by prescription. Commercial salt substitutes also contain considerable amounts of potassium (195 mg to 2,340 mg/1 teaspoon) (3). The estimated minimum requirement for healthy adults is 2,000 mg/day (5). The average U.S. dietary intake of potassium is approximately 2,500 mg/day (3).

RELEVANT RESEARCH

Potassium and Blood Pressure

- A meta-analysis report summarized the results of 33 randomized, clinical trials (a total of 2,609 subjects) examining potassium supplementation for hypertension. All trials included adult subjects ranging from ages 18 y to 79 y. Twenty trials included hypertensive subjects and 12 trials included normotensive subjects. Three of the studies were single-blind, and seven had no placebo control. The results from each study were pooled after weighting the results for individual studies by the inverse of its variance for blood pressure change. Potassium supplements were associated with a significant reduction in mean systolic and diastolic blood pressure (↓4.44 mm Hg, ↓2.45 mm Hg, respectively). After exclusion of a trial with extreme results, potassium supplementation was still associated with a significant reduction in systolic and diastolic blood pressure (↓3.11 mm Hg, ↓1.97 mm Hg, respectively). These effects appeared to be the greatest in studies where subjects had higher intakes of sodium (6).

- In a double-blind, placebo-controlled study, 300 normotensive women (mean age = 39 y) from the Nurses Health Study II whose reported intakes of potassium, calcium, and magnesium were between the 10th and 15th percentiles were randomized to receive one of five supplements for 16 weeks: (1) 40 mmol (1,564 mg) potassium; (2) 1,200 mg calcium; (3) 336 mg magnesium; (4) all three minerals together; or (5) a placebo. The mean differences among the treatment and placebo groups were significant for potassium supplements (−2.0 mm Hg systolic, −1.7 mm Hg diastolic). The administration of calcium and magnesium with potassium did not enhance the blood pressure-lowering effect of potassium alone (7).

- In a double-blind, placebo-controlled trial, 87 healthy African Americans (systolic pressure = 100 to 159, diastolic = 70 mm Hg to 94 mm Hg) were randomized to receive 80 mmol (3,127 mg) potassium or a placebo while following a low-potassium diet (32 mmol to 35 mmol/day) for 21 days. Nine blood pressure readings were taken during three visits during the trial. There were no differences in blood pressure between groups at the baseline. The potassium-supplemented group had significantly lower systolic (−6.9 mm Hg) and diastolic (−2.5 mm Hg) blood pressure compared to the placebo group (8).

- In a double-blind, placebo-controlled trial, 125 patients with untreated mild or borderline hypertension were randomly assigned to one of four treatments for six months: (1) 60 mmol (2,345 mg) potassium plus 1,000 mg calcium; (2) 60 mmol potassium plus 360 mg magnesium; (3) calcium plus magnesium; or (4) a placebo. Blood pressure measurements were taken at the baseline, and at three and six months of treatment. There were no significant differences in dietary intakes of potassium, calcium, or magnesium among groups during the study. The mean differences in changes in blood pressure between treatment and placebo groups were not significant. The authors concluded: "This trial provides little evidence of an important role of combinations of cation supplements in the treatment of mild or borderline hypertension" (9).

- In a double-blind, placebo-controlled, crossover study, 18 untreated elderly hypertensive patients with a systolic blood pressure > 160 and/or diastolic > 95 mm Hg received in random order 60 mmol (2,345 mg) potassium (potassium chloride) for four weeks and a placebo for four weeks. Dietary electrolyte intake was recorded during a four-week run-in period and during the study. After potassium supplementation, there was a significant drop in supine clinic blood pressure, standing, and 24-hour ambulatory systolic blood pressure compared to placebo phase. There was no effect in clinic standing diastolic blood pressure, 24-hour ambulatory diastolic blood pressure, or pulse rate. Plasma renin activity increased and body weight fell after potassium supplementation (10).

- A meta-analysis of 19 clinical trials from 1980 to 1989 (11 double-blind) involving 586 subjects (412 with essential hypertension) reported that oral potassium supplements significantly lowered systolic and diastolic blood pressure (–5.9 mm Hg and –3.4 mm Hg, respectively). Doses ranged from 40 mmol to 140 mmol (1,564 mg to 5,472 mg) potassium in studies lasting from 5 to 112 days. The magnitude of the blood pressure-lowering effect was greater in patients with high blood pressure and was more pronounced the longer the duration of supplementation. The authors concluded that an increase in potassium intake should be included in the recommendations for a non-pharmacological approach to the control of blood pressure in uncomplicated essential hypertension (11).

- In a randomized, multicenter trial (Dietary Approaches to Stop Hypertension, DASH), 459 subjects with systolic blood pressure < 160 mm Hg and diastolic blood pressures of 80 mm Hg to 95 mm Hg were randomized to one of three controlled diets for eight weeks: (1) control diet—low in fruits and vegetables and low-fat dairy, and a 37 percent fat diet typical of the average diet in the United States (average dietary potassium intake = 1,752 mg/day); (2) diet rich in fruits and vegetables (total dietary fat = 37 percent; average potassium intake = 4,101 mg/day); or (3) combination diet rich in fruits and vegetables and low-fat dairy products and with reduced saturated fat and total fat (total dietary fat = 25 percent; average potassium intake = 4,415 mg). Prior to the study, all subjects were fed control diets for three weeks. Sodium intake and body weight were maintained at constant levels. The combination diet resulted in a significant reduction in systolic (–5.0 mm Hg) and diastolic (–3.0 mm Hg) blood pressure compared to subjects on the control diet. The fruit and vegetable-rich diet resulted in a statistically significant reduction of systolic (–2.8 mm Hg) and diastolic (–1.1 mm Hg) blood pressure compared to the control diet. Among the 133 subjects with hypertension, the combination diet significantly reduced systolic and diastolic pressure by 11.4 and 5.5 mm Hg more, respectively, than the control diet. Subjects without hypertension also experienced significant reductions of systolic and diastolic blood pressure by 3.5 mm Hg and 2.1 mm Hg. The authors concluded that a diet rich in fruits, vegetables, and low-fat dairy foods and with reduced saturated and total fat can substantially lower blood pressure (12).

SAFETY

- High-dose potassium chloride prescriptions (6,000 mg to 12,000 mg KCl/day) have been associated with gastrointestinal lesions, hemorrhage, and obstruction, primarily in patients with delayed intestinal transit time (13).

- Potassium supplements when combined with angiotensin-converting enzyme inhibitors may cause hyperkalemia (14).

- Liberal use of potassium-containing salt-substitutes has caused hyperkalemia in patients with compromised cardiovascular or renal function who use diuretics (2).

REFERENCES

1. Oh MS. Water, electrolyte, and acid-base balance. In: Shils ME, Olson JA, Shike M, Ross AC, eds. *Modern Nutrition in Health and Disease.* 9th ed. Philadelphia, PA: Lea & Febiger; 1999:105–139.
2. Riccardella D, Dwyer J. Salt substitutes and medicinal potassium sources: risks and benefits. *J Am Diet Assoc.* 1985;85:471–474.
3. Tobian L. Dietary sodium chloride and potassium have effects on the pathophysiology of hypertension in humans and animals. *Am J Clin Nutr.* 1997;65:606S–611S.
4. Pennington JA. *Bowes and Church's Food Values of Portions Commonly Used.* 17th ed. Philadelphia, PA: Lippincott-Raven Publishers; 1998.
5. National Research Council, Subcommittee on the 10th Edition of the RDAs, Food and Nutrition Board, Commission on Life Sciences. *Recommended Dietary Allowances.* 10th ed. Washington, DC: National Academy Press; 1989.
6. Whelton PK, He J. Potassium in preventing and treating high blood pressure. *Semin Nephrol.* 1999;19:494–499.
7. Sacks FM, Willett WC, Smith A, et al. Effect on blood pressure of potassium, calcium, and magnesium in women with low habitual intake. *Hypertension.* 1998;31:131–138.
8. Brancati FL, Appel LJ, Seidler AJ, et al. Effect of potassium supplementation on blood pressure in African Americans on a low-potassium diet. A randomized, double-blind, placebo-controlled trial. *Arch Intern Med.* 1996;156:61–67.
9. Sacks FM, Brown LE, Appel L, et al. Combinations of potassium, calcium, and magnesium supplements in hypertension. *Hypertension.* 1995;26:950–956.
10. Fotherby MD, Potter JF. Potassium supplementation reduces clinic and ambulatory blood pressure in elderly hypertensive patients. *J Hypertens.* 1992;10:1403–1408.
11. Cappuccio FP, MacGregor GA. Does potassium supplementation lower blood pressure? A meta-analysis of published trials. *J Hypertens.* 1991;9:465–473.
12. Appel LJ, Moore TJ, Obarzanek E, et al. A clinical trial of the effects of dietary patterns on blood pressure. *N Engl J Med.* 1997;16:1117–1124.
13. McMahon FG, Akdamar K, Ryan JR, et al. Upper gastrointestinal lesions after potassium chloride supplements: a controlled clinical trial. *Lancet.* 1982;2:1059–1061.
14. Burnakis TG, Mioduch HJ. Combined therapy with captopril and potassium supplementation. A potential for hyperkalemia. *Arch Intern Med.* 1984;144:2371–2372.

P

Probiotics

See Acidophilus.

Pyridoxine

See Vitamin B$_6$ (Pyridoxine).

Pyruvate

Pyruvate, a 3-carbon molecule, is produced endogenously from phosphoenolpyruvate in the end stages of glycolysis. It can be reduced to lactate in the cytosol or decarboxylated to acetyl CoA in the mitochondria. Some researchers have hypothesized that pyruvate supplementation may spare oxidation of glucose, thus improving sports endurance by sparing glycogen. Preliminary investigations revealed pyruvate prevented the development of hepatic steatosis in rats receiving chronic ethanol feedings. These findings led to additional research testing pyruvate supplementation on fat metabolism in animals and humans (1, 2).

Media and Marketing Claims	Efficacy
Weight loss aid	?↑
Improves exercise endurance	↔
Lowers cholesterol	↔

Advisory

May be associated with flatus and diarrhea

Drug/Supplement Interactions

No reported adverse interactions

KEY POINTS

- In preliminary studies in small numbers of obese subjects mainly on very low-calorie diets, pyruvate enhanced weight and fat loss. These studies have been criticized for reliance on biolelectrical impedance, which is not generally regarded as an effective measure of body fat in obese subjects. Other studies, some published as abstracts (not discussed here), have reported enhanced weight loss in overweight subjects who ingested pyruvate.

- In two preliminary laboratory studies, seven days of supplementation with pyruvate and dihydroxyacetone improved exercise endurance in untrained subjects. However, pyruvate administered had no ergogenic effect on exercise in two studies of trained athletes. Much more research is needed before the claim that pyruvate enhances exercise endurance can be supported. In addition, athletes should be cautioned that pyruvate supplementation has been associated with gastrointestinal distress, which could interfere with sport performance.

- One preliminary study showed that pyruvate had no effect on blood lipids in hyperlipidemic subjects on low-fat diets, but another study reported pyruvate prevented lipids from increasing in subjects on high-fat diets. More research is needed to clarify these findings and to explore the possible mechanisms involved. It is not prudent to suggest that individuals take pyruvate supplements with the notion that it allows them to eat a high-fat diet without consequences.

- It is of note that commercially available pyruvate supplements do not contain dihydroxyacetone and are not available in the high doses used in many of the research studies.

FOOD SOURCES

Pyruvate is found in animal products; however, food sources have not been quantified.

DOSAGE INFORMATION/BIOAVAILABILITY

Pyruvate is sold in the form of sodium or calcium pyruvate in capsules or tablets supplying 0.5 g to 1 g per serving. This dose is considerably less than those used in research which typically provided 25 g to 50 g pyruvate in addition to dihydroxyacetone (another three-carbon metabolite of carbohydrate metabolism).

RELEVANT RESEARCH

Pyruvate and Weight Loss

- In a double-blind, placebo-controlled study, 26 healthy overweight men and women (body mass index [BMI] > 27) were randomized to receive 6 g pyruvate or a placebo daily for six weeks. All subjects participated in an exercise program consisting of a 45-minute to 60-minute aerobic/anaerobic routine three times weekly. Body composition was determined by bioelectrical impedance. (Researchers stated that they used a newer technology bioelectrical impedance that is more accurate than previous versions used by the Stanko et al. studies, described later.) All subjects were instructed by a dietitian to follow a 2,000-kcal controlled diet. There were no significant differences in dietary intake as assessed by food records between groups. After six weeks, there was a significant decrease in body weight (–1.2 kg), body fat (–2.5 kg) and percent body fat (23 percent pretrial vs 20.3 percent six weeks posttrial) in the pyruvate group. Profile of Mood States fatigue and vigor scores were significantly improved for the pyruvate group at week 6 (vigor) and weeks 4 and 6 (fatigue). There was no significant change in total lean body mass in the pyruvate group. The placebo group demonstrated significant improvements for POMS vigor at weeks 2 and 4, but no changes in body weight, body fat, or percent body fat (3).

- In a double-blind, placebo-controlled study, 53 overweight subjects (BMI > 25) were randomized to one of three groups for six weeks: (1) 6 g pyruvate (total of 10 capsules also containing zinc, vitamin B_6, chromium, cranberry powder, dehydroacetone, and cornsilk); (2) a placebo; and (3) control. The first two groups received dietary counseling, and all three groups engaged in supervised circuit training exercise three times per week. At study's end, subjects taking the pyruvate supplement experienced significant decreases in fat mass, percent body fat, and increases in lean body mass as measured by bioelectrical impedance. Despite the exercise regimen, the placebo and control groups had no significant changes in body composition. The authors suggested that the exercise protocol might not have been sufficient to induce weight changes. In addition, the pyruvate group, but not the control or placebo group, had improved scores on the Profile of Mood States fatigue and vigor ratings (4).

- In a randomized, placebo-controlled study, 13 obese women (average BMI = 38.9 kg/m^2) confined to a metabolic ward were given 16 g pyruvate and 12 g dihydroxyacetone (PD) or a placebo of 26 g polyglucose both as isocaloric substitutions for a portion of the carbohydrate content of the diet for 21 days. Subjects were instructed to control energy expenditure and to closely monitor dietary compliance. All subjects were fed 500-kcal hypocaloric, liquid diets (60 percent carbohydrate, 40 percent protein) for 21 days. Body composition as determined by bioelectrical impedance, energy deficit (calculated from metabolic rates measured by using a metabolic cart and compared to weight and fat loss), and nitrogen metabolism (assessed by analyzing all urine and stool samples for 21 days and estimating insensible nitrogen losses) were measured. The authors chose to use bioelectrical impedance because of previous research showing it to reliably measure changes in body composition in obese patients. Subjects receiving PD had significantly greater weight loss (6.5 kg vs 5.6 kg) and fat loss (4.3 kg vs 3.5 kg) than the placebo group subjects. There were no differences between groups in resting metabolic rate, nitrogen balance, and hematology indexes. The authors acknowledged: "With the small differences in body composition changes observed in the present study, the sensitivity of any technique available for measurement of body composition is in question. Therefore, our results must be considered preliminary and need corroboration by long-term, large-scale, clinical evaluations" (5).

- In a similar randomized, placebo-controlled study by the same investigators, 14 obese women confined to bed in a metabolic ward were given 30 g pyruvate or 22 g polyglucose as placebo as part of a 1,000-kcal hypocaloric, liquid diet (68 percent carbohydrate, 22 percent protein) for 21 days. Body composition, energy deficit, and nitrogen metabolism were measured using the same methods as the previously cited study. Subjects fed pyruvate had significantly greater weight loss (5.9 kg vs 4.3 kg) and fat loss (4.0 kg vs 2.7 kg) than the placebo group. Quality of weight loss (fat loss vs protein loss) was improved with pyruvate (6).

- In a placebo-controlled (not blinded) study by the same researchers, 17 obese women (weight ranging from 72.5 to 139.7 kg) confined to bed in a metabolic ward followed a hypoenergetic diet (1.3 MJ/day) for weight loss for three weeks and then were randomized to receive 15 g pyruvate and 75 g dihydroxyacetone (PD) or a placebo during refeeding with a hyperenergetic diet (1.5 × resting energy expenditure) for an additional three weeks. Using the same methods as the previous studies, resting energy expenditure, body composition by electric impedance, nitrogen balance, serum proteins, biochemical profile, thyroid hormones, and insulin were measured before and after refeeding. During the hypoenergetic diet, weight loss and fat loss were similar in both groups. During refeeding, both groups experienced weight gain; however, weight gain and body fat gain were significantly less in subjects receiving PD than in the placebo group. There were no differences in any other parameter measured (7).

Pyruvate and Exercise Endurance

- In a double-blind, placebo-controlled, crossover study, seven trained cyclists received in random order 7 g pyruvate (calcium pyruvate) or a placebo daily for one week each, with a two-week washout period. The researchers chose the dose based on the amount typically found in commercial supplements. Subjects cycled at 74 percent to 80 percent of their maximum oxygen consumption until exhaustion. There was no difference in performance times between the two trials. Measured blood indices (insulin, peptide C, glucose, lactate, glycerol, free fatty acids) were not affected. In a separate study reported in the same article, a range of pyruvate doses were administered to 9 recreational athletes to determine what dose might increase blood pyruvate concentration. The 7 g, 15 g, and the 25 g dose of pyruvate did not significantly affect blood levels of pyruvate, glucose, lactate, glycerol, or free fatty acids during a four-hour period following ingestion (8).

- In a double-blind, placebo-controlled study, 42 collegiate football players were randomly assigned to one of four treatments daily for five weeks: (1) creatine monohydrate; (2) calcium pyruvate; (3) combination (60 percent pyruvate plus 40 percent creatine); or (4) a placebo. Creatine alone and pyruvate alone were administered in three doses providing 0.22 g/kg/day (average dose for a 100-kg subject = 22 g). The combination product provided 0.13 and 0.09 g/kg/day for pyruvate and creatine, respectively. Exercise tests were performed before and after the supplementation period while subjects continued their normal training schedules. Body composition was assessed using hydrostatic weighing and measuring seven skinfold sites. Food diaries recorded at weeks 1 and 5 revealed no significant differences in total calories or macronutrients across time or among groups. Compared to the placebo and pyruvate alone, subjects receiving creatine and creatine plus pyruvate had significantly greater increases in body mass, lean body mass, one repetition maximum (RM) bench press, combined one RM squat and bench press, and static vertical jump power output. Percent body fat, fat mass, and cycle peak power, total work performed, blood lactate concentration, and ratings of perceived exertion during cycle ergometry did not differ among groups. In the pyruvate group, 6 of 11 subjects reported mild headaches that subsided after two weeks. The authors concluded that creatine supplementation appears to have beneficial effects on body composition and anaerobic exercise, but that pyruvate supplementation does not offer any additional advantages (9).

P

- In a double-blind, placebo-controlled, crossover design study, 10 untrained, free-living males on controlled diets (55 percent carbohydrate, 15 percent protein, 30 percent fat, 35 kcal/kg) were supplemented in random order with 25 g sodium pyruvate plus 75 g dihydroxyacetone (PD) added to pudding or 100 g polyglucose added to pudding (placebo) for 7 days each, with a 7- to 14-day washout period. Diets were administered at the research site (details of diet administration were not provided). Subjects performed submaximal exercise on an arm ergometer to exhaustion at the end of each seven-day diet. Muscle biopsies were taken before and immediately after exercise to obtain muscle glycogen. PD-supplemented subjects exercised significantly longer than placebo (160 minutes vs 133 minutes). Resting triceps muscle glycogen was significantly greater than during placebo administration but did not differ between trials at the point of exhaustion. Arterial and venous glucose difference (glucose extraction) was significantly greater before exercise and after 60 minutes of exercise, but not at exhaustion during PD supplementation compared to the placebo. Whole arm fractional glucose extraction (calculated by dividing arteriovenous concentration of glucose by arterial concentration of glucose) was significantly greater before exercise, after 60 minutes of exercise, and at exhaustion during PD supplementation than in placebo group measurements. There were no differences in respiratory exchange ratios, plasma free fatty acids, β-hydroxybutyrate, glycerol, catecholamines, and insulin between groups. Most subjects on the PD diet experienced flatus and borborygmus (intestinal noise). The authors hypothesized that pyruvate increased endurance by augmenting sources of carbohydrate for fuel used during exercise (10).

- In a similar double-blind, placebo-controlled, crossover study by the same research team, eight untrained, free-living male subjects on controlled high carbohydrate diets (70 percent carbohydrate, 18 percent protein, 12 percent fat, 35 kcal/kg) were supplemented in random order with 25 g sodium pyruvate plus 75 g dihydroxyacetone (PD) or 100 g polyglucose for 7 days each, with a 7- to 14-day washout period. All meals were given to the subjects at the research site, but were consumed on an out patient basis. After each diet, exercise to exhaustion on the cycle ergometer was performed at 70 percent VO_{2max}. Blood samples and muscle biopsies were taken. Endurance capacity was significantly improved after PD compared to placebo results (79 minutes vs 66 minutes). Whole-leg arterial and venous glucose difference (glucose extraction) was significantly greater at rest and after 30 minutes of exercise, but not at exhaustion during DP supplementation compared to use of the placebo. There were no differences between treatments on muscle glycogen content or other blood parameters. The authors concluded that a 20 percent increase in leg endurance following PD supplementation may have been caused by increased glucose availability for oxidation by exercising muscle (11).

Pyruvate and Blood Lipids

- In a randomized, placebo-controlled study, 34 free-living subjects with hyperlipidemia were placed on a low-fat, low-cholesterol diet for four weeks, followed by six more weeks of the same diet supplemented with 22–44 g pyruvate (7 percent of the diet) or 18 g to 35 g polyglucose. There were no significant differences between groups in dietary intake (assessed by three-day food records at weeks 0 and 6). Pyruvate supplementation had no effect on plasma total, LDL, and HDL cholesterol or triglycerides. However, pyruvate subjects experienced a mild but significant reduction in weight (–0.6 kg) and fat mass (–0.4 kg) compared to weights of the placebo group (12).

- In a randomized, placebo-controlled study, 40 subjects with hyperlipidemia were put on a high-fat (45 percent to 74 percent of energy, 18 percent to 20 percent saturated fat), high-cholesterol (560 mg to 620 mg), anabolic diet (0.11 MJ to 0.12 MJ/kg body weight) for four weeks, followed by six more weeks of supplementation of the same diet with 36 g to 53 g pyruvate or 21 g to 37 g polyglucose (placebo) as a portion of carbohydrate energy. Pyruvate supplementation resulted in a significant reduction of plasma total cholesterol by 4 percent and LDL cholesterol by 5 percent, compared to no change in placebo subjects. There were no differences between groups on triglyceride and HDL cholesterol levels. Pyruvate supplementation significantly lowered resting heart rate and blood pressure, causing the authors to speculate that pyruvate may have a positive inotropic effect on cardiac muscle (13).

SAFETY

- There are no long-term studies testing the safety of pyruvate supplementation greater than six weeks.
- Flatus, diarrhea, and borborygmus were reported in most subjects ingesting pyruvate and dihydroxyacetone.

REFERENCES

1. Sukula WR. Pyruvate: beyond the marketing hype. *Int J Sport Nutr.* 1998;8:241–249.
2. Ivy JL. Effect of pyruvate and dihydroxyacetone on metabolism and aerobic capacity. *Med Sci Sports Exerc.* 1998;30:837–843.
3. Kalman D, Colker CM, Wilets I, et al. The effects of pyruvate supplementation on body composition in overweight individuals. *Nutrition.* 1999;15:337–340.
4. Kalman D, Colker CM, Stark R, et al. Effect of pyruvate supplementation on body composition and mood. *Curr Ther Res.* 1998;59:793–802.
5. Stanko RT, Tietze DL, Arch JE. Body composition, energy utilization, and nitrogen metabolism with a severely restricted diet supplemented with dihydroxyacetone and pyruvate. *Am J Clin Nutr.* 1992;55:771–776.
6. Stanko RT, Tietze DL, Arch JE. Body composition, energy utilization, and nitrogen metabolism with a 4.25 MJ/day low-energy diet supplemented with pyruvate. *Am J Clin Nutr.* 1992;56:630–635.
7. Stanko RT, Arch JE. Inhibition of regain in body weight and fat with addition of 3-carbon compounds to the diet with hyperenergetic refeeding after weight reduction. *Int J Obes Relat Metab Disord.* 1996;20:925–930.
8. Morrison MA, Spriet LL, Dyck DJ. Pyruvate ingestion for seven days does not improve aerobic performance in well-trained individuals. *J Appl Physiol.* 2000;89:549–556.

P

9. Stone MH, Sanborn K, Smith LL, et al. Effects of in-season (5 weeks) creatine and pyruvate supplementation on anaerobic performance and body composition in American football players. *Int J Sport Nutr.* 1999;9:146–165.

10. Stanko RT, Robertson RJ, Spina RJ, et al. Enhancement of arm exercise endurance capacity with dihydroxyacetone and pyruvate. *J Appl Physiol.* 1990;68:119–124.

11. Stanko RT, Robertson RJ, Galbreath RW, et al. Enhanced leg exercise endurance with a high-carbohydrate diet and dihydroxyacetone and pyruvate. *J Appl Physiol.* 1990;69:1651–1656.

12. Stanko RT, Reynolds HR, Hoyson R, et al. Pyruvate supplementation of low-cholesterol, low-fat diet: effects on plasma lipid concentrations and body composition in hyperlipidemic patients. *Am J Clin Nutr.* 1994;59:423–427.

13. Stanko RT, Reynolds HR, Lonchar KD, et al. Plasma lipid concentrations in hyperlipidemic patients consuming a high-fat diet supplemented with pyruvate for 6 wk. *Am J Clin Nutr.* 1992;56:950–954.

Riboflavin

See Vitamin B$_2$ (Riboflavin).

Royal Jelly

Royal jelly is a milky substance secreted from the pharyngeal glands of young worker honeybees (*Apis mellifera*). During the early stages of growth, royal jelly is the food of female bee larvae, but only the queen bee continues to consume royal jelly while the other larvae become sexually immature worker bees. Because royal jelly causes the queen bee to become fertile, grow large, and live several years (compared to the lifespan of a few weeks for worker bees), some have extrapolated that royal jelly will have beneficial effects in humans.

Chemical analysis has shown that half the dry weight of royal jelly is protein, with the remainder made up of free amino acids, fatty acids, sugars, and vitamins and minerals (specific quantities not reported). Royalisin, a protein, and 10-hydroxy-2-decenoic acid, a fatty acid, have been identified in royal jelly as potential antibiotic agents (1–3).

Media and Marketing Claims	Efficacy
Fights infections	NR
Supports a healthy heart	NR
Reduces signs of aging	NR
Improves mental alertness	NR
Improves stamina and physical energy	NR
Reduces symptoms of depression	NR

Advisory

Contraindicated in individuals with asthma or atopy

Drug/Supplement Interactions

No reported adverse interactions

KEY POINTS

- Although it appears that certain components of royal jelly may have antibacterial properties, much more research needs to be conducted before claims that royal jelly fights infection can be substantiated. It is also worthy to note that royal jelly was bactericidal to *Lactobacillus* and *Bifidobacteria,* which are considered to be beneficial to intestinal health (*see* Acidophilus/*Lactobacillus Acidophilus* [LA]).

- Several poorly controlled trials reported in journals not accessible in English are used to support claims that royal jelly benefits the cardiovascular system. However, there is no evidence from well-controlled clinical trials that royal jelly improves cardiovascular disease risk factors.

- No peer-reviewed, controlled studies have evaluated the effects of royal jelly on aging, alertness, stamina, fatigue, or depression. Overall, there appears to be no substantive data to support supplementation with royal jelly.

- Given the number of asthmatic and anaphylactic reactions reported, royal jelly is contraindicated in individuals with a history of asthma or allergic reaction for which there is a genetic predisposition.

DOSAGE INFORMATION/BIOAVAILABILITY

Royal jelly is often combined with ginseng, raw honey, bee pollen, and B vitamins in the form of a capsule or tablet. Royal jelly is usually sold in 1-g tablets containing approximately 30 mg to 150 mg royal jelly. In addition, royal jelly is a popular ingredient added to fruit "smoothies."

RELEVANT RESEARCH

Royal Jelly and Immunity & Antibacterial Properties

- Royal jelly contains an antibacterial protein recently identified as royalisin (0.3 mg/g of royal jelly). In an *in vitro* study, royalisin isolated from royal jelly was reported to have potent antibacterial activity against Gram-positive (including *Clostridium, Corynebacterium, Leuconostoc, Staphylococcus, Lactobacillus, Bifidobacterium,* and *Streptococcus*) bacteria comparable with the effective concentrations of various antibiotics. (*Lactobacillus* and *Bifidobacterium* are considered beneficial bacteria in the colon.) Royalisin had no effect on Gram-negative bacteria. The authors propose using royalisin as an antibacterial compound to preserve food (1).

R

- A study in mice found that royal jelly (1 g/kg) significantly decreased serum levels of antigen-specific IgE and inhibited histamine release from mast cells, resulting in suppression of immediate hypersensitivity reactions of ear skin (4).

Royal Jelly and Cardiovascular Disease

- There are no peer-reviewed studies available in English on royal jelly and cardiovascular disease.

- A systematic review and meta-analysis were conducted examining the effect of royal jelly on atherosclerosis in 17 animal studies and 9 human trials (5 placebo-controlled) in European and Asian journals. In the animal studies, royal jelly significantly decreased serum and liver total lipids and cholesterol levels in rats and rabbits and also retarded the formation of atheromas in rabbits fed a high-fat diet. Meta-analysis of the controlled human trials reported that royal jelly (in doses ranging from 30 mg to 100 mg/day for three to six weeks) resulted in a significant reduction in total serum lipids and cholesterol levels and normalization of HDL and LDL in subjects with hyperlipidemia. The author hypothesized that royal jelly may decrease reabsorption of cholesterol in the gastrointestinal tract and increase its excretion in the bile. However, the studies evaluated did not control subjects' dietary intake, weight, or use of medications, which would have skewed the overall results (5). None of the studies included in this analysis were available in English for direct evaluation.

SAFETY

- There have been several reports of asthma attacks and anaphylaxis following ingestion of royal jelly in atopic individuals (6–8). Testing of allergic patients revealed that the symptoms were true IgE-mediated hypersensitivity reactions (9).

- According to a study of 461 subjects in Hong Kong who were reported royal jelly users, 9 subjects (7 percent) reported 14 adverse reactions such as eczema, rhinitis, acute asthma, uticaria. Subjects reporting adverse reactions also had a history of clinical allergies (10).

- Specific allergic symptoms include: rhinitis, acute asthma, eczema, conjunctivitis, pruritis, uticaria, and in some cases angioedema. Most symptoms appear within two hours of ingestion (8).

- One report of death occurred in an 11-year-old, atopic girl after ingesting 500 mg royal jelly (11).

- One report of hemorrhagic colitis occurred in a 53-year-old woman after taking royal jelly for 25 days (12).

REFERENCES

1. Fujiwara S, Imai J, Fujiwara M, et al. A potent antibacterial protein in royal jelly. *J Biol Chem.* 1990;265:11333–11337.

2. Vittek J. Effect of royal jelly on serum lipids in experimental animals and humans with atherosclerosis. *Experientia.* 1995;51:927–935.

3. Palma MS. Composition of freshly harvested Brazilian royal jelly: identification of carbohydrates from the sugar fraction. *J Agricultural Res.* 1992;31:42–44.

4. Oka H, Emori Y, Kobayashi N, et al. Suppression of allergic reactions by royal jelly in association with the restoration of macrophage function and the improvement of Th1/Th2 cell responses. *Int Immunolpharmacol.* 2001;1:521–532.

5. Leung R, Thien FCK, Baldo BA, et al. Royal jelly-induced asthma and anaphylaxis: clinical characteristics and immunologic correlations. *J Allergy Clin Immunol.* 1995;96:1004–1007.

6. Peacock S, Murray V, Turton C. Respiratory distress and royal jelly. *BMJ.* 1995;311:1472.

7. Larporte JR, Ibaanez L, Vendrell L, et al. Bronchospasm induced by royal jelly. *Allergy.* 1996;51:440.

8. Harwood M, Harding S, Beasley R, et al. Asthma following royal jelly. *NZ Med J.* 1996;109:325.

9. Thien FC, Leung R, Baldo BA, et al. Asthma and anaphylaxis induced by royal jelly. *Clin Exp Allergy.* 1996;26:216–222.

10. Leung R, Ho A, Chan J, et al. Royal jelly consumption and hypersensitivity in the community. *Clin Exp Allergy.* 1997;27:333–336.

11. Bullock RJ, Rohan A, Straatmans JA. Fatal royal jelly-induced asthma. *Med J Aust.* 1994;160:44.

12. Yonei Y, Shibagaki K, Tsukada N, et al. Case report: hemorrhagic colitis associated with royal jelly intake. *J Gastroenterol Hepatol.* 1997;12:495–499.

S-adenosylmethionine (SAM-e)

S-adenosylmethionine (SAM-e) was first discovered in the 1950s and about 20 years later was stabilized into a salt to become available for clinical investigation. SAM-e is synthesized in all living cells from methionine and adenine triphosphate (ATP) and is involved in a wide variety of metabolic reactions. The production of SAM-e is tied closely to folate and vitamin B_{12} metabolism. SAM-e functions primarily in the transferring of methyl groups to substrates such as nucleic acids, proteins, polysaccharides, fatty acids, and phospholipids. After donating its methyl group, SAM-e is converted into S-adenosylhomocysteine, which is hydrolyzed into adenosine and homocysteine. The homocysteine can be further converted into cysteine and indirectly into glutathione, both of which are intracellular antioxidants (1–4).

In Europe, where SAM-e is available as a drug, it has been investigated for its possible role in the management of osteoarthritis and depression. The mechanism of action behind the potential antiinflammatory and antidepressant effects of SAM-e are not fully understood. It has been hypothesized that SAM-e stimulates the production of proteoglycans in cartilage that may cushion joints. There are numerous theories on how SAM-e may affect depression, including increasing the synthesis of the neurotransmitters serotonin, dopamine, and norepinephrine. SAM-e became available in the United States in March 1999 and is now sold as a dietary supplement (1–4).

S

Media and Marketing Claims	Efficacy
Reduces pain from arthritis and rebuilds joints	?↑
May benefit fibromyalgia	↔
Antidepressant	?↑
Good for liver dysfunction	?↑

Advisory

- Mild gastrointestinal distress
- Associated with manic reaction in bipolar disorder patients

Drug/Supplement Interactions

- Intravenous SAM-e taken with clomipramine (antidepressant) resulted in serotonin syndrome in one report
- SAM-e taken with other antidepressants may speed onset of antidepressant action
- Possible interaction of SAM-e with Levodopa

KEY POINTS

- There is evidence from several controlled trials that SAM-e may relieve symptoms of osteoarthritis, at least as effectively as traditional nonsteroidal anti-inflammatory drugs (NSAIDS). Further, it appears to be better tolerated without the serious adverse effects on the gastrointestinal tract and cartilage that are associated with NSAID use. More clinical data are needed to determine if SAM-e actually supports cartilage regeneration.

- There is some evidence from a few trials that SAM-e may relieve pain in fibromyalgia patients, although not all research is in agreement. More controlled research in larger numbers of subjects is needed before supplementation can be recommended to this population.

- Several studies of intravenous and oral supplementation demonstrate that SAM-e exerts antidepressant activity, at least as effectively as some tricyclic medications. However, SAM-e has not been tested against selective serotonin reuptake inhibitors such as Prozac. Severely depressed patients should be under the care of a health professional and should not self-medicate with SAM-e unless directed by a physician.

- There is evidence from laboratory and some clinical trials that intravenous or oral SAM-e may protect against liver damage. Because more data are needed, patients with liver diseases should discuss SAM-e supplementation with their health care provider.

- It is of note that the doses of SAM-e used in clinical trials would cost consumers approximately $50 to $80 per month.

FOOD SOURCES

None

DOSAGE INFORMATION/BIOAVAILABILITY

SAM-e is sold in several forms wherein an additional compound (tosylate, disulfate tosylate, disulfate ditosylate, 1,4 butanedisulfate) is added to keep it stable. Manufacturers typically recommend taking anywhere from 400 mg to 1,200 mg per day. The cost for a month's supply of an active dose is approximately $50 to $80. In most studies researchers have used enteric coated tablets to promote maximum absorption. In a recent analysis of 13 brands of SAM-e by ConsumerLab.com, six did not contain the amount of SAM-e they purported to contain on the label (5).

In animal and small human studies, enteric-coated tablets of SAM-e raised plasma and synovial fluid levels of SAM-e (1). In one study, eight healthy men and women were given 400 mg SAM-e (in two enteric coated tablets) after an overnight fast. Blood samples were collected before, and three, six, and nine hours after consuming SAM-e. In women, after three and six hours, SAM-e concentrations were 6- and 3.5-fold higher than baseline values, respectively. In men, peak levels occurred after six hours (3.7- fold higher than baseline) (1, 6).

RELEVANT RESEARCH

SAM-e and Osteoarthritis

- In a double-blind, placebo-controlled study, 81 patients (ages 40 y to 85 y) with knee osteoarthritis were randomized to receive daily intravenous (i.v.) bolus of 400 mg SAM-e for five days followed by oral enteric tablets (200 mg × 3) for 23 days or an intravenous placebo for five days followed by oral placebo for 23 days. All subjects participated in a seven-day washout period before the study. Acetaminophen use was permitted and recorded throughout the study, but no other analgesic or antiarthritic medications were allowed. Six times during the study (enrollment, after washout, after second and fourth intravenous injection, and after 9 days and 23 days of oral therapy), patients completed the Stanford Health Assessment Questionnaire disability and pain scales and visual analogue scales for rest and walking pain. At each visit, patients also estimated the duration of morning stiffness and overall activity of arthritis and physicians performed an assessment of swelling, tenderness, and range of motion. Subjects were divided into two groups for statistical analysis: Group A—subjects with mild arthritis (n = 48) and Group B—subjects with more severe global arthritis (n = 33). In Group A, the SAM-e treated group had a significantly greater reduction in overall pain and rest pain, but no other differences in other parameters when compared to the placebo treated group. In Group B, the response to treatment did not differ between groups. However, the authors noted that baseline characteristics of Group B differed significantly and thus may have flawed the results. Four patients treated with SAM-e and one treated with placebo withdrew from the study due to adverse events (neurological symptoms and chest pain) during the intravenous treatment. There were no significant differences in laboratory studies (complete blood count, white cell differential count, urinalysis, stool hemoccult) between groups) (7).

- In a double-blind, comparative, multicenter study, 734 subjects with clinically diagnosed hip or knee osteoarthritis were randomly assigned to receive 1,200 mg SAM-e,

750 mg naproxen (nonsteroidal antiinflammatory), or a placebo daily for 30 days. Subjects were not permitted to use any pain medications during the study. All patients underwent clinical exams at the beginning, after two weeks, and at the end of treatment. The following parameters were assessed: (1) night pain and day pain; and (2) degree of difficulty carrying out specific activities, such as standing up from a chair, going upstairs, and walking on an even floor. At the end of the study, physicians and subjects each evaluated the efficacy and tolerability of treatments. Forty subjects withdrew from the study because of side-effects (10 withdrew from the SAM-e group, 17 from the naproxen group, and 13 from the placebo group). SAM-e and naproxen exerted the same analgesic activity, and both were significantly more effective than the placebo. The efficacy of SAM-e and naproxen were rated the same by subjects and physicians; both of them were rated as statistically superior to the placebo. The tolerability of SAM-e was significantly greater than for naproxen and did not differ from the placebo, according to both subject and physician evaluations. Side-effects (gastrointestinal, headache, dizziness, hypersomnia, insomnia) occurred in 28 percent of the SAM-e group, 47 percent of the naproxen group, and 25 percent of the placebo group (8).

- In a double-blind, comparative trial, 48 patients (mean age = 65 y) with diagnosed knee osteoarthrits were randomized to receive enteric-coated tablets of SAM-e (1,200 mg) or piroxicam (20 mg) (a nonsteroidal anti-inflammatory) for 84 days. A seven-day single-blind initial washout period was performed in order to exclude patients demonstrating a placebo-effect. Pain, active and passive motility, morning stiffness, and distance covered before the onset of pain were assessed at the beginning, at the end, and every 28 days of the study. The residual therapeutic activity of SAM-e and piroxicam was assessed for 56 days posttreatment. During this time, all subjects were given placebos and clinical parameters were reevaluated every 14 days. Forty-five patients completed the study. Both SAM-e and piroxicam demonstrated significant improvement in the total pain score after 28 days of treatment. The other clinical parameters (morning stiffness, distance walked before the onset of pain, active and passive motility) improved significantly in both groups after about day 56. There were no significant differences in efficacy or tolerability between groups. Clinical improvement was maintained significantly longer in patients treated with SAM-e than in patients taking piroxicam. The authors noted that the clinical effect of SAM-e appears to be delayed compared to piroxicam, but that its effect lasts longer after discontinuation of drug therapy (9).

- In a double-blind, comparative trial, 36 subjects (ages 56 y to 72 y) with osteoarthritis of the knee, hip, and/or spine were randomized to receive 1,200mg SAM-e or 150mg indomethacin daily for four weeks. Clinical parameters of pain and morning stiffness were assessed before and after 7, 14, 21 and 28 days of therapy. Subjects treated with SAM-e had significantly improved total scores obtained by the sum of all clinical findings compared to pretreatment values. Similar improvement was found in indomethacin-treated subjects. Laboratory parameters did not change in either group. Two adverse effects (nausea) occurred in the SAM-e group compared to seven adverse events in the indomethacin group (10).

- In a double-blind, comparative trial, 36 subjects (ages 37 y to 70 y) with osteoarthritis of the hip, knee, and/or spine were randomized to receive 1,200 mg SAM-e or 1,200 mg ibuprofen daily for four weeks. Morning stiffness, pain at rest, pain on motion, crepitus, swelling, and limitation of motion of the affected joints were assessed before and after 7, 14, 21, and 28 days of treatment. The mean clinical scores showed a significant improvement compared to baseline in both treatment groups. The improvement was equally evident at all sites of osteoarthritis. The weekly values of the clinical scores were similar in the SAM-e and ibuprofen-treated groups. Both treatments appeared to be well tolerated, and no subjects withdrew from the study. There were no abnormal laboratory values in either group at any stage of the study (11).

- In a double-blind, comparative, multicenter study, 150 subjects (ages 45 y to 75 y) with hip and knee osteoarthritis were randomized to receive 1,200 mg SAM-e or 1,200 mg ibuprofen daily for 30 days. There was an initial washout period of five days for all subjects. Subjective parameters of pain (rest pain, night pain, loading pain, active movement pain, passive movement pain, and muscle spasm) were recorded at baseline and at days 16 and 31. At the end of the trial, efficacy and tolerability were rated by both the physician and patient. Both groups reported improvement in subjective pain symptoms. Likewise, physician and subject evaluation of treatments were favorable for both SAM-e and ibuprofen. There were no differences in laboratory tests between groups. Minor side-effects were reported in 5 subjects treated with SAM-e and in 16 subjects taking ibuprofen (12).

SAM-e and Fibromyalgia

- In a double-blind, placebo-controlled study in Denmark, 44 patients with primary fibromyalgia were randomized to receive 800 mg SAM-e or a placebo daily for six weeks. Patients were discouraged from using analgesic or anti-inflammatory drugs. Patients were permitted to use a rescue remedy of acetaminophen if needed. Use of drugs was documented. There was no washout period. Tender point score, isokinetic muscle strength, disease activity, subjective symptoms (visual analog scale), mood parameters, and side-effects were evaluated. There were significant improvements in disease activity, pain experienced during the last week, fatigue, morning stiffness, and mood evaluated by Face Scale in the SAM-e treated subjects compared to the placebo. There were no differences between groups in the tender point score, isokinetic muscle strength, mood evaluated by the Beck Depression Inventory, and side-effects (13).

- In a double-blind, placebo-controlled, crossover study, 34 patients with primary fibromyalgia received intravenously 600 mg SAM-e or a placebo daily for 10 days. There were no significant differences in improvement in the primary outcome (tender point change between the two treatment groups). There was a trend toward improvement of subjective pain at rest, pain on movement, and overall well-being in the SAM-e group, but this was not significant. There was no effect on isokinetic muscle strength, Zerrsen self-assessment questionnaire, and mood evaluated by the face scale (14).

- In a double-blind, placebo-controlled, crossover study, 25 patients (ages 33 y to 55 y) with primary fibromyalgia were randomized to receive intravenously 200 mg SAM-e

S

or placebo daily for 21 days, followed by a two-week washout period before switching to the other treatment. Assessment of pain (counting the number of subjective painful areas and the number of muscular and tendinous tender points) and assessment of depression (using the Hamilton Depression Rating Scale and an Italian questionnaire for the self-evaluation of depression [SAD]) were performed at entry, at days 21 and 35, and at study's end. Six patients withdrew from the study for unexplained reasons. Two other subjects withdrew after developing abscesses at the injection site. SAM-e treatment resulted in a significant decrease in pain evaluated as the number of trigger points plus painful sites. Placebo treatment had no effect on these parameters. Scores on both the Hamilton and SAD scales decreased significantly after SAM-e treatment, but not with the placebo (15).

SAM-e and Depression

- Researchers performed a meta-analysis of double-blind, randomized trials investigating the effects of parenteral or oral SAM-e compared with placebo or tricyclic antidepressants (TCA) on depression between 1972 and 1992. Studies were only included if subjects had a diagnosis of depressive syndrome determined clinically or based on the Diagnostic and Statistical Manual of Mental Disorders, if efficacy was assessed using the Hamilton Depression Rating Scale before and after treatment, if the trial was less than 12 weeks long, if dosage of $\geq$ 200 mg/day by parenteral route and $\geq$ 1,600 mg day by oral route, and if data were reported in a way that would allow for quantification of the effect size. Six studies (n= 200 subjects) were selected for meta-analysis of SAM-e versus a placebo, with only three trials using oral SAM-e tablets. Four trials were selected for meta-analysis of SAM-e compared to TCAs (n = 201 subjects), with only two trials using oral SAM-e tablets. Results demonstrated a greater response rate with SAM-e compared to the placebo, with a global effect size ranging between 17 percent to 38 percent depending on the definition of response. SAM-e had an antidepressant effect comparable to standard TCAs. The authors noted that the heterogeneity of the placebo-controlled trials made interpretation of the data difficult (16).

- In a double-blind, placebo-controlled study, 80 women (ages 45 y to 59 y) clinically diagnosed as having DSM-III-R major depressive disorder or dysthmia between 6 and 36 months following either natural menopause or hysterectomy were randomized to receive 1,600 mg SAM-e or placebo daily for 30 days. All subjects were given placebos in an initial washout period of one week. Treatment efficacy was evaluated by administering the Hamilton Depression Rating Scale (HAM-D) and the Rome Depression Inventory (RDI) at baseline and at days 10 and 30. Additionally, patients were administered the Minnesota Multiphasic Personality Inventory (MMPI), at baseline and day 30. At the end of the study, clinicians evaluated improvement using the Clinician Global Impression Improvement Scale (CGI-I). Ten patients dropped out for reduced compliance in each treatment group (60 completed the study). There were no significant differences at baseline in HAM-D scores between groups. There was a significant improvement in depressive symptoms as measured by the HAM-D, RDI, MMPI, and CGI-I in subjects treated with SAM-e compared to subjects taking the placebo from day 10 of the study (17).

- In a double-blind, comparative study, 26 patients (mean age = 39 y) with a DSM-III-R diagnosis of major depression were randomized to receive 1,600 mg SAM-e or 250 mg desipramine daily for four weeks. Only 17 patients (11 taking SAM-e and 6 taking desipramine) completed at least two weeks of the study. At baseline and weekly throughout the study, each subject completed the Hamilton Depression Scale (HAM-D), the Systematic Assessment for Treatment Emergent Events, and the Beck Depression Inventory. A patient was classified as a responder if he or she showed a reduction of more than 50 percent on total HAM-D scores at week 4 from baseline. Based on this definition, 6 of 11 SAM-e patients and 2 of 6 desipramine patients were responders. Regardless of treatment, patients with a 50 percent decrease in their HAM-D score showed a significant increase in plasma SAM-e concentrations. The authors concluded that the correlation between plasma SAM-e levels and the degree of clinical improvement in depressed patients suggests that SAM-e may play an important role in regulating mood (18).

- In a double-blind, placebo-controlled trial, 18 male in-patients (mean age = 42 y) who met the DSM-III criteria for major depression that was unipolar, without psychotic features were randomized to receive SAM-e or placebo. The first five patients received gradually increasing doses of SAM-e (200 mg/day from days 1 to 7 to 1,600 mg/day days 7 to 21). The remaining subjects were given 1,600 mg SAM-e for the entire 21 days of the study. Hamilton Depression Ratings (HAM-D) and the Carroll Rating Scale for Depression (CRSD) were given at baseline and on days 3, 7, 14, and 21. Fifteen subjects completed the study. At baseline, there were no differences in HAM-D scores. Although both groups improved, by day 14 and 21, HAM-D scores in the SAM-e group were significantly improved compared to the placebo group. Regarding the CRSD, scores were not statistically different until the end of the study at which time the SAM-e-treated subjects had improved scores compared to the placebo group. One subject in the SAM-e group developed a manic episode on day 19 of the study. No other serious side-effects occurred (19).

SAM-e and Liver Function

- In a double-blind, placebo-controlled, multicenter trial in Spain, 123 patients (106 men, 17 women, average age = 51 y) with alcoholic liver cirrhosis were randomized to receive 1,200 mg SAM-e or a placebo daily for two years. Seventy-five patients were in Child class A, 40 in class B, and 8 in class C (class A indicates least severe liver disease and class C indicates more advanced liver disease). There were no significant differences between the two groups with regard to age, sex, previous episodes of major cirrhosis complications, Child classification, or liver function tests. The overall mortality/liver transplantation was not significantly different between the placebo group and the SAM-e group. However, when patients in Child C class (more advanced liver disease) were excluded from analysis, the overall mortality/transplantation rate was significantly reduced in the SAM-e treated subjects compared to the placebo group. In addition, the differences between the groups in the two-year survival curves (time to death or liver transplantation) were also significantly in favor of SAM-e (20).

S

- Two review articles discuss animal and human studies that reported parenteral SAM-e prevents or reverses hepatotoxicity due to drugs and chemicals such as alcohol, acetaminophen, steroids, and lead (21, 22). Researchers in one review discussed data indicating that patients with cirrhosis may have an acquired metabolic block in hepatic conversion of methionine to SAM-e, and they propose that exogenous SAM-e may be an essential nutrient in these patients to normalize overall hepatic transmethylation and transsulfuration activity (22).

- In one study of baboons, intravenous SAM-e attenuated alcohol induced liver injury (23).

SAFETY

- In one study, SAM-e (1,600 mg/day for 19 days) induced a manic episode in a 65-year-old male, depressed patient in a controlled trial. The subject had no prior history of mania. The authors noted that SAM-e triggering a switch into mania had been previously reported in two other studies (19).

- Mild gastrointestinal stress may occur with the onset of treatment (4).

- Toxicity studies in animals suggest that SAM-e is relatively nontoxic at high doses. SAM-e does not appear to affect brain waves or seizure threshold (4).

- There was one case report of a toxic drug interaction between injected SAM-e with clomipramine that resulted in serotonin syndrome (24). However, several trials have combined SAM-e with other tricyclic antidepressants with no such effect (4).

- Levodopa (drug for Parkinson's disease) may deplete SAM-e (25). Additionally, SAM-e has been found to induce Parkinson disease-like motor impairments in rodents (25). Until more information is available, individuals with Parkinson's disease should not self-supplement with SAM-e without physician approval.

REFERENCES

1. Stramentinoli G. Pharmacologic aspects of S-adenosylmethionine. *Am J Med.* 1987;83(suppl 5A):35–42.
2. Baldessarini RJ. Neuropharmacology of S-adenosyl-L-methionine. *Am J Med.* 1987;83(suppl 5A):95–103.
3. Bottiglieri T, Hyland K, Reynolds EH. The clinical potential of ademetionine (S-adeosylmethionine) in neurological disorders. *Drugs.* 1994;48:137–152.
4. Chavez M. SAMe: S-adenosylmethionine. *Am J Health Syst Pharm.* 2000;57:119–123.
5. ConsumerLab.com. "Product Review: SAMe" Available at http://www.consumerlab.com/results/same.asp. Accessed July 7, 2002.
6. Giulidori P, Stamentinoli G. A radioenzymatic method for S-adenosyl-L-methionine determination in biological fluids. *Anal Biochem.* 1984;137:217–220.
7. Bradley JD, Flusser D, Katz BP, et al. A randomized, double-blind, placebo-controlled trial of intravenous loading with S-adenosylmethionine (SAM) followed by oral SAM therapy in patients with knee osteoarthritis. *J Rheumatol.* 1994;21:905–911.

8. Caruso I, Pietrogrande V. Italian double-blind multicenter study comparing S-Adenosylmethionine, naproxen, and placebo in the treatment of degenerative joint disease. *Am J Med.* 1987;83(suppl 5A):66–71.

9. Maccagno A, Di Giorgio EE, Caston OL. Double-blind controlled clinical trial of oral S-adenosylmethionine versus piroxicam in knee osteoarthritis. *Am J Med.* 1987;83(suppl 5A):72–77.

10. Vetter G. Double-blind comparative clinical trial with S-adenosylmethionine and indomethacin in the treatment of osteoarthritis. *Am J Med.* 1987;83(suppl 5A):78–80.

11. Muller-Fassbender H. Double-blind clinical trial of S-adenosylmethionine versus ibuprofen in the treatment of osteoarthritis. *Am J Med.* 1987;83(suppl 5A):81–83.

12. Marcolongo R, Girodano N, Colombo B, et al. Double-blind, multicenter study of the activity of S-adenosylmethionine in hip and knee osteoarthritis. *Curr Ther Res.* 1985;37:82–94.

13. Jacobsen S, Danneskiold-Samsoe B, Andersen RB. Oral S-adensoylmethionine in primary fibromyalgia. Double-blind clinical evaluation. *Scand J Rheumatol.* 1991; 20:294–302.

14. Volkman H, Norregaard J, Jacobsen S, et al. Double-blind, placebo-controlled cross-over study of intravenous S-adenosyl-L-methionine in patients with fibromyalgia. *Scand J Rheumatol.* 1997;26:206–211.

15. Tavoni A, Vitali C, Bombardieri S, et al. Evaluation of S-adenosylmethionine in primary fibromyalgia. A double-blind crossover study. *Am J Med.* 1987;83(suppl 5A):107–110.

16. Bressa GM. S-adenosyl-l-methionine (SAMe) as antidepressant: meta-analysis of clinical studies. *Acta Neurol Scand.* 1994;154:7–14.

17. Salmaggi P, Bressa GM, Nicchia G, et al. Double-blind, placebo-controlled study of S-adenosyl-L-methionine in depressed postmenopausal women. *Psychother Psychosom.* 1993;59:34–40.

18. Bell KM, Potkin SG, Carreon D, et al. S-adenosylmethionine blood levels in major depression: changes with drug treatment. *Acta Neurol Scand Suppl.* 1994;154:15–18.

19. Kagan BL, Sultzer DL, Rosenlicht N, et al. Oral S-adenosylmethionine in depression: a randomized, double-blind, placebo-controlled trial. *Am J Psychiatry.* 1990;147:591–595.

20. Mato JM, Camara J, Fernandez de Paz J, et al. S-adenosylmethionine in alcoholic liver cirrhosis: a randomized, placebo-controlled double-blind, multicenter trial. *J Hepatol.* 1999;30:1081–1089.

21. Friedel HA, Goa KL, Benfield P. S-adenosyl-l-methionine. A review of its pharmacological properties and therapeutic potential in liver dysfunction and affective disorders in relation to its physiological role in cell metabolism. *Drugs.* 1989;38:389–416.

22. Chawla RK, Bonkovsky HL, Galambos JT. Biochemistry and pharmacology of S-adenosyl-l-methionine and rationale for its use in liver disease. *Drugs.* 1990;40:98–110.

23. Lieber CS, Casini A, DeCarli LM, et al. S-adenosyl-l-methionine attenuates alcohol liver injury in the baboon. *Hepatology.* 1990;11:165–172.

24. Iruela LM, Minguez L, Merino J, et al. Toxic interaction of S-adenosylmethionine and clomipramine. *Am J Psychol.* 1993;150:522.

25. Charlton CG, Crowell B. Parkinson's disease like effects of S-adenosyl-L-methionine: effects of L-dopa. *Pharmacol Biochem Behav.* 1992;43:423–431.

S

St. John's Wort (*Hypericum perforatum*)

St John's wort (SJW), a yellow-flowering plant, has been used in traditional folk medicine for hundreds of years to treat a variety of disorders. Recently, the herb has gained popularity as an herbal remedy for mild to moderate depression. The mechanism by which SJW might affect depression is unknown. One thought is that the herb may raise serotonin levels similar to serotonin reuptake inhibitors. It may also inhibit reuptake of monoamines, dopamine noradrenaline, and neurotransmitters GABA and glutamate (1). Another theory suggests that it may reduce cortisol levels. SJW contains many compounds including naphthodianthrones (hypericin and pseudohypericin), flavonoids (quercetin, quercitrin, hyperin), phloroglucinols (hyperforin and adhyperforin), essential oil, and xanthones (2). Although the active components have not been identified, some researchers believe its effects may be caused by hypericin, pseudohypericin, or hyperforin.

Media and Marketing Claims	Efficacy
Alleviates mild depression	?↑
Promotes emotional well-being	NR

Advisory

May cause photosensitivity, especially in fair-skinned individuals

Drug/Supplement Interactions

- Do not combine with antidepressant medications (tricyclics, serotonin reuptake inhibitors); possible dangerous additive effects
- Negative interaction with cyclosporin (immunosuppressant), decreases effectiveness
- Potentially decreases effectiveness of a variety of drugs metabolized via the cytochrome P450 enzyme pathway, including oral contraceptives, protease inhibitor indinavir (for HIV infections), theophylline (bronchodilator), digoxin, and numerous other drugs for epilepsy, heart disease, depression, immune suppression, psychosis

KEY POINTS

- Clinical trials in Europe have suggested that SJW may improve symptoms of mild to moderate depression compared to a placebo. And, it also may have similar benefits and fewer side-effects compared to antidepressants. Some have criticized that the dosages, preparations, and the inclusion criteria for patients have not been consistent. The NIH study in progress has attempted to correct for the limitations of these studies and should provide useful information that adds to the totality of the scientific data.

- Studies in patients with major depression are contradictory. Much more evidence is needed before SJW can be recommended as an alternative to antidepressants for severe depression. Severely depressed individuals should be under the care of a mental health professional.

- There is no evidence that SJW elevates mood or improves emotional well-being in individuals without clinical depression.

- SJW negatively interacts with a number of prescription drugs. Patients and physicians need to be aware of these interactions to prevent possible adverse effects.

FOOD SOURCES

None

DOSAGE INFORMATION/BIOAVAILABILITY

SJW dried extract is available in tablets, capsules, teas, powders, and tinctures. It is also commonly added to products that contain valerian root, kava or black cohosh. Labels suggest protecting the herb from heat or light to preserve its active components. Most clinical studies used 300 mg SJW extract as tablets (standardized to 0.3 percent hypericin) taken three times per day (900 mg extract total). In one study, ingestion of 300 mg to 900 mg SJW extract raised plasma levels of hypericin and pseudohypericin in 2.0 hours to 2.6 hours and 0.3 hours to 1.1 hours, respectively. Plasma levels reached a steady state after four days of supplementation (3).

RELEVANT RESEARCH

St. John's Wort and Mild to Moderate depression

- In a double-blind, parallel-design, multicenter study in Germany, 324 patients were randomized to receive 500 mg hypericum extract ZE 117 or 150 mg imipramine (antidepressant drug) for six weeks. Main outcome measures included: Hamilton Rating Scale for Depression (HAMD), clinical global impression scale (CGIS), and patient's global impression scale. Both groups improved on the main outcome measures, with no significant differences between groups. However, the mean score on the anxiety-somatization subscale of the HAMD reported a significant improvement with SJW compared to imipramine. Tolerability was also significantly better with SJW. The authors concluded that SJW is therapeutically equivalent to imipramine in treating mild to moderate depression, but the herb appears to be better tolerated (4).

- In a double-blind, placebo-controlled multicenter trial in Germany, 263 patients with moderate depression were randomized to receive 1,050 mg SJW extract (divided into three doses daily), 100 mg imipramine (in three doses), or a placebo daily for eight weeks. SJW was significantly more effective in reducing HAMD scores than the placebo, and as effective as imipramine. No differences between SJW and imipramine were found for Hamilton anxiety scores, clinical global impressions scales and the Zung self-rating depression scale. Quality of life was more improved with both active treatments compared to the placebo. The rate of adverse events was similar between SJW and the placebo, which was less than that of the imipramine group (5)

S

- In a double-blind, parallel-design study, 240 subjects were randomized to receive 500 mg SJW extract (hypericum Ze 117) or 40 mg of the serotonin reuptake inhibitor fluoxetine (prozac) for six weeks. Both groups had reductions in mean HAMD scores, with no significant differences between the treatments. However, SJW use was associated with a significantly superior score on the mean Clinical Global Impression Scale item I (severity) and also the responder rate. Incidence of adverse events was significantly lower with SJW (8 percent) compared to Prozac (23 percent) (6).

- In a double-blind, parallel design study, 30 outpatients with mild to moderate depression were randomized to receive 600 mg of standardized SJW (LI 160) or 50 mg sertraline (serotonin reuptake inhibitor) daily for one week, followed by 900 mg SJW or 75 mg sertraline daily for six weeks. Symptom severity levels as measured by HAMD and the Clinical Global Impression Scale were significantly reduced in both treatment groups. Clinical response (defined as greater than or equal to 50 percent reduction in HAMD scores) was observed in 47 percent of SJW subjects and 40 percent of sertraline subjects. Both treatments were well tolerated (7).

- In a double-blind, parallel, placebo-controlled study, 147 outpatients suffering from clinically diagnosed mild or moderate depression were randomized to receive one of three treatments: (1) a placebo, (2) 300 mg standardized SJW extract (5 percent hyperforin), or (3) 300 mg extract (0.5 percent hyperforin) for 42 days. Depressive symptoms were assessed using the HAMD on days 0, 7, 14, 28, and 42. Depression was also rated by the investigators at the beginning and end of the study using the Clinical Global Impression Scale. Extract containing 5 percent hyperforin was significantly superior to the placebo in alleviating depressive symptoms according to HAMD scores, whereas the clinical effects of 0.5 percent hyperforin extract were not different from the placebo group. The authors concluded that the therapeutic effect of SJW depends on its hyperforin content (8).

- In a double-blind, comparative study, 165 patients with mild to moderate depression were randomly assigned to receive 900 mg standardized SJW or 75 mg tricyclic amitriptyline (antidepressant) for six weeks. There were no significant differences between groups on the HAMD response rate, although there was a tendency for a better response in the amitriptyline group. Decreases in the total HAMD and Montgomery-Asberg scores showed a significant advantage for amitriptyline, but only at week 6. Fewer adverse events occurred with subjects using St. John's wort (37 percent of subjects) compared to amitriptyline (64 percent), specifically in relation to anticholinergic and central nervous system side-effects (dry mouth, drowsiness, dizziness). Other reported side-effects included headache, constipation, and nausea/vomiting. The author suggested that the superiority in tolerability of SJW could improve compliance in antidepressant pharmacotherapy (9).

- European researchers completed a meta-analysis of 23 randomized clinical trials of SJW lasting four to eight weeks in outpatients with mild or moderate depression (n = 1,757). Twenty trials used double-blind designs, 15 trials were placebo-controlled, and three trials compared SJW to tricyclic antidepressants. Daily doses of hypericin and the dose of the total extract varied considerably in the studies examined (0.4 mg to 2.7 mg and 300 to 1,000 mg, respectively). Most of the studies were conducted in Germany. The results reported that SJW extracts were significantly more effective than placebo and equally as effective as standard antidepressants. Side-effects (not specified) were seen in 19.8 percent of the patients using SJW compared to 52 percent of patients taking antidepressant drugs. The authors noted that the daily dose of SJW varied greatly among studies and classification of depressive disorders was not consistent. They concluded that future research should compare SJW with other antidepressants in well-defined groups of patients and should systematically evaluate the efficacy of different extracts and doses (10).

- The National Institutes of Health (NIH) is funding the first US multicenter study of SJW. The study began in January 1998 and results are expected to be available in 2002 (contact *www.clinicaltrials.gov*). Patients with major depression (n = 336) have been randomly assigned to receive 900 mg standardized SJW, a placebo, or a serotonin uptake inhibitor for eight weeks, and the regimen will be continued for an additional four months in patients who respond positively to SJW.

St John's Wort and Major Depression

- In a double-blind, placebo-controlled, multicenter study in the United States, 200 patients with major depression were randomized to receive either SJW extract (900 mg/day for four weeks, increased to 1,200 mg/day in the absence of response), or a placebo for eight weeks. All subjects completed a one-week, single-blind, run-in of placebo use prior to treatment. The main outcome measure was rate of change on the Hamilton Rating Scale for Depression (HAMD) and secondary measures included the Beck Depression Inventory (BDI), Hamilton Rating Scale for Anxiety (HAM-A), the Global Assessment of Function (GAF) scale, and the Clinical Global Impression-Severity and Improvement scales (CGI-S and CGI-I). There were no significant differences in any of the assessment scales. The proportion of subjects responding was not different between groups. The number reaching remission of illness was significantly higher with SJW (14.3 percent) than the placebo (4.9 percent) group, although overall numbers were considered low. Treatment was well tolerated, with the exception of significantly greater occurrence of headache with SJW compared to the placebo. The authors concluded that SJW was not effective for major depression in this study (11).

- In a double-blind, comparative, multicenter study, 209 clinically diagnosed severely depressed patients (ages 18 y to 70 y) were randomized to receive 1,800 mg standardized SJW extract divided into three doses or 150 mg imipramine (antidepressant)/day for six weeks. Response was defined as a reduction of at least 50 percent of the HAMD. Both treatments were effective, as measured by a reduction in the scale but not statistically equivalent within an *a priori* defined 25 percent interval of deviation (imipramine was more effective). Both treatments were statistically equivalent, as measured by global assessment of efficacy by the investigators and patients. The percentage of adverse effects (ie, dry mouth, gastric symptoms, sedation, sweating, constipation) was statistically significantly greater in imipramine-treated subjects (41 percent of subjects) than in SJW-treated subjects (23 percent). The authors acknowledged the need for more studies in this population but suggested that SJW may be an alternative to synthetic tricyclic antidepressant imipramine in the majority of severe forms of depression (12).

SAFETY

- There are no controlled studies conducted for longer than eight weeks testing the safety of SJW supplementation in humans. The risk of relapse and side-effects that may occur with long-term use is not known

- SJW appears to decrease the effectiveness of a number of prescription drugs. This negative drug interaction is believed to be due to SJW's inhibition of human cytochrome P450 enzymes (13). There have been several reports of organ rejection after transplant when SJW is combined with the immune suppressant drug cyclosporin A (14–18). In addition, SJW may decrease levels of digoxin for heart patients and indinavir used to treat HIV (19, 20). Following the release of reports of drug interactions, FDA warned health professionals of potential adverse effects of using SJW with other drugs that are metabolized via the P450 enzyme pathway. These drugs include: oral contraceptives, antiepileptics, anti-inflammatories, antidepressants, antivirals, benzodiazepines, beta-blockers, and several other drugs for cardiovascular diseases.

- Reported side-effects with SJW include gastrointestinal symptoms, dizziness, headache, allergic reactions, and fatigue (21, 22).

- The effects of taking SJW in addition to standard antidepressant medications have not been studied. It has been suggested that this combination could result in "serotonin syndrome," a condition characterized by flushing, lethargy, confusion, agitation, tremors, and sweating. A washout period of two weeks has been recommended to prevent the possible dangerous additive effects of psychoactive drugs and SJW (23).

- In livestock, SJW causes photosensitivity. Although this reaction has not been seen in humans, it may be advisable for people, especially fair-skinned individuals, to lessen sun exposure while taking this herb alone or in conjunction with photosensitizing drugs (22, 24).

- SJW was originally believed to act as an MAO inhibitor; however, this has not been demonstrated *in vivo*, and there have been no reported MOA-inhibitor associated hypertensive crises in humans using SJW, to date (25).

- Chronic administration of 900 mg/kg of a standardized SJW extract resulted in non-specific symptoms of toxicity in rats and dogs, including reduced body weight, slight pathological changes in liver and kidneys, and some histopathological changes in the adrenals. The no-effect single dose in mice and rats was reported to be greater than 5,000 mg/kg SJW extract (25).

REFERENCES

1. Nathan PJ. Hypericum perforatum (St John's Wort): a non-selective reuptake inhibitor? A review of the recent advances in its pharmacology. *J Psychopharmacol.* 2001;15:47–54.

2. Blumenthal M, ed. *The Complete German Commission E Monographs Therapeutic Guide to Herbal Medicines.* Austin, Tex: American Botanical Council; 1998.

3. Staffeldt B, Kerb R, Brockmoller J, et al. Pharmacokinetics of hypericin and pseudohypericin after oral intake of the *Hypericum perforatum* extract LI 160 in healthy volunteers. *J Geriatr Psychiatry Neurol.* 1994;7(suppl 1):S47–S53.

4. Woelk H. Comparison of St. John's wort and imipramine for treating depression: randomized controlled trial. *BMJ.* 2000;321:536–539.

5. Phipp M, Kohnen R, Hiller KO. Hypericum extract versus imipramine or placebo in patients with moderate depression: randomized multicenter study of treatment for eight weeks. *BMJ.* 2000;319:1534–1538.

6. Schrader E. Equivalence of St John's wort extract (Ze 117) and fluoxetine: a randomized, controlled study in mild-moderate depression. *Int Clin Psychopharmacol.* 2000;15:61–68.

7. Brenner R, Azbel V, Madhusoodanan S, et al. Comparison of an extract of hypericum (LI 160) and sertraline in the treatment of depression: a double-blind, randomized pilot study. *Clin Ther.* 2000;22:411–419.

8. Laakmann G, Schule C, Baghai T, et al. St. John's wort in mild to moderate depression: the relevance of hyperforin for the clinical efficacy. *Pharmacopsychiatry.* 1998;31(suppl 1):54–59.

9. Wheatley D. LI 160, an extract of St. John's wort, versus amitriptyline in mildly to moderately depressed outpatients—a controlled 6 week clinical trial. *Pharmacopsychiatry.* 1997;30(suppl 2):77–80.

10. Linde K, Ramirez G, Mulrow CD, et al. St John's wort for depression—an overview and meta-analysis of randomized clinical trials. *BMJ.* 1996;313:253–258.

11. Shelton RC, Keller MB, Gelenberg A, et al. Effectiveness of St John's wort in major depression: a randomized controlled trial. *JAMA* 2001;285:1978–1986.

12. Vorbach EU, Arnoldt KH, Hubner WD. Efficacy and tolerability of St. John's wort extract LI 160 versus imipramine in patients with severe depressive episodes according to ICD-10. *Pharmacopsychiatry.* 1997;30(suppl 2):81–85.

13. Obach RS. Inhibition of human cytochrome P450 enzymes by constituents of St John's wort, an herbal preparation used in the treatment of depression. *J Pharmacol Exp Ther.* 2000;294:88–95.

14. Karliova M, Treichel U, Malago M, et al. Interaction of Hypericum perforatum (St. John's wort) with cyclosporin A metabolism in a patient after liver transplantation. *J Hepatol.* 2000;33:853–855.

15. Mai I, Kruger H, Budde K, et al. Hazardous pharmacokinetic interaction of Saint John's wort (Hypericum perforatum) with the immunosuppressant cyclosporin. *Int J Clin Pharamcol Ther.* 2000;38:500–502.

16. Barone GW, Gurley BJ, Ketel BL, et al. Drug interaction between St. John's wort and cyclosporine. *Ann Pharmacother.* 2000;34:1014–1016.

17. Breidenbach T, Kliem V, Burg M, et al. Profound drop of cyclosporin A whole blood trough levels caused by St. John's wort (*Hypericum perforatum*). *Transplantation.* 2000;27:2229–2230.

18. Ruschitzkaa F, Meier PJ, Turina M, et al. Acute heart transplant rejection due to Saint John's wort. *Lancet.* 2000;355:1912.

S

19. Johne A, Brockmoller J, Bauer S, et al. Pharmacokinetic interaction of digoxin with an herbal extract from St John's wort (Hypericum perforatum). *Clin Pharmacol Ther.* 1999;66:338–345.
20. Piscitelli SC, Burstein AH, Chaitt D, et al. Indinavir concentrations and St John's wort. *Lancet.* 2000;355:547–548.
21. De Smet PA, Nolen WA. St John's wort as an antidepressant. *BMJ.* 1996;313:241–242.
22. Kupecz D. St John's wort: an alternative therapy in treating depression. *Nurse Pract.* 1998;23:110–112.
23. Gordon JB. SSRIs and St. John's wort: possible toxicity? *Am Fam Physician.* 1998;57:950, 953.
24. Brockmoller J, Reum T, Bauer S, et al. Hypericin and pseudohypericin: pharmacokinetics and effects on photosensitivity in humans. *Pharmacopsychiatry.* 1997;30(suppl 2):94–101.
25. Cott JM, Fugh-Berman A. Is St John's wort (*Hypericum perforatum*) an effective antidepressant? *J Nerv Ment Dis.* 1998;186:500–501.

Saw Palmetto (*Serenoa repens*)

Native to the southern regions of North America, the berries of the saw palmetto plant were used in the early part of the century to treat conditions such as cystitis and bronchitis. Possible active constituents in saw palmetto include free fatty acids, sitosterols, flavonoids, and polysaccharides. The liposterolic (fatty acids and sterols) extract of saw palmetto has been investigated for its potential role in treating benign prostatic hyperplasia (BPH). The mechanism of action of saw palmetto is not fully understood. One theory suggests that saw palmetto may benefit BPH by inhibiting 5a-reductase, thereby limiting the conversion of testosterone into dihydrotestosterone (DHT) (1, 2, 3). Because DHT is associated with hyperplasia, it has been implicated in the pathogenesis of BPH. Studies have also shown that saw palmetto inhibits the binding of DHT to androgen receptors in prostate cell lines, and that it may exert antioxidant and anti-inflammatory effects (4, 5, 6).

Media and Marketing Claims	Efficacy
Improves symptoms related to an enlarged prostate	?↑
Prevents prostate cancer	NR

Advisory

- Rarely, causes gastrointestinal discomfort
- Regular consultation with a physician is recommended for individuals taking this herb

Drug/Supplement Interactions

- No reported adverse interactions
- Theoretically, may interfere with hormone drug therapies

KEY POINTS

- Evidence from clinical trials is limited in terms of the short duration of studies and variability in study design, formulations, and reports of outcomes. The available research suggests that saw palmetto improves urologic symptoms and flow measures. When compared to standard therapy for BPH (finasteride), saw palmetto appears to have similar improvement in urinary tract symptoms and urinary flow and has less reported adverse effects. More research is needed using standardized supplements to determine long-term efficacy.

- The German Commission E monograph on saw palmetto states that the herb only relieves the symptoms associated with an enlarged prostate but does not reduce the enlargement.

- There is currently no evidence that saw palmetto prevents prostate cancer in humans.

FOOD SOURCES

None

DOSAGE INFORMATION/BIOAVAILABILITY

Saw palmetto is available in capsules, tablets, or tinctures from the liposterolic portion of the berry in hexane or ethanol extract. Labels suggest taking 160 mg to 320 mg of the extract daily (equivalent to 2 ml to 4 ml of tincture or 3 g to 4 g of dried berries). Some products are standardized to contain 85 percent to 95 percent fatty acids. Most studies used the liposterolic extract of *Serenoa repens (S repens)* available in Europe and the United States.

RELEVANT RESEARCH

Saw Palmetto and Benign Prostate Hyperplasia (BPH)

- In a systematic review of 18 randomized controlled trials (16 were double-blinded) of 2,939 subjects with BPH, reviewers found that subjects treated with saw palmetto (*S repens*) for at least 30 days had improvements in urinary tract symptom scores, nocturia, self-rating scores of urinary tract symptoms, peak urine flow, and residual urine volume compared to a placebo. Compared with subjects taking finasteride, subjects treated with saw palmetto had similar improvements in urinary tract symptom scores and peak urine flow and had a lower rate of erectile dysfunction. The authors noted that the results should be viewed with caution because many of the studies did not report outcome data and statistical information consistently (7).

- In a double-blind, placebo-controlled U.S. study, 44 men with symptomatic BPH, ages 45 y to 80 y were randomized to receive saw palmetto herbal blend (318 mg saw palmetto lipoidal extract plus 240 mg nettle root extract plus 480 mg pumpkin seed extract

S

plus 99 mg lemon bioflavonoid extract plus 570 IU vitamin A) or a placebo daily for six months. Endpoints included routine clinical measures (symptom score, uroflowmetry and postvoid residual urine volumes), blood analyses (prostate-specific antigen, sex hormones, and multiphasic analysis), prostate volumetrics by magnetic resonance imaging, and prostate biopsy. Both groups experienced clinical improvements, with a slight nonsignificant advantage with the saw palmetto blend group. There were no changes in prostate specific antigen or prostate volume in either group. A significant decrease in the percent prostate epithelium (from 17.8 percent at baseline to 10.7 percent at study's end) occurred after saw palmetto blend treatment. Histological studies also indicated a significant increase in percent of atrophic glands (from 25.2 percent to 40.9 percent) with saw palmetto. No adverse effects were noted (8).

SAFETY

- In the research cited, 320-mg doses of saw palmetto extracts were well tolerated for studies lasting up to six months. However, there are no controlled studies testing the safety of long-term supplementation.

- According to the German Commission E monograph on saw palmetto, in rare cases, this herb may be associated with gastrointestinal discomfort. The monograph also notes that consultation with a physician at regular intervals is recommended during use of this herb (9).

- In the cited studies, side-effects of saw palmetto use were generally mild and comparable with the placebo. Minor side-effects reported were primarily gastrointestinal including nausea, constipation, diarrhea, and vomiting (1.3 percent in men taking saw palmetto vs 0.9 percent in placebo subjects vs 1.5 percent in finasteride [drug for BPH] subjects) (7).

- Saw palmetto supplementation was reported as a possible cause of an intraoperative hemorrhage in a male patient undergoing surgery for a brain tumor. His abnormal bleeding time normalized a few days after he stopped taking the herb. This was the first report suggesting saw palmetto has anticoagulant effects (10).

REFERENCES

1. Niederprum HJ, Schweikert HU, Zanker KS. Testosterone 5a-reductase inhibition by free fatty acids from Sabal serrulata fruits. *Phytomedicine.* 1994;1:127–133.
2. Di Silverio F, Monti S, Sciarra A, et al. Effects of long-term treatment with *Serenoa repens* (Permixon) on the concentrations and regional distribution of androgens and epidermal growth factor in benign prostatic hyperplasia. *Prostate.* 1998;37:77–83.
3. Gerber GS. Saw palmetto for the treatment of men with lower urinary tract symptoms. *J Urol.* 2000;163:1408–1412.
4. Plosker GL, Brogden RN. *Serenoa repens* (Permixon). A review of its pharmacology and therapeutic efficacy in benign prostatic hyperplasia. *Drugs Aging.* 1996;9:379–395.

5. Ravenna L, Di Silverio F, Russo MA, et al. Effects of the lipidosterolic extract of *Serenoa repens* (Permixon) on human prostatic cell lines. *Prostate*. 1996;29:219–230.

6. Schulz V, Hansel R, Tyler VE. *Rational Phytotherapy: A Physician's Guide to Herbal Medicine*. 3rd ed. Berlin, Germany: Springler-Verlag, 1998.

7. Wilt TJ, Ishani A, Stark G, et al. Saw palmetto extracts for treatment of benign prostatic hyperplasia: a systematic review. *JAMA*. 1998;280:1604–1609.

8. Marks LS, Partin AW, Epstein JI, et al. Effects of saw palmetto herbal blend in men with symptomatic benign prostatic hyperplasia. *J Urol*. 2000;163:1451–1456.

9. Blumenthal M, ed. *The Complete German Commission E Monographs Therapeutic Guide to Herbal Medicines*. Austin, Tex: American Botanical Council; 1998.

10. Cheema P, El-Mefty O, Jazieh AR. Intraoperative hemorrhage associated with the use of extract of saw palmetto herb: a case report and review of literature. *J Intern Med*. 2001;250:167–169.

Selenium

Selenium, an essential trace mineral, was first recognized as important to human nutrition in the 1970s. As part of a number of selenoproteins in the body, selenium forms the active site of the potent antioxidant enzyme glutathione peroxidase. Functioning synergistically with vitamin E, selenium protects against cellular damage from oxygen radicals. Selenium also plays a role in the function of the thyroid and male reproductive system. Several organic and inorganic forms exist in nature: selenomethionine (predominant form in food); selenocysteine; and methylselenocysteine. Low selenium intakes caused by selenium deficient soil or total parenteral nutrition have been associated with Keshan disease (cardiomyopathy), aspermatogenesis, cataracts, and growth retardation. Although the functions and requirements of selenium are not fully understood, recent research has focused on the potential role of selenium in cancer and cardiovascular disease prevention (1).

Media and Marketing Claims	Efficacy
Protects against cancer	?↑
Reduces risk of cardiovascular disease	↔
Immunity-enhancing	NR
Improves athletic performance	↓

Advisory

Usually safe in doses of less than the Tolerable Upper Intake Level (UL): 400 µg selenium/day for adults

Drug/Supplement Interactions

Two reports of conflicting actions of selenium with the chemotherapeutic drug cisplatin (may protect against cytotoxicity of the drug or enhance cytotoxicity)

KEY POINTS

- Selenium is an essential trace mineral important in human health. Individuals should be encouraged to consume a balanced diet including foods rich in selenium (meat, seafood, whole grains). If dietary selenium is not adequate, a multivitamin/mineral supplying the adult RDA (55 µg) is suggested, and should not exceed the Tolerable Upper Intake Level (400 µg).

- Epidemiological research and evidence from a large multicenter trial suggest that selenium supplements may reduce cancer risk. Additional controlled clinical trials are needed to confirm the results of this study.

- Epidemiological studies are conflicting regarding the relationship of selenium status to heart disease. Again, controlled, clinical trials are required to determine the potential efficacy of selenium in preventing heart disease.

- Preliminary evidence from animal studies and one human study suggest that selenium may enhance lymphocyte function. More research is needed to determine the clinical benefit of selenium supplements in immune-compromised individuals.

- In the few studies reported, selenium does not enhance exercise performance. More evidence is needed on the role of selenium and exercise-induced oxidative stress in humans.

- It is important to note that most of the research on selenium is observational reports on the correlation of plasma selenium levels, not supplements, to a particular disease or condition in humans. More research specifically testing the efficacy and safety of selenium supplements is needed.

FOOD SOURCES

Because of the differences in the selenium content of soil, there is a wide variation in the selenium content of plant foods. Meats, seafood, and whole grains are good sources of selenium. The typical US diet supplies an average of 70 µg to 100 µg selenium/day (1).

Food	Selenium (µg/Serving)*
Tuna, canned in water (3 oz)	56
Beef, lean ground (4 oz)	18
Sunflower seeds, with hulls (1 c)	22
Chicken breast, skinless (½)	24
Egg (1)	16
Bread, whole wheat (1 slice)	9.5
Wheat germ, toasted (2 tbsp)	9.2
Cheese, cheddar (1½ oz)	6.0
Cocoa powder (1 tbsp)	0.8

Source: Data from USDA (2)
*Serving sizes calculated from values from Reference 2.

DOSAGE INFORMATION/BIOAVAILABILITY

Selenium is sold as inorganic sodium selenite or organic selenomethionine in tablets and capsules in doses ranging from 25 µg to 200 µg. High-selenium yeast (organic) is also available in capsules. Selenium is sold in individual supplements or as part of "antioxidant" formulas that also include vitamin E, C, and beta-carotene. The new RDA for selenium is 55 µg/day for both men and women (3). Most ingested selenium is almost completely absorbed. Excretion is the primary homeostatic mechanism for selenium (1).

RELEVANT RESEARCH

Selenium and Cancer

- In a double-blind, placebo-controlled, multicenter trial, 1,312 subjects aged 18 y to 80 y diagnosed with basal/squamous cell carcinomas of the skin were randomized to receive selenium enriched yeast (200 µg/day) or a low-selenium yeast placebo. Subjects were recruited from 1983 to 1990 and followed through 1993. Regular dermatologic exams and plasma selenium concentrations were recorded. Selenium did not affect the primary endpoint: incidence of recurrent skin carcinomas. However, selenium supplementation was correlated with significant reductions in secondary endpoints: mortality from all cancers combined (29 deaths in the selenium group vs 57 deaths in placebo group), incidence of all cancers combined (77 deaths in the selenium group vs 119 deaths in the placebo group), lung cancer, colorectal cancer, and prostate cancer. The blinded phase of the trial was stopped early because of the apparent reductions in mortality and cancer incidence with selenium treatment. The authors concluded: "These effects of selenium require confirmation in an independent trial of appropriate design before new public health recommendations can be made" (4). This study has been criticized for suggesting that selenium supplements have a greater effect on lung cancer reduction than smoking cessation does—a result that shows too strong an effect to be biologically plausible (5).

- Four trials are underway at the Arizona Cancer Center and Arizona College of Public Health to follow up the previous study. These trials will attempt to assess the effects of 200 µg selenium/day on the prevention and treatment of prostate cancer (6).

- In a double-blind, placebo-controlled study, 33 subjects with head and neck cancer were randomized to receive 200 µg/day of sodium selenite on the first day of treatment (eg, surgery, radiation, or both) for eight weeks. Immune functions were monitored. Selenium therapy resulted in significantly enhanced cell-mediated immune responsiveness as measured by the patient's lymphocyte response to stimulation with mitogen, to generate cytotoxic lymphocytes, and to destroy tumor cells. In contrast, the placebo group had a decline in immune responsiveness. Additionally, patients had significantly lower plasma selenium levels than healthy individuals, and patients in stages III or IV of disease had higher levels than those in stage II or IV (7).

- In a randomized controlled trial (Linxian study), 29,584 Chinese adults (aged 40 y to 69 y) were randomized to receive one of four dietary supplements for five years providing doses ranging from one to two times the US RDA: (1) beta-carotene, vitamin E, and selenium; (2) riboflavin and niacin; (3) vitamin C and molybdenum; or (4) retinol and zinc. Mortality and cancer incidence were assessed from March 1986 to May 1991. A total of 2,127 deaths occurred during the trial period (32 percent of all deaths were attributed to esophageal or stomach cancer). There was a significantly lower total mortality (relative risk = 0.91) among subjects supplemented with beta-carotene, vitamin E, and selenium. The reduction was mainly because of lower cancer rates, with the reduced risk beginning to arise about one to two years after the start of supplementation. No significant effects on mortality rates were apparent with the other three treatments. However, the design of this study does not permit the attribution of cancer reduction to selenium alone (8).

- Several epidemiological studies suggest an inverse relationship between selenium status and cancer incidence (9).

Selenium and Cardiovascular Disease

- In a nested, case-control study, prospective plasma samples were taken from subjects in the Physicians' Health Study. Within the study, 251 subjects who had myocardial infarctions (MI) were matched to healthy controls to explore whether plasma selenium predicted the risk of MI. There were no significant differences between groups for mean plasma selenium levels or in comparing highest to lowest quintiles of plasma levels after adjusting for other cardiovascular risk factors. According to the authors, "These data provide no evidence for an association between increased plasma selenium and reduced risk of MI at the current levels of selenium intake within the US" (10).

- In a prospective, cohort study, 3,387 Danish men aged 53 y to 74 y without cardiovascular disease were followed for three years. Subjects completed questionnaires, underwent clinical exams, and had blood samples drawn. Three years later data were collected on the number of ischemic heart disease (IHD) events. Men with serum selenium levels in the lowest tertile had a 70 percent increased risk of IHD (11).

- In a cross-sectional study of 1,132 Eastern Finnish men (mean age = 54 y), serum selenium concentrations had a strong significant inverse relationship with platelet aggregation and a weak positive relationship with plasma HDL cholesterol levels. Men with ischemic electrocardiogram findings during exercise had a lower mean selenium level than men with normal electrocardiograms (12).

- A review article summarized possible mechanisms whereby selenium may protect against heart disease including reduction of LDL oxidation, modulation of prostaglandin synthesis and platelet aggregation, and protection against toxic heavy metals. However, the author noted: "The therapeutic benefit of selenium administration in the prevention and treatment of cardiovascular diseases still remains insufficiently documented" (13).

Selenium and Immunity

- In a randomized, placebo-controlled study, 21 healthy subjects with selenium replete status (as indicated by plasma selenium levels) were randomized to receive 200 µg selenium/day as sodium selenite or a placebo for eight weeks. The ability of peripheral blood lymphocytes to develop into cytotoxic lymphocytes, destroy tumor cells, respond to stimulation with alloantigen, and affect the activity of natural killer cells was measured. Supplementation resulted in a 118 percent increase in cytotoxic lymphocyte-mediated tumor cytotoxicity and an 82.3 percent increase in natural killer cell activity compared to baseline values. Selenium supplements did not produce significant changes in plasma selenium levels. The authors concluded: "The results indicated that the immuno-enhancing effects of selenium in humans require supplementation above the replete levels produced by normal dietary intakes" (14).

- Selenium deficiency appears to have deleterious effects on the immune system in animal studies (15). For example, in one study, a benign form of a human enterovirus (coxsackievirus) became virulent in selenium-deficient mice (16). Several *in vitro* and animal studies have demonstrated that selenium may protect immune cells (lymphocytes) from oxidative damage and radiation (17), and enhance lymphocyte function (18, 19).

- Selenium deficiency has been reported in HIV-positive patients. A review article noted that selenium deficiency is a significant predictor of HIV-related mortality independent of CD4 and antiretroviral treatment (20).

- In a prospective, observational study, 134 surgical and medical intensive care unit (ICU) patients were assessed for plasma selenium concentrations and presence or absence of systemic inflammatory response syndrome (SIRS), sepsis, or direct ischemia-reperfusion during their ICU stay. Patients with SIRS had lower plasma selenium concentrations than those without SIRS. Plasma selenium was also lower in all patients with severe sepsis and septic shock, and in patients with ischemia-reperfusion from aortic cross-clamping. The frequency of ventilator associated pneumonia, organ system failure, and mortality was three-fold higher in patients with low plasma selenium concentrations at time of admission (= 0.70 µmol/L) than for the other patients. The authors concluded that the decrease in plasma selenium concentrations reached values observed in nutritional selenium deficiency and may be associated with the increase in morbidity and mortality of these patients (21).

Selenium and Exercise

- In a double-blind, placebo-controlled study, 24 healthy, untrained, male subjects were given 180 µg selenium (selenomethionine) or a placebo during a 10-week endurance training program (three times a week). A maximum endurance treadmill test was completed before and after the training. Maximal oxygen uptake and plasma and erythrocyte glutathione peroxidase activity were measured before and after the test. Training significantly increased plasma glutathione peroxidase activity and aerobic power and capacity. Selenium supplementation caused a significant increase in the basal plasma glutathione level but had no effect on physical performance parameters (22).

- Selenium and/or vitamin E deficient rats were found to have oxidative free radical generation in lung tissue as measured by electron spin resonance spectra. The oxidative generation increased when rats were subjected to exhaustive exercise. Selenium and/or vitamin E-supplemented rats did not experience free radical generation during exercise. The authors suggested that these supplements offer protection against exercise-induced oxidative stress (23).

SAFETY

- The Tolerable Upper Intake Level (UL), the highest amount likely to pose no adverse effects, is 400 µg/day (3).

- No serious adverse effects were reported with 200 µg selenium/day for several years (4).

- Doses above 750 µg/day were associated with loss of hair and nails in China, whereas an average consumption of 724 µg in high seleniferous areas of South Dakota and Wyoming showed no toxicity. Other symptoms of reported toxicity include nausea, diarrhea, irritability, peripheral neuropathy, and fatigue (1).

REFERENCES

1. Burk RF, Levander OA. Selenium. In: Shils ME, Olson JA, Shike M, Ross AC, eds. *Modern Nutrition in Health and Disease*. 9th ed. Baltimore, Md: Williams & Wilkins; 1999:265–276.
2. USDA nutrient data laboratory. Agricultural Research Service. Available at: http://www.nal.usda.gov/fnic/. Accessed July 3, 2002.
3. Food and Nutrition Board, Institute of Medicine. *Dietary reference Intakes: Vitamin C, Vitamin E, Selenium, and Carotenoids*. Washington, DC: National Academy Press; 2000.
4. Clark LC, Combs GF, Turnbull BW, et al. Effects of selenium supplementation for cancer prevention in patients with carcinoma of the skin. A randomized controlled trial. Nutritional Prevention of Cancer Study Group. *JAMA*. 1996;276:1957–1963.
5. Colditz GA. Selenium and cancer prevention. Promising results indicate further trials required. *JAMA*. 1996;276:1984–1985.
6. Clark LC, Marshall JR. Randomized, controlled chemoprevention trials in populations at very high risk for prostate cancer: elevated prostate-specific antigen and high-grade prostatic intraepithelial neoplasia. *Urology*. 2001;185–187.
7. Kiremidjian-Schumacher L, Roy M, Glickman R, et al. Selenium and immunocompetence in patients with head and neck cancer. *Biol Trace Elem Res*. 2000;73:97–111.
8. Blot WJ, Li JY, Taylor PR, et al. Nutrition intervention trials in Linxian, China: supplementation with specific vitamin/mineral combinations, cancer incidence, and disease-specific mortality in the general population. *J Natl Cancer Inst*. 1993;85:1483–1492.
9. Fleet JC. Dietary selenium repletion may reduce cancer incidence in people at high risk who live in areas with low soil selenium. *Nutr Rev*. 1997;55:277–279.
10. Salvini S, Hennekens CH, Morris JS, et al. Plasma levels of the antioxidant selenium and risk of myocardial infarction among U.S. physicians. *Am J Cardiol*. 1995;76:1218–1221.
11. Suadicani P, Hein HO, Gyntelberg F. Serum selenium concentration and risk of ischemic heart disease in a prospective cohort study of 3000 males. *Atherosclerosis*. 1992;96:33–42.

S

12. Salonen JT, Salonen R, Seppanen K, et al. Relationship of serum selenium and antioxidants to plasma lipoproteins, platelet aggregability and prevalent ischemic heart disease in Eastern Finnish men. *Atherosclerosis.* 1988;70:155–160.

13. Neve J. Selenium as a risk factor for cardiovascular diseases. *J Cardiovasc Risk.* 1996;3:42–47.

14. Kiremidjian-Schumacher L, Roy M, Wishe HI, et al. Supplementation with selenium and human immune cell functions. II. Effect on cytotoxic lymphocytes and natural killer cells. *Biol Trace Elem Res.* 1994;41:115–127.

15. Patterson BH, Levander OA. Naturally occurring selenium compounds in cancer chemoprevention trials: a workshop summary. *Cancer Epidemiol Biomarkers Prev.* 1997;6:63–69.

16. Beck MA, Kolbeck PC, Shi Q, et al. Increased virulence of a human enterovirus (coxsackievirus B3) in selenium-deficient mice. *J Infect Dis.* 1994;170:351–357.

17. Sun E, Xu H, Liu Q, et al. Effect of selenium in recovery of immunity damaged by H_2O_2 and ^{60}Co radiation. *Biol Trace Elem Res.* 1995;48:239–250.

18. Roy M, Kiremidjian-Schumacher L, Wishe HI, et al. Supplementation with selenium restores age-related decline in immune cell function. *Proc Soc Exp Biol Med.* 1995;209:369–375.

19. Kiremidjian-Schumacher L, Roy M, Wishe HI, et al. Regulation of cellular immune response by selenium. *Biol Trace Elem Res.* 1992;33:23–35.

20. Baum MK, Shor-Posner G. Micronutrient status in relationship to mortality in HIV-1 disease. *Nutr Rev.* 1998;56(1 pt 2):S135–S139.

21. Forceville X, Vitoux D, Gauzit R, et al. Selenium, systemic immune response syndrome, sepsis, and outcome in critically ill patients. *Crit Care Med.* 1998;26:1536–1544.

22. Tessier F, Margaritis I, Richard MJ, et al. Selenium and training effects on the glutathione system and aerobic performance. *Med Sci Sports Exerc.* 1995;27:390–396.

23. Reddy KV, Kumar TC, Prasad M, et al. Pulmonary lipid peroxidation and antioxidant defenses during exhaustive physical exercise: the role of vitamin E and selenium. *Nutrition.* 1998;14:448–451.

Shark Cartilage

Shark cartilage is thought to contain a substance that may inhibit angiogenesis (the formation of new blood vessels typically seen in malignant tumors). Because the shark skeleton is made up of cartilage (a nonvascularized tissue) and sharks rarely develop neoplasms, it has been hypothesized that consuming shark cartilage may help slow tumor growth. Although the active component(s) have not been identified, one recent study isolated a potent angiogenesis inhibitor composed of two single peptides from blue shark cartilage. One inhibitor, SCF2, appears to be a heat-stable proteoglycan that contains keratan sulfate units and peptides. From preliminary *in vitro* studies and a popular consumer book *Sharks Don't Get Cancer*, some extrapolated that shark cartilage could cure cancer in humans (1–3).

Note: Shark cartilage is also a source of chondroitin sulfate. (*See* Chondroitin Sulfate.)

Media and Marketing Claims	Efficacy
Cures cancer	NR

Caution

- Not enough data to evaluate safety
- One report of hepatitis associated with shark cartilage ingestion

Drug/Supplement Interactions

No reported adverse interactions

KEY POINTS

- There is currently no evidence from controlled trials that shark cartilage cures cancer in animals or humans. Although the media has reported on a few human trials in cancer patients outside the United States (1), these studies have not been published in peer-reviewed journals; thus, their validity is difficult to assess.

- *In vitro* and animal studies suggest that shark cartilage decreases tumor vascularization, however, these results provide limited evidence of its efficacy in humans. One of the first controlled human studies suggested that shark cartilage inhibits angiogenesis in healthy men with experimentally induced wounds. An open clinical trial of cancer patients did not show any benefit with supplementation, although controlled trials are needed to substantiate these results. In sum, clinical trials in large populations are needed to determine whether shark cartilage has an effect on cancer prognosis.

- The National Institutes of Health (NIH) National Center for Complementary and Alternative Medicine allocated $1 million in March 1998 to be distributed through the National Cancer Institute's nationwide system of oncology groups for trials of shark or bovine cartilage for cancer treatment. Two double-blind, placebo-controlled, randomized studies and one open trial are in progress. One study is examining shark cartilage extract in patients receiving chemotherapy and radiation for non-small cell lung cancer. Another is testing shark cartilage in patients with metastatic kidney cancer. The third, open phase II study, is investigating shark cartilage in patients with relapsing or refractory multiple myeloma. These studies will add more evidence to determine the efficacy and safety of shark cartilage in cancer patients. (Check *www.clinicaltrials.gov* for updates.)

FOOD SOURCES

None

DOSAGE INFORMATION/BIOAVAILABILITY

Shark cartilage is sold in capsules, tablets, and powder form. Manufacturers' labels suggest taking 5-mg to 20-g doses three to four times a day. Manufacturers suggest mixing the powder with water and taking it orally or as an enema. Some of the potentially active components of shark cartilage are only recently being investigated, and therefore the intestinal absorption of crude shark cartilage extract needs to be studied.

RELEVANT RESEARCH

Shark Cartilage and Angiogenesis/Cancer

- In a placebo-controlled study, 29 healthy male subjects were randomized into three groups for 23 days: (1) 7 mL liquid shark cartilage extract; (2) 21 mL liquid shark cartilage extract; or (3) placebo. On day 12, a polyvinyl alcohol sponge threaded in a perforated silicone tubing was inserted subcutaneously in the arm and removed on day 23. Researchers indirectly measured angiogenesis by assessing of endothelial cell density with factor VIII immunostaining on histological sections of the implant. Mean endothelial cell density was significantly lower in groups that had received either dose of shark cartilage extract. There were no differences among groups in side-effects, blood chemistry, urine analysis, or bleeding times. The authors concluded: "These results demonstrate that the liquid cartilage extract contains an antiangiogenic component bioavailable in humans by oral administration. This is the first report of an inhibition of wound angiogenesis in healthy men." (4)

- In an open clinical trial, 60 patients with advanced previously treated cancer (breast, colorectal, lung, prostate, non-Hodgkin lymphoma, brain, and unknown primary tumor) were given 1 g shark cartilage/kg/day divided into three doses for 12 weeks. Evaluation of extent of disease, quality of life score, and hematologic, biochemical, and selected immune function were determined at baseline, and after 6 and 12 weeks. Thirteen patients were lost to follow-up or refused treatment, 5 patients were taken off the study because of adverse gastrointestinal side-effects (nausea, vomiting, or constipation) or intolerance to shark cartilage, and 5 patients died of progressive disease during the study. No complete or partial positive responses were noted. Twenty percent of the 50 assessable patients (or 16.7 percent of the 60 intent-to-treat patients) had stable disease for 12 weeks or more. The authors concluded: "Under the specific conditions of this study, shark cartilage as a single agent was inactive in patients with advanced-stage cancer and had no salutary effect on quality of life. The 16.7 percent rate of stable disease was similar to results in patients with advanced cancer treated with supportive care alone" (5). However, the results of this study should be viewed with caution because it lacked standard controls (placebo and blinding).

- In a study of mice with induced renal tumors, oral shark cartilage had no significant effect in the rate of development of dysplastic renal tubules in mice receiving shark cartilage vs control animals. However, use of shark cartilage significantly delayed development of papillary and solid tumors compared to the rate for controls (6).

- In an animal study, mice implanted with tumors in the rear feet (SCCVII carcinoma) were injected with shark cartilage extracts in doses ranging from 5 mg to 100 mg per mouse daily for 25 days postimplantation of the primary tumor. None of the shark cartilage doses tested had any effect on attenuating the growth of the primary tumor, nor

S

did it inhibit the development of metastases to the lungs, assessed at autopsy. Compared to controls, shark cartilage-treated mice had no signs of adverse toxicity as measured by changes in body weight and lethality. The authors concluded: "Our results offer no support for the proposed use of shark cartilage extracts as an anticancer therapy" (7).

- In an *ex vivo* study, crude extracts of shark cartilage were incubated with rabbit corneas that contained implanted tumors. After 19 days, the maximum blood vessel lengths of the tumors were measured. Corneas treated with shark cartilage showed sparse vascularization and average vessel length was 75 percent shorter than in the controls. The authors concluded that shark cartilage extract from basking sharks strongly inhibited tumor-induced neovascularization *in vitro* (8).

- Other animal and *in vitro* studies have shown shark cartilage extract to have an antiangiogenic and anti-inflammatory effect (2, 9–12).

SAFETY

- There is limited research extending beyond 12 weeks testing the safety of shark cartilage supplementation in humans. One open study reported 21 adverse effects, most of which were gastroenterologic (nausea, vomiting, constipation). However, because this trial was not placebo-controlled, it is also likely that the adverse events were caused by cancer treatments (5).

- There is one case report of hepatitis attributed to seven weeks of shark cartilage supplementation in a 57-year-old man (dose not specified) (13).

REFERENCES

1. Hunt TJ, Connelly JF. Shark cartilage for cancer treatment. *Am J Health Syst Pharm.* 1995;52:1756, 1760.
2. Sheu JR, Fu CC, Tsai ML, et al. Effect of U-995, a potent shark cartilage-derived angiogenesis inhibitor, on anti-angiogenesis and anti-tumor activities. *Anticancer Res.* 1998;18:4435–4441.
3. Liang JH, Wong KP. The characterization of angiogenesis inhibitor from shark cartilage. *Adv Exp Med Biol.* 2000;476:209–223.
4. Berbari P, Thibodeau A, Germain L, et al. Antiangiogenic effects of the oral administration of liquid cartilage extract in humans. *J Surg Res.* 1999;87:108–113.
5. Miller DR, Anderson GT, Stark JJ, et al. PhaseI/II trial of the safety and efficacy of shark cartilage in the treatment of advanced cancer. *J Clin Oncol.* 1998;16:3649–3655.
6. Barber R, Delahunt B, Grebe SK, et al. Oral shark cartilage does not abolish carcinogenesis but delays tumor progression in a murine model. *Anticancer Res.* 2001;21:1065–1069.
7. Horsman MR, Alsner J, Overgaard J. The effect of shark cartilage extracts on the growth and metastatic spread of the SCCVII carcinoma. *Acta Oncol.* 1998;37:441–445.

S

8. Lee A, Langer R. Shark cartilage contains inhibitors of tumor angiogenesis. *Science.* 1983;221:1185–1187.

9. Dupont E, Savard PE, Jourdain C, et al. Antiangiogenic properties of a novel shark cartilage extract: potential role in the treatment of psoriasis. *J Cutan Med Surg.* 1998;2:146–152.

10. McGuire TR, Kazakoff PW, Hoie EB, et al. Antiproliferative activity of shark cartilage with and without tumor necrosis factor-a in human umbilical vein endothelium. *Pharmacotherapy.* 1996;16:237–244.

11. Fontenele JB, Araujo GB, de Alencar JW, et al. The analgesic and anti-inflammatory effects of shark cartilage are due to a peptide molecule and are nitric oxide (NO) system dependent. *Biol Pharm Bull.* 1997;20:1151–1154.

12. Fontenele JB, Viana GS, Xavier-Filho J, et al. Anti-inflammatory and analgesic activity of a water-soluble fraction from shark cartilage. *Braz J Med Biol Res.* 1996;29:643–646.

13. Ahsar B, Vargo E. Shark-cartilage induced hepatitis. *Ann Intern Med.* 1996;125:780–781.

Sodium Bicarbonate

Sodium bicarbonate (baking soda) is an alkaline salt that buffers metabolic acids in the body. Because exhaustion during high-intensity exercise has been attributed to lactic acidosis and an increase in hydrogen ion (H^+), bicarbonate supplementation has been proposed to enhance the buffering capacity of the blood. Metabolic demands of high-intensity activity are met mainly by the anaerobic breakdown of glucose resulting in the production of metabolic acids (lactic acid), which decrease the pH of exercising muscle. It is thought that bicarbonate may reduce the acidity of muscle cells by drawing out H^+ and lactic acid. Theoretically, increasing the body's buffering capacity may delay the onset of fatigue and improve exercise performance (1).

Media and Marketing Claims	Efficacy
Enhances power and strength	?↑

Advisory

- Potential side-effects include cramps, bloating, and diarrhea
- Not for use by those with sodium restrictions

Drug/Supplement Interactions

No reported adverse interactions

KEY POINTS

- Laboratory studies of high-intensity exercise show that sodium bicarbonate (300 mg/kg) may exert an ergogenic effect under conditions of anaerobic exercise lasting from one to seven minutes. In contrast, there are relatively few field studies testing the effectiveness of sodium bicarbonate supplementation in specific sports.

- Sodium bicarbonate supplementation is not recommended for recreational athletes because of possible gastrointestinal side-effects and because its potential benefits are limited to near maximal exercise lasting one to seven minutes. One review summarized: "The use of $NaHCO_3$ loading while engaging in sustained exercise at much lower intensities for more than 10 minutes should not be practiced." Additionally, chronic sodium bicarbonate supplementation is not recommended for any individual because of the high sodium load.

FOOD SOURCES

Sodium bicarbonate is household baking soda.

DOSAGE INFORMATION/BIOAVAILABILITY

Sodium bicarbonate is sold in capsules, usually with other alkaline salts (sodium phosphate and sodium citrate). Most products recommend taking 15 g to 22 g sodium bicarbonate with water one to two hours before exercise.

RELEVANT RESEARCH

Sodium Bicarbonate and Exercise Performance

- In a meta-analysis, 29 randomized, placebo-controlled, double-blind trials (total n = 285 subjects) supplementing bicarbonate during anaerobic exercise (sprints on a cycle or row ergometer, or track run) were analyzed. Only 3 percent of the subjects were female. Studies provided bicarbonate in dosages ranging from 100 mg to 400 mg sodium bicarbonate/kg body weight ($\approx$ 7 g to 28 g for a 70-kg person) via capsules, solution, or intravenous injection. The time interval for ingestion ranged from a bolus dose to ingestion throughout a three-hour time period immediately before exercise or up to three hours prior to exercise. The main endpoints assessed in most of the trials included time to exhaustion, changes in power over a given period of time, and total work accomplished during a period of time. Sixteen of the trials included in the analysis showed no effect with treatment compared to 19 studies that reported benefits. Sodium bicarbonate ingestion resulted in a more alkaline blood pH, with the dosage only moderately related to the increase in pH and HCO_3. Overall, there was a positive effect on performance with bicarbonate (weighted mean effect size = 0.44), indicating that the mean performance of the bicarbonate trials was 0.44 standard deviations better than the placebo trial. However, the range of effect was large. The authors attributed this to differing dosages, intensity and duration of exercise, and conditions of ingestion. Studies involving performance trials with a large anaerobic segment, large doses of bicarbonate, or repetitive work bouts showed the most powerful ergogenic effect. The authors noted that some studies failed to provide complete information on methodologies, particularly ingestion information of bicarbonate and accompanying fluids (2).

- One review article reported that while there is evidence in laboratory studies that the administration of sodium bicarbonate improves high power performance, only one out of five field studies reported a beneficial effect (3).

- Another review article concluded that bicarbonate (300 mg/kg) loading delays fatigue during exhaustive exercise lasting one to seven minutes, but that studies employing other exercise protocols and lower dosages have not consistently improved performance (1).

SAFETY

- Ingestion of sodium bicarbonate is contraindicated for individuals with sodium intake restriction. A typical dose (15 g to 22 g) contains 4 g to 6 g sodium.

- Doses of 300 mg/kg body weight have not been associated with any reported serious adverse effects.

- However, some subjects report gastrointestinal distress, including diarrhea, cramps, and bloating after ingestion. This is attributed to the sodium load, which pulls additional fluid into the intestine to create an isotonic solution. Drinking sufficient water may alleviate these side-effects (1).

REFERENCES

1. Linderman JK, Gosselink KL. The effects of sodium bicarbonate ingestion on exercise performance. *Sports Med.* 1994;18:75–80.
2. Matson LG, Tran ZV. Effects of sodium bicarbonate ingestion on anaerobic performance: a meta-analytic review. *Int J Sport Nutr.* 1993;3:2–28.
3. Horswill CA. Effects of bicarbonate, citrate, and phosphate loading on performance. *Int J Sport Nutr.* 1995;5:S111–S119.

Soy Protein and Isoflavones

S

Soy protein and isoflavones (a type of flavonoid found primarily in soy products) are found naturally in food and packaged in supplements. They are being investigated for their potential protective role in heart disease, cancer, menopause, and osteoporosis. Isoflavones are naturally occurring weak estrogens (also called phytoestrogens) that may exert both estrogenic and antiestrogenic properties. Genistein, daidzein, and glycetein are the principle isoflavones in the soybean (1).

FDA reviewed research and approved the health claim for soy foods and supplements that dietary intake of 25 g soy protein per day had a cholesterol-lowering effect. FDA permits health claims for soy products that allow foods and supplements containing 6.25 g soy protein (or one-fourth of the 25-g amount shown in studies to have a cholesterol-lowering effect) to carry statements about the role of soy protein in reducing the risk of coronary heart disease in conjunction with a diet low in saturated fat and cholesterol (2).

Media and Marketing Claims	Efficacy
Lowers cholesterol	↑
Reduces risk of breast and prostate cancer	NR
Treats menopause symptoms	NR
Reduces risk of osteoporosis	NR

Advisory

- Should not be used by women with breast cancer until more data are gathered
- Ipriflavone, a synthetic isoflavone dietary supplement, may be associated with lymphocytopenia

Drug/Supplement Interactions

- Soy supplements may reduce the absorption of thyroid replacement drugs (levothyroxine) when taken concurrently
- Theoretically, the potential estrogenic properties of soy could interfere with estrogen replacement therapy
- May reduce absorption of thyroid replacement drugs (levothyroxine)

KEY POINTS

- There is evidence that soy protein may lower cholesterol levels in individuals with hypercholesterolemia but apparently has less of an effect in individuals with normal cholesterol levels. Whether these effects are specifically related to isoflavones or other compounds in soy protein (eg, saponins, phytic acid) or an interaction between soy protein and isoflavones needs further study. Therefore, at present, soy foods are preferable to concentrated supplements of isolated genistein or daidzein.

- The potential relationship between soy protein and specific isoflavones in human cancer is inconclusive. *In vitro* and animal studies are promising; however, studies specifically testing soy protein supplements or genistein in cancer prevention studies or cancer treatment in humans are lacking. In one animal study, genistein appeared to stimulate mammary cancer growth in ovariectomized mice. The notion that age at administration may be a critical factor in how soy protein or isoflavones affect cancer is intriguing and requires further study. Currently, several trials are underway testing the effects of soy on the development of prostate cancer.

- Preliminary research is conflicting regarding the effect of soy protein supplementation on hot flashes. Some studies reported a significant placebo response, and thus, the effectiveness of soy was difficult to assess. Most of the positive studies reported only minimal reductions in hot flashes. Although the data are insufficient to suggest soy

S

protein as an alternative to hormone replacement therapy, soy foods are nutritious and clearly play a role in a healthful eating plan for both women and men.

- Preliminary research from one study suggests that soy protein containing isoflavones (2.25 mg isoflavones/g protein) increases lumbar bone density and may attenuate losses in postmenopausal women. Currently, a number of studies are underway testing the effect of soy protein or isoflavone supplements on bone health. Earlier studies using the synthetic isoflavone, ipriflavone, have shown a reduction in bone loss in postmenopausal women. However, a large-scale, well-controlled trial of ipriflavone supplements reported no benefit in women with osteoporosis and was associated with significant decreases in lymphocyte concentrations. In general, however, whole soy foods are preferred over supplements because many soy products such as whole soybeans, tofu prepared with calcium salts, and fortified soy milk are also good sources of calcium, which plays a role in preserving bone density.

- Although people in certain cultures have been consuming soy foods for centuries, the efficacy and safety of concentrated sources of isolated isoflavones in pill form is not known. As with other phytochemicals, the composition of isoflavones in plants with other nutrients and numerous other phytochemicals occur in certain proportions. Until the research is clear, soy products such as soy milk and soy-based beverages, tofu, and whole soybeans will continue to be the preferred source of soy protein, isoflavones, and other potentially bioactive compounds in the diet.

FOOD SOURCES

Food	Soy Protein (g) (3)	Genistein (mg)	Daidzein (mg) (4)
Natto (fermented soybeans) (½ c)	15	32	23
Flour, soy (½ c)	22	94	56
Milk, soy (1 c)	7	6	4
Nuts, soy, roasted (2 tbsp)	5	26	16
Protein isolates, soy (isolated soy protein—92% protein)	23 (1 oz)*	51 (½ c)*	19 (½ c)*
Soybeans (½ c)	11	6	20
Tempeh (½ c)	16	32	23
Soy protein, dry textured (½ c) (70% protein)	11 (6)	72	43
Tofu (4 oz)	17	19	9

Soy protein gram amounts adapted from USDA (4) and US Soyfoods Directory (5).
*Amounts in parentheses = serving sizes.

Most soy products (soybean, tofu, soy milk, tempeh, soy flour) contain isoflavones; however, soy foods undergoing processing techniques that use excessive water, alcohol, or organic washings have few isoflavones. For example, textured soy protein or soy protein concentrates made by aqueous alcohol extraction are very low in isoflavones because the isoflavones are soluble in alcohol and are thus removed during processing. Lowering of isoflavone contents of some soy products may result from dilution of added ingredients (ie, water in soy milk). Soy oil and soy sauce contain no appreciable soy protein or isoflavones (6).

In general, a 7-g to 10-g serving of soy protein supplies 30 mg to 50 mg isoflavones (1 mg to 2 mg genistein/g soy protein). Three servings of soy foods (ie, 2 c soy milk, 4 oz tofu) provide approximately 20 g to 30 g soy protein.

In the United States, the average daily intake of genistein is 1 mg to 2 mg compared to 20 mg to 80 mg in Japan (7).

DOSAGE INFORMATION/BIOAVAILABILITY

Soy protein powders provide 1 mg to 10 mg isoflavones in 1.0 g to 3.5 g of soy protein. A typical serving of a commercial soy protein supplement provides approximately 20 g to 25 g protein. Soy isoflavones are available in tablets or capsules, powders, drinks, and bars. Genistein supplements provide 30 mg to 55 mg genistein. Mixed isoflavonoid supplements typically provide 25 mg to 100 mg total isoflavones. The bioavailability of isoflavones apparently varies from 13 percent to 35 percent depending on gut microflora (8). Ingestion of 60 g soy protein resulted in increased plasma concentrations of genistein (plasma peak after 6 to 8 hours) and daidzein (plasma peak after 1.5 hours) (9).

RELEVANT RESEARCH

Soy Protein/Isoflavones and Cardiovascular Disease

- A meta-analysis of 38 controlled clinical trials (n = 730 subjects) evaluated the effects of soy protein consumption on serum lipid levels in humans. Twenty studies used isolated soy protein, 15 used textured soy protein, and 3 used a combination of the two. There was a significant association between soy protein intake (average intake = 47 g/day) and improved serum lipids. Thirty-four of 38 trials reported decreases in serum cholesterol. Overall, daily soy protein consumption was associated with a 9.3 percent decrease in total cholesterol, 12.9 percent decrease in LDL cholesterol, and 10.5 percent decrease in serum triglycerides. There was an insignificant increase in HDL cholesterol (10).

- In a double-blind, placebo-controlled trial, 213 male and female, healthy (normotensive, normolipidemic) subjects (ages 50 y to 75 y) were randomized to receive either soy protein isolate (40 g soy protein, 118 mg isoflavones) or placebo (casein) daily for three months. One-hundred seventy-nine subjects completed the study. Dietary compliance was measured by urinary phytoestrogen levels. Blood pressure, lipids, hormone profiles, vascular function, and endothelial function were assessed. Soy was associated with a significant reduction in mean blood pressure ($\downarrow$ 4.2 mm Hg) compared to placebo. Soy also resulted in significant reductions in low- to high-density lipoprotein ratios and triglycerides (TG), but also resulted in an increase in lipoprotein a (Lp(a)). Both groups experienced improved total, LDL, and HDL cholesterol with no significant differences between groups. There were no significant changes in any hormonal level (FSH, LH, testosterone) in males or females in either group. Arterial function also did not differ between groups, as both groups improved. Peripheral vascular resistance significantly improved with soy, whereas flow-mediated vasodilation (measure of endothelial function) actually declined in male subjects consuming soy compared to a placebo. The authors noted that soy supplementation had both beneficial (improved blood pressure, cholesterol ratios, TG, peripheral vascular resistance) and negative cardiovascular effects (increase in Lp(a) and decline in endothelial function in men) (11).

- In a double-blind, placebo-controlled trial, 104 postmenopausal women were randomized to receive 60 g isolated soy protein or a placebo (caseinate) daily for 12 weeks. Seventy-seven subjects (44 were dyslipidemic) completed the trial. Both the soy and placebo groups experienced significant reductions in total and LDL cholesterol, but only soy had a significant reduction on apolipoprotein B and the LDL/HDL ratios. Lipoprotein (a) plasma levels were not significantly changed by either treatment. The authors concluded that isolated soy protein is slightly better than caseinate in favorably modifying the lipoprotein metabolism of postmenopausal women, and this effect is greatest in those with hypercholesterolemia (12).

- In a double-blind, parallel design trial, 156 men and women with hypercholesterolemia who had been given instruction in a National Cholesterol Education Program Step I diet were randomized for nine weeks to one of five daily diets: 25 g isolated soy protein with 3, 27, 37, or 62 mg isoflavones, or 25 g casein (for isoflavone-free comparison). Compared with casein, soy protein with 62 mg of isoflavones significantly lowered total and LDL cholesterol levels by 4 percent and 6 percent, respectively. Soy protein with 37 mg isoflavones reduced total and LDL cholesterol by 8 percent. There was a dose-response effect of increasing amounts of isoflavones on total and LDL cholesterol levels. Triglycerides and HDL cholesterol were not affected. Soy protein with only 3 mg isoflavones had no significant effect on lipid levels (13).

- In a double-blind, placebo-controlled trial, 156 subjects with hypercholesterolemia on a National Cholesterol Education Program (NCEP) Step I cholesterol-lowering diet were randomized to consume one of five beverages for nine weeks: (1) 25 g soy protein containing 62 mg isoflavones, (2) 25 g soy protein containing 37 mg isoflavones, (3) 25 g soy protein containing 27 mg isoflavones, (4) 25 g soy protein containing 3 mg isoflavones, or (5) a placebo beverage (25 g casein, 0 mg isoflavones). Prior to randomization to treatment, subjects completed a four-week run-in using the NCEP step 1 diet. In subjects with a baseline LDL > 160 mg/dL, LDL cholesterol was significantly reduced by 10 percent in those subjects ingesting the 62-mg isoflavone dose and by 10 percent in subjects ingesting the 37-mg isoflavone dose compared to the placebo, but not with lower levels of isoflavone. In subjects with baseline LDL between 140 mg/dL and 160 mg/dL, there was no significant effect on cholesterol with any soy protein beverage (14).

- In a placebo-controlled, single-blinded, crossover study, 21 healthy, normocholesterolemic perimenopausal and menopausal women were assigned in random order to receive 80 mg isoflavones (45 mg genistein) without soy protein or a placebo for five weeks each. A second isoflavone five-week period was added at the end of the study. Four weeks prior to the study, subjects were counseled by a dietitian to follow a base-line diet (less than 30 percent fat, rich in whole grains, fruits, and vegetables, and no soy or legumes). During the study, background diets were closely monitored by a dietitian. Laboratory measures were taken at the baseline and at the end of the treatment and placebo periods. Isoflavone treatment resulted in a significant 26 percent improvement in systemic arterial compliance (arterial elasticity) compared to the placebo. Arterial pressure and plasma lipids were not affected. The authors concluded: "One important measure of arterial health, systemic arterial compliance, was significantly improved in perimenopausal and menopausal women taking soy isoflavones to about the same extent as is achieved with hormone replacement therapy" (15).

- In a controlled study, 60 ovariectomized monkeys were assigned to one of three groups for 12 weeks and fed diets containing: (1) casein-lactalbumin (CAS) as the protein source; (2) CAS plus a semipurified extract of soy, rich in isoflavones; or (3) intact soy protein. The intact soy group had significantly lower plasma total, LDL, and HDL cholesterol than the CAS group. The semipurified extract of soy did not have the same effects as intact soy protein on plasma lipids (16).

- Two review articles discussed potential mechanisms by which soy protein and/or isoflavones may reduce risk of heart disease. Animal and *in vitro* studies have demonstrated that soy may: (1) increase bile acid excretion, (2) promote estrogenic activity, (3) improve vascular reactivity, and (4) inhibit LDL cholesterol oxidation and exhibit antioxidant activity. Alternatively, soy protein may displace foods high in saturated fat and cholesterol and thus have an indirect effect on lowering blood cholesterol levels (17, 18).

Soy Protein/Isoflavones and Cancer

- Several epidemiological studies have found that consumption of soy foods is associated with lower risk of breast, colon, and prostate cancers in China and Japan. Consumption of nonfermented soy products (soy milk and tofu) tended to be either protective or not associated with cancer risk, whereas no consistent pattern was apparent with fermented soy foods (miso). In the studies that demonstrated a protective effect, a single serving of soy (½ c tofu or 1 c soy milk) was associated with reduced cancer risk (19).

- Several animal and *in vitro* studies have shown that genistein inhibits growth of a wide range of cancerous cell lines including breast, colon, lung, leukemia, and prostate cells. Specifically, genistein inhibits protein tyrosine kinases, DNA topoisomerases, and other critical enzymes involved in cell growth and signal transduction (19, 20).

- Rats treated neonatally or prepubertally with genistein had a longer latency before the appearance of experimentally induced mammary tumors and a reduction in tumor number compared to control rats. Rats given genistein after 35 days of age showed less reduction in breast cancer risk. However, in a study of ovariectomized mice, genistein increased cell proliferation of human breast cancer cell xenografts compared to the control diet (21).

- One article noted that most *in vitro* studies have used concentrations of isoflavones in excess of 10 µM, a blood level greater than the 1 µmol to 5 µmol blood level that can be achieved even with high soy consumption (a soy beverage providing 42 mg genistein and 27 mg daidzein raised plasma levels of isoflavones from 0.55 µmol to 0.86 µmol after two weeks). However, one study did report that nontransformed human mammary epithelial cells are far more sensitive to genistein at lower concentrations (0.5 µmol to 1.0 µmol), implying that genistein may have a greater chemopreventive effect before tumor cell phenotype is acquired. The authors concluded that although the plasma genistein levels achievable with soy food feeding are unlikely to be sufficient to inhibit the growth of mature, established breast cancer cells by chemotherapeutic-like mechanisms, these levels potentially could have a chemopreventive effect by regulating the proliferation of epithelial cells in the breast (22).

Soy Protein/Isoflavones and Menopause

- In a double-blind, placebo-controlled study, 69 menopausal women were randomized to one of three groups for 24 weeks to receive: (1) isolated soy protein with 80.4 mg isoflavones/day; (2) isolated soy protein with 4.4 mg of isoflavones/day; or (3) whey protein control. A menopausal index assessed changes in hot flashes and night sweats and other symptoms at baseline, week 12 and week 24. There were no differences between groups in hot flash or night sweat frequency. However, there was a significant decrease in hot flash and night sweat frequency with time in all treatment groups. The authors concluded that this indicated a placebo effect or simply an improvement in symptoms during the course of the trial (23).

- In a double-blind, placebo-controlled, multicenter study, 177 postmenopausal women (mean age = 55 y) who were experiencing five or more hot flashes per day were randomized to receive either soy isoflavone extract (total of 50 mg genistin and daidzin per day) or a placebo daily for 12 weeks. Both groups experienced relief of vasomotor symptoms; however, the soy group had significant reductions in hot flashes during the first two weeks whereas the placebo group had no relief until week 4. Throughout 12 weeks, the soy group had greater reductions in frequency and severity of hot flashes, but this difference did not reach significance. Examination of endometrial thickness by ultrasound, lipoproteins, bone markers, sex hormone-binding globulin and follicle-stimulating hormone, and vaginal cytology did not change in either group (24).

- In a double-blind, placebo-controlled, crossover study, 177 breast cancer survivors with substantial hot flashes receive in random order soy tablets (150 mg soy isoflavones—similar to amount in three glasses of soy milk) and a placebo each daily for four weeks, following a one-week baseline period with no treatment, but no washout. Patients completed a daily questionnaire documenting hot flash frequency and intensity, and perceived side effects. At the end of the study, use of soy tablets had no effect on hot flashes (25).

- In a double-blind, placebo-controlled study, two groups of postmenopausal women were randomized to the control group (n = 19) and given a placebo or to the treated group (n = 20) and given 400 mg/day standardized soy extract (50 mg isoflavones).

S

After six weeks, conjugated equine estrogens were given to each subject for four weeks. At the end of this period, soy and placebo treatment were stopped, and subjects were given medroxyprogesterone acetate with the estrogen daily until week 12. At week 6, when compared to pretreatment data, a significant reduction in the mean number of hot flashes per week and severity of hot flashes was observed in subjects receiving soy, whereas a greater effect of relief was observed in both soy and placebo groups during estrogen therapy. No soy-related changes were observed in vaginal cytology, endometrial thickness, uterine artery pulsatility index, or metabolic and hormonal parameters. The authors concluded that soy appears to be a safe and effective treatment for relief of hot flashes in women who refuse or have contraindications for hormone replacement therapy (26).

- In a double-blind, placebo-controlled study, 104 postmenopausal women were randomized to receive 60 g soy protein isolate containing 40 g protein and 76 mg isoflavones daily or a placebo (60 g casein, no isoflavones) for 12 weeks. Twenty-five patients dropped out of the study (11 in the soy group, 14 in the placebo group) because of gastrointestinal side-effects such as constipation and bloating. Changes from baseline in self-reported mean number of moderate to severe hot flashes and night sweats were measured during treatment. Compared to ingesting the placebo, subjects consuming soy protein reported significantly fewer mean number of hot flashes per 24 hours after 4, 8, and 12 weeks. Specifically, soy resulted in a 26 percent reduction in the mean number of hot flashes by week 3, a 33 percent reduction by week 4, and a 45 percent reduction in hot flashes compared to 30 percent reduction in the placebo group by week 12. The overall rates of adverse effects were similar for soy and casein-placebo (27).

- In a controlled study, 97 free-living post-menopausal women were randomly assigned to a group provided with soy foods substituting approximately one-third of total caloric intake (textured soy protein, dry whole soy beans providing a total of 165 mg isoflavones/day) or a control group that was instructed to eat as usual for four weeks. Soy foods were provided by the researchers. Changes in follicle stimulating hormone (FSH), leutinizing hormone (LH), sex hormone-binding globulin, and vaginal cytology were measured to assess estrogenic response. FSH and LH did not decrease and sex hormone binding globulin did not increase in the soy group as hypothesized. The authors concluded: "A four-week, soy-supplemented diet was expected to have estrogenic effects on the liver and pituitary in postmenopausal women, but estrogenic effects were not seen. At most, there was a small estrogenic effect on vaginal cytology" (28).

Soy Protein/Isoflavones/Ipriflavone and Osteoporosis

- In a double-blind, placebo-controlled study, 69 perimenopausal subjects were randomly assigned to one of three groups for 24 weeks: (1) soy protein isolate with isoflavones (80.4 mg/day); (2) soy protein isolate with poor isoflavone content; or (3) control (whey protein). Treatment was given in the form of a muffin and protein powder to be mixed into a drink. Subjects were told to stop taking any of their own supplements and were provided with a vitamin and mineral supplement containing 160 mg calcium (all treatments provided 650 mg calcium daily). Lumbar spine bone mineral density (BMD) and bone mineral content (BMC) were assessed at baseline and at the end of the trial. Change in BMD did not occur in either soy group, but significant BMD losses occurred in the control group. When various factors were taken into account (such as body composition, alcohol intake, smoking history, and hormone levels), the soy protein with isoflavones had a significant positive effect on the percentage of change (loss) in both BMD and BMC (29).

- In a double-blind, placebo-controlled study, 66 free-living, hypercholesterolemic, postmenopausal women were randomized to one of three groups for six months to receive: (1) NCEP Step I diet with 40 g protein/day from casein and nonfat dry milk, (2) NCEP Step I diet with 40 g protein from isolated soy protein containing 1.39 mg isoflavones/g protein, or (3) NCEP Step 1 diet with 40 g isolated soy protein containing 2.2 mg isoflavones/g protein. Prior to randomization, all subjects followed a 14-day run-in period on the NCEP Step I diet. Total and regional bone mineral content and density of the lumbar spine, proximal femur and total body were assessed by dual-energy x-ray absorptiometry at the baseline and after six months. Blood lipids were also analyzed at the baseline and every two weeks during the study. Of the skeletal sites tested, lumbar-spine bone mineral content and density increased significantly after six months of treatment with soy protein containing 2.2 mg isoflavones/g protein compared to the control group. The lower dose (1.39 mg isoflavones/g) was not associated with any significant changes in bone density. Both soy protein treatments were associated with a significant increase in HDL cholesterol and improvement in the ratio of total to HDL cholesterol compared to control (30).

- Several studies conducted in Europe and Asia found ipriflavone (600 mg), a synthetic isoflavone derivative available as a dietary supplement, reduced bone loss in animal models of experimental osteoporosis and in postmenopausal women (31–34).

- In a double-blind, placebo-controlled, multicenter study in Europe, 475 postmenopausal women with osteoporosis of the lumbar spine were randomized to receive 600 mg ipriflavone or a placebo daily for three years. Both groups received 500 mg calcium/day. Spine, hip, and forearm BMD were assessed by dual-energy radiograph absorptiometry, and biomarkers of bone resorption were measured every six months. The number of new vertebral fractures was assessed each year. There were no differences in the yearly percentage of change in BMD at any site compared to baseline between groups. There were also no differences in biochemical markers and vertebral fractures. Subjects receiving ipriflavone had a significant reduction in lymphocyte concentrations that began six months after treatment. Thirty-one subjects developed lymphocytopenia, which returned to normal levels in 81 percent of the subjects after two years (35).

- In a double-blind, placebo-controlled, multicenter study in Italy, 198 postmenopausal women (aged 50 y to 65 y) with vertebral bone density below the mean value for normal were randomized to receive 600 mg ipriflavone or a placebo for two years. All subjects also received a daily calcium supplement of 1 g as calcium carbonate.

One-hundred thirty-four subjects completed the trial. Bone density and markers of bone turnover were measured at the baseline and every six months. Analysis of liver and kidney function and routine hematological blood tests were measured before and at the end of treatment. There was a significant increase in vertebral bone density in the ipriflavone-treated women with average percent changes of +1.4 after one year, and +1 percent after two years. The difference in bone density between the placebo and ipriflavone groups was significant. Urinary hydroxyproline was significantly decreased in ipriflavone-treated subjects, suggestive of a reduction in bone turnover rate. Patient compliance assessed by residual tablet count, revealed a drug intake of > 80 percent after two years in 92 percent of all subjects (32).

SAFETY

- Soy foods have been consumed in Asian cultures for centuries. However, the detailed studies to assess long-term safety of isoflavone supplements or high intakes of isolated soy protein are needed to explore potential safety issues.

- There is some concern that soy protein and isoflavones, which possess weak estrogenic activity, may stimulate cancer proliferation in women with breast cancer (36, 37). Genistein administered to ovariectomized mice with experimentally induced breast cancer stimulated tumor growth (21, 38). Until more research is available, women with breast cancer should consult with their oncologist and avoid using soy protein and concentrated isoflavone supplements.

- Soy protein supplementation appears to slightly alter thyroid hormones (39, 40). In one case report, a 45-year-old woman with hypothyroidism required unusually high doses of levothyroxine to achieve suppressive levels of free thryoxine (T(4)) and thyroid-stimulating hormone (TSH). The patient had been taking her thyroid medication with a soy protein supplement drink. Taking the soy protein drink at a different time improved her thyroid levels (41).

- Some individuals exhibit soy protein allergy to soybeans and soy foods, although the incidence is rare.

- In a case report, daily consumption of a soy protein supplement drink decreased absorption of levothyroxine in a 45-year-old woman with a history of thyroidectomy. Higher doses of the thyroid replacement drug were needed to achieve therapeutic serum thryroid hormone levels. In light of this report, individuals on thyroid replacement therapy should get their physician's approval before taking soy supplements. (42)

REFERENCES

1. Anderson RL, Wolf WJ. Compositional changes in trypsin inhibitors, phytic acid, saponins, and isoflavones related to soybean processing. *J Nutr.* 1995;125:581S–588S.
2. FDA Proposed Rule. Food labeling: health claims; soy protein and coronary heart disease. *Fed Regist.* November 10, 1998;63:62977–63015.

S

3. USDA nutrient data laboratory. Agricultural Research Service. Available at: http://www.nal.usda.gov/fnic/cgi-bin/nut_search.pl. Accessed August 23, 1999.

4. Kirk P, Patterson RE, Lampe J. Development of a soy food frequency questionnaire to estimate isoflavone consumption in US adults. *J Am Diet Assoc.* 1999;99:558–563.

5. U.S. Soyfoods Directory. Soyfoods descriptions. Available at: http://www.soyfoods.com/soyfoodsdescriptions/TexturedSoyProtein.html. Accessed August 23, 1999.

6. Lusas EW, Riaz MN. Soy protein products: processing and use. *J Nutr.* 1995;125:573S–580S.

7. Barnes S, Peterson TG, Coward L. Rationale for the use of genistein-containing soy matrices in chemoprevention trials for breast and prostate cancer. *J Cell Biochem Suppl.* 1995;22:181–187.

8. Xu X, Harris KS, Wang HJ, et al. Bioavailability of soybean isoflavones depends upon gut microflora in women. *J Nutr.* 1995;125:2307–2315.

9. Watanabe S, Yamaguchi M, Sobue T, et al. Pharmacokinetics of soybean isoflavones in plasma, urine, and feces of men after ingestion of 60 g baked soybean powder (Kinako). *J Nutr.* 1998;128:1710–1715.

10. Anderson JW, Johnstone BM, Cook-Newell ME. Meta-analysis of the effects of soy protein intake on serum lipids. *N Engl J Med.* 1995;333:276–282.

11. Teeded HJ, Dalais FS, Kosopoulos D, et al. Dietary soy has both beneficial and potentially adverse cardiovascular effects: a placebo-controlled study in men and postmenopausal women. *J Clin Endocrinol Metab.* 2001;86:3053–3060.

12. Vigna GB, Pansini F, Bonaccorsi G, et al. Plasma lipoproteins in soy-treated postmenopausal women: a double-blind, placebo-controlled trial. *Nutr Metab Cardiovasc Dis.* 2000;10:315–322.

13. Crouse JR, Morgan T, Terry JG, et al. A randomized trial comparing the effect of casein with that of soy protein containing varying amounts of isoflavones on plasma concentrations of lipids and lipoproteins. *Arch Intern Med.* 1999;159:2070–2076.

14. Crouse JR III. Soy protein containing isoflavones reduces plasma concentrations of lipids. *Arch Intern Med.* In press.

15. Nestel PJ, Yamashita T, Pomeroy S, et al. Soy isoflavones improve systemic arterial compliance but not plasma lipids in menopausal and perimenopausal women. *Arterioscler Thromb Vasc Biol.* 1997;17:3392–3398.

16. Greaves KA, Parks JS, Williams JK, et al. Intact dietary soy protein, but not adding an isoflavone-rich soy extract to casein, improves plasma lipids in ovariectomized cynomolgus monkeys. *J Nutr.* 1999;129:1585–1592.

17. Lichtenstein AH. Soy protein, isoflavones, and cardiovascular disease risk. *J Nutr.* 1998;128:1589–1592.

18. Potter SM. Soy protein and cardiovascular disease: the impact of bioactive components in soy. *Nutr Rev.* 1998;56:231–235.

19. Messina MJ, Persky V, Setchell KD, et al. Soy intake and cancer risk: a review of the *in vitro* and *in vivo* data. *Nutr Cancer.* 1994;21:113–131.

20. Barnes S. Effect of genistein on *in vitro* and *in vivo* models of cancer. *J Nutr.* 1995;125:777S–783S.

S

21. Barnes S. The chemopreventive properties of soy isoflavonoids in animal models of breast cancer. *Breast Cancer Res Treat.* 1997;46:169–179.
22. Barnes S, Sfakianos J, Coward L, et al. Soy isoflavonoids and cancer prevention. Underlying biochemical and pharmacological issues. *Adv Exp Med Biol.* 1996;401:87–100.
23. St Germain A, Peterson CT, Robinson JG, et al. Isoflavone-rich or isoflavone-poor soy protein does not reduce menopausal symptoms during 24 weeks of treatment. *Menopause.* 2001;8:17–26.
24. Upmalis DH, Lobo R, Bradley L, et al. Vasomotor symptom relief by soy isoflavone extract tablets in postmenopausal women: a multicenter, double-blind, randomized, placebo-controlled study. *Menopause.* 2000;7:236–242.
25. Quella SK, Loprinzi CL, Barton DL, et al. Evaluation of soy phytoestrogens for the treatment of hot flashes in breast cancer survivors: a North Central Cancer Treatment Group Trial. *J Clin Oncol.* 2000;18:2793–2793.
26. Scambia G, Mango D, Signorile PG. Clinical effects of a standardized soy extract in postmenopausal women: a pilot study. *Menopause.*2000;7:105–111.
27. Albertazzi P, Pansini F, Bonaccorsi G, et al. The effect of dietary soy supplementation on hot flushes. *Obstet Gynecol.* 1998;91:6–11.
28. Baird DD, Umbach DM, Lansdell L, et al. Dietary intervention study to assess estrogenicity of dietary soy among postmenopausal women. *J Clin Endocrinol Metab.* 1995;80:1685–1690.
29. Alekel DL, St Germain A, Peterson CT, et al. Isoflavone-rich soy protein attenuates bone loss in the lumbar spine of perimenopausal women. *Am J Clin Nutr.* 2000;72:844–852.
30. Potter SM, Baum JA, Teng H, et al. Soy protein and isoflavones: their effects on blood lipids and bone density in postmenopausal women. *Am J Clin Nutr.* 1998;68:1375S—1379S.
31. Brandi ML. Natural and synthetic isoflavones in the prevention and treatment of chronic diseases. *Calcif Tissue Int.* 1997;61:5–8.
32. Agnusdei D, Crepaldi G, Isaia G, et al. A double-blind, placebo-controlled trial of ipriflavone for prevention of postmenopausal spinal bone loss. *Calcif Tissue Int.* 1997;61:142–147.
33. Agnusdei D, Bufalino L. Efficacy of ipriflavone in established osteoporosis and long-term safety. *Calcif Tissue Int.* 1997;61(suppl 1):S23—S27.
34. Agnusdei D, Gennari C, Bufalino L. Prevention of early postmenopausal bone loss using low doses of conjugated estrogens and the non-hormonal, bone-active drug ipriflavone. *Osteoporos Int.* 1995;5:462–466.
35. Alexandersen P, ET AL. Ipriflavone in the treatment of postmenopausal osteoporosis. *JAMA.* 2001;285:1482–1488.
36. McMichael-Phillips DF, Harding C, Morton M, et al. Effects of soy-protein supplementation on epithelial proliferation in the histologically normal human breast. *Am J Clin Nutr.* 1998;68:1431S—1435S.
37. Petrakis NL, Barnes S, King EB, et al. Stimulatory influence of soy protein isolate on breast secretion in pre- and postmenopausal women. *Cancer Epidemiol Biomarkers Prev.* 1996;5:785–794.

38. Hsieh CY, Santell RC, Haslam SZ, et al. Estrogenic effects of genistein on the growth of estrogen-receptor-positive human breast cancer (MCF-7) cells in vitro and in vivo. *Cancer Res.* 1998;58:3833–3838.
39. Persky VW, Turyk ME, Wang L, et al. Effect of soy protein on endogenous hormones in postmenopausal women. *Am J Clin Nutr.* 2002;75:145–153.
40. Divi RL, Chang HC, Doerge DR. Anti-thyroid isoflavones from soybeans: isolation, characterization, and mechanism of action. *Biochem Pharmacol.* 1997;54:1087–1096.
41. Bell DS, Ovalle F. Use of soy protein and resultant need for increased dose of levothyroxine. *Endocr Pract.* 2001;7:193–194.
42. Bell DS, Ovalle F. Use of soy protein supplement and resultant need for decreased dose of levothryoxine. *Endoc Pract.* 2001; 7:193–194.

Spirulina/Blue-Green Algae

One of many forms of blue-green algae, spirulina (*Spirulina platensis* or *Spirulina maxima*) is a multicellular organism classified as a group of cyanobacteria. Spirulina grows wild in highly alkaline lakes. Other forms of algae used in supplements include *Aphanizomenon flos aquae* (blue-green algae) and *Chlorella pyrenoidosa* (green algae). The characteristic blue-green color in spirulina is because of the chlorophyll and phycocyanin content. These pigments and other compounds (glycolipids and sulfolipids) have been studied for their potential anti-inflammatory, antioxidant, and antiviral properties. Spirulina (platensis) has a history of use in an African village in Chad where dried cakes of spirulina (called *dihe*) are harvested from Lake Chad and are eaten with meals and in sauces. Spirulina (maxima) is also found abundantly in Lake Texcoco near Mexico City. It is thought that spirulina was harvested, dried, and sold for human consumption by the Aztecs during the time of Spanish conquest (1–4).

Dried spirulina contains 60 percent to 70 percent protein, 10 percent to 20 percent carbohydrates, 9 percent to 14 percent lipids (including gamma-linolenic acid and some cholesterol), 4 percent nucleic acids, and 4 percent to 6 percent ash (minerals). In general, microalga are viewed as having a protein quality value greater than other vegetable sources, but poorer than animal sources because alga are somewhat deficient in methionine, cysteine, and lysine (2). Spirulina is also a source of beta-carotene and iron. Originally thought to be a source of vitamin B_{12}, B_{12} analogues present in algae are not considered biologically active (5). Spirulina has been commercialized in feed for animals, as a coloring agent in Japanese foods, and for use in dietary supplements (1–3, 6, 7).

Media and Marketing Claims	Efficacy
Improves immunity	NR
Lowers cholesterol	NR
Reduces cancer risks	NR
Improves intestinal health	NR

S

Advisory

No reported serious adverse effects

Drug/Supplement Interactions

No reported adverse interactions

KEY POINTS

- Like other microbial cells, spirulina is a source of protein, and some vitamins and minerals. These nutrients are found in concentrated amounts, which is why companies promote spirulina as a "superfood." As a protein source, however, spirulina is considerably more expensive than an equivalent amount of protein from eggs, dairy, meat, or soy products. Although rich in certain nutrients, spirulina supplements are not a substitute for the fiber and variety of nutrients and phytochemicals in the five to nine servings of fruits and vegetables recommended for daily consumption by the National Cancer Institute and Food Guide Pyramid. Consumers must decide whether the cost differential is worth supplementing with spirulina.

- There is preliminary evidence from *in vitro* and animal studies suggesting that isolated sulfolipids and sulfated polysaccharides in spirulina provide immune-enhancing and antiviral activity. Controlled clinical trials are needed to determine whether spirulina enhances immune function and resistance to infection in humans.

- Preliminary studies in rodents have reported a lipid-lowering effect with high doses of spirulina. Controlled clinical trials are needed to determine whether this effect is apparent in humans.

- There is preliminary evidence from one human study in India and from animal studies suggesting that spirulina inhibits oral cancers. Additional controlled clinical trials are needed.

- Research on spirulina's effect on digestion and elimination is lacking. However, some strains promote the growth of lactic acid bacteria *in vitro*, which may have a positive effect on the gastrointestinal tract. (*See* Acidophilus for effects on intestinal health.)

FOOD SOURCES

Spirulina (dried cakes) harvested from Lake Chad is consumed in Africa.

DOSAGE INFORMATION/BIOAVAILABILITY

Spirulina is available in tablets, capsules, powders, and in processed foods such as snack bars providing approximately 500 mg per dose. Product labels recommend consuming 3 g to 10 g of the algae per day. Spirulina, along with other microalgae, are cultivated both in man-made environments (photostats) and in naturally occurring environments (2). Ten grams of dried spirulina contains 29 kcal, 0.7 g fat, 5.7 g protein, 2.4 g carbohydrates, 5.7 RE (57 IU) vitamin A, 0.24 mg thiamin, 0.38 mg riboflavin, 1.3 mg niacin, 0.4 mg vitamin B_6, 0 mg vitamin B_{12}, 9.4 µg folate, 1 mg vitamin C, 0.5 mg vitamin E, 104 mg sodium, 136 mg potassium, 12 mg calcium, 20 mg magnesium, 2.8 mg iron, and 0.2 mg zinc (8). Manufacturers' analyses report variable levels of these nutrients, and some report significantly higher levels of vitamin A, iron, and calcium for the same quantity of spirulina.

Note: Spirulina is not a reliable source of vitamin B_{12}, as described later.

The bioavailability of carotenes from spirulina is comparable to other food sources such as carrots (9). In East Indian children with vitamin A deficiency, spirulina (2 g/day) raised serum retinol levels significantly (9). Studies in rats suggest that beta-carotene from spirulina is absorbed and thus can be a source of vitamin A (10). In addition, the absorption of iron from spirulina was lower than that of ferrous sulfate from whole egg, but higher than that from whole wheat (11).

Initial analysis of the vitamin B_{12} content of spirulina using bioassay methods presented values that were not accurate. More sensitive measures (radioassays and newer microbiological methods) have produced data indicating that much of the vitamin B_{12} amounts previously reported were actually B_{12} analogues (2). Vitamin B_{12} analogues are not believed to possess biological activity in humans (12).

RELEVANT RESEARCH

Spirulina and Immunity

- In one animal study, spirulina enhanced humoral and cell-mediated immune functions in chickens (13). In another study, spirulina stimulated macrophage function, phagocytosis, and interleukin-1 in mice (14).

- A sulfated polysaccharide (calcium spirulan) isolated from spirulina was found to inhibit herpes simplex virus type 1, human cytomegalovirus, measles virus, mumps virus, influenza A virus and human immune-deficiency virus (HIV) *in vitro* (15, 16).

- Sulfolipids isolated from blue-green algae (type not specified) demonstrated anti-HIV activity *in vitro* (17).

Spirulina and Cholesterol

- Animal studies conducted by one research group found a hypocholesterolemic effect of *Spirulina platensis* (18, 19). In one study, spirulina prevented the fructose-induced increase in liver triglyceride levels in rats fed a 60 percent fructose diet (20).

Spirulina and Cancer

- In a placebo-controlled, single-blind (details of blinding of subjects not sufficiently described) study, 87 tobacco-chewing subjects from a fishing village in India with oral leukoplakias were randomized to receive 1 g *Spirulina fusiformis* (containing 2 mg beta-carotene, 4 mg total carotenes, 1 µg vitamin B_{12}, 1 mg iron, 0.35 mg zinc, and 0.06 mg vitamin B-complex) or a placebo daily for one year. Subjects were advised to stop using tobacco and alcohol. Subjects had normal plasma concentrations of vitamin A at the baseline and did not suffer from vitamin A deficiency. Biopsies from lesions were

S

taken at baseline and at the end of the study. Subjects were assessed every two months by a dentist and physician who were blinded to treatment groups. Complete response was defined as total disappearance of the lesions. The complete response rates of homogenous lesions were 11 percent with the placebo and 57 percent with spirulina; the difference was statistically significant. None of the nodular and ulcerated leukoplakias (n = 4) responded to treatment. There was no difference between groups in plasma retinol, beta-carotene, and alpha-tocopherol. The authors summarized: "More human trials with hard endpoints in different settings and different populations are required to further establish the effectiveness of spirulina algae before any conclusions can be made" (21).

- Spirulina extracts have been shown to inhibit chemically-induced buccal cancers in animal studies by one group of investigators (22–24).

Spirulina and Intestinal Health

- An *in vitro* study reported that spirulina (platensis) promoted the growth of lactic acid bacteria (*Lactobacillus bulgaricus, L casei, L acidophilus, L lactis, Streptococcus thermophilus*) in media with pH adjusted to 5.3, 6.3, and 7.0. The authors concluded that further experiments in animals and humans are needed to determine whether spirulina may be used as a type of prebiotic to improve lactic acid bacteria colonization and human health (25).

SAFETY

- Spirulina fed at high levels to mice (10, 20, and 30 percent of diet) for 13 weeks had no adverse affects on behavior, food and water intake, growth or survival, blood chemistries, and gross or microscopic findings from postmortem examinations. The algae levels tested were higher than any anticipated human consumption (26). In addition, reproductive toxicity and mutagenicity tests in rodents reported no toxic effects with spirulina (27, 28).

- Some blue-green algae (such as *Aphanizomenon flos aquae*, but not *Spirulina platensis, maxima, or fusiformis*) contain toxins that could pose a danger if they are inadvertently included in supplements when alga are taken from natural water sources. Ingestion could cause allergic reactions, mild liver enzyme elevation, and gastroenteritis in humans (29). Manufacturers have drafted voluntary guidelines to detect and control exposure to cyanotoxins in supplements (2).

- Individuals following vegan and macrobiotic diets should not rely on spirulina as their sole source of vitamin B_{12} because vitamin B_{12} found in algae may not have adequate biological activity. In one study, vitamin B_{12}-deficient vegetarian children did not respond to therapy with spirulina compared to improvements seen in children consuming the vitamin from fish sources (5).

- Although no long-term studies have evaluated the safety of spirulina, this algae along with others has been ingested in different areas of the world as a food for hundreds of years with few reports of adverse effects (1, 2).

REFERENCES

1. Ciferri O. Spirulina, the edible microorganism. *Microbiol Rev.* 1983;47:551–578.
2. Kay RA. Microalgae as food and supplement. *Crit Rev Food Sci Nutr.* 1991;30:555–573.
3. Maranesi M, Barzanti V, Carenini G, et al. Nutritional studies on *Spirulina maxima. Acta Vitaminol Enzymol.* 1984;6:295–304.
4. Romay C, Armesto J, Remirez D, et al. Antioxidant and anti-inflammatory properties of C-phycocyanin from blue-green algae. *Inflamm Res.* 1998;47:36–41.
5. Dagnelie PC, van Staveren WA, van den Berg H. Vitamin B_{12} from algae appears not to be bioavailable. *Am J Clin Nutr.* 1991;53:695–697.
6. Ciferri O, Tiboni O. The biochemistry and industrial potential of spirulina. *Annu Rev Microbiol.* 1985;39:503–526.
7. Clement G, Giddey C, Menzi R. Amino acid composition and nutritive value of the alga spirulina maxima. *J Sci Food Agric.* 1967;18:497–501.
8. Pennington JAT. *Bowes and Church's Food Values of Portions Commonly Used.* 17th ed. Philadelphia, Pa: Lippincott-Raven Publishers; 1998.
9. Annapurna V, Shah N, Bhaskaram P, et al. Bioavailability of Spirulina carotenes in preschool children. *J Clin Biochem Nutr.* 1991;10:145–151.
10. Annapurna VV, Deosthale YG, Bamji MS. Spirulina as a source of vitamin A. *Plant Foods Hum Nutr.* 1991;41:125–134.
11. Kapoor R, Mehta U. Iron bioavailability from *Spirulina platensis,* whole egg, and whole wheat. *Indian J Exp Biol.* 1992;30:904–907.
12. Herbert V, Drivas G. Spirulina and vitamin B12. *JAMA.* 1982;248:3096–3097.
13. Qureshi MA, Garlich JD, Kidd MT. Dietary *Spirulina platensis* enhances humoral and cell-mediated immune functions in chickens. *Immunopharmacol Immunotoxicol.* 1996;18:465–476.
14. Hayashi O, Katoh T, Okuwaki Y. Enhancement of antibody production in mice by dietary *Spirulina platensis. J Nutr Sci Vitaminol (Tokyo).* 1994;40:431–441.
15. Hayashi K, Hayashi T, Kojima I. A natural sulfated polysaccharide, calcium spirulan, isolated from *Spirulina platensis: in vitro* and *ex vivo* evaluation of anti-herpes simplex virus and anti-human immunodeficiency virus activities. *AIDS Res Hum Retroviruses.* 1996;12:1463–1471.
16. Hayashi T, Hayashi K, Maeda M, et al. Calcium spirulan, an inhibitor of enveloped virus replication, from blue-green alga *Spirulina platensis. J Nat Prod.* 1996;59:83–87.
17. Gustafson KR, Cardellina JH, Fuller RW, et al. AIDS-Antiviral sulfolipids from cyanobacteria (blue-green algae). *J Natl Cancer Inst.* 1989;81:1254–1258.
18. Devi MA, Venkataraman IV. Hypocholesterolemic effect of blue green algae *Spirulina platensis* in albino rats. *Nutr Rep Intl.* 1983;28:519–530.
19. Devi MA, Venkataraman IV, Rajasekaran T. Hypocholesterolemic effect of diets containing algae on albino rats. *Nutr Rep Intl.* 1983;20:83–90.
20. Gonzalez de Rivera C, Miranda-Zamora R, Diaz-Zagoya JC, et al. Preventive effect of *Spirulina maxima* on the fatty liver induced by a fructose-rich diet in the rat, a preliminary report. *Life Sci.* 1993;53:57–61.
21. Mathew B, Sankaranarayanan R, Nair PP, et al. Evaluation of chemoprevention of oral cancer with *Spirulina fusiformis. Nutr Cancer.* 1995;24:197–202.

S

22. Schwartz J, Shklar G. Regression of experimental hamster cancer by beta-carotene and algae extracts. *J Oral Maxillofac Surg.* 1987;45:510–515.

23. Schwartz J, Shklar G, Reid S, et al. Prevention of experimental oral cancer by extracts of Spirulina-Dunaliella algae. *Nutr Cancer.* 1988;11:127–134.

24. Shklar G, Schwartz J. Tumor necrosis factor in experimental cancer regression with alpha-tocopherol, beta-carotene, canthaxanthin and algae extract. *Eur J Cancer Clin Oncol.* 1988;24: 839–850.

25. Parada JL, Zulpa de Caire G, Zaccaro de Mule MC, et al. Lactic acid bacteria growth promoters from *Spirulina platensis. Int J Food Microbiol.* 1998;45:225–228.

26. Salazar M, Martinez E, Madrigal E, et al. Subchronic toxicity study in mice fed *Spirulina maxima. J Ethnopharmacol.* 1998;62:235–241.

27. Chamorro G, Salazar M. Dominant lethal study of *Spirulina maxima* in male and female rats after short-term feeding. *Phytother Res.* 1996;10:28–32.

28. Chamorro G, Salazar S, Favila-Castillo L, et al. Reproductive and peri- and postnatal evaluation of *Spirulina maxima* in mice. *J Appl Phycol.* 1997;9:107–112.

29. Spoerke DG, Rumack BH. Blue-green algae poisoning. *J Emerg Med.* 1985;2:353–355.

Valerian *(Valeriana officinalis)*

Valerian, the common name for plants belonging to the genus *Valeriana,* has been used for centuries as a sleep aid. *Valeriana officinalis* is the species most often used for traditional medicinal purposes. Originally carried on the US National Formulary, valerian was omitted in the 1950s because of increased use of barbiturates. In Europe, it is widely prescribed for its mild sedative effects. Valerian is thought to act by depressing the central nervous system and promoting muscle relaxation. Although the active components have not been identified, researchers have suggested that the valepotriates, volatile oils (valerenic acid), or a combination of these may be responsible for the sedative properties. The valeprotriate and volatile oil levels have been found to vary considerably in the native plant and different types of preparations (1, 2).

Media and Marketing Claims	Efficacy
Enhances sleep	?↑
Reduces stress and anxiety	NR

Advisory

- May be associated with serious withdrawal symptoms if abruptly discontinued; doses should be tapered slowly
- Possible morning drowsiness with high doses (≥900 mg)
- Users should avoid driving/operating heavy machinery until they are comfortable with dosage
- Not for individuals with liver disease because of liver toxicity risk

Drug/Supplement Interactions

- Potential dangerous interaction if taken with barbiturates or other sleep medications
- Potential to increase sedative effect of anesthetics; may increase anesthetic requirements with long-term use. Tapering the dose of valerian several weeks before an individual's surgery may be advisable

KEY POINTS

- Preliminary research suggests valerian may improve sleep quality. In one study, valerian was more effective in self-described irregular sleepers than in "good sleepers." However, one reviewer cautioned: "It is difficult to adequately quantify the sleep promoting effects of valerian based on these trials because the study designs, subject characteristics, dosage, and content of the various preparations differed" (2).

- At this time, no studies have compared the effects of valerian to sleep-promoting drugs (benzodiazepines, barbiturates). There is currently no evidence that valerian is habit-forming, as is the case for some sedative medications.

- The sedative effects of valerian were too mild to be picked up by EEG studies. If valerian is in fact this mild, the same effects could also be potentially be produced by engaging in soothing activities such as taking a bath, or listening to relaxing music.

- More clinical trials are needed to evaluate the potential role of valerian in reducing every day tension and anxiety.

- Overall, much more controlled research is needed to examine the efficacy, long-term safety, and potential active components of valerian.

FOOD SOURCES

None

DOSAGE INFORMATION/BIOAVAILABILITY

Valerian is sold as capsules, tablets, teas, and tinctures. Many products are standardized to different levels of valerenic acid. Some labels recommend taking 200 to 1,500 mg one hour before bedtime or during "stressful" days. It is often combined with other herbs such as kava, skullcap, passion flower, chamomile, and hops. The unpleasant smell associated with aqueous valerian results from enzyme hydrolysis of some of the plant components (2).

RELEVANT RESEARCH

Valerian and Sleep

- Researchers conducted a systematic review of clinical trials of valerian extract with subjects experiencing insomnia. Nine randomized, placebo-controlled, double-blind studies using single preparations of valerian were examined for methodological quality. The authors reported that the study findings were contradictory and had many inconsistencies between trials in terms of patients, experimental design and procedures, and methodological quality. They concluded that evidence for valerian as a treatment for insomnia is inconclusive and more rigorous trials are needed (3).

- In a double-blind, placebo-controlled, randomized, crossover study, 16 subjects with previously established psychophysiological insomnia (ages 22 y to 55 y) had their sleep assessed after a single dose and a multiple dose of valerian (14 days). Subjects received 600 mg valerian extract doses one hour before bedtime. During the study, subjects underwent eight polysomnographic recordings. The main outcome was effect on sleep efficiency (total sleep time/time in bed × 100). Other objective parameters measuring sleep structure were assessed (sleep time, sleep onset latency, slow wave sleep, REM sleep). In addition, subjective parameters of sleep quality were assessed (morning feeling, daytime performance, perceived sleep time). A single dose of valerian had no effect on polysomnography readings or subjective sleep parameters. After the multiple-dose treatment, sleep efficiency was significantly increased for both the placebo and valerian treatments compared to baseline polysomnography, indicating a placebo effect. However, slow-wave sleep latency was significantly reduced with valerian, shifting it to the beginning of the sleep period. The authors suggested that this result may indicate a reconstruction of slow wave sleep back to its proper physiological place. Overall, however, the authors concluded that in comparison to the immediate effects of other sleep inducing substances such as benzodiazepines, the influence of valerian on sleep is slight and delayed. The authors concluded that valerian will therefore hardly prove effective for patients with acute, reactive sleep disturbances who need rapid recovery from their complaints (4).

- Two single-blind, placebo-controlled, crossover design trails examined the effect of a single dose of valerian and hops on the central nervous system in 12 healthy subjects. The first trial used 500 mg valerian plus 120 mg hops vs a placebo. The second trial in the same volunteers used a higher dose, 1,500 mg valerian and 360 mg hops daily vs a placebo. Subjects underwent electroencephalograph (EEG) studies prior to, one, two, and four hours after herb ingestion during rest and under mental demand. EEG changes during the low-dose phase were not significantly different from placebo, except for a reduction of alpha- and beta-1 waves four hours after intake. The high-dose phase had significant increases in the delta waves, decreases in alpha, and a weak decrease in beta waves. No significant differences were noted between the herbs and the placebo during mental performance tests. The authors concluded that the EEG was able to show slight but clear visible effects on the nervous system especially after the high dosage (5).

- In a double-blind, placebo-controlled trial, 14 elderly poor sleepers were randomized to receive 1,215 mg valerian extract (divided into three doses) or a placebo for seven days. Sleep polysomnography was conducted on three nights, at one week intervals (before, during, and after treatment) in a sleep laboratory. Valerian treated subjects had an increase in slow-wave sleep and a decrease in sleep stage 1 compared to the placebo. (Slow wave sleep appears to be involved in restoration and growth and in maintaining

V

general health.) There was no effect on REM sleep, sleep onset time, or time awake after sleep onset. There was also no effect on self-rated sleep quality (6).

- In a double-blind, placebo-controlled study, seven subjects (mean age 45 y) with self-reported insomnia received in random order a placebo, 450 mg valerian extract, and 900 mg valerian extract before bedtime for four nights each during 12 nights at home. Subjective sleep ratings were assessed by a questionnaire and movement was recorded by wrist-worn activity meters. There was a significant decrease in sleep latency (time to sleep onset) with valerian (15.8 ± 2.2 minutes vs 9.0 ± 1.5 minutes). Valerian produced more stable sleep the first quarter of the night but had no effect on the rest of the night. Valerian had no effect on total sleep time, the number of minutes of movement, or the total number of movements. The 900 mg dose had no added benefit, but was associated with next morning sleepiness (7).

- In a double-blind, placebo-controlled study, 128 subjects were given valerian extract (400 mg) prepared in the laboratory, a commercial valerian product (400 mg valerian plus hop flower extract), or a placebo in random order before bedtime during nine nonconsecutive nights at home. Subjects completed postsleep questionnaires after each morning. Valerian extract significantly decreased subjective sleep latency scores and improved sleep quality. When subjects were divided into self-reported "poor" vs "good" sleepers, valerian extract significantly improved sleep quality in poor sleepers compared to the placebo, but not for good sleepers. The commercial valerian had no effect on any sleep parameter except a significant increase in reports of next-morning "hangovers." There was no change in night awakenings, hangover effect, or dream recall. The authors could not explain the discrepancy between valerian treatments (8).

- Ten subjects from the above study slept for four nights in a sleep laboratory while undergoing electroencephalograph (EEG) studies. Subjects received 400 mg valerian extract and a placebo for two nights each. Valerian had no effect on EEG parameters or subjective evaluation of sleep (8).

- In a placebo-controlled, double-blind, crossover study, 27 patients with self-reported sleep difficulties were given 400 mg of a commercial standardized valerian extract or a placebo for one night each, with no washout period. Subjects were randomized with regard to which treatment was taken first. The morning after taking the final dose, subjects rated their sleep and the two preparations. The difference between ratings of the two preparations was statistically significant as 21 of 27 subjects rated valerian as better than the control). No adverse effects were reported (9).

Valerian and Anxiety

- In a double-blind, 2 × 2 factorial design study, 50 healthy subjects were randomly assigned to receive 100 mg valerian extract, 20 mg propranolol (beta-blocker), valerian plus propranolol, or a placebo. Ninety minutes after administration, subjects were asked to stand up and complete as many arithmetic calculations as possible in front of a group. Changes in physiological activation (pulse frequency), in performance, and in mood variables were assessed before and after the test. As expected, both propranolol treatments prevented the normal increase in pulse induced by the social stress

V

situation. Valerian had no effect on pulse frequency, but did lead to less intensive subjective feelings of somatic arousal compared to the placebo. The authors concluded that valerian influences feelings of somatic arousal despite high physiological activation during an induced stress situation (10).

SAFETY

- There are no long-term trials testing the safety of valerian in humans. Data from short-term studies suggest that valerian preparations are well-tolerated (2).

- Some subjects have reported feeling drowsy the morning following ingestion of higher doses of valerian (900 mg). However, a randomized, controlled, double-blind trial of 102 subjects reported that a single or repeated evening administration of 600 mg valerian extract had no relevant negative impact on reaction time, alertness, and concentration the morning after intake (11).

- One review suggested that valerian be tapered several weeks before surgery, due to the potential excessive sedation when combined with anesthetics. Additionally, long-term use of valerian could increase anesthesia requirements (12).

- In a case study, a man with a history of coronary artery disease, hypertension, and congestive heart failure experienced cardiac complications and delirium after abruptly stopping valerian. He had been self-medicating with valerian (530 mg to 2 g per dose) five times daily for several years to aid sleep. The authors cautioned that valerian may be associated with serious withdrawal symptoms when abruptly discontinued (13).

- Valerian should not be used concomitantly with barbiturates and benzodiazepine because excessive sedative effects may occur (14).

- The herb has been linked to a few cases of liver damage, which has been attributed to contamination (15). In light of the dearth of safety data, valerian preparations should be avoided by individuals with liver disease (2).

- Some valepotriates have demonstrated cytotoxic activity *in vitro*, but this has not been observed *in vivo*. This may be because of poor absorption and distribution, and instability of valepotriates (2).

REFERENCES

1. Wagner J, Wagner ML, Hening WA. Beyond benzodiazepines: alternative pharmacologic agents for the treatment of insomnia. *Ann Pharmacother.* 1998;32:680–691.
2. Houghton PJ. The biological activity of valerian and related plants. *J Ethnopharmacol.* 1988;22:121–142.
3. Stevinson C, Ernst E. Valerian for insomnia: a systematic review of randomized clinical trials. *Sleep Med.* 2000;1:91–99.
4. Donath F, Quispe S, Diefenbach K, et al. Critical evaluation of the effect of valerian extract on sleep structure and sleep quality. *Pharmacopsychiatry.* 2000;33:47–53.

5. Vonderheid-Guth B, Todorova A, Brattstrom A, et al. Pharmacodynamic effects of valerian and hops extract combination (Ze 91019) on the quantitative-topogrophical EEG in healthy volunteers. *Eur J Med Res.* 2000;5:139–144.

6. Schulz H, Stolz C, Muller J. The effect of valerian extract on sleep polygraphy in poor sleepers: a pilot study. *Pharmacopsychiatry.* 1994;27:147–151.

7. Leathwood PD, Chauffard F. Aqueous extract of valerian reduces latency to fall asleep in man. *Planta Med.* 1985;51:144–148.

8. Leathwood PD, Chauffard F, Heck E, et al. Aqueous extract of valerian root (*Valeriana officinalis L*) improves sleep quality in man. *Pharmacol Biochem Behav.* 1982;17:65–71.

9. Lindahl O, Lindwall L. Double blind study of a valerian preparation. *Pharmacol Biochem Behav.* 1989;32:1065–1066.

10. Kohnen R, Oswald WD. The effects of valerian, propranolol, and their combination on activation, performance, and mood of healthy volunteers under social stress conditions. *Pharmacopsychiatry.* 1988;21:447–448.

11. Kuhlmann J, Berger W, Podzuweit H, et al. The influence of valerian treatment on "reaction time, alertness and concentration in volunteers." *Pharmacopsychiatry.* 1999;32:235–241.

12. Ang-Lee, MK, Moss J, Yuan CS. Herbal medicines and perioperative care. *JAMA.* 2001;286:208–216.

13. Carges HP, Varia I, Doraiswamy PM. Cardiac complications and delirium associated with valerian root withdrawal. *JAMA.* 1998;280:1566–1567.

14. Miller LG. Herbal medicinals: selected clinical considerations focusing on known or potential drug-herb interactions. *Arch Intern Med.* 1998;158:2200–2211.

15. Shepherd C. Sleep disorders. Liver damage warning with insomnia remedy. *BMJ.* 1993;306:1477.

Valine

See Branched-Chain Amino Acids (BCAAs).

Vanadium

Vanadium (vanadyl sulfate, or VS) is a trace mineral present in nature and mammalian cells. Because the physiological role is not clearly defined, vanadium is presently not deemed essential in human nutrition. Vanadium deficiency has not been identified in humans but has been reported in goats and rats. Research in the last 30 years has found that vanadium exists in several forms each with varying actions. Because animal studies have shown vanadium helps facilitate glucose uptake into muscle and converts glucose into fat, researchers are investigating the potential role of vanadium supplements in the management of diabetes (1–3).

Media and Marketing Claims	Efficacy
Reduces the need for insulin	?↑
Increases muscle mass	↓
Maximizes strength	↓

Advisory

Tolerable Upper Intake Level (UL): from foods and supplements, 1.8 mg elemental vanadium/day

Drug/Supplement Interactions

- Vanadyl sulfate may have blood-thinning effects, and thus, may interact with anticoagulant drugs
- Potential additive effect on lowering blood glucose levels if combined with diabetes medications

KEY POINTS

- According to preliminary findings in very small numbers of patients, VS appears to improve insulin sensitivity mainly in subjects with type 2 diabetes. However, according to one review article: "It is still too early to conclude whether vanadium salts will be used therapeutically in the future care of diabetes. It is more likely that vanadium research will assist in a better understanding of the backup systems involved, and eventually lead to the development of more potent and less toxic vanadium substitutes" (1).
- Preliminary research shows VS has little or no effect on strength training and body composition. Much more research is needed to validate VS supplementation in athletes.
- At this time, routine supplementation of vanadium is not supported by scientific evidence. Supplements containing high amounts of vanadium should be avoided because of potential toxicity.

FOOD SOURCES

The average American diet provides 15 µg to 30 µg vanadium/day. Rich sources of vanadium are shellfish, parsley, mushrooms, and dill seed (4). Vanadium is also present in wine (2 µg/kg to 17 µg/kg) (5).

DOSAGE INFORMATION/BIOAVAILABILITY

Vanadium is sold in the form of vanadyl sulfate (VS) or vanadate providing 7 mg to 15 mg/capsule (≈1 mg to 5 mg elemental vanadium). Some manufacturers suggest taking very high doses of vanadium (15 mg to 60 mg vanadyl sulfate/day or about 5 mg to 20 mg elemental vanadium). Although the metabolism of vanadium is not well understood, it is estimated that 5 percent to 30 percent is absorbed from the intestine where it binds to iron-containing proteins in the blood (4).

A biological role of vanadium has not been identified; therefore, the National Academy of Sciences have not set an RDA or AI (adequate intake) levels (3).

RELEVANT RESEARCH

VS and Diabetes

- In a single-blind, placebo-controlled (not randomized) study, eight patients with type 2 diabetes mellitus received 100 mg VS daily for four weeks. Six patients continued the study and received a placebo for an additional four weeks. Daily glucose tests were self-recorded and four euglycemic-hyperinsulinemic clamps were administered before, during, and after the study. VS was associated with a significant 20 percent decrease in fasting glucose compared to no effect during the placebo phase. VS also caused a decrease in hepatic glucose output during hyperinsulinemia that was sustained through the placebo phase. There was no effect on peripheral (muscle) insulin resistance, glycogen synthesis, glycolysis, or lipolysis. The authors concluded: "VS resulted in modest reductions of fasting plasma glucose and hepatic insulin resistance" (6).

- Five type 2 and five type 1 diabetic patients were given 125 mg sodium metavanadate/day for two weeks in a four-week study. Subjects recorded blood glucose four times daily, as well as insulin dosage and diet throughout the study. Glucose metabolism measured by a two-step euglycemic-hyperinsulinemic clamp was not significantly increased by vanadate in type 1 patients, but improved by 29 percent during low-dose insulin infusion, and 39 percent in high-dose insulin infusion in type 2 patients. Basal hepatic glucose production and suppression of hepatic glucose production were unaffected by vanadate; however, there was a decrease in insulin requirements in type 1 subjects. Cholesterol levels were significantly reduced in all subjects. The authors concluded: "Vanadate or related agents may have a potential role as adjunctive therapy in patients with diabetes mellitus" (7).

- In a single-blind, placebo-controlled study, seven type 2 diabetic obese subjects and six nondiabetic obese subjects underwent euglycemic-hyperinsulinemic clamps after two weeks of placebo and after three weeks of 100 mg VS/day. All subjects were instructed to keep diet and exercise constant, but this was not monitored. Glucose turnover, glycolysis, glycogen synthesis, and carbohydrate and lipid oxidation were measured. Significant reductions in fasting plasma glucose and HbA_{1c} were seen in type 2 diabetic subjects using VS, but not in nondiabetic controls. However, HbA_{1c} has a turnover rate of 60 to 90 days and the duration of VS supplementation was only 21 days; thus, it would not reflect an effect of VS. The glucose infusion rate required to maintain euglycemia significantly increased in type 2 diabetic subjects while they took VS, but not controls. This improvement in insulin sensitivity was attributed to a significant increase of glucose disposal and enhanced suppression of hepatic glucose output in these subjects. VS also was associated with a significant suppression of plasma free fatty acids and lipid oxidation during clamps. Transient gastrointestinal symptoms (nausea,

V

mild diarrhea, cramps) were experienced by all subjects during VS supplementation. The authors concluded: "VS does not alter insulin sensitivity in nondiabetic subjects, but it does improve both hepatic and skeletal muscle insulin sensitivity in NIDDM [type 2] subjects in part by enhancing insulin's inhibitory effect on lipolysis. These data suggest that VS may improve a defect in insulin signaling specific to type NIDMM" (8).

- Another study of similar design found that three weeks of 100 mg VS/day improved hepatic and peripheral insulin sensitivity in six type 2 diabetic subjects. These effects were sustained for up to two weeks after subjects discontinued VS supplements (9).

- A review article summarized research in animals suggesting that vanadate and vanadyl mimic the action of insulin and appear to be effective treatment for animal models of both type 1 and type 2 diabetes (10).

VS and Weight Training

- In a double-blind, placebo-controlled trial, 40 trained subjects were randomly assigned to receive 0.5 mg vanadyl sulfate/kg/day or a placebo for 12 weeks. Subjects were pair-matched based on sex, age, weight, height, and training program. Measurements included body weight, skinfold thickness, body circumference, and 1- and 10-repetition maximum tests for the bench press and leg extension at weeks 0, 4, 8, and 12. Blood tests and a subjective questionnaire were also given. Thirty-one subjects completed the trial (two subjects in the VS group withdrew as a result of excessive tiredness and mood changes). Anthropometric measures and body composition did not differ between the groups. Both groups improved performance but the only significant effect of treatment was a treatment × time interaction in the leg extension, which the authors attributed to the vanadyl subjects having a lower performance at the baseline. The authors concluded: "Vanadyl sulfate was ineffective in changing body composition in weight training athletes, and any modest performance-enhancing effect requires further investigation" (11).

SAFETY

- Tolerable Upper Intake Level for vanadium from foods and supplements is 1.8 mg elemental vanadium/day based on renal toxicity data (3).

- Vanadium can be a relatively toxic element. The high amounts of vanadium used in the human studies discussed here were pharmacological doses that have been associated with toxicity in animals. These doses far exceed amounts available from the diet.

- Toxicity studies in animals have shown that inorganic vanadium can induce hematological and biochemical changes; reproductive and developmental toxicity; excess vanadium retention in bone, kidney, and liver; and pro-oxidative effects on glutathione, ascorbic acid, lipids, and NADPH (12). More recent data have shown that organic vanadium compounds are much safer than inorganic vanandium salts and do not cause gastrointestinal discomfort, or liver or kidney toxicity (13).

- Side-effects associated with VS therapy in the studies discussed here included cramping, diarrhea, and abdominal pain. When 12 subjects were given 22.5 mg vanadium for five months, similar gastrointestinal disturbances were reported (4).

- Excess vanadium consumption (4 mg to 18 mg, 6 weeks to 10 weeks) may cause green discoloration of the green tongue (4).

- The safety of 0.5 mg/kg/day in 31 weight-training athletes was assessed throughout 12 weeks. VS had no effect on hematological indexes, blood viscosity, and biochemistry (14).

REFERENCES

1. Shechter Y, Li J, Meyerovitch J, et al. Insulin-like actions of vanadate are mediated in an insulin-receptor-independent manner via non-receptor protein tyrosine kinases and protein phosphotyrosine phosphates. *Mol Cell Biochem.* 1995;153:39–49.
2. Moore RJ, Friedl KE. Physiology of nutritional supplements: Chromium picolinate and vanadyl sulfate. *Natl Strength Cond Assoc J.* 1992;14:47–51.
3. Institute of Medicine, Food and Nutrition Board. *Dietary Reference Intakes for Vitamin A, Vitamin K, Chromium, Copper, Iodine, Iron, Manganese, Molybdenum, Nickel, Silicon, Vanadium, and Zinc.* Washington, DC: National Academy Press; 2001.
4. Nielsen FH. Ultratrace Minerals. In: Shils ME, Olson JA, Shike M, Ross AC, eds. *Modern Nutrition in Health and Disease.* 9th ed. Baltimore, Md: Williams & Wilkins; 1999:286–288.
5. Teissedre PL, Krosniak M, Portet K, et al. Vanadium levels in French and Californian wines: influence on vanadium dietary intake. *Food Addit Contam.* 1998;15:585–591.
6. Boden G, Chen X, Ruiz J, et al. Effects of vanadyl sulfate on carbohydrate and lipid metabolism in patients with non-insulin-dependent diabetes mellitus. *Metabolism.* 1996;45:1130–1135.
7. Goldfine AB, Simonson DC, Folli F, et al. Metabolic effects of sodium metavanadate in humans with insulin-dependent and non-insulin-dependent diabetes mellitus *in vivo* and *in vitro* studies. *J Clin Endocrinol Metab.* 1995;80:3311–3320.
8. Halberstam M, Cohen N, Shlimovich P, et al. Oral vanadyl sulfate improves insulin sensitivity in NIDDM but not in obese nondiabetic subjects. *Diabetes.* 1996;45:659–666.
9. Cohen N, Halberstam M, Shlimovich P, et al. Oral vanadyl sulfate improves hepatic and peripheral insulin sensitivity in patients with non-insulin-dependent diabetes mellitus. *J Clin Invest.* 1995;95:2501–2509.
10. Goldfine AB, Simonson DC, Folli F, et al. *In vivo* and *in vitro* studies of vanadate in human and rodent diabetes mellitus. *Mol Cell Biochem.* 1995;153:217–231.
11. Fawcett JP, Farquhar SJ, Walker RJ, et al. The effect of oral vanadyl sulfate on body composition and performance in weight-training athletes. *Int J Sport Nutr.* 1996;6:382–390.
12. Domingo JL, Gomez M, Sanchez DJ, et al. Toxicology of vanadium compounds in diabetic rats: the action of chelating agents on vanadium accumulation. *Mol Cell Biochem.* 1995;153:233–240.

V

13. Srivastava AK. Anti-diabetic and toxic effects of vanadium compounds. *Mol Cell Biochem.* 2000;206:177–182.

14. Fawcett JP, Farquhar SJ, Thou T, et al. Oral vanadyl sulphate does not affect blood cells, viscosity, or biochemistry in humans. *Pharmacol Toxicol.* 1997;80:202–206.

Vitamin A/Beta-Carotene

Beta-carotene, a precursor to vitamin A, is the most abundant provitamin-A carotenoid found in fruits and vegetables. Carotenoids act as electron-transport agents during photosynthesis and also protect plants from oxygen radicals. Of the approximately 600 carotenoids that have been identified, only 50 show provitamin A activity (1). Approximately six of the many carotenoids in nature are found in significant amounts in human plasma (1). Other provitamin A carotenoids that have been studied in depth include alpha-carotene and beta-cryptoxanthin (lutein and lycopene are carotenoids that are not converted into vitamin A) (2). Beta-carotene and other carotenoids are being investigated for their possible antioxidant activity in cancer, cardiovascular diseases, and other conditions of oxidative stress (3). The National Academy of Sciences Food and Nutrition Board (FNB) panel on Antioxidants and Related Compounds reviewed data to determine whether dietary reference intakes (DRI) could be set for beta-carotene and other carotenoids. The panel concluded that no value could be determined at this time to set required levels of intake. However, the panel did support recommendations to increase intake of carotenoid-rich fruits and vegetables (4).

Vitamin A is the general term used to describe retinoids that have the biologic activity of retinol. This fat-soluble, essential vitamin exists in three oxidative states: retinol (alcohol), retinal (aldehyde), and retinoic acid. Vitamin A plays a role in cell differentiation and morphogenesis, thus affecting growth, reproduction, bone development, skin, and immunity. As part of rhodopsin, the retinal form of vitamin A has a major function in vision (1).

Media and Marketing Claims	Efficacy
Beta-carotene	
Reduces risk of cancer	↔
Prevents cardiovascular disease	↓
Enhances immunity	NR
Improves vision and reduces cataract formation	NR
Reverses aging of skin	NR
Vitamin A	
Enhances immunity	?↑
Improves vision (if deficient)	↑
Treats skin disorders (prescription vitamin A analogues)	↑
Reverses aging of skin	NR

V

Advisory

- Beta-carotene supplements may increase risk of lung cancer and fatal heart disease and intracerebral hemorrhage in middle-aged, male smokers
- Vitamin A, but not beta-carotene, is toxic in doses 10 times the RDA
- The Tolerable Upper Intake Level (UL) for adult men and women is 3,000 µg/day (10,000 IU) preformed vitamin A.
- Teratogenic; the UL is 3,000 µg preformed vitamin A/day for pregnant women, and 2,000 µg/day for pregnant teenagers.

Drug/Supplement Interactions

- HMG-CoA reductase inhibitors (ie, Lipitor, Lovastatin, Fluvastatin) used to reduce cholesterol and oral contraceptives are associated with increased blood levels of vitamin A. Vitamin A levels may need to be monitored if individual is combining vitamin A supplements with these drugs
- Isotretinoin (Accutane) is similar in structure to vitamin A. Using vitamin A supplements with this drug may result in toxicity
- Antacids (ie, Prevacid, Prilosec) may interfere with vitamin A/beta-carotene absorption

KEY POINTS

- Beta-carotene supplements have not reduced the risk of cancer at most sites, and there is evidence of an increase in risk for lung cancer among smokers and asbestos workers receiving beta-carotene supplements. Many researchers agree that nutrients in food work synergistically and that the cancer-protective effects of diets rich in carotenoid-containing fruits and vegetables are not because of any one carotenoid.

- Similarly, beta-carotene supplements have not demonstrated any benefit in preventing or treating cardiovascular disease and in fact may increase risk of death from myocardial infarction in male smokers with a history of heart disease and intracerebral hemorrhage in male smokers without a history of stroke.

- Vitamin A deficiency has a negative effect on immune status. However, most studies evaluating the effects of beta-carotene supplements on immune function showed no benefit. Although patients with AIDS tend to have reduced plasma carotenoid levels, more research is needed to determine whether beta-carotene supplements improve overall health and survival in these patients.

- The role of vitamin A in vision is well known. An overt deficiency of vitamin A can result in night or permanent blindness. The role of beta-carotene in reducing incidence of cataracts and ARM is less well-understood, though preliminary evidence is not suggestive of a benefit. Other carotenoids (lutein, xeaxanthin) are being investigated for their potential protective effect on degenerative vision disorders.

- High doses of synthetic vitamin A are currently used in prescription medications to treat acne (isotretinoin) and other skin disorders. While using these medications, patients are closely monitored for adverse affects by their physician. Self-dosing with

V

equivalent amounts of over-the-counter vitamin A is not recommended because of the severe side-effects associated with pharmacological doses. Although topical vitamin A analogues (tretinoin or Retin A) are used in the treatment of acne, blemishes, and wrinkles, there is no evidence that oral vitamin A or beta-carotene supplements reverse the signs of aging.

- At this time, there is much controversy surrounding the benefits and possible adverse effects of supplementing with beta-carotene and/or other carotenoids. The FNB report on carotenoids concluded that beta-carotene supplements are not advisable, other than as a provitamin A source and to control vitamin A deficiency in at-risk populations. Until further evidence is gathered, individuals should be encouraged to consume a variety of fruits and vegetables rich in carotenoids (*see* Food Sources).

FOOD SOURCES

Good sources of preformed vitamin A include liver, eggs, and fortified milk. Rich sources of beta-carotene are found in bright orange and yellow fruits and vegetables. Data for the specific carotenoid contents of foods are limited because calculation methods are fairly new (5, 6). Mild heat treatment, blenderizing, and dietary fat enhance carotenoid absorption, whereas soluble fiber interferes with carotenoid uptake (7).

Food (mg/3.5 oz) (6)	β-carotene	α-carotene	β-cryptoxanthin	Lutein and Zeaxanthin	Lycopene
Apricot	176	—	—	—	8.64
Beet greens	25.6	0.03	—	—	—
Broccoli	13.0	—	—	18.0	—
Carrot	98.0	37.0	—	—	—
Collard greens	54.0	—	—	—	—
Corn	0.51	0.50	—	7.8	—
Mango	13.0	0.01	0.54	—	—
Spinach, raw	41.0	—	—	102.0	—
Juice, tomato, canned	9.0	—	—	—	8.58

Source: Data from Mangels AR, et al. (6)

Food	Vitamin A	RE = IU
Liver, beef (3.5 oz)	10,602	37,679
Potato, sweet (1)	2,487	24,877
Carrot (1)	2,025	20,253
Spinach (½ c)	737	7,371
Mango (1)	805	8,061
Papaya (1)	85	863
Milk, nonfat (1 c)	149	500
Egg (1)	84	280

Source: Data from Pennington JAT (8)

DOSAGE INFORMATION/BIOAVAILABILITY

The RDA for vitamin A is 900 μg (3,000 IU) for men and 700 μg (2,333 IU) for women (4). This differs from the previous 1989 RDA for vitamin A of 1,000 RE (5,000 IU) for men and 800 RE (4,000 IU) for women (9). The National Academy of Sciences Food and Nutrition Board (FNB) did not set a DRI for beta-carotene or other carotenoids (4). The report did note that the National Cancer Institute's recommendations for five fruits and vegetables daily would provide approximately 5 mg to 6 mg/day provitamin A carotenoids, and that this amount from foods is similar to the quantity needed to maintain plasma beta-carotene levels in the range associated with a lower risk of various chronic diseases (4).

Beta-carotene is sold individually or with other carotenoids or with vitamin C or E in doses ranging from 15,000 IU to 50,000 IU (≈ 90 mg to 300 mg beta-carotene). Beta-carotene is bottled in either the synthetic form (all-*trans* beta-carotene) or the natural form (all-*trans* beta-carotene and 9-*cis*-beta-carotene) derived from *Dunaliella* alga. Most studies have used the synthetic form of beta-carotene. Beta-carotene from supplements has a much higher bioavailability than from foods. For instance, 30 mg/day of supplemental all-*trans*-beta-carotene increased plasma beta-carotene levels five times more than beta-carotene from carrots (4).

Although the synthetic all-*trans* beta-carotene may be more efficiently absorbed, the tendency of the synthetic form to alter normal serum *trans/cis* ratios in favor of the *trans* isomer may not be a beneficial effect (10).

Vitamin A is available in single preparations or multivitamin/mineral supplements typically providing 5,000 IU to 10,000 IU (≈ 1,500 μg to 3,000 μg vitamin A) as retinol or retinyl palmitate.

Many supplements contain both retinyl palmitate and beta-carotene, which are represented on the label as "total vitamin A activity." Although most supplement labels list vitamin A and beta-carotene in international units (IU), the preferred unit of measure is micrograms or retinol activity equivalents (RAE), where

> 1 RAE* = 1 μg retinol
> = 12 μg of all-*trans*-beta-carotene
> = 24 μg all other provitamin A carotenoids
> 1 IU vitamin A activity = 0.3 μg of all-*trans*-retinol
> = 3.6 μg all-*trans*-beta-carotene
> = 7.2 μg other provitamin A carotenoids

RELEVANT RESEARCH

Beta-Carotene's Effect on Plasma Carotenoids

- A four-year, placebo-controlled study of 108 subjects supplemented with 25 mg beta-carotene resulted in a 151 percent increase in serum beta-carotene but did not signif-

---

* RAE is the new interconversion unit used in place of Retinol Equivalent (RE) used in the 1989 RDA values.

icantly change serum retinol, alpha-tocopherol, or other serum carotenoids (lycopene, lutein, or alpha-carotene) (11).

- A five-year study supplementing 259 subjects with 50 mg beta-carotene daily increased beta- and alpha-carotene plasma concentrations by 9- to 10-fold and 2-fold, respectively. Supplementation had no effect on plasma lycopene, lutein/zeaxanthin, retinol, or alpha-tocopherol levels (12). Beta-carotene from a single ingestion of 12-mg to 30-mg supplements raised plasma levels higher than a similar amount of beta-carotene in carrots (13, 14).

Beta-Carotene/Vitamin A and Cancer

- Several observational and intervention studies have examined the effects of dietary beta-carotene and beta-carotene supplements (and other micronutrients) in cancer prevention. These studies were developed because of the large epidemiological evidence that high intakes of fruits and vegetables are associated with reduced risk of cancer at several sites, and because of the known biological properties of beta-carotene. Both epidemiological and intervention trials are described here.

Breast Cancer

- In a prospective cohort study in The Netherlands, 65,573 women were followed for 4.3 years for incidence of breast cancer. After adjusting for risk factors, breast cancer risk was not influenced by the intake of beta-carotene, vitamin E, fiber, vitamin C supplements, vegetables, or potatoes. For dietary retinol, a weak positive association was observed (15).

- In a population-based, case-control study, 3,543 subjects with breast cancer and 9,406 controls were evaluated for food and supplement use. Eating carrots or spinach more than two times per week compared to eating none was associated with a 44 percent reduced risk of breast cancer. However, there was no association between estimated preformed vitamin A intake from foods and supplements and risk of breast cancer across all categories of intake (16).

- In a retrospective cohort study, 273 women with breast cancer and 371 matched controls were interviewed about their diet at different ages throughout their life. Women were at lower risk of developing breast cancer with increasing levels of reported dietary intake of beta-carotene (17).

- In a case-control study, biopsies of breast tissue were taken from 46 patients with breast cancer and 63 controls. There was an insignificant inverse relationship between breast adipose concentrations of retinoids and carotenoids and risk of breast cancer. There was also an insignificant positive association between dietary intake (including supplements) of preformed vitamin A and retinol concentrations in breast tissue. There was no relation between dietary carotenoids and carotenoid levels in breast tissue. The authors concluded that the finding of an inverse association between adipose retinoids and carotenoids and beta-carotene is intriguing but requires further studies with larger sample sizes (18).

Beta-carotene and Other Cancers in Women

- In the double-blind, placebo-controlled, Women's Health Study, 29,876 women (aged > 45 y) were randomized to receive beta-carotene (50 mg on alternate days), vitamin E, aspirin, or a placebo. The beta-carotene arm was terminated early after a median treatment duration of 2.1 years plus two years follow up. Beta-carotene had no effect on cancer incidence, nor did it have any significant effects for any site-specific cancer. Additionally, beta-carotene had no effect on all cause mortality or cardiovascular disease incidence (19)

Lung Cancer

- In the Alpha-Tocopherol Beta-Carotene (ATBC) Cancer Prevention Study, 29,133 male cigarette smokers aged 50 y to 69 y were randomized to receive 20 mg beta-carotene, 50 mg alpha-tocopherol, both vitamins, or a placebo for five to eight years. Beta-carotene did not cause a decrease in cancer at any site and was associated with a significant 18 percent increased risk in lung cancer (number of cases: 474 vs 402). However, lower lung cancer rates were observed in men in the placebo group who had higher amounts of both serum and dietary beta-carotene and vitamin E at the baseline (20).

- In a follow-up analysis, results from the ATBC Cancer Prevention Study were examined to determine whether the pattern of intervention effects across subgroups would provide further interpretation of the main ATBC study results. The beta-carotene effect appeared stronger in subjects who smoked ± 20 cigarettes/day than in those who smoked five to 19 cigarettes daily and in those with higher alcohol intake (> 11 g ethanol/day). The authors concluded: "Beta-carotene at pharmacologic levels may modestly increase lung cancer incidence in cigarette smokers, and this effect may be associated with heavier smoking and higher alcohol intake" (21).

- In the prospective, double-blind, placebo-controlled Beta-Carotene and Retinol Efficacy Trial (CARET), 18,314 men and women at risk of developing lung cancer (asbestos workers and smokers) were randomized to receive 30 mg beta-carotene plus 25,000 IU vitamin A (retinyl palmitate) or a placebo. The study was stopped 21 months early because of "clear evidence of no benefit and substantial evidence of possible harm." An analysis of subgroups revealed a greater risk of lung cancer in subjects in the highest quartile of alcohol intake. The authors noted that the excess lung cancer incidence and mortality with beta-carotene and vitamin A were highly consistent with the results found in the ATBC study (22).

Colon Cancer

- In the ATBC study (see above for details), beta-carotene supplements (50 mg for 5 y to 8 y) had no effect on colorectal cancer incidence (23).

- In a double-blind, placebo-controlled study, 18 patients with resected colonic polyps and 19 patients with colon cancer were randomized to receive 30 mg beta-carotene/day or a placebo for three months. Blood samples of T-lymphocyte subsets were taken before and at the end of the study and compared to 14 healthy control subjects. Initially, there were no differences in total leukocyte counts, percentage of lymphocytes, and various subsets of lymphocytes between the three groups, although the cancer patients had lower percentages of CD4 and interleukin-2 receptor-positive cells (IL-2R+). After three months of beta-carotene supplementation, IL-2R+ T-lymphocytes and CD4+ lymphocytes were significantly increased only in cancer patients. There were no changes in patients with resected polyps when compared to controls. The authors concluded: "Beta-carotene increased the number of IL-2R+ T lymphocytes and CD4+ lymphocytes, which in turn may produce IL-2 only in patients with cancer who may already have some deficiency in their immune system. This increase in activated T lymphocytes may mediate cytotoxic reactions to cancer cells via cytokine production [stimulate an immune reaction against tumor cells]" (24).

- An *in vitro* study of two colon cancer cell lines found alpha and beta-carotene significantly inhibited cancer growth by decreasing cell viability, DNA synthesis, and cell proliferation. A higher dose of retinoic acid (active metabolite of vitamin A) was needed to produce the same results as the alpha- and beta-carotene. The authors concluded that the potential antitumor activity of carotenoids may be independent of their provitamin A activity (25).

Oral Cancer

- In a prospective cohort study (ATBC Cancer Prevention Study), 409 male smokers were randomized to receive 20 mg beta-carotene, 50 mg vitamin E, a mixture of both, or a placebo daily for five to seven years. There was no significant difference between groups in the prevalence of oral mucosal lesions or in the cells of unkeratinized epithelium of the tongue (26).

- In a double-blind, placebo-controlled study, 264 patients who had been curatively treated for a recent early-stage squamous cell carcinoma of the oral cavity, pharynx, or larynx were randomly assigned to receive 50 mg beta-carotene or a placebo daily for up to 90 months. After a median follow-up of 51 months, there were no differences between groups in the development of a second primary tumor plus local recurrence. When analyzed by specific site of cancer, beta-carotene had no effect on second occurrence of head and neck cancer or lung cancer. The vitamin also had no effect on total mortality (27).

Beta-carotene and Skin Cancer

- In a double-blind, placebo-controlled Physician's Health Study, 22,071 healthy male physicians (aged 40 y to 82 y) were randomized to receive 50 mg beta-carotene or placebo every other day for 12 years. After adjusting for age and aspirin assignment, beta-carotene supplements had no significant effect on incidence of nonmelanoma skin cancer (basal cell carcinoma and squamous cell carcinoma). There was also no evidence of a harmful or beneficial effect of beta-carotene on skin cancer incidence when subjects were separated by smoking status (current, past, or never) (28).

Beta-Carotene and Cardiovascular Disease

- In a prospective, double-blind, placebo-controlled study, 27,271 male smokers from the ATBC Cancer Prevention Study with no history of myocardial infarction were randomized to receive 20 mg beta-carotene, 50 mg alpha-tocopherol, a mixture of both, or a placebo daily for five to eight years. The endpoint was the first nonfatal or fatal major coronary event. Beta-carotene supplementation had no significant effect on the incidence of nonfatal or fatal coronary events compared to other groups. Vitamin E supplementation decreased nonfatal coronary events by 4 percent and decreased the incidence of fatal disease by 8 percent. Neither supplement had any effect on incidence of myocardial infarction. The authors concluded: "Supplementation with beta-carotene has no primary preventive effect on major coronary events" (29).

- In a double-blind, placebo-controlled study, a subgroup of 1,862 male smokers with previous myocardial infarction from the ATBC Cancer Prevention Study were randomized to receive 20 mg beta-carotene, 50 mg alpha-tocopherol, both, or a placebo daily for an average of five years. There were no significant differences in the number of major coronary events between any supplementation group and the placebo group. There were statistically significantly more deaths from coronary heart disease in the beta carotene and the combined alpha-tocopherol and beta-carotene groups than the placebo group, but no significant increase in the alpha-tocopherol group. The authors concluded that alpha-tocopherol or beta-carotene supplements are not recommended in male smokers with heart disease (30).

- In a prospective, double-blind, placebo-controlled study, 1,759 male smokers with angina pectoris from the ATBC Cancer Prevention Study were randomized to receive 20 mg beta-carotene, 50 mg vitamin E, mixture of both, or a placebo daily for five to seven years. Recurrence of angina pectoris at annual follow-up visits, progression from mild to severe angina, and incidence of major coronary events were measured. There were no significant differences between groups. The authors concluded: "There was no evidence of beneficial effects for alpha-tocopherol or beta-carotene supplements in male smokers with angina pectoris, indicating no basis for therapeutic or preventive use of these agents in such patients" (31).

- In a double-blind, placebo-controlled study, nine women were randomized to receive a low carotenoid diet plus 0.5 mg/day beta-carotene or a carotenoid-depleting diet without supplements for 60 days while living in a metabolic research unit where exercise, diet, and activities were controlled. All subjects subsequently received 0.5 mg beta-carotene during days 60 to 100, and an additional 0.5 mg mixed carotenoid supplement during days 100 to 120. Concentrations of malondialdehyde-thiobarbituric acid (MDA-TBA) (a marker of lipid peroxidation) were analyzed during each phase of supplementation. At the start of the study, there were no differences between groups in MDA-TBA levels. In the first 60 days, the MDA-TBA values for the placebo group were significantly higher than the treatment group. During days 60 to 100 when both groups received beta-carotene, MDA-TBA levels were significantly lowered in the placebo group to the point where they matched the treatment group. The authors concluded that carotenoids prevent lipid peroxidation *in vivo* but that the antioxidant effect may be more effective when subjects are in a depleted condition or are suffering from a condition caused by lipid peroxidation. They suggested that further research is needed to identify the mechanism by which carotenoids prevent lipid peroxidation and the amount needed for normal activity (32).

Beta-Carotene and Immunity

- In a double-blind, placebo-controlled study, 58 healthy subjects older than 65 y were randomized to receive 8.2 mg beta-carotene, 13.3 mg lycopene, or a placebo daily for 12 weeks. Markers of immune function (T-cell subsets and the expression of functionally associated cell surface molecules, lectin-stimulated lymphocyte proliferation) were measured at baseline and at 12 weeks. No significant differences were seen in any of the immunity parameters measured in any group (33).

- In a double-blind, placebo-controlled study, 54 healthy, elderly men randomly selected from the Physician's Health Study were randomized to receive 50 mg beta-carotene every other day for 10 to 12 years. In a second study, 25 elderly women were given 90 mg beta-carotene/day for three weeks. Subjects taking supplements from both studies had greater plasma beta-carotene levels than placebo subjects. Delayed hypersensitivity skin test responses given pre- and postintervention did not differ between beta-carotene and placebo groups in either the short-term or long-term study. Short-term or long-term beta-carotene had no effect on T cell-mediated immune responses as measured by lymphocyte proliferation, interleukin-2 and prostaglandin E2 production, and composition of lymphocyte subsets (34).

- In a double-blind, placebo-controlled, crossover study, 25 healthy male nonsmokers were randomly assigned to receive 15 mg beta-carotene daily or a placebo for 26 days each. After beta-carotene supplementation, there were significant increases in plasma beta-carotene levels. There was a significant association of beta-carotene supplementation with an elevated expression of peripheral blood monocyte surface molecules (involved in initiating immune responses) and with an increase in the secretion of TNF-alpha (plays a role in host resistance to infection) by blood monocytes. The authors concluded: "Moderate increases in the dietary intake of beta-carotene can enhance cell-mediated immune responses within a relatively short period of time, providing a potential mechanism for the anticarcinogenic properties attributed to beta-carotene" (35).

- In a controlled depletion-repletion study, nine healthy women living in a metabolic unit for 100 days were fed a basal diet supplemented with 1.5 mg beta-carotene for 4 days (baseline), followed by the basal diet without supplements for 68 days (depletion), followed by 15 mg beta-carotene/day for the last 28 days (repletion). Neither beta-carotene depletion nor repletion significantly affected proliferation of peripheral blood mononuclear cells cultured with phytohemagglutinin or concanavalin A, *in vitro* production of interleukin 2 receptor, or the concentration of circulating lymphocytes and their subsets. The authors concluded that in healthy adults consuming adequate vitamin A, beta-carotene depletion had no apparent adverse effects and that modest beta-carotene supplementation had no beneficial effects (36).

- In a single-blind, placebo-controlled trial, 20 healthy male nonsmokers were randomized to receive 60 mg beta-carotene/day or a placebo for 44 weeks. The beta-carotene concentrations of plasma and mononuclear cells rose four and three times the baseline levels after two and four weeks, respectively. The CD4-CD8 ratio increased after nine months of beta-carotene supplementation. There was no change in natural killer cells, virgin T cells, memory T cells, and cytotoxic T cells. The authors speculated that beta-carotene supplementation could potentially benefit AIDS patients because a decrease in the CD4-CD8 ratio is often observed in this disease (37). Because this study was not double-blinded, the results must be viewed with caution.

- In a double-blind, placebo-controlled study, 17 HIV-infected subjects were randomized to receive 180 mg beta-carotene or a placebo for four weeks. Supplementation statistically significantly increased total white blood cells and CD4 lymphocyte count percentages (38).

Beta-Carotene and Cataracts/Age Related Maculopathy (ARM)

- In a double-blind, placebo-controlled study, a random sample of 1,828 male smokers from the ATBC Cancer Prevention Study were randomized to receive 20 mg beta-carotene, 50 mg alpha-tocopherol, a mixture of both, or a placebo daily for five to eight years. Supplementation did not affect the end-of-trial prevalence of nuclear, cortical, or posterior subcapsular cataract, or affect the median lens opacity meter value (measure of cataract severity). The authors concluded that supplementation with beta-carotene or alpha-tocopherol did not influence cataract prevalence in middle-aged smoking men (39).

- In a double-blind, placebo-controlled study, a subgroup of 941 male smokers from the ATBC Cancer Prevention Study were randomized to receive 20 mg beta-carotene, 50 mg alpha-tocopherol, a mixture of both, or a placebo daily for five to eight years. An ophthalmologic exam was performed on subjects at the end of the trial. There were 269 cases of age-related maculopathy (ARM), and no benefit of beta-carotene or vitamin E supplements (40).

- Other dietary carotenoids such as lutein and zeaxanthin may have a potential benefit in degenerative disorders of vision. Intake of spinach and collard greens (rich in lutein and zeaxanthin) were strongly associated with reduced risk of ARM in one epidemiological study (1).

Vitamin A and Skin

- Natural and synthetic analogues of vitamin A (isotretinoin, etretinate, aciretin) have been used successfully in the treatment of skin disorders, including acne vulgaris and psoriasis (41). Individuals undergoing retinoid therapy are monitored for adverse effects typical of hypervitaminosis A, including liver toxicity, abnormal lipid profiles, teratogenic effects, and mucocutaneous side-effects (42).

SAFETY

- The Tolerable Upper Intake Level (UL), the highest dose likely not to pose a risk, is 3,000 µg/day (10,000 IU) preformed vitamin A for adult men and women. There is no established UL for carotenoids.

- Acute, high doses of vitamin A (> 200,000 µg in adults) are associated with nausea, vomiting, increased cerebrospinal pressure, vertigo, blurred vision, and muscular uncoordination. The median lethal dose (LD_{50}) of vitamin A extrapolated from studies in monkeys is 500 mg (500,000 µg) for a 70-kg adult (1).

- Chronic toxicity can result from ingested doses 10 times the RDA causing alopecia, ataxia, bone and muscle pain, cheilitis, conjunctivitis, headache, hepatotoxicity, hyperlipemia, membrane dryness, pruritus, skin disorders, and visual impairment (1).

- Teratogenic comment: the UL is 3,000 µg preformed vitamin A/day for pregnant women, and 2,800 µg/day for pregnant teenagers.

- Vitamin A and other retinoids are teratogenic in experimental animals and women. Ingestion of 20,000 IU (6,000 µg) during early pregnancy can cause spontaneous abortion and birth defects. Healthy pregnant women eating well-balanced diets containing fruits and vegetables do not need supplemental vitamin A. However, if a supplement is required it should not exceed 10,000 IU (3,000 µg) during pregnancy (1).

- There are no known acute negative effects with high doses of beta-carotene. High doses may cause hypercarotenemia, resulting in an orange-yellow tint of the skin (1).

- Long-term ingestion of high dose beta-carotene supplements was associated with increased lung cancer risk in men who smoke and asbestos workers and increased death in male smokers with heart disease, and increased risk of intracerebral hemorrhage in smokers without a history of stroke (20–22, 30, 43).

- Although some researchers have cautioned that pharmacological doses of one or two carotenoids may have negative consequences such as lowering levels of other plasma carotenoids, evidence from two long-term studies reported no adverse effects of beta-carotene supplements on plasma vitamin E and five other carotenoids (11, 12).

REFERENCES

1. Shils ME, Olson JA, Shike M, Ross AC, eds. *Modern Nutrition in Health and Disease.* 9th ed. Baltimore, Md: Williams & Wilkins; 1999.
2. Vainio H, Rautalahti M. An international evaluation of the cancer preventive potential of carotenoids. *Cancer Epidemiol Biomarkers Prev.* 1998;7:725–728.
3. Mayne ST. Beta-carotene, carotenoids, and disease prevention in humans. *FASEB J.* 1996;10:690–701.
4. Food and Nutrition Board, Institute of Medicine. *Dietary Reference Intakes: Vitamin C, Vitamin E, Selenium, and Carotenoids.* Washington, DC: National Academy Press; 2000.
5. Chug-Ahuja, Holden JM, Beecher GR, et al. The development and application of a carotenoid database for fruits, vegetables, and selected multicomponent foods. *J Am Diet Assoc.* 1993;93:318–323.

6. Mangels AR, et al. Carotenoid content of fruits and vegetables: an evaluation of analytic data. *J Am Diet Assoc.* 1993;93:284–296.

7. Rock CL. Carotenoids: Biology and Treatment. *Pharmacol Ther.* 1997;75:185–197.

8. Pennington JAT. *Bowes and Church's Food Values of Portions Commonly Used.* 17th ed. Philadelphia, Pa: Lippincott-Raven Publishers; 1998.

9. National Research Council, Subcommittee on the 10th Edition of the RDAs, Food and Nutrition Board, Commission of Life Sciences. *Recommended Dietary Allowances.* 10th ed. Washington, DC: National Academy Press; 1989.

10. Patrick L. Beta-carotene: the controversy continues. *Altern Med Rev.* 2000;5:530–545.

11. Nierenberg DW, Dain BJ, Mott LA, et al. Effects of 4 y of oral supplementation with beta-carotene on serum concentrations of retinol, tocopherol, and five carotenoids. *Am J Clin Nutr.* 1997;66:315–319.

12. Mayne ST, Cartmel B, Silva F, et al. Effect of supplemental beta-carotene on plasma concentrations of carotenoids, retinol, and alpha-tocopherol in humans. *Am J Clin Nutr.* 1998;68:642–647.

13. Brown ED, Micozzi MS, Craft NE, et al. Plasma carotenoids in normal men after a single ingestion of vegetables or purified beta-carotene. *Am J Clin Nutr.* 1989;49:1258–1265.

14. Micozzi MS, Brown ED, Edwards BK, et al. Plasma carotenoid response to chronic intake of selected foods and beta-carotene supplements in men. *Am J Clin Nutr.* 1992;55:1120–1125.

15. Verhoeven DT, Assen N, Goldbohm RA, et al. Vitamin C and E, retinol, beta-carotene, and dietary fiber in relation to breast cancer risk: a prospective cohort study. *Br J Cancer.* 1997;75:149–155.

16. Longnecker MP, Newcomb PA, Mittendorf R, et al. Intake of carrots, spinach, and supplements containing vitamin A in relation to risk of breast cancer. *Cancer Epidemiol Biomarkers Prev.* 1997;6:887–892.

17. Jumaan AO, Holmberg L, Zack M, et al. Beta-carotene intake and risk of post-menopausal breast cancer. *Epidemiology.* 1999;10:49–53.

18. Zhang S, Tang G, Russell RM, et al. Measurement of retinoids and carotenoids in breast adipose tissue and a comparison of concentrations in breast cancer cases and control subjects. *Am J Clin Nutr.* 1997;66:626–632.

19. Lee IM, Cook NR, Manson JE, et al. Beta-carotene supplementation and incidence of cancer and cardiovascular disease: the Women's Health Study. *J Natl Cancer Inst.* 1999;91:2102–2106.

20. Albanes D, Heinonen OP, Huttunen JK, et al. Effects of alpha-tocopherol and beta-carotene supplements on cancer incidence in the Alpha-Tocopherol Beta-Carotene Cancer Prevention Study. *Am J Clin Nutr.* 1995;62:1427S—1430S.

21. Albanes D, Heinonen OP, Taylor PR, et al. Alpha-tocopherol and beta-carotene supplements and lung cancer incidence in the Alpha-Tocopherol, Beta-Carotene cancer prevention study: effects of base-line characteristics and study compliance. *J Natl Cancer Inst.* 1996;88:1560–1570.

22. Omenn GS, Goodman GE, Thornquist MD, et al. Risk factors for lung cancer and for intervention effects in CARET, the Beta-Carotene and Retinol Efficacy Trial. *J Natl Cancer Inst.* 1996;88:1550–1559.

V

23. Albanes D, Malila N, Taylor PR, et al. Effects of supplemental alpha-tocopherol and beta-carotene on colorectal cancer: results from a controlled trial (Finland). *Cancer Causes Control.* 2000;11:197–205.

24. Kazi N, Radvany R, Oldham T, et al. Immunomodulatory effect of beta-carotene on T lymphocyte subsets in patients with resected colonic polyps and cancer. *Nutr Cancer.* 1997;28:140–145.

25. Onogi N, Okuno M, Matsushima-Nishiwaki R, et al. Antiproliferative effect of carotenoids on human colon cancer cells without conversion to retinoic acid. *Nutr Cancer.* 1998;32:20–24.

26. Liede K, Hietanen J, Saxen L, et al. Long-term supplementation with alpha-tocopherol and beta-carotene and prevalence of oral mucosal lesions in smokers. *Oral Dis.* 1998;4:78–83.

27. Mayne ST, Cartmel B, Baum M, et al. Randomized trial of supplemental beta-carotene to prevent second head and neck cancer. *Cancer Res.* 2001;61:1457–1463.

28. Frieling UM, Schaumberg DA, Kupper TS, et al. A randomized, 12-year primary-prevention trial of beta carotene supplementation for nonmelanoma skin cancer in the physician's health study. *Arch Dermatol.* 2000;136:179–184.

29. Virtamo J, Rapola JM, Ripatti S, et al. Effect of vitamin E and beta-carotene on the incidence of primary nonfatal myocardial infarction and fatal coronary heart disease. *Arch Intern Med.* 1998;158:668–675.

30. Rapola JM, Virtamo J, Ripatti S, et al. Randomized trial of alpha-tocopherol and beta-carotene supplements on incidence of major coronary events in men with previous myocardial infarction. *Lancet.* 1997;349:1715–1720.

31. Rapola JM, Virtamo J, Ripatti S, et al. Effects of alpha tocopherol and beta carotene supplements on symptoms, progression, and prognosis of angina pectoris. *Heart.* 1998;79:454–458.

32. Dixon ZR, Shie FS, Warden BA, et al. The effect of a low carotenoid diet on malondialdehyde-thiobarbituric acid (MDA-TBA) concentrations in women: a placebo-controlled, double-blind study. *J Am Coll Nutr.* 1998;17:54–58.

33. Corridan BM, O'Donoghue M, Hughes DA, et al. Low-dose supplementation with lycopene or beta-carotene does not enhance cell-mediated immunity in healthy free-living elderly humans. *Eur J Clin Nutr.* 2001;55:627–635.

34. Santos MS, Leka LS, Ribaya-Mercado JD, et al. Short- and long-term beta-carotene supplementation do not influence T cell-mediated immunity in healthy elderly persons. *Am J Clin Nutr.* 1997;66:917–924.

35. Hughes DA, Wright AJ, Finglas PM, et al. The effect of beta-carotene supplementation on the immune function of blood monocytes from healthy male nonsmokers. *J Lab Clin Med.* 1997;129:309–317.

36. Daudu PA, Kelley DS, Taylor PC, et al. Effect of a low-beta-carotene diet on the immune functions of adult women. *Am J Clin Nutr.* 1994;60:969–972.

37. Murata T, Tamai H, Morinobu T, et al. Effect of long-term administration of beta-carotene on lymphocyte subsets in humans. *Am J Clin Nutr.* 1994;60:597–602.

38. Coodley GO, Nelson HD, Loveless MO, et al. Beta-carotene in HIV infection. *J Acquir Immune Defic Syndr.* 1993;6:272–276.

V

39. Teikari JM, Virtamo J, Rautalahti M, et al. Long-term supplementation with alpha-tocopherol and beta-carotene and age-related cataract. *Acta Ophthalmol Scand.* 1997;75:634–640.

40. Teikari JM, Laatikainen L, Virtamo J, et al. Six-year supplementation with alpha-tocopherol and beta-carotene and age-related maculopathy. *Acta Ophthalmol Scand.* 1998;76:224–229.

41. Hartmann D, Bollag W. Historical aspects of the oral use of retinoids in acne. *J Dermatol.* 1993;20:674–678.

42. David M, Hodak E, Lowe NJ. Adverse effects of retinoids. *Med Toxicol Adverse Drug Exp.* 1988;3:273–288.

43. Leppala JM, Virtamo J, Fogelholm R, et al. Controlled trial of alpha-tocopherol and beta-carotene supplements on stroke incidence and mortality in male smokers. *Arterioscler Thromb Vasc Biol.* 2000;20:230–235.

Vitamin B$_1$ (Thiamin)

The water-soluble vitamin thiamin, as part of thiamin pyrophosphate (TPP) and thiamin triphosphate (TTP), acts as a coenzyme in the metabolism of carbohydrates and branched-chain amino acids. Thiamin works synergistically with lipoic acid, niacin (NAD+), and pantothenic acid in energy production. The body contains a total of 30 mg of thiamin (80 percent as TPP) with higher concentrations found in muscles including the heart, and in the liver, kidneys, and brain. Because thiamin is not stored in large amounts in any tissue, a continuous dietary supply is needed to prevent deficiency. Beriberi, the clinical deficiency of thiamin, is characterized by peripheral neuropathy, muscle atrophy, and/or cardiovascular problems (edema, cardiomegaly, congestive heart failure). Although an overt deficiency is rare in most people, the elderly, alcoholics, dialysis patients, and patients in hypermetabolic states are at increased risk (1).

Media and Marketing Claims	Efficacy
Increases energy and prevents fatigue	NR
Reduces dementia in Alzheimer's disease patients	↔
Reduces stress	NR
Prevents canker sores	NR

Advisory

- No reported serious adverse effects
- Tolerable Upper Intake Level (UL) has not been established

Drug/Supplement Interactions

Loop diuretics (furosemide) increase urinary thiamin losses and may result in thiamin deficiency

V

KEY POINTS

- There is little evidence from well-controlled studies suggesting that thiamin supplements reduce fatigue and increase the perception of "energy" in healthy individuals without thiamin deficiency. In one small study, a high dose of a thiamin derivative did not result in an improvement in physical performance.

- The elderly may be at risk for a number of nutritional deficiencies including thiamin deficiency. Preliminary research in Alzheimer's patients on high-dose thiamin therapy is equivocal. Elderly patients may need to modify their diet to ensure adequate consumption of thiamin (and other B vitamins) and if intake is low, a multivitamin/mineral supplement providing 100 percent of the RDA would be helpful.

- Although thiamin and other B-vitamin requirements increase with intense physical exertion or physical trauma, there is currently no controlled research indicating that thiamin supplements improve the body's ability to cope with daily emotional stress or anxiety.

- There is preliminary evidence that a subclinical thiamin deficiency is associated with recurrent mouth ulcers. Research is needed to determine the possible role of thiamin supplements in ameliorating this condition.

FOOD SOURCES

Meat, legumes, whole grains (germ), and seeds are good sources of thiamin. Thiamin is easily oxidized by heat (cooking, baking, pasteurization, spray-drying milk), sulfites (in dried fruit), irradiation, refining whole wheat, and sodium bicarbonate (added to canned legumes) (1). In addition, the presence of thiaminases present in raw fish (sushi) and rice bran or thiamin antagonists in tea, coffee, and rice bran interfere with thiamin absorption (1).

Food	Thiamin (mg)
Pork loin (3.5 oz)	0.92
Peas, green (½ c)	0.23
Rice, brown (1 c)	0.19
Beans, pinto (½ c)	0.16
Potato, baked	0.16
Peanuts (1 oz)	0.12
Chicken breast (3.5 oz)	0.07
Beef, ground, lean (3.5 oz)	0.05
Broccoli (½ c)	0.04

Source: Data from Pennington (2)

DOSAGE INFORMATION/BIOAVAILABILITY

The adult RDA is 1.1 mg for adult women and 1.2 for men (3). Thiamin is available in multivitamin/mineral supplements, B-complex supplements, and single preparations in the form of thiamin hydrochloride in dosages ranging from 1 mg to 500 mg. Some studies have used a fat-soluble thiamin derivative (thiamin tetrahydrofurfuryl disulfide) that is absorbed more efficiently than the water-soluble form and is readily converted into thiamin (4). Ingested thiamin is fairly well absorbed and is converted to phosphorylated forms (TPP and TTP) (1). Thiamin status depends on its bioavailability from foods, alcohol consumption, presence of antithiamin factors, and folate and protein status (1).

RELEVANT RESEARCH

Thiamin and Exercise

- In a short-term, double-blind, placebo-controlled, crossover study, 14 subjects were randomized to receive 1,000 mg of a thiamin derivative (thiamin tetrahydrofurfuryl disulfide) or a placebo for four days each. There was a 10-day washout between trials. On day 3, subjects completed a progressive exercise test to exhaustion on a cycle ergometer to determine $VO_{2submax}$, VO_{2peak}, lactate concentration, lactate threshold, and heart rate. On day 4 subjects performed a maximal timed trial on the cycle. There were no significant differences between trials on any of the parameters measured (4).

Thiamin for the Elderly and Dementia

- There have been several reports of low plasma and brain thiamin levels in patients with Alzheimer's disease and frontal lobe degeneration of the non-Alzheimer's type (5–7).
- In a double-blind, placebo-controlled study, 76 elderly subjects (35 subjects with two low erythrocyte concentrations of TPP measured three months apart and 41 subjects with one low TPP level) were randomly assigned to ingest 10 mg thiamin daily or a placebo for three months. Blood pressure, hand-grip strength, height, weight, and BMI were measured before and after the study. Cognition, functional ability, and general health were assessed by the Mini-Mental State Examination, the 45-point Frenchay Activities Index, and the Nottingham Health Profile, respectively. Daily alcohol and food intake was assessed as part of a dietary survey with a validated food frequency questionnaire. Treatment was associated with a significant increase in erythrocyte TPP concentrations compared to the placebo. Average daily alcohol intake was significantly higher in subjects with persistently low TPP levels than in those with only one low TPP level. Only thiamin-treated subjects with persistently low TPP levels (n = 18) showed subjective benefits with significant improvements in quality of life, and significant decreases in systolic blood pressure and weight compared to placebo subjects with persistently low TPP (n = 17). There was an insignificant trend toward self-reported improvements in sleep and energy with thiamin supplement use. There was no effect on grip strength, functional ability, cognition, or general health. The authors concluded that the community-dwelling elderly population may benefit from thiamin supplementation or dietary modification (8).
- In a double-blind, placebo-controlled, crossover trial, 18 patients with Alzheimer's-type dementia were randomized to receive 3,000 mg thiamin daily or a placebo for one

V

month each with no washout period. A second single-blinded experiment was performed using 4,000 mg to 8,000 mg thiamin/day for 5 to 13 months in 17 patients (6 from the first trial). Doses were increased monthly throughout this second trial. Neuropsychological tests (Alzheimer's Disease Assessment Scale, ADAS; Mini-Mental State Examination, MMSE), electrocardiogram, complete blood count, and liver function tests were performed at the baseline and at the end of each treatment phase in the first trial and every four weeks in the second trial. A physician assessment (Clinical Global Impression of Change, CGIC) was included only in the second experiment. In the first experiment, a statistically significant improvement in ADAS scores occurred in the thiamin condition compared to the placebo after one month. Placebo scores, but not thiamin treatment scores, on ADAS and MMSE were significantly worse after one month compared to the baseline. In the second trial, high-dose thiamin significantly improved ADAS scores compared to the baseline at months 1, 6, and 7. MMSE scores did not differ. CGIC scores tended to improve but did not reach significance. There were no noted adverse effects with high dose thiamin other than mild intestinal upset with the 7,000-mg dose. The authors concluded: "We advise caution in over-interpretation of these data in order to avoid raising public expectations. In our opinion, high-dose thiamin offers only a mildly beneficial symptomatic therapy, and the ultimate treatment of Alzheimer's disease will await better understanding of the underlying mechanisms in order to develop a therapy that halts or prevents structural damage to the brain" (9).

- In a double-blind, placebo-controlled study, 10 subjects with Alzheimer's-type dementia were given 3,000 mg thiamin or a placebo daily for 12 months. In both groups, MMSE scores, verbal learning, and naming scores decreased significantly throughout the study period. There were no differences between the groups at any point during the study. The authors concluded: "These results do not support the hypothesis that long-term administration of thiamin at 3 g/day might slow the progression of dementia of the Alzheimer's type" (10).

- In a double-blind, placebo-controlled, crossover study, 11 moderately impaired patients with "probable Alzheimer's disease" were given 3,000 mg thiamin or a placebo (niacinamide) for three months each. Patients were well-nourished with no evidence of thiamin deficiency. There was a significant improvement in global cognitive scores on the MMSE with thiamin therapy compared to a niacinamide placebo. There was no effect on behavioral ratings or the subjective judgment of clinical state between therapies (11).

Thiamin and Mouth Ulcers

- Low erythrocyte thiamin levels have been associated with recurrent aphthous stomatitis (mouth ulcers) independent of age, sex, or underlying disease causing the stomatitis (12).

- A study of 60 patients with recurrent mouth ulcers found that 28.2 percent were deficient in at least one of the following: thiamin, riboflavin, and pyridoxine. Replacement therapy of these vitamins was given to a group of deficient and nondeficient patients for one month. At the end of the study and three months after, subjects with a deficiency had a significant sustained clinical improvement. The authors suggested that vitamin B_1, B_2, and B_6 deficiency may be a possible precipitating factor in recurrent aphthous ulceration. However, the study design does not permit attribution of the benefits to thiamin supplements alone (13).

SAFETY

- Thiamin in excessive doses is rapidly cleared by the kidneys and has no apparent toxic effects (1). The Tolerable Upper Intake Level (UL) has not been set due to lack of data for quantitative risk assessment.

- The LD_{50} in mice and dogs is 125 mg to 350 mg/kg body weight.

REFERENCES

1. Tanphaichitr V. Thiamin. In: Shils ME, Olson JA, Shike M, Ross AC, eds. *Modern Nutrition in Health and Disease.* 9th ed. Baltimore, Md: Williams & Wilkins; 1999:381–389.
2. Pennington JAT. *Bowes & Church's Food Values of Portions Commonly Used.* 17th ed. Philadelphia, Pa: Lippincott; 1998.
3. Institute of Medicine, Food and Nutrition Board. *Dietary Reference Intakes for Thiamin, Riboflavin, Niacin, Vitamin B-6, Folate, Vitamin B-12, Pantothenic Acid, Biotin, and Choline.* Washington, DC: National Academy Press; 1998.
4. Webster MJ, Scheett TP, Doyle MR, et al. The effect of a thiamin derivative on exercise performance. *Eur J Appl Physiol.* 1997;75:520–524.
5. Gold M, Hauser RA, Chen MF. Plasma thiamine deficiency associated with Alzheimer's disease but not Parkinson's disease. *Metab Brain Dis.* 1998;13:43–53.
6. Bettendorff L, Mastrogiacomo F, Wins P, et al. Low thiamine diphosphate levels in brains of patients with frontal lobe degeneration of the non-Alzheimer's type. *J Neurochem.* 1997;69:2005–2010.
7. Mastrogiacomo F, Bettendorff L, Grisar T, et al. Brain thiamine, its phosphate esters, and its metabolizing enzymes in Alzheimer's disease. *Ann Neurol.* 1996;39:585–591.
8. Wilkinson TJ, Hanger HC, Elmslie J, et al. The response to treatment of subclinical thiamine deficiency in the elderly. *Am J Clin Nutr.* 1997;66:925–928.
9. Meador K, Loring D, Nichols M, et al. Preliminary findings of high-dose thiamine in dementia of Alzheimer's type. *J Geriatr Psychiatry Neurol.* 1993;6:222–229.
10. Nolan KA, Black RS, Sheu KF, et al. A trial of thiamine in Alzheimer's disease. *Arch Neurol.* 1991;48:81–83.
11. Blass JP, Gleason P, Brush D, et al. Thiamine and Alzheimer's disease. A pilot study. *Arch Neurol.* 1988;45:833–835.
12. Haisraeli-Shalish M, Livneh A, Katz J, et al. Recurrent aphthous stomatitis and thiamine deficiency. *Oral Surg Oral Med Oral Pathol Oral Radiol Endod.* 1996;82:634–636.
13. Nolan A, McIntosh WB, Allam BF, et al. Recurrent aphthous ulceration: vitamin B1, B2 and B6 status and response to replacement therapy. *J Oral Pathol Med.* 1991;20:389–391.

V

Vitamin B$_2$ (Riboflavin)

As part of the coenzymes FAD (flavin adenine dinucleotide) and FMN (flavin adenine mononucleotide), riboflavin is involved in numerous oxidation/reduction reactions. Riboflavin, along with other water-soluble B vitamins, is used in the oxidation of glucose and fatty acids to produce ATP. FAD and FMN also act together to convert vitamin B$_6$ to its functional coenzyme, which then converts tryptophan into niacin. The thyroid gland is responsible for regulating an enzyme that phosphorylates riboflavin to its active form. Although rare in Western cultures, riboflavin deficiency is characterized by photophobia, vascularization of the cornea, magenta tongue, cheilitis, and seborrheic dermatitis of the nose and scrotum. The elderly and alcoholics are at increased risk for subclinical riboflavin deficiency (1, 2). Less than five percent of individuals in all genders and lifestage groups have intakes less than the Estimated Average Requirement for riboflavin (3).

Media and Marketing Claims	Efficacy
Prevents migraine headaches	NR
Increases energy	NR

Advisory

- No reported serious adverse effects
- Tolerable Upper Intake Level (UL) is not yet established

Drug/Supplement Interactions

No reported adverse interactions

KEY POINTS

- A preliminary controlled study in 55 subjects suggested that high-dose riboflavin reduces the frequency, incidence, and duration of migraine headaches in the short term. Additional studies are needed to examine the potential beneficial role of riboflavin in migraine headaches.

- Riboflavin is necessary for energy production; however, there is no evidence that healthy individuals have increased "energy" or less fatigue from supplements.

FOOD SOURCES

Good sources of riboflavin include dairy products, meats, eggs, and green leafy vegetables. Although riboflavin is heat stable, it is easily destroyed by light and alkali (baking soda). Sixty percent of the vitamin is lost during milling of flour. However, breads and cereals are enriched to replace losses (1, 2).

Food	Riboflavin (mg)
Milk, nonfat (1 c)	0.34
Egg (1)	0.26
Spinach (½ c)	0.21
Spaghetti (1 c)	0.14
Salmon (3.5 oz)	0.11
Chicken (½ breast)	0.11
Broccoli, (½ c)	0.09

Source: Data from Pennington JAT (4)

DOSAGE INFORMATION/BIOAVAILABILITY

The RDA for riboflavin is 1.3 mg/day for men and 1.1 mg/day for women (3). Riboflavin is available in multivitamin/mineral supplements, B-complex supplements, and individual preparations as pure riboflavin in dosages ranging from 1.1 mg to 100 mg. One study reported that the maximal amount of riboflavin absorbed from a single dose (40 mg to 60 mg) in eight healthy subjects was 27 mg (5). However, even though intestinal absorption of riboflavin is a saturable process, there is evidence that prolonged retention of the vitamin in the small intestine can increase the total amount absorbed (6).

RELEVANT RESEARCH

Riboflavin and Migraine

- In a double-blind, placebo-controlled trial, 55 patients with migraine were randomized to receive 400 mg riboflavin or a placebo for three months. All patients received a placebo for one month prior to the study. There was a significant reduction in attack frequency, number of headache days, and duration of migraines with riboflavin treatment compared to the placebo. In a comparison the proportion of subjects with favorable responses, the riboflavin group (59 percent improved) had a statistically greater improvement compared to placebo (15 percent improved). The authors concluded that because of its apparent tolerability, low cost, and potential benefit, riboflavin is a candidate for a comparative trial using an established prophylactic migraine drug (6).

- In a comparative study (not blinded or randomized), 26 subjects with migraine history received either beta-blocker drugs or 400 mg riboflavin for four months. Auditory-evoked cortical potentials were recorded at least three days before or after an attack (the intensity of evoked cortical potentials usually increases in migraine). None of the subjects had received prophylactic migraine therapy for at least one month before the first recording. After treatment with beta-blockers, the intensity dependence of the auditory evoked cortical potentials (IDAP) was significantly decreased, and this correlated with a significant clinical improvement. After riboflavin treatment, there was no change in IDAP. Headache frequency decreased significantly in both groups.

V

When clinical efficacy (expressed as change in headache frequency) was compared with IDAP change, there was a positive correlation with beta-blockers, but not with riboflavin. However, this study was not blinded or randomized, so the results may be biased and should be viewed with caution (7).

SAFETY

- Because excess riboflavin is excreted by the kidneys, toxicity is very low (1, 8).
- Due to lack of data, a Tolerable Upper Intake Level (UL) has not been determined for riboflavin (3).

REFERENCES

1. McCormick DB. Riboflavin. In: Shils ME, Olson JA, Shike M, Ross AC, eds. *Modern Nutrition in Health and Disease.* 9th ed. Baltimore, Md: Williams & Wilkins; 1999:391–399.
2. Madigan SM, Tracey F, McNulty H, et al. Riboflavin and vitamin B-6 intakes and status and biochemical response to riboflavin supplementation in free-living elderly people. *Am J Clin Nutr.* 1998;68:389–395.
3. Institute of Medicine, Food and Nutrition Board. *Dietary Reference Intakes for Thiamin, Riboflavin, Niacin, Vitamin B-6, Folate, Vitamin B-12, Pantothenic Acid, Biotin, and Choline.* Washington, DC: National Academy Press; 1999.
4. Pennington JAT. *Bowes and Church's Food Values of Portions Commonly Used.* 17th ed. Philadelphia, Pa: Lippincott; 1998.
5. Zempleni J, Galloway JR, McCormick DB. Pharmacokinetics of orally and intravenously administered riboflavin in healthy humans. *Am J Clin Nutr.* 1996;63:54–66.
6. Schoenen J, Jacquy J, Lenaerts M. Effectiveness of high-dose riboflavin in migraine prophylaxis. A randomized controlled trial. *Neurology.* 1998;50:466–470.
7. Sandor PS, Afra J, Ambrosini A, et al. Prophylactic treatment of migraine with beta-blockers and riboflavin: differential effects on the intensity dependence of auditory evoked cortical potentials. *Headache.* 2000;40:30–35.
8. Bates CJ. Bioavailability of riboflavin. *Eur J Clin Nutr.* 1997;51(suppl 1):S38–S42.

Vitamin B₃ (Niacin)

Niacin is the collective term used to describe nicotinic acid and nicotinamide (or nicotinate and niacinamide, respectively). The metabolically active forms of niacin are the coenzymes: nicotinamide adenine dinucleotide (NAD) and NAD phosphate (NADP). Hundreds of enzymes are dependent on NAD and NADP in the synthesis and/or degradation of carbohydrates, fatty acids, and amino acids. The classic deficiency of niacin, pellagra, is characterized by dermatitis, diarrhea, and dementia, commonly referred to as the three Ds. Nicotinic acid has been used as an effective therapy for lowering blood lipids since 1955 (1).

Media and Marketing Claims	Efficacy
Lowers cholesterol (nicotinic acid)	↑
May prevent development of diabetes (nicotinamide)	↔
Improves arthritis symptoms	NR

Advisory

- The Tolerable Upper Intake Level (UL) is 35 mg niacin equivalents/day
- Pharmacological doses of niacin should only be used while under the care of a physician due to potential serious adverse effects

Drug/Supplement Interactions

- May interfere with diabetic medications
- May increase risk of myopathy if combined with lovastatin (HMG-CoA reductase inhibitor for hypercholesterolemia)
- May increase levels of carbamazepine (antiseizure drug)

KEY POINTS

- High-dose niacin (nicotinic acid) is an accepted medical therapy for treating hyperlipidemia. Nicotinamide does not produce lipid-lowering effects. Nicotinic acid therapy has been found to significantly lower the risk of cardiovascular disease endpoints and all-cause mortality. Because of the side-effects and risk of hepatoxicity, patients should be under medical supervision while they are taking gram quantities of niacin. Self-administration of nicotinic acid is not recommended.

- According to animal studies, nicotinamide has a protective effect on beta-cells in the pancreas. Although a meta-analysis of 16 clinical trials also reported a protective effect on beta-cells with nicotinamide, there was no improvement in glycemic control in patients with diagnosed type 1 diabetes. Trials are underway investigating the effects of nicotinamide therapy in individuals at risk for developing type 1 diabetes. Of the completed clinical studies, one reported no benefit in preventing or delaying diabetes onset. More research is needed to clarify possible benefits, dosage, and safety of using nicotinamide in the possible prevention of type 1 diabetes for individuals at risk. The efficacy of nicotinic acid in patients with established diabetes is unclear. Although nicotinic acid can be effective in treating dyslipidemia, it may also worsen glycemic control.

- There is preliminary research suggesting a possible benefit of nicotinamide therapy for osteoarthritis. Large, controlled clinical trials are needed to verify these results.

- For most individuals, a balanced diet in accordance with the Food Guide Pyramid should provide sufficient niacin to meet daily recommendations. Pharmacological doses of either nicotinic acid or niacinamide should only be taken while people are under the care of a physician.

V

FOOD SOURCES

Meats, fish, legumes, some cereals, and products containing enriched flours (breads, cereals, pastas) are good sources of niacin (1 mg to 40 mg/100 g). Coffee beans also have a high niacin content (40 mg/100 g). Niacin is unique in that the essential amino acid tryptophan, a niacin precursor, can contribute significantly to meeting dietary niacin requirements. Therefore, a diet containing 100 g protein (approximately 1 percent tryptophan) and no preformed niacin could meet the RDA (1, 2).

Food	Niacin (mg)
Chicken breast (½)	11.8
Tuna, canned (3 oz)	11.3
Beef, ground, lean (3.5 oz)	4.3
Peanuts, roasted (1 oz)	3.8
Avocado (1 medium)	3.3
Bagel (3½ in)	3.2
Potato, baked, no skin (medium)	2.2
Beans, navy (1 c)	1.3
Mango (1)	1.2
Milk, nonfat (1 c)	0.2

Source: Data from Pennington JAT (3)

DOSAGE INFORMATION/BIOAVAILABILITY

The RDA for niacin is represented as milligrams of Niacin Equivalents (NE) because tryptophan can contribute to total niacin intake. The revised RDA is 16 mg NE for adult men and 14 mg NE for adult women, with a Tolerable Upper Intake Level (UL) set at 35 mg NE/day for adults older than 18 years (4). Niacin is available in single preparation supplements or in multivitamin/mineral or B-complex supplements as nicotinic acid (nicotinate) or nicotinamide (niacinamide) supplements in doses ranging from 14 mg to 1,000 mg. In many foods, niacin has low bioavailability because it is bound to macromolecules of carbohydrate or protein. Food processing or mild alkaline treatment during cooking releases much of the bound niacin (1, 4).

RELEVANT RESEARCH

Niacin (Nicotinic Acid/Nicotinate) and Cardiovascular Disease

- Nicotinic acid at pharmacologic doses (1 g to 3 g/day divided into three or four doses) is well known as a drug used to decrease levels of triglycerides, and total and LDL cholesterol, and increase HDL cholesterol levels. Despite extensive research demonstrating the lipid-lowering activity of nicotinic acid, the mechanism of action is not known. These large doses have been associated with flushing of the skin (vasodilation), hyperuricemia, abnormal liver function, and hyperglycemia and should be administered under the supervision of a physician. Nicotinamide does not affect blood lipids or cause these side-effects (1).

- One review article summarized six major randomized, placebo-controlled trials of niacin with cardiovascular endpoints. The Coronary Drug Project (n = 8,341 men) reported significant decreases in recurrent myocardial infarction and cerebrovascular events with niacin monotherapy (3 g/day). The other five trials used varying combinations of niacin with other pharmacologic agents. These trials reported significant reductions in coronary and total mortality, coronary events, and angiographic progression of atherosclerosis in all trials except for one in patients with normal blood cholesterol levels at entry. According to the author, "The use of niacin to prevent or treat atherosclerotic cardiovascular disease is based on strong and consistent evidence from clinical trials" (5).

Niacin and Diabetes

- In animal studies, high doses of nicotinamide have prevented or delayed the development of disease in spontaneously diabetic nonobese mice (a model of human type 1 diabetes). In laboratory studies, nicotinamide has demonstrated a protective effect on beta-cells (insulin-producing cells in the pancreas). On the basis of the positive outcome of animal experiments, several placebo-controlled trials are being conducted in Europe to test whether niacin therapy delays the development of type 1 diabetes in individuals at high risk (6). One forthcoming trial (European Nicotinamide Diabetes Intervention Trial—ENDIT) will examine whether nicotinamide will reduce the rate of progression of type 1 diabetes in individuals at high risk of developing the disease (7).

- In a placebo-controlled trial (Deutsche Nicotinamide Intervention Study), 55 individuals (aged 3 y to 12 y) at risk of developing type I diabetes were randomized to receive 1.2 g/m body surface area sustained-release nicotinamide or a placebo for a maximum of 3.8 years. Subjects at risk for developing diabetes were identified by screening siblings (aged 3 y to 12 y) of patients with type 1 diabetes for the presence of high titer islet cell antibodies. Rates of diabetes onset were similar in both groups. The trial was terminated after the eleventh case of diabetes showed that no reduction of the cumulative diabetes incidence was detectable after three years. The authors concluded: "In this subgroup of diabetes-prone individuals at very high risk and with an assumed rapid disease progression, nicotinamide treatment did not cause a major decrease or delay of diabetes development" (5).

- A 1996 meta-analysis of 16 trials (10 randomized, 5 of which were placebo-controlled) testing nicotinamide treatment in patients with recent-onset type 1 diabetes reported no differences in the insulin dose required or glycosylated hemoglobin values between treated and control patients. However, after one year of diagnosis, baseline C-peptide (measure of pancreatic beta-cell function) was significantly higher in nicotinamide-treated patients than in controls. This statistical difference was present when the five placebo-controlled trials only were analyzed. There were few adverse effects (2 of 291 subjects reported skin rash, 2 subjects experienced recurrent hypoglycemia, and 2 sub-

V

jects experienced transient elevation in transaminase). The authors concluded: "Since adverse effects were negligible, we suggest that prolonged use of nicotinamide after IDDM diagnosis should be tested to see whether residual beta-cell function can be preserved for longer periods" (8).

- In a controlled, crossover trial, 13 dyslipidemic patients with type 2 diabetes were assigned in random order to receive nicotinic acid (1.5 g three times daily) or no therapy for eight weeks each. Compared with control, nicotinic acid supplements significantly reduced blood lipids; however, therapy resulted in a deterioration of glycemic control (16 percent increase in plasma glucose, 21 percent increase in glycosylated hemoglobin levels, and glycosuria in some patients). The authors concluded: "Despite improvement in lipid and lipoprotein concentrations, because of worsening hyperglycemia and the development of hyperuricemia, nicotinic acid must be used with caution in patients with non-insulin-dependent diabetes. We suggest that the drug not be used as a first-line hypolipidemic drug in patients with non-insulin dependent diabetes mellitus" (9).

- In a single-blind, placebo-controlled study, 18 type 2 diabetes patients of normal body weight unresponsive to sulfonylureas were randomized to receive one of three treatments for six months: (1) insulin plus 1.5 g nicotinamide, (2) insulin plus a placebo, or (3) current sulfonylureas plus nicotinamide. Subjects were evaluated for C-peptide, glycosylated hemoglobin, and fasting daily blood glucose levels before and at the end of the study. Compared with group 2, C-peptide release increased in both groups 1 and 3. Multiple regression analysis revealed that nicotinamide administration was the only significant factor for the improvement in C-peptide release (10).

Niacin and Arthritis

- In a double-blind, placebo-controlled trial, 72 patients with osteoarthritis were randomized to receive 3 mg nicotinamide (divided into six doses) or a placebo daily for 12 weeks. Global arthritis impact and pain, joint range of motion and flexibility, erythrocyte sedimentation rate, complete blood count, liver function tests, cholesterol, uric acid, and fasting blood sugar were measured. There was a statistically significant 29 percent improvement in global arthritis impact with nicotinamide compared to a worsening of 10 percent with the placebo. There were no differences in pain levels between groups. There was a statistically significant 13 percent reduction of anti-inflammatory medication use, reduced erythrocyte sedimentation, and increased joint mobility associated with nicotinamide treatment. Nicotinamide had no effect on fasting blood glucose, uric acid, cholesterol, or hematological values. The authors concluded that nicotinamide may play a role in the treatment of osteroarthritis and that more extensive evaluation is warranted (11).

SAFETY

- The Tolerable Upper Intake Level (UL) is 35 mg Niacin Equivalents/day for adults more than 18 years old (4).

- High doses of nicotinic acid can cause skin flushing and pruritis, gastrointestinal discomfort, and abnormal liver function tests. Taking regular niacin with meals in divided doses or with aspirin may reduce flushing (12). Individuals taking high-dose nicotinic acid should be monitored by their physician because of these serious adverse effects (13). In contrast, nicotinamide has not been associated with vasodilative effects.

- Although sustained or time-released niacin (nicotinic acid) supplements reduce skin flushing, they have been associated with liver toxicity (14). However, a new prescription time-released niacin preparation approved by the FDA for treating lipid disorders was reported to be safe and well-tolerated at doses of 2,000 mg/day in a two-year study (15).

- High doses of nicotinamide may be associated with reversible liver toxicity and liver enzyme abnormalities. It has also inconsistently been associated with minor insulin resistance (16).

- Niacin therapy should not be used by patients with active peptic ulcers or gastroesophageal reflux, liver disease, or alcohol abuse (13).

- The oral median lethal dose (LD$_{50}$) for the rat is 4.5 g to 5.2 g/kg for nicotinic acid and 3.5 g/kg nicotinamide (1).

- An acute oral dose of nicotinamide (2 g) was associated with an increase in insulin resistance in patients at risk for developing type 1 diabetes (17). Nicotinic acid caused deterioration of glycemic control in type 2 diabetes patients (9).

REFERENCES

1. Cervantes-Laurean D, McElvaney NG, Moss J. Niacin. In: Shils ME, Olson JA, Shike M, eds. *Modern Nutrition in Health and Disease.* 9th ed. Baltimore, Md: Williams & Wilkins; 1999:401–411.
2. van den Berg H. Bioavailability of niacin. *Eur J Clin Nutr.* 1997;51(suppl 1):S64—S65.
3. Pennington JAT. *Bowes and Church's Food Values of Portions Commonly Used.* 17th ed. Philadelphia, Pa: Lippincott-Raven Publishers; 1998.
4. Institute of Medicine, Food and Nutrition Board. *Dietary Reference Intakes for Thiamin, Riboflavin, Niacin, Vitamin B-6, Folate, Vitamin B-12, Pantothenic Acid, Biotin, and Choline.* Washington, DC: National Academy Press; 1998.
5. Guyton JR. Effect of niacin on atherosclerotic cardiovascular disease. *Am J Cardiol.* 1998;82(12A):18U–23U.
6. Lampeter EF, Klinghammer A, Scherbaum WA, et al. The Deutsche Nicotinamide Intervention Study: An attempt to prevent type I diabetes. Denis Group. *Diabetes.* 1998;47:980–984.
7. Schatz DA, Bingley PJ. Update on major trials for the prevention of type 1 diabetes mellitus: the American Diabetes Prevention Trial (DPT-1) and the European Nicotinamide Diabetes Intervention Trial (ENDIT). *J Pediatr Endocrinol Metab.* 2001;14:619–622.
8. Pozzilli P, Browne PD, Kolb H. Meta-analysis of nicotinamide treatment in patients with recent-onset IDDM. The Nicotinamide Trialists. *Diabetes Care.* 1996;19:1357–1363.

V

9. Garg A, Grundy SM. Nicotinic acid as therapy for dyslipidemia in non-insulin-dependent diabetes mellitus. *JAMA*. 1990;264:723–726.

10. Polo V, Saibene A, Pontiroli AE. Nicotinamide improves insulin secretion and metabolic control in lean type 2 diabetic patients with secondary failure to sulphonylureas. *Acta Diabetol*. 1998;35:61–64.

11. Jonas WB, Rapoza CP, Blair WF. The effect of niacinamide on osteoarthritis: a pilot study. *Inflamm Res*. 1996;45:330–334.

12. Jungnickel PW, Maloley PA, Vander Tuin EL, et al. Effect of two aspirin pretreatment regimens on niacin-induced cutaneous reactions. *J Gen Intern Med*. 1997;12:591–596.

13. Schuna AA. Safe use of niacin. *Am J Health Syst Pharm*. 1997;54:2803.

14. Henkin Y, Oberman A, Hurst DC, et al. Niacin revisited: clinical observations on an important but underutilized drug. *Am J Med*. 1991;91:239–246.

15. Capuzzi DM, Guyton JR, Morgan JM, et al. Efficacy and safety of an extended-release niacin (Niaspan): A long-term study. *Am J Cardiol*. 1998;82(12A):74U—81U.

16. Knip M, Douek IF, Moore WP, et al. Safety of high-dose nicotinamide: a review. *Diabetologia*. 2000;43:1337–1345.

17. Greenbaum CJ, Kahn SE, Palmer JP. Nicotinamide's effect on glucose metabolism in subjects at risk for IDDM. *Diabetes*. 1996;45:1631–1634.

Vitamin B_6 (Pyridoxine)

Vitamin B_6 is the collective term used to describe pyridoxine (found in plant foods), and the phosphorylated forms pyridoxal and pyridoxamine (found in animal foods). The coenzyme forms of B_6 are pyridoxal 5'phosphate (PLP) and pyridoxamine 5'phosphate (PMP). PLP, the active form, is involved in more than 100 enzymatic reactions. After absorption, the liver releases vitamin B_6 as pyridoxal into the blood plasma with the majority bound to hemoglobin in red blood cells. The other major pool of vitamin B_6 is found in the muscle, where PLP is bound to glycogen phosphorylase. Vitamin B_6 plays a role in the synthesis, catabolism, and transport of amino acids, gluconeogenesis, niacin formation, neurotransmitter synthesis, erythrocyte metabolism, hormone modulation, and lipid metabolism (1, 2).

Media and Marketing Claims	Efficacy
Relieves pain of carpal tunnel syndrome	↔
Relieves symptoms of PMS	↔
Reduces risk of cardiovascular disease	?↑
Beneficial for asthmatics	↓
Treats autism	↔

Advisory

• The Tolerable Upper Intake Level (UL) is 100 mg/day for adults

- Long-term use of very high doses (500 mg to 5,000 mg/day) is associated with nerve damage

Drug/Supplement Interactions

The following drugs all interfere with vitamin B_6 status: Isoniazid (antibiotic); hydralazine (for hypertension); phenelzine, cycloserine (antibiotic); penicillamine (for Wilson's disease); conjugated estrogens (oral contraceptives); theophylline (bronchodilator); corticosteroids (anti-inflammatory); erythromycin (antibiotic); gentamicin, neomycin, sulfonamides (antibiotics), alcohol and caffeine. Alternatively, high-dose supplements could potentially interfere with these drugs.

KEY POINTS

- Vitamin B_6 supplementation for carpal tunnel sydrome remains controversial. Most of the studies to date were small, uncontrolled, and lacked randomization and double-blind design. Large, well-controlled studies are required before recommendations can be made.

- Evidence from studies using high-dose supplements of vitamin B_6 in subjects with PMS is equivocal. Although there is evidence of some beneficial effects, most positive trials have been criticized for poor quality. One researcher concluded: "Physicians recommending vitamin B_6 should convey appropriate precautions to their patients, as popular lore holds that this vitamin is unharmful and of likely benefit."

- Epidemiololgical data suggest that low serum levels of vitamin B_6 are associated with increased CVD risk. An intake of 3 mg/day of vitamin B_6 was associated with lower risk of heart attack in women. Controlled clinical trials are required to fully evaluate the effect of vitamin B_6 supplements on cardiovascular risk factors and CVD incidence.

- Asthma patients taking theophylline, a vitamin B_6 antagonist, may have reduced vitamin B_6 status. High-dose supplementation does not appear to improve asthmatic symptoms.

- Studies suggesting the efficacy of vitamin B_6 for autistic disorder have been criticized for serious methodological flaws. A well-controlled, small study did not support the use of vitamin B_6 in treating autism. Again, larger, controlled trials are needed to substantiate this finding.

- Individuals who may be at risk for low vitamin B_6 status (*see* Safety) should be encouraged to consume whole grains, legumes, and nuts rich in vitamin B_6 as part of a varied, healthy eating plan. Vitamin supplements may be used if needs are not met through diet, but care must be taken not to exceed the adult UL of 100 mg/day.

V

FOOD SOURCES

Good food sources of vitamin B_6 are whole grains, legumes, nuts, meat, and poultry. Most of the vitamin is removed from the grain during milling and processing.

Food Vitamin B6 (mg)*

Food	Vitamin B6 (mg)
Beans, garbanzo (½ c)	0.535
Seeds, sunflower (⅓ c)	0.459
Banana (1 medium)	0.369
Avocado (½ c)	0.332
Potato, baked, with skin (½ c)	0.701
Soybeans (½ c)	0.295
Rice, brown (½ c)	0.231
Beef, ground (3 oz)	0.224
Carrots, raw, chopped (½ c)	0.109
Peas, frozen (½ c)	0.088
Milk, nonfat (8 oz)	0.012
Peaches, canned (½ c)	0.011

*Serving sizes are calculated from values from USDA home page, www.nal.usda.gov/fnic

DOSAGE INFORMATION/BIOAVAILABILITY

The RDA for adults is 1.3 mg for men and women 19 y to 50 y, 1.5 mg for women older than 50 y, and 1.7 for men older than 50 y (3). The typical intake of vitamin B_6 for men is approximately 2 mg and for women, 1.5 mg (3). The average bioavailability of vitamin B_6 is 75 percent from most foods (1). Vitamin B_6 is sold in capsules or tablets in the form of pyridoxine hydrochloride or PLP. Supplements range in doses from 10, 50, 100, and 250, up to 500 mg per pill.

RELEVANT RESEARCH

B_6 and Carpal Tunnel Syndrome (CTS)

- In a cross-sectional study, 125 randomly selected active workers underwent electrodiagnostic testing for CTS and were assessed for vitamin B_6 status. Vitamin B_6 status (red blood cell and plasma levels) was unrelated to self-reported symptoms of CTS, electrophysiologically determined nerve function, and CTS (defined by self-report and electrophysiological results). The authors concluded: "Empiric prescription of vitamin B_6 to patients with CTS is unwarranted and potentially hazardous" (4).

- In a cross-sectional study, 441 self-selected subjects from six industries and a university setting participated in study comparing plasma vitamin B_6 concentrations to the prevalence and severity of nerve slowing, self-reported hand/wrist symptoms, and the prevalence of CTS. Dietary vitamin B_6 intake was not assessed. There were no significant differences in plasma PLP concentrations between subjects with no CTS symptoms (controls) and subjects with nerve slowing, CTS symptoms, or both. However, in male nonvitamin users, higher PLP levels were associated with reduced prevalence and frequency of CTS symptoms (5). The design, data analyses, and discussion of results in this study have been criticized by other researchers (6). However, the study is included here because it is cited to support marketing claims.

- In an uncontrolled, unblinded study, the role of vitamin B_6 supplementation in 20 patients having CTS was examined by measuring clinical and electrophysiological parameters before and after three months of vitamin B_6 supplementation (200 mg pyridoxine HCl). Electroencephalograms (EEG) and motor latency (common screening test for CTS) were not affected by vitamin B_6 therapy. However, pain scores and sensory latency were improved by vitamin B_6. There were no reported neurological side-effects associated with dosage (7). Because this study lacked proper controls, the results are difficult to evaluate. It is included here because it is cited to support marketing claims.

- There has been considerable debate regarding the efficacy of vitamin B_6 for CTS (6, 8, 9). A review article concluded that the literature has not provided convincing evidence for the use of vitamin B_6 as the sole treatment for patients with CTS. However, the authors noted that vitamin B_6 may be of value as adjunct therapy because of its potential benefit on pain perception and increasing pain threshold (10).

B_6 and Premenstrual Syndrome (PMS)

- A meta-analysis of 10 randomized, placebo-controlled, double-blinded studies that examined supplemental vitamin B_6 (50 mg to 600 mg/day) for PMS reported a relief in overall PMS and depressive PMS symptoms. However, of the 10 studies, only 1 was scored by the authors as high-quality, and this trial reported no effect of B_6 on PMS. The remaining nine studies were considered to be poor quality (11).

- A review article summarized 12 controlled trials on supplemental vitamin B_6 (ranging from 50 mg to 500 mg/day) in the treatment of PMS. The authors noted that the major drawbacks of the trials were the limited number of subjects and varying dosages. They concluded that the existing evidence of positive effects of vitamin B_6 is weak and that well-designed trials are needed to change this view (12).

- In a double-blind, placebo-controlled, crossover study, 63 women aged 18 y to 49 y were randomized to receive 50 mg pyridoxine or a placebo for three months each (no washout period). Subjects kept a daily menstrual diary grading the severity of nine symptoms one month prior to baseline followed by six months treatment. Only 32 subjects completed the entire study. Of these women, a significant benefit of pyridoxine was observed on emotional symptoms (depression, irritability, tiredness), but not on any other PMS symptoms measured (13).

- In a double-blind, placebo-controlled study, 55 women with self-reported moderate to severe PMS were randomly assigned to receive 150 mg pyridoxine or a placebo for two months. Subjects kept daily logs one month prior to the baseline, followed by two months of treatment. Vitamin B_6 improved autonomic symptoms (dizziness, vomiting) and behavioral symptoms; however it did not improve symptoms of depression and anxiety during the premenstrual phase. The authors concluded: "Because depression and anxiety are more likely than other premenstrual symptoms, such as water retention, to interfere with daily activities, we conclude that B_6 is not the treatment of choice for the symptoms most women present" (14).

V

- In a retrospective study, the effect of pyridoxine was assessed by the response to treatment (defined as "none," "partial," or "good") in 630 PMS patients attending a PMS clinic during the period of 1976 to 1983. The daily doses of pyridoxine varied from 40 mg to 100 mg during the early years to 120 mg to 200 mg in the later years examined. The response to treatment was "good" (no significant residual complaints) in 40 percent of patients treated with 100 mg to 150 mg vitamin B_6, and 60 percent in patients treated with 160 mg to 200 mg. No symptoms of peripheral neuropathy were noted (15).

- In a double-blind, placebo-controlled, crossover study, 44 women (average age = 32 y) were given in random order one of four treatments for one menstrual cycle: (1) 200 mg magnesium (oxide); (2) 50 mg vitamin B_6; 3) magnesium with B_6; or (4) a placebo. During the study, each subject recorded daily symptoms on a five-point scale in a menstrual diary of 30 symptoms that were grouped into categories (anxiety, craving, depression, hydration, other). Urinary magnesium output was not affected by treatment, suggesting poor absorption of the magnesium. There were no overall differences in symptoms among the treatments; however, a modest significant reduction in premenstrual anxiety-related symptoms was associated with the magnesium plus B_6 combination (16).

B_6 and Cardiovascular Disease

- In the Nurse's Health cohort study, 80,082 women with no history of heart disease, diabetes, or cancer filled out dietary questionnaires in 1980 and every two years through 1994. After correcting for cardiovascular risk factors, fiber, vitamin E, and saturated fat, trans fat, and polyunsaturated fat intake, the risk of myocardial infarction was lowest among women with the highest intakes of folate and vitamin B_6 from food and supplements. The lowest risk was seen among women whose vitamin B_6 intake was above 3 mg/day (17).

- In a prospective case-cohort, Atherosclerosis Risk in Communities (ARIC) study, a sample of middle-aged adults was assessed for coronary heart disease risk during an average of 3.3 years. Heart disease was negatively associated with plasma vitamin B_6 (PLP) in both sexes. After correcting for a number of risk factors (age, sex, race, field center, smoking, cholesterol levels, hypertension, diabetes, dietary vitamin intake), plasma PLP still had this association. The authors concluded: "Our findings point more strongly to the possibility that vitamin B_6 offers independent protection" (18).

- In a case-control study, 22 vitamin B_6-deficient asthma patients using theophylline (B_6 antagonist) and 24 matched controls with normal vitamin B_6 status were given oral methionine load tests. Methionine loading resulted in significantly higher homocysteine and cystathionine concentrations in vitamin B_6-deficient patients than in controls. All subjects were then supplemented with 20 mg vitamin B_6/day for six weeks. Supplementation significantly reduced homocysteine levels in deficient subjects but did not affect controls. The authors concluded: "A vitamin B_6 deficiency may contribute to impaired transsulfuration and an abnormal methionine load test, which is associated with premature vascular disease" (19).

- A meta-analysis of 12 randomized trials of vitamin supplements' effect on homocysteine levels reported that although folic acid and vitamin B$_{12}$ reduced homocysteine levels, vitamin B$_6$ did not have any significant effect (20).

B$_6$ and Asthma

- It has been suggested that vitamin B$_6$ corrects an abnormality in tryptophan metabolism seen in patients with asthma (21).

- In a double-blind, placebo-controlled study, 31 patients taking steroid medication for asthma were randomized to receive 300 mg pyridoxine or a placebo daily for nine weeks. There was no difference between groups on pulmonary function tests, asthma symptom scores, 24-hour urinary 5-hydroxy-indole acetic acid (serotonin metabolite), skin test reactivity, and blood serotonin levels. Patients treated with the bronchodilator theophylline had lower plasma pyridoxine levels at the baseline than did nonmedicated subjects. The authors concluded; "Prescription or usage of oral pyridoxine for the treatment of asthma cannot be justified in such patients" (21).

- In a double-blind, placebo-controlled, crossover study, 20 healthy subjects were put on theophylline and received in random order 15 mg pyridoxine hydrochloride or a placebo for seven weeks each, with a six-week washout period. Evaluation of central nervous system (CNS) stimulation and side-effects were recorded at the baseline, after a two-week run-in period, after a series of tests (hand steadiness, electrophysiological tests, the Sternberg Test of information processing), after the administration of a single 7-mg/kg dose of rapid-release theophylline, and after four weeks of 8 mg/kg of slow-release theophylline. Five subjects did not complete the study because of theophylline-associated headaches. During vitamin B$_6$ supplementation, subjects had significantly reduced theophylline-related hand tremors after a single dose of theophylline and a similar but insignificant trend was observed with repeated doses when compared to the placebo. Compared to the placebo, vitamin B$_6$ supplementation had no significant effect on CNS symptoms, electroencephalography, the Sternberg Test of information processing, or questionnaires of sleep quality and daytime sleepiness (22).

B$_6$ and Autism

- In a double-blind, placebo-controlled, crossover study, 10 children with autism were randomized to receive pyridoxine (30 mg/kg) and magnesium (10 mg/kg) supplements or a placebo for four weeks each. The mean dose ingested was 638.9 mg of pyridoxine and 216 mg magnesium oxide. Prior to the study, subjects took a two-week supply of a placebo and baseline parameters were measured. Teachers, parents, and clinicians evaluated autistic behavior with the Children's Psychiatric Rating Scale (CPRS), the Clinical Global Impression Scale, and the NIMH Global Obsessive Compulsive Scale. Pyridoxine and magnesium supplements had no effect on autistic behavior compared to the placebo. During the placebo run-in phase of the study, 5 of 10 subjects had a 30 percent greater reduction in CPRS scores. The authors concluded that their study "raises the issue of whether a 'placebo' or 'study' effect may be present in patients with autism disorder" (23).

V

- A critical analysis of 12 studies using vitamin B$_6$ and magnesium combinations for autistic patients was reported. Although most of the research reported favorable responses to vitamin treatment, the authors noted that these findings need to be interpreted with caution because of methodological shortcomings in many of the studies. Specific problems included: imprecise outcome measures, small samples, repeat use of the same subjects in more than one study, lack of adjustment for regression effects in measuring improvement, and failure to collect long-term follow-up data (24).

SAFETY

- The Tolerable Upper Intake Level (UL) for vitamin B$_6$, the highest amount likely to pose no risk for most people, is 100 mg/day for adults, 80 mg/day for children 14 y to 18 y, 60 mg/day for 9 y to 13 y, 40 mg/day for 4 y to 8 y (3).

- Large populations of CTS subjects using 100 mg to 150 mg/day vitamin B$_6$ have reported little or no toxicity in 5- to 10-year studies. However, neurological symptoms (numbness, tingling, bone pain, muscle weakness) were reported in 103 of 172 (60 percent) of women supplementing with an average dose of Vitamin B$_6$ = 117 mg daily for three years. After six months cessation, symptoms were reversed and serum B$_6$ levels returned to normal (25). Another articled reported that women chronically self-medicating with 500 mg to 5,000 mg/day for PMS developed peripheral neuropathy during a one- to three-year period (26).

- The following drugs are vitamin B$_6$ antagonists: Isoniazid (antibiotic), hydralazine (for hypertension), phenelzine, cycloserine (antibiotic), penicillamine (for Wilson's disease), ethinylestradiol, mestranol (contraceptives), theophylline (bronchodilator), corticosteroids (anti-inflammatory), erythromycin (antibiotic), gentamicin (antibiotic), neomycin (antibiotic), sulfonamides (antibiotic), alcohol, and caffeine. Adding 10 mg/day vitamin B$_6$ may correct for losses associated with long-term use of these drugs. Alternatively, large doses of vitamin B$_6$ (500 mg to 1,000 mg/day) may affect the metabolism of these drugs (1). Consult with a physician regarding these drug-nutrient interactions.

REFERENCES

1. Leklem JE. Vitamin B$_6$. In: Shils ME, Olson JA, Shike M, Ross AC, eds. *Modern Nutrition in Health and Disease*. 9th ed. Baltimore, Md: Williams & Wilkins; 1999;413–421.
2. Linder MC, ed. *Nutritional Biochemistry and Metabolism*. 2nd ed. New York, NY: Elsevier; 1991.
3. Institute of Medicine, Food and Nutrition Board. *Dietary Reference Intakes for Thiamin, Riboflavin, Niacin, Vitamin B-6, Folate, Vitamin B-12, Pantothenic Acid, Biotin, and Choline*. Washington, DC: National Academy Press; 1998.
4. Franzblau A, Rock CL, Werner RA, et al. The relationship of vitamin B6 status to median nerve function and carpal tunnel syndrome among active industrial workers. *J Occup Environ Med*. 1996;38:485–491.

5. Keniston RC, Nathan PA, Leklem JE, et al. Vitamin B$_6$, vitamin C, and carpal tunnel syndrome. A cross-sectional study of 441 adults. *J Occup Environ Med.* 1997;39:949–959.

6. Franzblau A, Rock CL, Werner RA, et al. Vitamin B$_6$, vitamin C, and carpal tunnel syndrome [letter]. *J Occup Environ Med.* 1998;40:305–309.

7. Bernstein Al, Dinesen JS. Brief communication: effect of pharmacologic doses of vitamin B$_6$ on carpal tunnel syndrome, electroencephalographic results, and pain. *J Am Coll Nutr.* 1993;12:73–76.

8. Keniston RC, Leklem JE, Nathan PA. Vitamin B$_6$ in carpal tunnel syndrome [letter]. *J Occup Environ Med.* 1996;38:959–960.

9. Keniston RC, Leklem JE, Nathan PA. Vitamin B$_6$ in carpal tunnel syndrome. *J Occup Environ Med.* 1996;38:959–960.

10. Jacobson MD, Plancher KD, Kleinman WB. Vitamin B$_6$ (pyridoxine) therapy for carpal tunnel syndrome. *Hand Clin.* 1996;12:253–257.

11. Wyatt KM, Dimmock PW, Jones PW. Poor-quality studies suggest that vitamin B$_6$ use is beneficial in premenstrual syndrome. *BMJ.* 1999;318:1375–1381.

12. Kleijnen J, Ter Riet G, Knipschild P. Vitamin B$_6$ in the treatment of the premenstrual syndrome—a review. *Br J Obstet Gynaecol.* 1990;97:847–852.

13. Doll H, Brown S, Thurston A, et al. Pyridoxine (vitamin B$_6$) and the premenstrual syndrome: a randomized crossover trial. *J R Coll Gen Pract.* 1989;39:364–368.

14. Kendall KE, Schnurr PP. The effects of vitamin B$_6$ supplementation on premenstrual symptoms. *Obstet Gynecol.* 1987;70:145–149.

15. Brush MG, Bennett T, Hansen K. Pyridoxine in the treatment of premenstrual syndrome: a retrospective survey in 630 patients. *Br J Clin Pract.* 1988;42:448–452.

16. De Souza MC, Walker AF, Robinson PA, et al. A synergistic effect of a daily supplement for one month of 200 mg magnesium plus 50 mg vitamin B$_6$ for the relief of anxiety-related premenstrual symptoms: a randomized, double-blind, crossover study. *J Womens Health Gend Based Med.* 2000;9:131–139.

17. Rimm EB, Willett WC, Hu FB, et al. Folate and vitamin B$_6$ from diet and supplements in relation to risk of coronary heart disease among women. *JAMA.* 1998;279:359–364.

18. Folsom AR, Nieto FJ, McGovern PG, et al. Prospective study of coronary heart disease incidence in relation to fasting total homocysteine, related genetic polymorphisms, and B vitamins: the Atherosclerosis Risk in Communities (ARIC) study. *Circulation.* 1998;98:204–210.

19. Ubbink JB, van der Merwe A, Delport R, et al. The effect of subnormal vitamin B-6 status on homocystein metabolism. *J Clin Invest.* 1996;98:177–184.

20. Clarke R, Armitage J. Vitamin supplements and cardiovascular risk: review of the randomized trials of homocysteine-lowering vitamin supplements. *Semin Thromb Hemost.* 2000;26:341–348.

21. Sur S, Camara M, Buchmeier A, et al. Double-blind trial of pyridoxine (vitamin B$_6$) in the treatment of steroid-dependent asthma. *Ann Allergy.* 1993;70:147–152.

22. Bartel PR, Ubbink JB, Delport R, et al. Vitamin B$_6$ supplementation and theophylline-related effects in humans. *Am J Clin Nutr.* 1994;60:93–99.

23. Findling RL, Maxwell K, Scotese-Wojtila L, et al. High-dose pyridoxine and magnesium administration in children with autistic disorder: an absence of salutary effects in a double-blind, placebo-controlled study. *J Autism Dev Disord.* 1997;27:467–479.

V

24. Pfeiffer SI, Norton J, Nelson L, et al. Efficacy of vitamin B_6 and magnesium in the treatment of autism: a methodology review and summary of outcomes. *J Autism Dev Disord.* 1995;25:481–493.

25. Dalton K, Dalton MJ. Characteristics of pyridoxine overdose neuropathy syndrome. *Acta Neurol Scand.* 1987;76:8–11.

26. Bernstein AL. Vitamin B_6 in clinical neurology. *Ann N Y Acad Sci.* 1990;585:250–260.

Vitamin B_{12} (Cobalamin)

Vitamin B_{12} is a water-soluble vitamin containing cobalt. The active forms of vitamin B_{12}, methylcobalamin and adenosylcobalamin, function as part of the enzymes methionine synthetase and methylmalonyl-CoA mutase, respectively. As part of methionine synthetase, methylcobalamin is used to regenerate the folate cofactor back to tetrahydrofolate, allowing folate to biosynthesize purines and pyrimidines necessary for DNA formation. Additionally, methylcobalamin recycles homocysteine to methionine providing methyl groups necessary for the biosynthesis of many structures including myelin. The mutase allows catabolism of odd-chain length fatty acids and some amino acids (1, 2).

A deficiency of vitamin B_{12} impairs these enzymatic reactions. Pernicious anemia, characterized by neurological damage and megaloblastic anemia, is the classic B_{12} deficiency that occurs when there is a lack of intrinsic factor secretion (IF). However, a more prevalent cause of mild deficiency is because of food-bound cobalamin malabsorption. This malabsorption, the inability to absorb food-bound but not free cobalamin, occurs in 10 percent to 30 percent of people over the age of 50 y because of achlorhydria (3). Therefore, neuropsychiatric symptoms may be present without overt macrocytic anemia or reduced serum cobalamin levels. Those at risk for B_{12} deficiency include the elderly, chronic alcohol abusers, patients on long-term therapy with gastric acid inhibitors, vegans, patients with partial gastrectomy, atrophic gastritis, autoimmune disorders (type 1 diabetes, AIDS/HIV, and thyroid disorders), dementia, and patients undergoing nitrous oxide anaesthesia (1, 2, 4).

Media and Marketing Claims	Efficacy
B_{12} supplements are needed for the elderly who are often deficient	↑
May help symptoms of dementia	NR
Improves sleep quality	NR
Improves neurological function in AIDS	NR
Reduces risk of cardiovascular disease	NR
Helpful for diabetics	NR
Increases energy	NR

Advisory

- No reported serious adverse effects
- No Tolerable Upper Intake Level (UL) established

Drug/Supplement Interactions

- Several drugs may interfere with vitamin B$_{12}$ absorption and lower blood levels: AZT (HIV therapy); antacids (only food-bound B$_{12}$, not supplemental); clofibrate (for hypercholesterolemia)' colchicines (for gout); cycloserine, erythromycin (antibiotics); isoniazid (antibiotic for tuberculosis); metformin (for diabetes); aldomet (antihypertensive); neomycin (antibiotic prior to surgery); nitrous oxide (anesthetic gas); oral contraceptives; sulfanamides (antibiotic); tetracycline (antibiotic)
- Supplemental vitamin C or iron may interfere with the bioavailability of vitamin B$_{12}$

KEY POINTS

- Individuals > 50 y are at increased risk for preclinical vitamin B$_{12}$ deficiency because of possible malabsorption of food-bound cobalamin. Classic deficiency symptoms such as pernicious anemia are not usually present in this population. In the National Academy of Sciences Food and Nutrition Board's dietary reference intakes (DRIs) for B$_{12}$ released in 1998, it is advised that individuals more than 50 years old meet the RDA mainly by consuming foods fortified with vitamin B$_{12}$ or a B$_{12}$-containing supplement (3). One review article noted that for those with a documented deficiency, large amounts of oral vitamin B$_{12}$ (100 µg to 1,000 µg/day) are effective; thus, the quantity usually found in multivitamin supplements (< 6 µg) is not adequate. At the current time, there is some controversy regarding the most effective method of screening for deficiency and the minimum effective dose of oral vitamin B$_{12}$ needed to correct deficiency in elderly subjects.

- Vitamin B$_{12}$ deficiency can progress to produce signs of dementia. Controlled studies verifying clinical improvement in dementia because of vitamin B$_{12}$ supplementation are lacking. The role of supplements in treating Alzheimer's-type dementia or neurological disturbances unrelated to deficiency has not been adequately tested in controlled trials. However, the NAS recommends that those older than 50 y consume the RDA for vitamin B$_{12}$ from fortified foods or vitamin supplements. Because individuals with Alzheimer's disease and dementia are typically elderly, they are included in this recommendation.

- The first randomized, placebo-controlled study of vitamin B$_{12}$ in subjects with delayed sleep phase syndrome reported no benefit. This conflicted with previous open trials and case studies of B$_{12}$ (not described here). Additional controlled research is needed to determine what role, if any, vitamin B$_{12}$ plays in sleep disorders.

- There is a lack of controlled trials on the effect of B$_{12}$ supplements on AIDS-related dementia. However, because decreased blood cobalamin levels occur in 20 percent of patients with AIDS and drugs used to treat the infection may lower B$_{12}$ levels, this population should be evaluated for vitamin B$_{12}$ deficiency and treated if needed.

- Because vitamin B$_{12}$ reduces serum levels of homocysteine (a possible risk factor for cardiovascular disease) the vitamin may be indirectly involved in cardiovascular health. Though many researchers have demonstrated a link between elevated homocysteine levels and heart disease, it is of note that the American Heart Association cur-

V

rently does not recognize homocysteine levels as an independent risk factor for cardiovascular disease. Controlled trials are needed to determine whether vitamin B_{12} supplements reduce cardiovascular risk and mortality, particularly in patients with hyperhomocysteinemia.

- Increased homocysteine levels have been associated in some studies with diabetic complications in type 2 diabetics. Long-term, controlled trials of vitamin B_{12} are needed to determine whether, in fact, lowering homocysteine concentrations reduces the risk of developing and/or helps treat neuropathy, nephropathy and other chronic conditions related to diabetes..

- Vitamin B_{12} injections were historically given to patients complaining of fatigue. There is a lack of evidence from controlled trials verifying this effect in subjects with normal cobalamin status.

- Overall, healthy individuals aged < 50 y who eat a diet including animal products or an adequate amount of foods fortified with vitamin B_{12} do not require B_{12} supplements. However, vegans and healthy people aged > 50 y may need to take a vitamin B_{12} supplement, especially those not consuming enough B_{12}-fortified foods to meet the RDA.

FOOD SOURCES

Vitamin B_{12} is only present in significant quantities in animal foods. Fermented soybeans and legumes contain an insignificant amount of vitamin B_{12}. Seaweed has some vitamin B_{12}-like activity; however, it is not thought to be bioavailable. The function and effects of cobalamin analogues present in foods are not known.

Food	Vitamin B12 (μg)
Oysters (6)	14.34
Crab, Alaskan (3 oz)	9.78
Beef, ground (3.5 oz)	2.90
Salmon, Atlantic (3 oz)	2.38
Egg (1)	0.56
Chicken (½ breast)	0.29
Milk, nonfat (1 c)	0.10

Source: Data is from Pennington JAT (5)

DOSAGE INFORMATION/BIOAVAILABILITY

The adult RDA for men and women is 2.4 μg daily (3). The average daily intake is estimated to be 5.0 μg in the United States (1). Vitamin B_{12} is available as cyanocobalamin (not active) and methylcobalamin (active form) in tablets and capsules in doses ranging from 2 μg to 1,000 μg. It is included in multivitamin/mineral and B-complex formulations.

V

The absorption of vitamin B_{12} is dependent on the presence of intestinal intrinsic factor. In healthy subjects, a maximal amount of 1.5 µg to 2.0 µg of dietary and supplemental vitamin B_{12} is absorbed per meal with the intrinsic factor system. Approximately 1 percent of high doses of supplemental vitamin B_{12} can be absorbed by passive diffusion, which does not require intrinsic factor (2). The methylcobalamin form is thought to be more efficiently absorbed and used than the cyanocobalamin form (6). In one study, vitamin B_{12} was destroyed and therefore was not bioavailable if coingested with supplemental vitamin C or iron (7).

Correction of documented vitamin B_{12} deficiency because of lack of intrinsic factor is routinely treated with parenteral cobalamin. In one study of individuals with B_{12} deficiency, however, 2 mg of cyanocobalamin administered orally on a daily basis was as effective as 1 mg administered intramuscularly on a monthly basis (8). One reviewer considered the route of oral cobalamin for deficiency states "an underused alternative to parenteral treatment" (9).

RELEVANT RESEARCH

Vitamin B₁₂ Deficiency in the Elderly

- Approximately 10 percent to 30 percent of the population older than 50 y have vitamin B_{12} deficiency (3) diagnosed by elevated methylmalonic acid with or without elevated total homocysteine concentrations in combination with low or low-normal B_{12} levels. Deficiency is most often because of food-cobalamin malabsorption caused by atrophic gastritis (most often due to *Heliobacter pylori*) and hypochlorhydria. Clinical signs and symptoms of deficiency in elderly patients can be masked by the presence of other conditions, making diagnosis and responses to therapy difficult to evaluate. Some experts raised concerns that the federally mandated food folate-fortification program could present a problem in the elderly because folate reduces hyperhomocysteinemia (a diagnostic marker of B_{12} deficiency) and thus could mask macrocytic anemia (10, 11).

Vitamin B₁₂ and Dementia in the Elderly

- In some reports, low serum cobalamin levels have been associated with Alzheimer's disease and dementia, but the data are not consistent (12–14). However, normal serum cobalamin concentrations do not rule out the possibility of deficiency (1, 15).

- In a prospective (not blinded or a placebo-controlled) study, 16 patients with low blood cobalamin levels but no outward symptoms of deficiency had hematological, neurological, and metabolic tests before and after eight weekly cyanocobalamin injections (1,000 µg) followed by monthly treatments for four more months. Nine patients had Alzheimer's disease (AD), 1 had possible AD, 3 had non-Alzheimer-type dementia, and 3 had nondementia disorders. Eight of the patients had impaired DNA synthesis in bone marrow cells (deoxyuridine suppression test) and 7 subjects had elevated serum methylmalonic acid. Eleven of the subjects had mild neurological abnormalities such as peripheral neuropathy and unsteady gait. Seven subjects had food-bound cobalamin malabsorption (egg yolk-cobalamin absorption test), whereas only 1 sub-

V

ject had classical malabsorption of free cobalamin detected by the Schilling's test. Vitamin B_{12} injections improved the mild metabolic abnormalities associated with deficiency, but had no consistent improvement in cognitive function in the 13 subjects with dementia (16).

- In an open, prospective study, 181 patients (mean age = 77.5 y) with diagnosed dementia were evaluated and had their serum vitamin B_{12} levels measured. The frequency of vitamin B_{12} deficiency defined as < 200 pg/mL was 25 percent (46 of 181; 36 subjects without anemia or macrocytosis). Treatment outcome of vitamin B_{12} injections (1 mg repeated five times at intervals of five days and a maintenance dose of 1 mg every three months) was obtained in 19 of 46 patients throughout 3 to 24 months. Sixteen of these 19 patients had persistent declines in mental functioning at follow-up visits despite cobalamin injections. Of the three patients that showed some improvement, all had mild dementia with a history of less than two years. The authors concluded that true vitamin B_{12} dementia is rare but that screening for low serum B_{12} levels should be considered in patients with recent onset of mild mental status changes (17).

Vitamin B_{12} and Sleep Disorders

- In a double-blind, placebo-controlled study, 50 patients with delayed sleep phase syndrome aged 13 y to 55 y were randomized to receive 3,000 µg methylcobalamin or a placebo divided into three oral doses daily for four weeks. There were no significant differences between groups in subjective evaluations of mood or drowsiness during the daytime or night sleep by sleep-log evaluation (18).

Vitamin B_{12} and HIV/AIDS

- Several studies have reported vitamin B_{12} malabsorption and deficiency in patients diagnosed as HIV-positive (19, 20). Low serum cobalamin levels were associated with faster progression of HIV type 1 disease as determined by CD4 cell count and the AIDS index (21, 22).

- In an *in vitro* study, methylcobalamin inhibited HIV-1 infection of healthy human blood monocytes and lymphocytes (23).

Vitamin B_{12} and Cardiovascular Disease

- A number of studies have reported that the B vitamins, in particular, supplemental vitamin B_{12} ($\approx$ 0.5 mg/day) and folic acid (0.5 mg to 5 mg/day), are associated with reductions in homocysteine levels (a risk factor for heart disease) by up to 30 percent (24).

- In a double-blinded, placebo-controlled trial, 89 men with coronary heart disease were randomized to receive 5 mg folic acid plus 1 mg vitamin B_{12} or a placebo daily for eight weeks. Brachial artery flow-mediated dilatation (endothelium dependent) and nitroglycerin-induced dilatation (endothelium independent) were measured before and after treatment. After treatment, flow-mediated dilatation was significantly improved after supplementation with the vitamins, but not with a placebo. The vitamins had no effect on nitroglycerin-induced dilatation. Additionally, the B vitamins were significantly associated with reductions in plasma total homocysteine, protein-bound homocysteine, and free homocysteine, and elevations in serum folate and vitamin B_{12}. In regression analysis, the improved flow-mediated dilatation was significantly correlated with reduction in free plasma homocysteine. From this the authors concluded that folic acid and B_{12} supplementation appears to improve vascular endothelial function, and this effect is likely mediated through reduced free homocysteine levels (25).

Vitamin B_{12} and Diabetes

- Increased homocysteine levels have been associated in some studies with complications such as neuropathy and nephropathy in type 2 diabetics (26–28). Because vitamin B_{12} appears to lower homocysteine levels, some propose that supplemental B12 may reduce the risk of developing these conditions.

- In a double-blind, placebo-controlled study, 50 Saudi Arabian patients with diabetic neuropathy (11 subjects with type 1 and 39 subjects with type 2 diabetes) were randomized to receive 1,500 mg methylcobalamin divided into three doses or a placebo daily for four months. The researchers did not evaluate vitamin B_{12} status. Clinical and neurophysiological (nerve conduction studies) were completed before and at the end of the study. There was a significant improvement in the somatic and autonomic symptoms with regression of signs of neuropathy after vitamin B_{12} treatment. However, motor and sensory nerve conduction studies showed no improvement (29).

SAFETY

- The Tolerable Upper Intake Level (UL) for vitamin B_{12} has not been determined due to low toxicity. Currently, no adverse effects have been associated with excess B12 intake from food or supplements in healthy people. (3).

- Individuals with vitamin B_{12} deficiency and who are at risk for Leber's optic atrophy (genetic disorder caused by chronic cyanide intoxication) should not be treated with the cyanocobalamin form of B_{12}, because it can increase the risk of neurological damage. Hydroxocobalamin is a cyanide antagonist and, thus, is not associated with adverse effects in this population (3).

REFERENCES

1. Weir DG, Scott JM. Vitamin B_{12} Cobalamin. In: Shils ME, Olson JA, Shike M, Ross AC, eds. *Modern Nutrition in Health and Disease.* 9th ed. Baltimore, Md: Williams & Wilkins; 1999:447–459.
2. Scott JM. Bioavailability of vitamin B_{12}. *Eur J Clin Nutr.* 1997;51(suppl 1):S49–S53.
3. Institute of Medicine, Food and Nutrition Board. *Dietary Reference Intakes for Thiamin, Riboflavin, Niacin, Vitamin B-6, Folate, Vitamin B-12, Pantothenic Acid, Biotin, and Choline.* Washington, DC: National Academy Press; 1998.

4. Nilsson-Ehle H. Age-related changes in cobalamin (vitamin B_{12}) handling. Implications for therapy. *Drugs Aging.* 1998;12:277–292.

5. Pennington JAT. *Bowes and Church's Food Values of Portions Commonly Used.* 17th ed. Philadelphia, Pa: Lippincott-Raven Publishers; 1998.

6. Anonymous. Methylcobalamin. *Altern Med Rev.* 1998;3:461–463.

7. Herbert V. The elderly need oral vitamin B-12. *Am J Clin Nutr.* 1998;67:739–752.

8. Kuzminski AM, Del Giacco EJ, Allen RH, et al. Effective treatment of cobalamin deficiency with oral cobalamin. *Blood.* 1998;92:1191–1198.

9. Delva MD. Vitamin B_{12} replacement. To B_{12} or not to B_{12}. *Can Fam Physician.* 1997;43:917–922.

10. Stabler SP, Lindenbaum J, Allen RH. Vitamin B-12 deficiency in the elderly: current dilemmas. *Am J Clin Nutr.* 1997;66:741–749.

11. Carmel R. Cobalamin, the stomach, and aging. *Am J Clin Nutr.* 1997;66:750–759.

12. Cole MG, Prchal JF. Low serum vitamin B_{12} in Alzheimer type dementia. *Age Ageing.* 1984;13:101–105.

13. Basun H, Fratiglioni L, Winblad B. Cobalamin levels are not reduced in Alzheimer's disease: results from a population based study. *J Am Geriatr Soc.* 1994;42:132–136.

14. Bell IR, Edman JS, Marby DW, et al. Vitamin B_{12} and folate status in acute geropsychiatric inpatients: affective and cognitive characteristics of a vitamin nondeficient population. *Biol Psychiatry.* 1990;27:125–137.

15. Hutto BR. Folate and cobalamin in psychiatric illness. *Compr Psychiatry.* 1997;38:305–314.

16. Carmel R, Gott PS, Waters CH, et al. The frequently low cobalamin levels in dementia usually signify treatable metabolic, neurologic and electrophysiologic abnormalities. *Eur J Haematol.* 1995;54:245–253.

17. Cunha UG, Rocha FL, Peixoto JM, et al. Vitamin B-12 deficiency and dementia. *Int Psychogeriatr.* 1995;7:85–88.

18. Okawa M, Takahashi K, Egashira K, et al. Vitamin B_{12} treatment for delayed sleep phase syndrome: a multi-center double-blind study. *Psychiatry Clin Neurosci.* 1997;51:275–279.

19. Paltiel O, Falutz J, Veilleux M, et al. Clinical correlates of subnormal vitamin B_{12} levels in patients infected with the human immunodeficiency virus. *Am J Hematol.* 1995;49:318–322.

20. Herzlich BC, Schiano TD, Moussa Z, et al. Decreased intrinsic factor secretion in AIDS: relation to parietal cell acid secretory capacity and vitamin B_{12} malabsorption. *Am J Gastroenterol.* 1992;87:1781–1788.

21. Tang AM, Graham NM, Chandra RK, et al. Low serum vitamin B-12 concentrations are associated with faster human immunodeficiency virus type 1 (HIV-1) disease progression. *J Nutr.* 1997;127:345–351.

22. Baum MK, Shor-Posner G, Lu Y, et al. Micronutrients and HIV-1 disease progression. *AIDS.* 1995;9:1051–1056.

23. Weinberg JB, Sauls DL, Misukonis MA, et al. Inhibition of productive human immunodeficiency virus-1 infection by cobalamins. *Blood.* 1995;86:1281–1287.

24. Clarke R, Armitage J. Vitamin supplements and cardiovascular risk: review of the randomized trials of homocysteine-lowering vitamin supplements. *Semin Thromb Hemost.* 2000;26:341–348.

25. Chambers JC, Ueland PM, Obeid OA, et al. Improved vascular endothelial function after oral B vitamins: an effect mediated through reduced concentrations of free plasma homocysteine. *Circulation.* 2000;102:2479–2483.

26. Ambrosch A, Dierkes J, Lobmann R, et al. Relation between homocysteinaemia and diabetic neuropathy in patients with type 2 diabetes mellitus. *Diabet Med.* 2001;18:185–192.

27. Buysschaert M, Dramais AS, Wallemacq PE, et al. Hyperhomocyteinemia in type 2 diabetes: relationship to macroangiopathy, nephropathy, and insulin resistance. *Diabetes Care.* 2000;23:1816–1822.

28. Stabler SP, Estacio R, Jeffers BW, et al. Total homocysteine is associated with nephropathy in non-insulin-dependent diabetes mellitus. *Metabolism.* 1999;48:1096–1101.

29. Yaqub BA, Siddique A, Sulimani R. Effects of methylcobalamin on diabetic neuropathy. *Clin Neurol Neurosurg.* 1992;94:105–111.

Vitamin C

Vitamin C is the term used to describe two biologically active forms of the nutrient: ascorbic acid (reduced form) and dehydroascorbic acid (oxidized form). Vitamin C acts as an electron donor for eight enzymes. Specifically, vitamin C is involved in reactions needed to synthesize collagen, neurotransmitters (dopamine, tyramine), carnitine, tyrosine, and catecholamines. Vitamin C's electron-donating function also makes it an effective antioxidant. The vitamin scavenges reactive oxygen species, singlet oxygen, hypochlorite, and hydroxyl, peroxyl, superoxide, peroxynitrite, nitroxide radicals. High tissue levels of ascorbate provide significant antioxidant protection in the eye, neutrophils, semen, and lipoproteins. The vitamin may also provide indirect antioxidant protection by regenerating other antioxidants including glutathione and vitamin E. Of particular interest is how supplementing doses of vitamin C may play a beneficial role in conditions and diseases resulting from oxidative damage. (1, 2).

Media and Marketing Claims	Efficacy
Treats the common cold	↔
Reduces symptoms of asthma	↔
Needed for immunity	?↑
Enhances exercise performance by increasing oxidative stress	↓
Reduces risk of heart disease	NR
Protects against cancer	?↑
Reduces risk of cataracts	?↑

V

Advisory

- The Tolerable Upper Intake Level (UL) for adults is 2,000 mg/day
- Diarrhea and cramping may occur with doses above the UL
- Not to be used by individuals with hematochromatosis (iron overload)
- Individuals with renal disorders may have increased risk of oxalate kidney stone formation with excess vitamin C
- May interfere with some blood and diagnostic tests

Drug/Supplement Interactions

- Increases iron absorption (ferric acid)
- May prolong clearance time for acetaminophen
- May increase activity of anticoagulants
- May interfere with activity of vitamin B_{12}, although doses up to 4 g/day do not induce B_{12} deficiency
- Excessive intake may interfere with copper metabolism
- When taken with aluminum-containing antacids, may increase aluminum absorption
- Aspirin, corticosteroids, and indomethacin (NSAID) increase urinary vitamin C losses

KEY POINTS

- According to research to date, subpopulations tend to have low plasma vitamin C levels, particularly men, elderly, smokers, individuals with diabetes, and oral contraceptive users. These individuals should be encouraged to increase their consumption of vitamin C-rich foods and beverages. For those who fail to consume adequate vitamin C through the diet, a vitamin C supplement (200 mg to 500 mg) may be appropriate to raise plasma levels.

- After 30 years of research testing vitamin C and rhinovirus treatment, results are equivocal. However, it is possible that some further protection may be offered by supplements to individuals with low plasma vitamin C stores or in subjects undergoing oxidative stress from physical exercise (ultramarathon runners).

- Similarly, the results from clinical studies of the effects of vitamin C on asthma are equivocal. Additional research is needed in this area. Asthmatic individuals should be encouraged to increase dietary sources of vitamin C.

- There is evidence that vitamin C has a positive effect on some markers of immune function.

- The National Academy of Sciences Food and Nutrition Board's report on antioxidant requirements stated that there is no evidence that people undergoing physical and mental stress have increased vitamin C needs. In regard to reducing exercise-induced oxidative damage, more research is needed to determine whether single preparations of vitamin C supplements affect markers of oxidative status and whether this improves performance and long-term health in athletes. Limited evidence suggests a potential role for vitamin C supplementation in reducing upper respiratory tract infections in ultraendurance athletes.

- According to epidemiological research, there appears to be an inverse correlation between vitamin C levels and cardiovascular disease. However, epidemiological evidence can only suggest associations rather than cause and effect. Sufficient data from controlled clinical trials are lacking; thus, more research is needed in this area. Again, consumption of vitamin C-rich fruits and vegetables should be encouraged in individuals with heart disease.

- There is a preponderance of epidemiological evidence linking fruit and vegetable intake to lower rates of cancer. There appears to be a possible protective effect of vitamin C intake and certain cancers; however, well-controlled clinical research is needed to further examine the potential role of vitamin C supplementation in cancer prevention.

- Epidemiological data suggest that vitamin C supplements may reduce cataract risk. Controlled clinical trials are needed to determine whether the supplements offer a protective effect.

FOOD SOURCES

Food	Vitamin C (mg)
Papaya (1 medium)	188
Strawberries (1 c)	84
Orange, navel (1)	75
Broccoli (½ c)	58
Mango (1)	57
Brussel sprouts (½ c)	48
Sweet pepper, raw (½ c)	45
Grapefruit (½ medium)	42
Raspberries (1 c)	31
Pineapple (1 c)	24
Potato, baked, with skin	26
Tomato (1 medium)	23

Source: Data is from Pennington JAT (3)

V

The average daily dietary vitamin C intake in the United States is 90 mg/day for women and 105 mg/day for men (2). Although many Americans do not consume enough fruits and vegetables, eating at least five servings of fruits and vegetables per day, as recommended by the National Cancer Institute and the Food Guide Pyramid, may provide more than 200 mg vitamin C (1). To maximize the amount of vitamin C in foods, it is important to be aware that vitamin C content is reduced by cooking, exposing foods to air and light, and prolonging storage and transport of fresh fruits and vegetables.

DOSAGE INFORMATION/BIOAVAILABILITY

Vitamin C is available in tablets, capsules, chewable tablets, and powders ranging from 60 mg to 1,000 mg/serving. Vitamin C is sold in a variety of forms including pure ascorbic acid, vitamin C from rose hips, chelated to sodium or other minerals, or bound to bioflavonoids. One study found vitamin C supplements from pure ascorbic acid were more bioavailable than other, more expensive commercial vitamin C preparations (4). Bioavailability of vitamin C from foods and from supplements is not significantly different (2). Plasma vitamin C concentrations in people who regularly consume vitamin C supplements are about 60 percent to 70 percent higher than in those who do not take supplements (5).

The National Academy of Sciences Food and Nutrition Board released dietary reference intakes (DRIs) for vitamin C in 2000. The new adult RDA for vitamin C is 75 mg/day for women and 90 mg/day for men (2). The report also stated that smokers require an additional 35 mg/day in order to obtain a steady-state ascorbate body pool similar to nonsmokers. These values were based on the amount of vitamin C intake needed to maintain near-maximal neutrophil concentrations with minimal urinary excretion of ascorbate.

The effectiveness of mega-dosing on tissue saturation has been the subject of debate (6, 7). Some researchers report that tissue and plasma saturation levels of vitamin C are reached with an approximate intake of 200 mg to 300 mg/day (8, 9). However, it has also been suggested that a daily intake near 1,000 mg is necessary to maintain plasma vitamin C levels at high concentrations (75 μmol to 80 μmol) (5). Maximal absorption is achieved by ingesting several spaced doses of less than 1,000 mg rather than one large dose (1).

RELEVANT RESEARCH

Vitamin C and the Common Cold

- Many review articles and meta-analyses have been written since Linus Pauling first published his research in the 1970s suggesting that 1 g vitamin C reduced rhinovirus symptoms in school children in a skiing camp in the Swiss Alps (10).

- In 1975, Thomas Chalmers published a meta-analysis of seven placebo-controlled trials stating vitamin C was not beneficial in treating the common cold (11).

- A retrospective analysis of Chalmers' review found that 1 g to 6 g/day of vitamin C did result in a significant decrease in the duration of cold episodes. Chalmers' analysis was criticized for including studies that employed low levels of supplemental vitamin C (25 mg to 50 mg/day) (12).

- In a more recent meta-analysis (1997), the six largest vitamin C supplementation (≥ 1 g/day) studies of more than 5,000 episodes of rhinovirus found no benefit of vitamin C compared to a placebo (13).

- A review of three studies investigating the common cold incidence following heavy physical stress (ski camp in the Swiss Alps, military training, and 90-km running race), found a considerable reduction of cold occurrence in groups supplemented with 600 mg to 1,000 mg vitamin C/day. The pooled risk ratios of common cold infection in these studies was 0.50 in favor of vitamin C-supplemented subjects (14).

- In a double-blind, placebo-controlled study, 92 ultramarathon runners and 92 controls (nonrunners) were supplemented with either 600 mg vitamin C or a placebo for 21 days prior to an ultramarathon race. (Controls did not run the race). Symptoms of upper respiratory tract (URT) infection were monitored for 14 days after the race. Sixty-eight percent of the runners in the placebo group reported development of symptoms of URT infection, which was significantly more than vitamin C-supplemented runners. The duration and severity of URT symptoms reported in vitamin C-nonrunning controls was significantly lower than nonrunning controls taking placebos (15).

Vitamin C for Asthma and Pulmonary Function

- A study of 2,526 adults randomly selected from the first National Health and Nutrition Examination Survey (NHANES I) between 1971 and 1974 found that dietary vitamin C was positively and significantly associated with forced expiratory volume (FEV_1) of the lung. The authors hypothesized that vitamin C intake may have a protective effect on pulmonary function (16).

- A case-control study, nested in a cross-sectional study of a random sample of adults in Scotland found that low intakes of vitamin C and manganese were associated with greater than a 5-fold increased risk of bronchial reactivity. The authors concluded: "This study provides evidence that diet may have a modulatory effect on bronchial reactivity and is consistent with the hypothesis that the observed reduction in antioxidant intake in the British diet over the last 25 years has been a factor in the increase in the prevalence of asthma over this period" (17).

- In a double-blind, placebo-controlled, crossover trial, 47 streetworkers of Mexico City were to receive in random order: antioxidant supplements (650 mg vitamin C plus 75 mg vitamin E plus 15 mg beta-carotene) and a placebo for about 2.5 months each (March to August 1996). Pulmonary function tests were done twice per week at the end of the workday. During the first phase, ozone levels were inversely associated with measures of lung function in the placebo group, but not in the antioxidant group. During the second phase, similar results were observed, but the lung function decrements were less pronounced in the placebo group. The authors suggested that the prior antioxidant supplementation might have provided residual protection for the lungs in placebo subjects in the second phase. The design of this study does not answer whether vitamin C, vitamin E, beta-carotene, or the combination of antioxidants improved lung function (18)

- In a double-blind, placebo-controlled, crossover study, 20 patients (aged 7 y to 28 y) with exercise-induced asthma (EIA) ingested in random order 2 g of vitamin C or a placebo one hour before a seven-minute treadmill exercise. Vitamin C had no effect on pulmonary function at rest. In 9 of 20 patients, a protective effect of vitamin C on

V

hyper-reactive airways was recorded. The authors concluded that the efficacy of vitamin C in preventing EIA cannot be predicted (19).

- In a review of 21 studies on the role of vitamin C on asthma and allergy, evidence was conflicting. The authors noted that the majority of studies were short-term and only assessed immediate effects of vitamin C supplementation. They concluded that long-term supplementation with vitamin C and delayed effects need to be studied (20).

Vitamin C and Immune Function

- In a single-blind, comparative trial, 30 healthy subjects were randomized to receive one of three treatments daily for 28 days: (1) 1,000 mg vitamin C, (2) 400 mg vitamin E, or (3) both vitamin C and E. Plasma concentrations of alpha-tocopherol, ascorbate, and lipid peroxides, as well as the production of cytokines by peripheral mononuclear cells (PMBC) were measured before, during, and one week after the study end. Production of interleukin-1 beta and tumor necrosis factor-alpha (TNF-apha) in the group supplemented with both vitamin C and E were significantly higher than the groups given vitamin E or C alone. The enhancing effect of supplementation with a combination of vitamins E and C was significantly correlated with peak plasma alpha-tocopherol and ascorbate levels and the lowest plasma lipid peroxide concentrations on day 14. In addition, an *in vitro* experiment with PBMCs showed that vitamins E and C reduced polysaccharide-induced prostaglandin E2 production and enhanced TNF-alpha production (21).

- In a double-blind, placebo-controlled trial, 57 elderly patients admitted to the hospital with acute respiratory infections (bronchitis and bronchopneumonia) were randomized to receive 200 mg vitamin/day or a placebo. Patients were assessed biochemically on admission and at weeks 2 and 4 in the study. Severity of illness was scored on a scale of 1 to 10 on three main diagnostic features of respiratory infections: cough; breathlessness; and radiological evidence of chest infection. Supplementation led to a significant increase in plasma and white blood cell vitamin C concentrations. When evaluated using a clinical scoring system based on major symptoms, vitamin C-supplemented subjects fared significantly better than did the placebo group, with a pronounced effect seen in the most serious cases (22).

- In a controlled trial, the effects of moderate vitamin C deficiency on immune function and oxidative damage were measured in eight healthy men (aged 25 y to 43 y) who consumed 5 mg to 250 mg/day ascorbic acid during 92 days on a metabolic unit. With ascorbic acid intakes of 5 mg, 10 mg, or 20 mg/day, subjects attained a state of moderate vitamin C deficiency (ascorbic acid concentrations in plasma, leukocytes, semen, and buccal cells dropped to less than 50 percent of the baseline, with no scorbutic symptoms observed). No changes in cell proliferation, erythrocyte antioxidant enzymes, and DNA strand breaks were observed. However, blood levels of glutathione and NAD(P) decreased during deficiency, as did delayed hypersensitivity responsiveness. Measures of oxidative damage (oxidatively modified DNA base, 8-hydroxy deoxyguanosine in sperm DNA, and fecapentaenes—ubiquitous fecal mutagens) were also increased during vitamin C depletion. The authors concluded that moderate vitamin C deficiency in the absence of scurvy results in alteration of antioxidant chemistries and may permit increased oxidative damage (23).

Vitamin C and Exercise-Induced Oxidative Stress

- In a placebo-controlled (not blinded) study, nine trained subjects participated in all three phases in random order: (1) exercise with placebo for one day, (2) exercise with 1 g vitamin C for one day, and (3) exercise following two weeks of vitamin C supplementation. Plasma thiobarbituric acid reacting substance (TBARS), a pro-oxidant biomarker, and oxygen radical absorbance capacity (ORAC), a measure of total antioxidant activity, were measured before and after 30 minutes of submaximal exercise on a treadmill. TBARS and ORAC did not differ among treatments at rest. Following exercise, vitamin C supplements attenuated the exercise-induced oxidative stress when taken for one day but not for two weeks. Oxidative stress was highest during the placebo trial. The authors concluded that further research is needed to explain these results and the effects of vitamin C supplementation on oxidative stress during exercise (24).

- In a double-blind, placebo-controlled study, 12 experienced marathon runners were randomized to receive 1 g vitamin C/day or a placebo for eight days. Blood samples were taken before and six hours after subjects completed a 2.5-hour treadmill run at 75 percent to 80 percent VO_{2max}. Vitamin C had no effect on hormonal (cortisol, catecholamines) or immune measures (leukocyte subsets, interleukin-6, natural killer cell activity, lymphocyte proliferation, granulocyte phagocytosis and activated oxidative burst) during recovery (25).

- In a double-blind, placebo-controlled study, 16 ultramarathon athletes were randomized to receive vitamin C (2×500 mg/day) or a placebo for seven days prior to a 90 km run, as well as on race day and two days following the run. Blood was drawn 16 hours before the race and at 30 minutes, 24 hours, and 48 hours after finishing. Prerace vitamin C levels in the supplemented group were unchanged after the race, while an increase was observed in the placebo group immediately postrace, and then returned to baseline after 24 hours. Immediately after the run, both groups experienced elevations in circulating neutrophils, monocytes and platelets, interleukin-6, cortisol, C-reactive protein (CRP), and creatine kinase. However, in the vitamin C supplemented group, CRP levels were significantly higher at each time point and cortisol levels were significantly lower only 30 minutes postrace. The authors concluded that these observations suggest that vitamin C may blunt the adaptive mobilization of the vitamin from adrenals during exercise-induced oxidative stress and may be associated with an enhancement of the acute phase protein response and attenuation of the exercise-induced increase in cortisol (26).

- In a double-blind, placebo-controlled trial of 184 healthy subjects, vitamin C (500 mg/day) had no significant effect or interaction effect on oxidative DNA damage as measured by urinary 8-hydroxy-2'deoxyguanosine (8-OhdG). However, fruit and

V

vegetable intake (at least three servings daily) was associated with lower oxidative damage (27).

Vitamin C and Cardiovascular Disease

- A systematic review was undertaken of all ecological, case-control, and prospective studies from 1980 to 1996 examining vitamin C intake or status with cardiovascular disease. For coronary heart disease 4 of 7 ecological, 1 of 4 case-control, and 3 of 12 cohort studies found a significant protective effect. For total circulatory disease, 2 of 3 cohort studies reported a significant protective correlation with vitamin C intake. For strokes, 2 of 2 epidemiological studies, 0 of 1 case-control study, and 2 of 7 cohort studies found a significant protective effect (28).

- An epidemiological study of 1,605 randomly selected Finnish men aged 42, 48, 54, or 60 y without cardiovascular disease found a higher incidence of myocardial infarction correlated with low plasma vitamin C levels (29). Another study of a randomly selected cohort of 730 elderly people revealed that subjects with the lowest vitamin C status had a higher mortality rate from stroke, but not mortality from coronary heart disease (30).

- A systematic review of cross-sectional and prospective studies from 1980 to 1996 on vitamin C and blood pressure was undertaken. Ten of 14 cross-sectional studies reported an inverse association between plasma vitamin C and blood pressure. Three of four reported an inverse relationship with dietary vitamin C intake. The authors noted that none of the cross-sectional studies adequately controlled for potential confounding dietary factors. Of four randomized, controlled trials, only one reported a significant decrease in blood pressure with vitamin C supplementation (250 to 1,000 mg), whereas two studies were considered "uninterpretable" (31).

- In a double-blind, placebo-controlled, crossover study, 40 men and women (ages 60 y to 80 y) were given in random order 500 mg vitamin C and a placebo for three months each, with a one-week washout period. Blood pressure and blood values were taken at baseline and at the end of each phase. Blood pressure measured at the clinic did not differ between groups. However, daytime ambulatory blood pressure showed a small, but significant, reduction in systolic, but not diastolic, pressure with vitamin C. Regression analysis revealed that the higher the baseline daytime pressure, the greater the fall in blood pressure observed with vitamin C. There were no differences between groups in cholesterol levels, although when women were analyzed alone, there was a significant rise in HDL cholesterol with vitamin C supplementation (32).

- Animal and human studies have investigated the role of vitamin C in cholesterol metabolism, in the maintenance of vascular integrity, in the synthesis of prostacyclin (vasodilator and antiplatelet agent), and its antioxidant role in lipid oxidation (via reductive regeneration of vitamin E). A comprehensive review article noted that although there appears to be a possible protective association between vitamin C and CVD, conclusive evidence is lacking. The author notes that human data have been inconsistent, but "taken together indicate that for individuals with high cholesterol concentrations (> 200 mg/dL) and less than full tissue saturation [of vitamin C], increasing the concentration of vitamin C may have a salutary effect on total cholesterol" (33).

Vitamin C and Cancer

- Cancer mortality was investigated within the 25-year Seven Countries Study. Vitamin C intake was inversely correlated with stomach cancer mortality even after correcting for smoking and sodium and nitrate intake (34). Review articles have also summarized evidence that suggests lower risk of esophagus, oral cavity, and pharynx cancers with vitamin C intake ($\approx$ 70 mg to 100 mg/day) (8). However, in the Linxian Nutrition Intervention Trial, supplementation of 120 mg vitamin C and 30 µg molybdenum for five years did not reduce mortality from stomach cancer in 29,584 Chinese subjects (35).

- Studies of vitamin C intake and breast cancer have reported conflicting results. A meta-analysis of 12 case-control studies showed vitamin C intake was inversely related to breast cancer risk (36).

- A review article specifically addressing supplement use and epidemiological research on cancer risk reported an inverse relationship between bladder cancer and vitamin C supplements in case-control studies (37).

Vitamin C and Cataracts

- In the Nurses' Health Study, 50,828 women aged 45 y to 67 y were evaluated for incidence of cataract extraction during an eight-year prospective study. Those who reported using vitamin C supplements for 10 or more years had a significant 45 percent reduction in cataract risk. In nonsupplement users, dietary vitamin C intake had no correlation with risk (38).

- In a cross-sectional study, a subset of 240 women with very high or very low vitamin C intakes were selected from the Nurses' Health Study cohort (no history of diabetes or diagnosed cataract). All subjects received a detailed eye exam. Women who took vitamin C supplements for 10 or more years (n = 26) had a significant 77 percent lower incidence of early age-related lens opacities and a significant 83 percent lower incidence of moderate lens opacities at any lens compared to women not taking vitamin C (n = 141). Of the 26 women who used supplements for 10 or more years, 4 had an average dose of < 400 mg/day, 12 had an average dose 400 mg to 700 mg/day, and 10 had an average dose of > 700 mg/day. However, use of supplements for less than 10 years had no statistical effect on the overall incidence of lens opacities (39).

- According to a review of five epidemiological studies (including the Nurse's Health Study) on cataract risk: "All have shown some evidence of protective effects, either for vitamin C specifically, or for vitamins in general" (8).

SAFETY

- The Tolerable Upper Intake Level (UL), the highest intake that is likely to pose no risk of adverse effects, is set at 2,000 mg/day from food and supplements. This level was selected because higher doses are associated with gastrointestinal distress (2).

V

- Vitamin C is generally considered safe even in large doses because of the efficiency of excess excretion by the kidneys. Several double-blind, controlled trials supplementing up to 10 g vitamin C daily for more than one year or up to 5 g/day for more than three years reported no serious adverse effects (40).

- Diarrhea and nausea can occur with very large doses because of the osmotic effects of the unabsorbed vitamin. These side-effects may be minimized by a gradual increase in vitamin C dose over time (1, 2).

- Because vitamin C facilitates nonheme iron absorption, large supplemental doses should be avoided by individuals with hemachromatosis (1, 2).

- Excess amounts of vitamin C in urine and feces from supplementation can interfere with certain diagnostic tests such as glycosuria and fecal occult blood. Additionally, excess vitamin C can interfere with blood tests based on redox chemistry including cholesterol and glucose (1).

- Large doses of vitamin C may interfere with anticoagulant medications (1). However, in healthy males, 2 g had no effect on hemostatic parameters (41).

- It is generally accepted that high vitamin C intakes do not cause kidney stone formation. In the Health Professional's Follow-Up Study, a cohort of 45,251 men age 40 y to 75 y with no history of kidney stones found no association between high daily intake of vitamin C (> 1,500 mg) and the risk of stone formation even when consumed in large doses (42). However, individuals with recurrent kidney stones or disease are advised not to supplement with doses exceeding 100 mg/day (5).

- There has been recent concern about the possible pro-oxidant effects of high doses of vitamin C, after publication of a non-peer-reviewed study published as a correspondence letter in *Nature*. According to the placebo-controlled study, 500 mg vitamin C supplementation increased 8-oxoadenine (marker of DNA damage) and decreased 8-oxoguanine levels in DNA isolated from lymphocytes. The authors concluded: "Our discovery of an increase in a potentially mutagenic lesion, 8-oxo-adenine, following a typical vitamin C supplementation should therefore be of some concern, although at doses of < 500 mg/day the antioxidant effect may predominate" (43). However, some researchers have suggested that the results and conclusions drawn from this study were widely misinterpreted because a reduction in 8-oxoguanine levels has been associated with lower mutation rates (4). Overall, experimental, epidemiological, and clinical studies do not suggest that high doses of vitamin C are linked to an increased risk for oxidative DNA damage or to an elevated risk of cancer (2, 5).

REFERENCES

1. Jacob RA. Vitamin C. In: Shils ME, Olson JA, Shike M, Ross AC, eds. *Modern Nutrition in Health and Disease.* 9th ed. Baltimore, Md: Williams & Wilkins; 1999:467–483.
2. Food and Nutrition Board, Institute of Medicine. *Dietary Reference Intakes: Vitamin C, Vitamin E, Selenium, and Carotenoids.* Washington, DC: National Academy Press; 2000.

3. Pennington JAT. *Bowes & Church's Food Values of Portions Commonly Used.* 17th ed. Philadelphia, Pa: Lippincott; 1998.

4. Johnston CS, Luo B. Comparison of the absorption and excretion of three commercially available sources of vitamin C. *J Am Diet Assoc.* 1994;94:779–781.

5. Johnston CS. Biomarkers for establishing a Tolerable Upper Intake Level for Vitamin C. *Nutr Rev.* 1999;57:71–77.

6. Shane B. Vitamin C pharmacokinetics: it's deja vu all over again. *Am J Clin Nutr.* 1997;66:1061–1062.

7. Blanchard J, Tozer TN, Rowland M. Pharmacokinetic perspectives on megadoses of ascorbic acid. *Am J Clin Nutr.* 1997;66:1165–1171.

8. Weber P, Bendich A, Schalch W. Vitamin C and human health—a review of recent data relevant to human requirements. *Int J Vitam Nutr Res.* 1996;66:19–30.

9. Levine M, Dhariwal KR, Welch RW, et al. Determination of optimal vitamin C requirements in humans. *Am J Clin Nutr.* 1995;62(6 suppl):1347S–1356S.

10. Hemila H. Vitamin C supplementation and the common cold—was Linus Pauling right or wrong? *Int J Vitam Nutr Res.* 1997;67:329–335.

11. Chalmers TC. Effects of ascorbic acid on the common cold. An evaluation of the evidence. *Am J Med.* 1975;58:532–536.

12. Hemila H, Herman ZS. Vitamin C and the common cold: a retrospective analysis of Chalmers' review. *J Am Coll Nutr.* 1995;14:116–123.

13. Hemila H. Vitamin C intake and susceptibility to the common cold. *Br J Nutr.* 1997;77:59–72.

14. Hemila H. Vitamin C and common cold incidence: a review of studies with subjects under heavy physical stress. *Int J Sports Med.* 1996;17:379–383.

15. Peters EM, Goetzsche JM, Grobbelaar B, et al. Vitamin C supplementation reduces the incidence of postrace symptoms of upper-respiratory-tract infection in ultramarathon runners. *Am J Clin Nutr.* 1993;57:170–174.

16. Schwartz J, Weiss ST. Relationship between dietary vitamin C intake and pulmonary function in the First National Health and Nutrition Examination Survey (NHANES I). *Am J Clin Nutr.* 1994;59:110–114.

17. Soutar A, Seaton A, Brown K. Bronchial reactivity and dietary antioxidants. *Thorax.* 1997;52:166–170.

18. Romieu I, Meneses F, Ramirez M, et al. Antioxidant supplementation and respiratory functions among workers exposed to high levels of ozone. *Am J Respir Crit Care Med.* 1998;158:226–232.

19. Cohen HA, Neuman I, Nahum H. Blocking effect of vitamin C in exercise-induced asthma. *Arch Pediatr Adolesc Med.* 1997;151:367–370.

20. Bielory L, Gandhi R. Asthma and vitamin C. *Ann Allergy.* 1994;73:89–96.

21. Jeng KC, Yang CS, Siu WY, et al. Supplementation with vitamins C and E enhances cytokine production by peripheral blood mononuclear cells in healthy adults. *Am J Clin Nutr.* 1996;64:960–965.

22. Hunt C, Chakravorty NK, Annan G, et al. The clinical effects of vitamin C supplementation in elderly hospitalized patients with acute respiratory infections. *Int J Vitam Nutr Res.* 1994;64:212–219.

V

23. Jacob RA, Kelley DS, Pianalto FS, et al. Immunocompetence and oxidant defense during ascorbate depletion in healthy men. *Am J Clin Nutr.* 1991;54(6 suppl):1302S–1309S.

24. Alessio HM, Goldfarb AH, Cao G. Exercise-induced oxidative stress before and after vitamin C supplementation. *Int J Sport Nutr.* 1997;7:1–9.

25. Nieman DC, Henson DA, Butterworth DE, et al. Vitamin C supplementation does not alter the immune response to 2.5 hours of running. *Int J Sport Nutr.* 1997;7:173–184.

26. Peters EM, Anderson R, Theron AJ. Attenuation of increase in circulating cortisol and enhancement of the acute phase protein response in vitamin C-supplemented ultra-marathoners. *Int J Sports Med.* 2001;22:120–126.

27. Huang HY, Helzlsouer KJ, Appel LJ, et al. The effects of vitamin C and vitamin E on oxidative DNA damage: results from a randomized controlled trial. *Cancer Epidemiol Biomarkers Prev.* 2000;9:647–652.

28. Ness AR, Powles JW, Khaw KT. Vitamin C and cardiovascular disease: a systematic review. *J Cardiovasc Risk.* 1996;3:513–521.

29. Nyyssonen K, Parviainen MT, Salonen R, et al. Vitamin C deficiency and risk of myocardial infarction: prospective population study of men from eastern Finland. *BMJ.* 1997;314:634–638.

30. Gale CR, Martyn CN, Winter PD, et al. Vitamin C and risk of death from stroke and coronary heart disease in a cohort of elderly people. *BMJ.* 1995;310:1563–1566.

31. Ness AR, Chee D, Elliott P. Vitamin C and blood pressure—an overview. *J Hum Hypertens.* 1997;11:343–350.

32. Fotherby MD, Williams JC, Forster LA, et al. Effect of vitamin C on ambulatory blood pressure and plasma lipids in older persons. *J Hypertens.* 2000;18:411–415.

33. Simon JA. Vitamin C and cardiovascular disease: a review. *J Am Coll Nutr.* 1992;11:107–125.

34. Ocke MC, Kromhout D, Menotti A, et al. Average intake of antioxidant (pro)vitamins and subsequent cancer mortality in the 16 cohorts of the Seven Countries Study. *Int J Cancer.* 1995;61:480–484.

35. Blot WJ, Li JY, Taylor PR, et al. Nutrition intervention trials in Linxian, China: supplementation with specific vitamin/mineral combinations, cancer incidence, and disease-specific mortality in the general population. *J Natl Cancer Inst.* 1993;85:1483–1492.

36. Howe GR, Hirohata T, Hislop TG, et al. Dietary factors and risk of breast cancer: combined analysis of 12 case-control studies. *J Natl Cancer Inst.* 1990;82:561–569.

37. Patterson RE, White E, Kristal AR, et al. Vitamin supplements and cancer risk: the epidemiologic evidence. *Cancer Causes Control.* 1997;8:786–802.

38. Hankinson SE, Stampfer MJ, Seddon JM, et al. Nutrient intake and cataract extraction in women: a prospective study. *BMJ.* 1992;305:335–339.

39. Jacques PF, Taylor A, Hankinson SE, et al. Long-term vitamin C supplement use and prevalence of early age-related lens opacities. *Am J Clin Nutr.* 1997;66:911–916.

40. Bendich A, Langseth L. The health effects of vitamin C supplementation: a review. *J Am Coll Nutr.* 1995;14:124–136.

41. Curhan GC, Willett WC, Rimm EB, et al. A prospective study of the intake of vitamins C and B6, and the risk of kidney stones in men. *J Urol.* 1996;155:1847–1851.

42. Tofler GH, Stec JJ, Stubbe I, et al. The effect of vitamin C supplementation on coagulability and lipid levels in healthy male subjects. *Thromb Res.* 2000;100:35–41.

43. Podmore ED, Griffiths HR, Herbert KE, et al. Vitamin C exhibits pro-oxidant properties. *Nature.* 1998;329:559.

Vitamin D

Vitamin D, considered both a hormone and a vitamin, functions primarily to maintain calcium homeostasis. Vitamin D is produced endogenously when ultraviolet light reacts with 7-dehydrocholesterol in the skin to produce cholecalciferol or vitamin D_3. In the liver, vitamin D_3 is hydroxylated into 25-hydroxy vitamin D_3, the most abundant form in the body. This compound is further hydroxylated in the kidneys to produce the active form, 1, 25-dihydroxy vitamin D3. (Two other equivalent terms for 1,25-dihydroxy vitamin D_3 are 1, 25-dihydroxy cholecalciferol and/or 1, $25(OH)_2D_3$.) When serum calcium levels decline, the activated vitamin D increases calcium and phosphorus absorption in the intestine, increases resorption of calcium in the kidneys, and stimulates bone mineral release (1, 2). Defects in vitamin D metabolism, lack of sun exposure, insufficient dietary intake, or a combination of these can result in rickets (children) or osteomalacia (adults). Vitamin D deficiency is fairly common among the elderly population, specifically the homebound and institutionalized (3–5).

Media and Marketing Claims	Efficacy
Necessary for bone health	↑
Improves calcium absorption	↑
Reduces risk of colon and breast cancer	↔

Advisory

- The Tolerable Upper Intake Level (UL) is 2,000 IU or 50 µg/day)
- People who use many supplements containing vitamin D and who consume high intakes of fish or fortified milk may be at risk for vitamin D toxicity
- Excessive intakes of vitamin D can result in hypercalcemia, hypercalciuria, calcification of bone and soft tissues

Drug/Supplement Interactions

- Estrogen therapy may increase blood levels of vitamin D and enhance calcium absorption
- Vitamin D may decrease the effectiveness of verapamil (calcium channel blocker for hypertension)
- The following drugs may increase risk of bone loss by interfering with the absorption and activity of vitamin D: anticonvulsant drugs, bile acid sequestrants (for hypercholesterolemia), cimetidine (antacid), corticosteroids (anti-inflammatory), heparin (anticoagulant), isoniazid (antibiotic), mineral oil, neomycin (antibacterial)

V

KEY POINTS

- Vitamin D is necessary for bone health. When taken with calcium, vitamin D appears to minimize losses of bone mineral density (BMD) and possibly the incidence of fractures. Substantial reductions in fracture rates have been found with combined therapy with calcium and vitamin D, but it is not clear which is the principal active agent or whether, in fact, the combination is optimal in fracture prevention (1).

- Vitamin D is necessary for efficient calcium absorption. Inadequate dietary vitamin D, insufficient exposure to sunlight, impaired activation of vitamin D, or defects in vitamin D metabolism interfere with calcium absorption. It is estimated that only 10 percent of dietary calcium is absorbed when vitamin D is deficient (24). More research is needed to determine the strength of the causal relationships between the two nutrients.

- Epidemiological studies have shown an inconsistent relationship between dietary vitamin D to reduced colorectal cancer risk. Data from some of these studies suggest a possible protective effect of total vitamin D intake (dietary and supplemental) against colorectal cancer. However, it is not known if these effects are because of vitamin D alone or multivitamin use. *In vitro* and animal data suggest that vitamin D may possibly reduce the risk of certain cancers, including mammary tumors. Vitamin D analogues are currently being tested in laboratory studies and in patients having advanced cancer. Controlled clinical trials of sufficient size are needed to clarify the potential protective role of supplemental vitamin D in cancer prevention.

- Vitamin D status may be compromised in elderly, institutionalized patients, and individuals with malabsorption disorders as in liver failure, Celiac sprue, Crohn's disease, and Whipple's disease. If sun exposure and dietary vitamin D intakes are low despite dietary counseling, this population may require supplemental vitamin D to help meet the recommended Adequate Intake (AI).

FOOD SOURCES

Food sources of vitamin D are limited. Egg yolks, liver, fish oils, fatty fish, fortified milk (100 IU/cup), and fortified breakfast cereals (40 IU to 80 IU/serving) are the best sources (6, 7). The Vitamin D content of fortified milk has been reported to vary (8). Estimates of U.S. dietary intake of vitamin D are not available due to variability of vitamin D in fortified foods and because U.S. surveys have not measured vitamin D intake (9).

DOSAGE INFORMATION/BIOAVAILABILITY

The Adequate Intake (AI) for vitamin D is 200 IU (5 μg) for adults younger than 50 y, 400 IU (10 μg) for adults 51 y to 70 y, and 600 IU (15 μg) for adults 70 y and older (9).

Vitamin D_3 (cholecalciferol) or vitamin D_2 (ergocalciferol) supplements are sold in single preparations or multivitamin/mineral supplements usually providing 200 IU to 400 IU (5 μg to 10 μg). (1 μg = 40 IU) In general, vitamin D_3 supplements raise blood levels of vitamin D_3 and 25-hydroxy vitamin D (measure of vitamin D status) (10). In one study, vitamin D_3 supplements increased serum 25-hydroxy vitamin D levels greater than vitamin D_2 supplements (11).

RELEVANT RESEARCH

Vitamin D Deficiency

- In an observational study, 290 patients (mean age = 62 y) on a general medical ward in Boston were assessed for hypovitaminosis D. Fifty-seven percent of the patients were considered vitamin D-deficient (assessed by serum 25-hydroxy vitamin D concentrations), of which 22 percent were severely deficient. In a subgroup of patients < 65 years (n = 77), incidence of deficiency was 42 percent. In the overall sample, 69 percent of the subjects did not consume the adequate intake (AI) for vitamin D for their age, and 43 percent of the patients with adequate consumption were vitamin D deficient (12).

Vitamin D (Alone or with Calcium) and Bone Health

- In a double-blind, placebo-controlled study, 389 male and female subjects > 65 years were randomized to receive 500 mg calcium plus 700 IU (17.5 µg) vitamin D_3 or a placebo daily for three years. There was a significant difference between the treatment and placebo groups at the femoral neck, spine and total-body BMD (assessed by dual-energy x-ray absorptiometry) after one year, but it remained significant only for total body BMD in the following two years. Of the 37 subjects who experienced nonvertebral fractures, significantly more were in the placebo group (n = 26) compared to the vitamin D-calcium-supplemented group (n = 11) (13).

- In a double-blind, placebo-controlled, prospective study, 2,578 free-living Dutch men and women > 70 y were randomly assigned to receive 400 IU (10 µg) vitamin D_3 or a placebo daily for a maximum of 3.5 years. All subjects had a mean dietary calcium intake of 868 mg/day. Vitamin D supplemented subjects had higher mean serum 25-hydroxy vitamin D levels than the placebo group. However, there were no differences in incidence of hip fractures or other peripheral fractures (14).

- In a double-blind, placebo-controlled trial, 348 Dutch women > 70 y were randomized to receive 400 IU (10 µg) vitamin D_3 or a placebo daily for two years. BMD was assessed by either single-photon absorptiometry (distal radius) or dual-energy X-ray absorptiometry (femoral neck and femoral trochanter). Supplements significantly increased serum 25-hydroxy vitamin D and 1, 25- dihydroxy vitamin D levels and urinary calcium/creatinine ratios, and significantly decreased parathyroid hormone (PTH) compared to placebo. (PTH levels are elevated during vitamin D deficiency.) There were no changes in biochemical markers of bone turnover between groups. Vitamin D-supplemented subjects had significantly increased BMD in the femoral neck, but not in the femoral trochanter or distal radius (15).

- In a double-blind, comparative study, 247 healthy postmenopausal women living in Boston were randomized to receive 100 IU (2.5 µg) vitamin D_3 or 700 IU (17.5 µg)

V

vitamin D_3 daily for two years. All women received 500 mg supplemental calcium as calcium citrate malate. Average dietary intake of vitamin D for all subjects was 100 IU (2.5 µg). Both treatment groups lost BMD from the femoral neck, but the high-dose vitamin D-supplemented group lost significantly less than the group receiving the lower dose. There were no changes in spinal and whole-body bone densities (assessed by dual-energy X-ray absorptiometry) between groups (16).

- In a double-blind, placebo-controlled trial, 249 healthy, postmenopausal women were randomized to receive 400 IU (10 µg) vitamin D_3 or a placebo daily for one year. Usual dietary intake of vitamin D was 100 IU (2.5 µg) for both groups. All subjects received 377 mg supplemental calcium as calcium citrate malate. BMD was measured at six-month intervals when serum 25-hydroxy vitamin D is highest (summer/fall) and lowest (winter/spring). Both groups had an increase in spinal BMD in the summer/fall. Both groups had losses in spinal BMD in the winter/spring, but the vitamin D supplemented group had significantly less bone loss and a significant overall improvement in spinal BMD. During the winter/spring months, 25-hydroxy vitamin D levels were lower and PTH levels were higher in the placebo than in the vitamin D group. The authors concluded: "At latitude 42 degrees [Boston], healthy postmenopausal women with vitamin D intakes of 100 IU [2.5 µg] daily can reduce late wintertime bone loss and improve net bone density of the spine over one year by increasing their intake to 500 IU [12.5 µg] daily. A long-term benefit of preventing vitamin D insufficiency in the winter seems likely although it remains to be shown" (17).

- In a meta-analysis report, researchers evaluated randomized, controlled trials lasting at least six months to determine whether vitamin D was more effective than no therapy or calcium supplementation alone in the management of corticosteroid-induced osteoporosis. Of nine trials, there was a moderate, significant benefit of vitamin D plus calcium compared to no therapy or calcium use alone (18).

- In a follow-up study of 295 healthy men and women who had completed a three-year controlled trial of calcium and vitamin D supplementation, BMD (at the spinal and femoral neck in men and at all sites in women) was lost after two years poststudy without treatment (19).

Vitamin D and Cancer

- In a prospective cohort study (Iowa-Women's Health Study), 34,702 postmenopausal women were assessed for colorectal cancer over a nine-year period. There was an insignificant association between high intakes of vitamin D and reduced risk of rectal cancer (20). In the Nurse's Health prospective cohort study (n = 84,448 women) there was an inverse association between intake of total vitamin D from foods and supplements (mean intake of highest vitamin D quintile = 728 IU [18.3 µg], vs lowest quintile = 55 IU [1.4 µg]) and risk of colorectal cancer during 12 years. Calcium intake was not associated with a lower risk of colorectal cancer. The authors concluded factors other than vitamin D in multivitamin supplements may account for this protective effect (21).

V

- In the Health Professional's Follow-Up Study, another prospective cohort study (n = 47,935 men), there was an inverse relationship between intake of supplemental vitamin D from multivitamins and colon cancer risk, but not with dietary vitamin D. The authors postulated that the reduction in risk could be attributed to multivitamin use rather than vitamin D alone (22).

- In a prospective case-control study, 95,000 cancer-free women were assessed for vitamin D status between 1964 and 1972. By 1991, 2,131 women developed breast cancer. A random sample of 96 women over 55 y with cancer were matched to controls. Prior to diagnosis, serum 1, 25 dihydroxy-vitamin D levels were measured in all subjects. The researchers chose to measure 1, 25 dihydroxy-vitamin D because this form has been recognized as a modulator of cell proliferation and differentiation in laboratory studies. (Note: This measure has little value in detecting vitamin D deficiency.) There was no relationship between breast cancer incidence and prediagnostic serum vitamin D levels (23).

- An *in vitro* study showed that vitamin D_3 inhibited cell proliferation and induced apoptosis (programmed cell death) in breast cancer, prostate cancer, and human osteosarcoma cell lines (24). Other *in vitro* and animal studies have also demonstrated these effects in mammary tumors (25, 26).

SAFETY

- The Tolerable Upper Intake Level (UL) for adults is 2,000 IU vitamin D (50 µg) (9).
- People who use many supplements containing vitamin D and who consume high intakes of fish or fortified milk, may be at risk for vitamin D toxicity (9).
- Excessive intakes of vitamin D are associated with hypercalcemia, hypercalciuria, calcification of bone and soft tissues including the kidney (kidney stones), lungs, and the tympanic membrane of the ear, which can result in deafness (7).

REFERENCES

1. Jones G, Strugnell SA, DeLuca HF. Current understanding of the molecular actions of vitamin D. *Physiol Rev.* 1998;78:1193–1231.
2. Reid IR. The roles of calcium and vitamin D in the prevention of osteoporosis. *Endocrinol Metab Clin North Am.* 1998;27:389–398.
3. Compston JE. Vitamin D deficiency: time for action. Evidence supports routine supplementation for elderly people and others at risk. *BMJ.* 1998;317:1466–1467.
4. Gloth FM III, Gundberg CM, Hollis BW, et al. Vitamin D deficiency in homebound elderly persons. *JAMA.* 1995;274:1683–1686.
5. Jacques PF, Felson DT, Tucker KL, et al. Plasma 25-hydroxy vitamin D and its determinants in an elderly population sample. *Am J Clin Nutr.* 1997;66:929–936.

V

6. Pennington JAT. *Bowes and Church's Food Values of Portions Commonly Used.* 17th ed. Philadelphia, Pa: Lippincott; 1998.

7. Linder MC. Nutrition and Metabolism of Vitamins. In: Linder MC, ed. *Nutritional Biochemistry and Metabolism with Clinical Applications.* 2nd ed. New York, NY: Elsevier; 1991:111–189.

8. Holick MF, Shao Q, Liu WW, et al. The vitamin D content of fortified milk and infant formula. *N Engl J Med.* 1992;326:1178–1181.

9. Institute of Medicine, Food and Nutrition Board. *Dietary Reference Intakes for Calcium, Phosphorus, Magnesium, Vitamin D, and Fluoride.* Washington, DC: National Academy Press; 1997.

10. Barger-Lux MJ, Heaney RP, Dowell S, et al. Vitamin D and its major metabolites: serum levels after graded oral dosing in healthy men. *Osteoporos Int.* 1998;8:222–230.

11. Trang HM, Cole DE, Rubin LA, et al. Evidence that vitamin D_3 increases serum 25-hydroxy vitamin D more efficiently than does vitamin D_2. *Am J Clin Nutr.* 1998;68:854–858.

12. Thomas MK, Lloyd-Jones DM, Thadhani RI, et al. Hypovitaminosis D in medical inpatients. *N Engl J Med.* 1998;338:777–783.

13. Dawson-Hughes B, Harris SS, Krall EA, et al. Effect of calcium and vitamin D supplementation on bone density in men and women 65 years of age or older. *N Engl J Med.* 1997;337:670–676.

14. Lips P, Graafmans WC, Ooms ME, et al. Vitamin D supplementation and fracture incidence in elderly persons. A randomized, placebo-controlled clinical trial. *Ann Intern Med.* 1996;124:400–406.

15. Ooms ME, Roos JC, Bezemer PD, et al. Prevention of bone loss by vitamin D supplementation in elderly women: a randomized double-blind trial. *J Clin Endocrinol Metab.* 1995;80:1052–1058.

16. Dawson-Hughes B, Harris SS, Krall EA, et al. Rates of bone loss in postmenopausal women randomly assigned to one of two dosages of vitamin D. *Am J Clin Nutr.* 1995;61:1140–1145.

17. Dawson-Hughes B, Dallal GE, Krall EA, et al. Effect of vitamin D supplementation on wintertime and overall bone loss in healthy postmenopausal women. *Ann Intern Med.* 1991;115:505–512.

18. Amin S, LaValley MP, Simms RW, et al. The role of vitamin D in corticosteroid-induced osteoporosis: a meta-analytic approach. *Arthritis Rheum.* 1999;42:1740–1751.

19. Dawson-Hughes B, Harris SS, Krall EA, et al. Effect of withdrawal of calcium and vitamin D supplements on bone mass in elderly men and women. *Am J Clin Nutr.* 2000;72:745–750.

20. Zheng W, Anderson KE, Kushi LH, et al. A prospective cohort study of intake of calcium, vitamin D, and other micronutrients in relation to incidence of rectal cancer among postmenopausal women. *Cancer Epidemiol Biomarkers Prev.* 1998;7:221–225.

21. Martinez ME, Giovannucci EL, Colditz GA, et al. Calcium, vitamin D, and the occurrence of colorectal cancer among women. *J Natl Cancer Inst.* 1996;88:1375–1382.

22. Kearney J, Giovannucci E, Rimm EB, et al. Calcium, vitamin D, and dairy foods and the occurrence of colon cancer in men. *Am J Epidemiol.* 1996;143:907–917.

V

23. Hiatt RA, Krieger N, Lobaugh B, et al. Prediagnostic serum vitamin D and breast cancer. *J Natl Cancer Inst.* 1998;90:461–463.
24. Fife RS, Sledge GW Jr, Proctor C. Effects of vitamin D_3 on proliferation of cancer cells in vitro. *Cancer Lett.* 1997;120:65–69.
25. Welsh J. Vitamin D compounds as potential therapeutics for estrogen-independent breast cancer. *Nutrition.* 1997;13:915–917.
26. Koren R, Hadari-Naor I, Zuck E, et al. Vitamin D is a prooxidant in breast cancer cells. *Cancer Res.* 2001;61:1439–1444.

Vitamin E

Vitamin E is an essential fat-soluble vitamin necessary in human health. The term vitamin E is the generic description for all tocopherol (alpha, beta, gamma, delta) and tocotrienol derivatives having the biologic activity of alpha-tocopherol. There are eight naturally occurring vitamin E compounds in plants and numerous stereoisomers of synthetic vitamin E. However, according to the Food and Nutrition Board 2000 report on antioxidants, vitamin E is only defined as alpha-tocopherol. Alpha-tocopherol is the most abundant and active of all the forms. It is also the primary form found in animal tissue, most concentrated in the plasma, liver, and adipose tissue. In foods, alpha- and gamma-tocopherols are generally the only isomers that have vitamin E activity (1–3).

Vitamin E deficiency is rare in healthy people but may occur in patients with genetic abnormalities, fat malabsorption syndromes, cystic fibrosis, pancreatic insufficiency, short bowel syndrome, chronic steatorrhea, and patients receiving total parenteral nutrition (TPN). Deficiency symptoms include peripheral neuropathy, hemolytic anemia, skeletal myopathy, ataxia, and retinopathy (1–3).

The main function of vitamin E is as a biologic antioxidant protecting cellular membranes from oxidative damage from peroxyl, hydroxyl, and superoxide radicals. In this role, it is critical in preventing the oxidation and peroxidation of polyunsaturated fatty acids (PUFAs) in and on the plasma membranes of cells. A number of other functions of vitamin E have been identified in experimental studies that explain how the vitamin may be involved in protecting against heart disease. *In vitro* studies show that vitamin E inhibits low-density lipoprotein (LDL) oxidation. Oxidation of LDL is believed to contribute to cardiovascular disease. Vitamin E also inhibits protein kinase C activity (involved in smooth muscle cell proliferation and differentiation), thrombin formation (a hormone that stimulates aggregation), and intercellular and vascular adhesion molecules. Vitamin E also appears to enhance the expression of the rate-limiting enzymes cytosolic phopholipase A_2 and cyclooxygenase-1. This results in the release of prostacyclin, a potent vasodilator and inhibitor of platelet aggregation in humans (1–3).

Vitamin E supplements have become popular among the public because of a number of *in vitro* and some clinical studies suggesting that vitamin E in doses higher than achievable from the diet may have beneficial effects in cardiovascular disease, cancer, immune response, and other conditions related to oxidative stress.

V

Media and Marketing Claims	Efficacy
Prevents heart disease and heart attack	↔
Prevents cancer	↔
Improves immunity in elderly	?↑
Slows progression of neuropsychiatric disorders	?↑
Improves lung function	?↑
Prevents cataracts	?↑
Improves blood sugar level in diabetics	?↑
Enhances exercise performance	NR

Advisory

The Tolerable Upper Intake Level (UL) for adults is 1,000 mg of any form of supplemental alpha tocopherol/day (equivalent to 1,500 IU natural, 1,100 IU synthetic)

Drug/Supplement Interactions

- May have an additive effect when combined with anticoagulant drugs (wafarin, heparin, aspirin) and other blood-thinning dietary supplements (eg, fish oil, ginkgo, garlic)
- The following may interfere with vitamin E absorption: bile acid sequestrants such as colestipol (for hypercholesterolemia), isoniazid (antibiotic), mineral oil
- May enhance the effects and reduce the dosage needed of cyclosporine (immune suppressant used to prevent transplant rejection)
- May potentially reduce cardiotoxicity associated with doxorubicin (chemotherapeutic drug)
- May increase blood levels of griseofulvin (antifungal for ringworm)

KEY POINTS

- Evidence from epidemiological studies suggests that dietary and supplemental vitamin E intakes are inversely related to risk of cardiovascular disease. Of four large-scale controlled trials, three did not show any risk reduction (the ATBC study using 50-mg doses in male smokers, HOPE study using 268 mg in high-risk patients, and GISSI study using 300 mg in high-risk patients). However, in the CHAOS study, patients with angiographically proven coronary artery disease had large reductions in risk of heart attack with either 268-mg or 567-mg doses. It has been suggested that a possible reason for the differing results may have to do with the level of atherosclerosis of the subjects. It is possible that the CHAOS participants had far less advanced lesions than those in the other study subjects (3). More research is needed to clarify how vitamin E may affect heart disease depending on the level of disease progression.

- At this time, there is much controversy surrounding recommending high-dose vitamin E supplements for cardiovascular patients. The 1999 American Heart Association consensus statement on vitamin E recognizes the benefits of vitamin E supplementation as promising, but not proven (4). The Food and Nutrition Board's 2001 report on antioxidants stated: "A large and growing body of experimental evidence suggests that high intakes of vitamin E may lower the risk of some chronic diseases, especially heart disease. However, the limited and discordant clinical trial evidence available precludes recommendations at this time. . ." (3).

- Observational studies of vitamin E supplements and recent experimental trials provide little support for a strong protective role for vitamin E against cancer. If vitamin E is protective against cancer, it may be that the protection is derived from the synergistic effects of the vitamin in combination with other cancer-protective nutrients and phytochemicals found in foods. Because liberal consumption of fruits and vegetables is associated with reduced cancer risk, individuals should be encouraged to eat vitamin E-rich fruits, vegetables, nuts, and seeds as part of a balanced diet.

- There is preliminary evidence that high-dose vitamin E supplements improve some immune function parameters in elderly subjects. The elderly population should be encouraged to consume vitamin E-rich plant foods and take a supplement if people's intake is not meeting the RDA. Although high-dose supplements have not shown any adverse effects in elderly subjects and may be of benefit, more research is needed before specific recommendations can be made to this population.

- There is preliminary evidence that high doses of vitamin E may slow progression of Alzheimer's disease and reduce tardive dyskinesia, which requires further study.

- There is preliminary evidence that dietary vitamin E is associated with improved lung function in elderly subjects. Results from the ATBC study are not suggestive of a benefit of vitamin E supplements in male smokers with chronic obstructive pulmonary disease. More research is needed to determine the potential role of vitamin E in lung function.

- According to observational studies, reduced incidence of cataracts is associated with reported vitamin E supplement use and with higher plasma concentrations of vitamin E. A clinical trial in male smokers (ATBC study) did not report any protection with 50 mg alpha-tocopherol. However, additional large clinical trials in different groups of subjects are needed to determine the potential role of vitamin E in cataract formation.

- Preliminary studies have shown improved metabolic parameters of patients with diabetes taking high doses of vitamin E. Additional controlled research is needed before recommendations can be made for this population.

- Although some studies reported that vitamin E supplements reduced oxidative damage from exercise, the overall effect on exercise performance has not been ergogenic. However, preliminary research under high altitude conditions is suggestive of a potential benefit with vitamin E supplements and requires further study.

V

FOOD SOURCES

The tocopherol content of the diet varies depending on time of harvest of vitamin E containing plants, processing, storage, and food preparation techniques. Nearly two-thirds of the vitamin E is lost during production of commercial oils. Furthermore, removing the germ from wheat and bleaching also destroys vitamin E. The average daily intake for vitamin E in the United States is estimated at 7 mg to 11 mg for men and 7 mg for women primarily from vegetable and seed oils used in salad oils and margarine. Coconut and fish oils are poor sources (some fish oil supplements add vitamin E) (1, 2).

Food	Alpha-tocopherol (mg)
Wheat germ oil (1 tbsp)	27.0
Kernels, sunflower seed (1 oz)	14.0
Oil, sunflower (1 tbsp)	7.0
Hazelnuts/filberts (1 oz)	6.8
Oil, cottonseed (1 tbsp)	5.3
Wheat germ (2 tbsp)	4.9
Papaya (1)	3.4
Cereals, fortified (1 c)	3.0–30.0
Peanut butter (2 tbsp)	3.0
Oil, canola (1 tbsp)	2.9
Avocado (1)	2.3
Mango (1)	2.3
Nuts, Brazil (1 oz)	2.2
Mustard greens (½ c)	1.4
Broccoli (½ c)	1.3
Butter (1 tbsp)	0.2

Source: Data is from Pennington JAT (4)

DOSAGE INFORMATION/BIOAVAILABILITY

Vitamin E is available in single preparations, in antioxidant "cocktails," or in multivitamin/mineral supplements in doses ranging from 10 IU to 800 IU. Mixed tocopherol and tocotrienol supplements are also available. Both natural and synthetic forms of vitamin E are sold in the free form or bound to succinate or acetate. Natural vitamin E is derived from plant raw materials after several chemical processing steps and is designated on labels as *d*-alpha-tocopherol (or RRR-alpha-tocopherol). Synthetic vitamin E is designated as *d,l*-alpha-tocopherol (or *all-rac*-alpha-tocopherol). To date, most of the studies examining the benefits of vitamin E supplements have employed the synthetic *d,l*-alpha-tocopherol form.*

Several studies have shown that the natural form is absorbed more efficiently and is more biologically active than synthetic vitamin E (1, 6, 7). The absorption rate of dietary alpha-tocopherol ranges from 50 percent to 70 percent. However, absorption decreases to less than 10 percent with pharmacological doses (200 mg) (2). There is a dose-dependent increase in serum, erythrocyte, and platelet vitamin E levels with vitamin E supplementation (1).

---

*The RRR- and *all-rac*-alpha-tocopherol are the correct terms for *d* and *d,l*-alpha-tocopherol, respectively, even though the *d* and *d,l* designations are sometimes used on supplement labels.

The 1989 RDA was originally given in RRR-alpha-tocopherol equivalents (TE) expressed as milligrams (8). However, the new Dietary Reference Intakes (DRIs) for vitamin E are based on alpha-tocopherol only and do not include amounts obtained from the other seven naturally occurring forms historically called vitamin E (β, γ, δ, and the four tocotrienols). These other forms are not counted as contributing to requirements for vitamin E because they are not converted to alpha-tocopherol in humans and are not easily recognized by the alpha-tocopherol transfer protein in the liver. The new RDA for vitamin E is 15 mg/day (22 IU) of alpha-tocopherol for women and men (3).

Supplement labels typically express vitamin E in International Units (IU), even though the DRIs are stated in milligrams. To determine the number of milligrams of alpha-tocopherol in a supplement or food expressed in IUs, use the following conversion factors (3):

If the form of vitamin E is "natural" (*d*-alpha-tocopherol or RRR-alpha-tocopherol), multiply IUs by 0.67. For example, 30 IU of natural vitamin E = 20 mg alpha-tocopherol (30 × 0.67).

If the form of vitamin E is "synthetic" (*d,l*-alpha-tocopherol or *all-rac*-alpha-tocopherol) multiply IUs by 0.45. For example, 30 IU of synthetic vitamin E = 13.5 mg alpha-tocopherol (30 × 0.45).

RELEVANT RESEARCH

Vitamin E and Cardiovascular Disease

- Epidemiological studies generally show an inverse relationship between vitamin E intake from food or supplements and coronary heart disease (9, 10). Three large, prospective epidemiology studies (the Nurses Health Study, the Health Professionals Follow Up Study, and the Established Populations for Epidemiologic Studies of the Elderly) reported that subjects who had used vitamin E supplements (> 100 IU (≈ 66 mg) for two or more years) had approximately 40 percent lower rates of coronary heart disease (1, 11–13).

- A meta-analysis pooling the four randomized trials (see subsequent trial descriptions for details of these studies) completed in Europe and America (total number of subjects = 51,000) reported no effect of vitamin E on cardiovascular or ischemic heart disease mortality and nonfatal myocardial infarction (14).

- In a double-blind, placebo-controlled study conducted in 19 countries (Heart Outcomes Prevention Evaluation—HOPE), 2,545 women and 6,996 men (age > 55 y) at high risk for cardiovascular events were randomized to receive 400 IU (268 mg)/day of natural source vitamin E or a placebo. After 4.5 years, vitamin E had no effect on total mortality, cardiovascular death, myocardial infarction, or stroke. There were also no significant differences between groups in secondary cardiovascular outcomes (unstable angina, congestive heart failure, revascularization or amputation, diabetes complications, cancer). The study is continuing to identify whether there is a protective effect with longer duration (15).

- In a large-scale, open label, Italian study (GISSI Prevenzione Study), 11,324 patients surviving recent (≤ 3 months) myocardial infarction were randomly assigned to one

V

of four groups for 3.5 years: (1) 1 g n-3 supplements; (2) 300 mg vitamin E; (3) both; or (4) neither supplement. The main endpoint was combined occurrence of death, nonfatal myocardial infarction, or nonfatal stroke. Vitamin E had no effect, although fish oil use resulted in significant reductions in the main endpoint and total mortality. There was no additional benefit of the combined vitamin E and n-3 supplements. The results of this study would have been strengthened if it had been double-blinded (16).

- In a double-blind, placebo-controlled trial, 27,271 Finnish male smokers from the Alpha Tocopherol Beta Carotene (ATBC) cancer prevention study (aged 50 y to 69 y) with no history of myocardial infarction (MI) were randomized to receive 50 mg alpha tocopherol, 20 mg beta-carotene, both supplements, or a placebo for five to eight years. The following variables were controlled in the statistical analysis: smoking, age, blood pressure, alcohol intake, BMI, activity level, diet, history of angina and diabetes, and serum concentrations of vitamin E and beta-carotene. Neither supplement affected the incidence of nonfatal MI. There was an insignificant 8 percent decrease in the incidence of fatal coronary disease with vitamin E supplementation. The authors concluded that: "Supplementation with a small dose of vitamin E has only a marginal effect on the incidence of fatal coronary heart disease in male smokers with no history of MI, but no influence on nonfatal MI" (17).

- In a double-blind, placebo-controlled trial, 1,862 male smokers with a history of myocardial infarction in the ATBC study were randomized to receive 50 mg alpha-tocopherol, 20 mg beta-carotene, both, or a placebo for five to eight years. During follow-up, 424 major coronary events occurred. There were no significant differences in the number of coronary events between any supplementation group and the placebo group. There were significantly more deaths in the beta-carotene and mixed supplement group than in the placebo group but no increase in subjects supplemented with vitamin E alone (18). (*See* Vitamin A/Beta-Carotene.)

- In a double-blind, placebo-controlled trial, 1,795 male smokers with angina in the ATBC study were randomized to receive 50 mg alpha-tocopherol, 20 mg beta-carotene, both supplements, or a placebo for five to eight years. Recurrence of angina at annual follow-up visits, progression of angina, and incidence of major coronary events were the main outcome measures. After 4 and 5.5 years, there were no significant differences in progression to severe angina or risk of coronary events between groups. The authors concluded: "There was no evidence of beneficial effects for alpha-tocopherol or beta carotene supplements in male smokers with angina pectoris, indicating no basis for therapeutic or preventive use of these agents in such patients" (19).

- In a double-blind, placebo-controlled study (Cambridge Heart Antioxidant Study-CHAOS), 2,002 patients with angiographically proven atherosclerosis were randomized to receive alpha-tocopherol (800 IU [≈ 528 mg] for 546 patients, 400 IU [≈ 264 mg] for remainder) or a placebo daily for a median of 510 days. Plasma alpha-tocopherol concentrations rose in vitamin E-supplemented subjects, but not in placebo subjects. In vitamin E-supplemented subjects, there was a significant 77 percent reduction in the risk of nonfatal MI compared to the placebo (14 vs 41 incidents). However, there was an insignificant excess of cardiovascular deaths in the vitamin E group (27 vs 23). The authors concluded: "In patients with symptomatic coronary atherosclerosis, alpha-tocopherol treatment substantially reduces the risk of nonfatal MI, with beneficial effects apparent after 1 year of treatment. The effect of alpha-tocopherol treatment on cardiovascular deaths requires further study" (20).

- In a short-term, double-blind, placebo-controlled study, 40 men with mildly elevated cholesterol were randomized to receive 80 mg alpha-tocopherol plus 140 mg tocotrienol or a single supplement of 80 mg alpha-tocopherol for six weeks. There were no significant differences between groups in LDL or HDL cholesterol, triglycerides, lipoprotein A, or lipid peroxide concentrations (21).

Vitamin E and Cancer

- In an observational study (American Cancer Society's Cancer Prevention Study II cohort), 711,891 men and women completed a health questionnaire in 1982 and were followed for 14 years for mortality. During that time, 4,404 deaths from colorectal cancer occurred. After adjustment for risk factors of colorectal cancer, regular use of vitamin E or C supplements was not associated with a decreased risk (22).

- In a double-blind, placebo-controlled study, 29,133 male smokers in the ATBC Cancer Prevention Study were randomized to receive 50 mg alpha-tocopherol, 20 mg beta-carotene, both, or a placebo daily for five to eight years. During that time 135 subjects developed colorectal cancers that were histologically confirmed. Colorectal cancer incidence was lower in the vitamin E group, but this difference did not reach statistical significance (23).

- In the ATBC study, vitamin E supplements were associated with significantly fewer incident cases of prostate cancer (99 cases vs 151 cases). There was an insignificant reduction in colorectal cancers (68 cases vs 81) and an insignificant increased risk in stomach cancer (70 cases vs 56) (24). A follow-up analysis of patients who developed prostate cancer showed no significant associations between baseline serum alpha-tocopherol or dietary vitamin E and prostate cancer (25).

- In the double-blind, placebo-controlled ATBC study, 2,132 men were identified as having atrophic gastritis. Of these subjects, 1,344 had upper gastrointestinal endoscopy after a median of 5.1 years of supplementation with vitamin E, beta-carotene, both, or a placebo. Neither supplement had any association with the end-of-trial prevalence of gastric neoplasias after adjustment for other possible risk factors. This effect was not modified by baseline serum or dietary intake of vitamins, or presence of *Helicobacter pylori* infection (26).

- In the ATBC study, 409 male smokers aged 55 y to 74 y were examined for oral mucosal lesions. There were no significant differences among the study groups either in prevalence of oral mucosal lesions or in the cells of unkeratinized epithelium (27).

Vitamin E and Immunity in the Elderly

- In a double-blind, placebo-controlled study, 161 healthy elderly subjects (aged 65 y to 80 y) were randomized to receive either vitamin E (either 50 mg or 100 mg) or a placebo daily for six months. Cellular immune responsiveness (CIR) was measured *in vivo* by delayed-type hypersensitivity (DTH) skin tests and *in vitro* by measuring the peripheral mononuclear cell production of interleukin 2 (IL-2), interferon-gamma (a T helper cell type 1 cytokine), interleukin-4 (a typical T helper cell type 2 cytokine) after stimulation with phytohemagglutinin. Both DTH scores and IL-2 production showed a trend toward increased responsiveness with increasing doses of vitamin E, but this trend was not significant. In a subgroup analysis, elderly subjects who were apparently healthy but had a low DTH response or were less physically active at baseline had an enhanced DTH response after a six-month supplementation with 100 mg vitamin E compared with use of a placebo. However, this difference was not significant when adjusted for multiple comparisons. No effect of 100 mg vitamin E was observed on T helper cell type 1 and type 2 cytokine production. The authors concluded that before vitamin E supplement use is widely proposed, new clinical trials should be conducted that show that vitamin E, possibly via an improvement of cellular immune responsiveness, is effective in reducing the morbidity of infectious diseases (28).

- In a double-blind, placebo-controlled study, 88 healthy subjects (> 65 y) were randomly assigned to one of four groups for 235 days: (1) 60 mg vitamin E, (2) 200 mg vitamin E, (3) 800 mg vitamin E, or (4) a placebo. All subjects had normal serum vitamin E concentrations at the baseline. Delayed-type hypersensitivity skin response (DTH); antibody response to hepatitis B, tetanus and diphtheria, and pneumococcal vaccines; and autoantibodies to DNA and thyroglobulin were assessed before and after supplementation. Supplementation with vitamin E for four months improved certain clinically relevant indexes of cell-mediated immunity. Subjects taking 200 mg had a 65 percent increase in DTH and a 6-fold increase in antibody titer to hepatitis B compared to placebo (17 percent and 3-fold, respectively), 60 mg (41 percent and 3-fold, respectively), 800 mg (49 percent and 2.5-fold, respectively). The subjects taking 200 mg also had a significant increase in antibody titer to tetanus vaccine. Subjects with the highest tertile of serum alpha-tocopherol concentrations after supplementation had significantly higher antibody response to hepatitis B and DTH. All findings were significant. Vitamin E had no effect on antibody titer to diphtheria and did not change immunoglobulin levels or T- and B-cell levels. There were no adverse effects observed (29).

- In a double-blind, placebo-controlled trial, 83 healthy subjects (> 65 y) were randomized to receive 100 mg alpha-tocopherol or a placebo daily for three months. Cellular immune responsiveness was measured by the *in vitro* response of peripheral blood mononuclear cells (PBMC) to the mitogens concanavalin A and phytohemagglutinin. Additionally, the humoral immune response was tested by measuring immunoglobulin antibody concentrations (IgG4 and IgA) against common antigens. Vitamin E supplementation was associated with a significant 51 percent increase in plasma levels of alpha-tocopherol compared to no change in the placebo group. No significant changes were observed in cellular immune responsiveness in either group. There was no effect of vitamin E on immunoglobulin levels. However, in the control group, there was a small but significant increase in certain immunoglobulin levels against antigens. The authors concluded that 100 mg of vitamin E did not appear to have a beneficial effect on the overall immune response in elderly subjects (30).

Vitamin E and Neuropsychiatric Disorders

- In a double-blind, placebo-controlled study (Alzheimer's Disease Cooperative Study), 341 patients with Alzheimer's disease were randomized to receive one of four treatments daily for two years: (1) 2,000 IU (1,320 mg) alpha-tocopherol; (2) 10 mg selegiline (selective MAO inhibitor); (3) both alpha-tocopherol and selegiline; or (4) a placebo. The primary outcome was the time to the occurrence of any of the following: death, institutionalization, loss of the ability to perform basic activities of daily living, or severe dementia. Despite randomization, the baseline score on the Mini-Mental State Examination was higher in the placebo group than in any of the other three groups, and this variable was predictive of the primary outcome. In the unadjusted analyses, there were no significant differences in the outcomes among the four groups. After adjustment, there were significant delays in the time to the primary outcome for patients treated with vitamin E (670 days), selegiline (655 days), and combination therapy (585 days) compared to the placebo (440 days) (31).

- In a double-blind, placebo-controlled study, 35 patients with tardive dyskinesia (29 diagnosed with schizophrenia, 6 diagnosed with mood disorder) were randomized to receive 1,600 IU (1,056 mg) alpha-tocopherol or a placebo for two months. Patients were assessed using the Abnormal Involuntary Movement Scale (AIMS) and Brief Psychiatric Rating Scale. In a subgroup of 23 patients, instrumental measurements of dyskinesia were assessed. There was a significant reduction of dyskinesia in the vitamin E group, but not the placebo group, on both the AIMS and the instrumental assessments. The overall reduction in AIMS was 24 percent in the vitamin E group. Of the vitamin E-treated subjects, there was a greater reduction in mean AIMS score (35 percent) in a subgroup of patients with TD for five years or less compared with the reduction (11 percent) in patients with TD for greater than five years. No changes in parkinsonism (tremor, muscle rigidity) were observed (32).

- In a double-blind, placebo-controlled study, 40 patients with tardive dyskinesia (TD) were randomized to receive 1,600 IU (1,056 mg) alpha-tocopherol or a placebo for 36 weeks. Using the AIMS score to measure TD severity, there was a significant difference in mean scores, in favor of vitamin E, beginning at 10 weeks and continuing to the end of the study (33).

Vitamin E and Lung Function

- In an observational study, dietary intakes of vitamin E and C and lung function were assessed in 178 elderly subjects (70 y to 96 y) selected on the basis of reported respiratory symptoms. After adjustment for age, gender, height, smoking, total energy intake, and vitamin C intake, vitamin E intake was significantly associated with FEV_1 (forced expiratory volume) and forced vital capacity (FVC). For every extra milligram increase in vitamin E in the daily diet, FEV_1 increased by an estimated 42 mL and FVC by an estimated 54 mL (34).

V

- In a double-blind, placebo-controlled study, 38 Dutch cyclists were randomized to receive 100 mg vitamin E plus 500 mg vitamin C daily for 15 weeks. Lung function was measured before and after each outdoor training session on several occasions (n = 380) during the summer of 1996. Daily environmental ozone concentrations averaged 77 μg/m. Ozone exposure in areas where cyclists trained was associated with a decrease in lung function (as assessed by FEV_1 and FVC) in both groups. In subjects supplemented with vitamin C and E, the effect of ozone on lung function was significantly less than in subjects receiving the placebo. The authors concluded that antioxidant supplementation confers partial protection against the acute effects of ozone on FEV_1 and FVC in cyclists. Because of the study design, it is impossible to determine whether the effects were because of vitamin E, C, or both (35).

- In the ATBC study, 50 mg/day alpha-tocopherol did not influence symptoms of chronic obstructive pulmonary disorders in middle-aged male smokers, but there was a reported beneficial effect of dietary intake of fruits and vegetables rich in vitamin E and beta-carotene (36). In addition, results from the ATBC study did not report a reduction in lung cancer with vitamin E supplements (37).

Vitamin E and Cataracts/Age-Related Maculopathy (ARM)

- In a prospective study (Nurses' Health Study cohort), 478 nondiabetic women aged 53 y to 73 y were given several food frequency questionnaires over the course of 13 years to 15 years. The prevalence of nuclear lens opacities was significantly lower with increasing duration of use of vitamin C, E, and multivitamins. However, only vitamin C supplement use remained significantly associated with nuclear opacities after mutual adjustment for use of vitamin E or multivitamin. Plasma vitamins C and E were also inversely related to prevalence of age-related nuclear lens opacities (38).

- In a prospective epidemiological study (Beaver Dam Eye Study), nuclear opacity was assessed in 1,354 subjects (aged 43 y to 84 y) using lens photographs taken at the baseline and at a five-year follow-up. After five years, 246 subjects developed a nuclear cataract in at least one eye. Antioxidant intakes were assessed using a food frequency questionnaire at the baseline (assessing intake during the previous year and 10 years prior to the baseline). Median intake of vitamin E was 3.7 mg in the lowest quintile and was 28.3 mg in the highest quintile. In the overall group, nuclear cataracts were not significantly related to intake of vitamin E or C. However, these vitamins were inversely associated with opacities in subjects who had other risk factors for cataracts. Lutein was the only carotenoid associated with a significant reduction in cataract incidence (39). In a subgroup of the Beaver Dam Eye Study, serum tocopherols (alpha plus gamma) were inversely related to the incidence of cataracts (after adjusting for age, smoking, serum cholesterol, heavy drinking, adiposity, and dietary linoleic acid intake) (40).

- In a prospective epidemiological study (Longitudinal Study of Cataract), 764 subjects were assessed for dietary intake, use of vitamin supplements, and plasma levels of vitamin E at the baseline and at yearly follow-up visits. The risk of nuclear opacification at follow-up was decreased by 31 percent in regular users of multivitamin supplements, by 57 percent in vitamin E supplement users, and by 42 percent in subjects with higher plasma levels of vitamin E. The authors concluded: "Because these data are based on observational studies only, the results are suggestive but inconclusive" (41).

- In a random sample of 1,828 participants from the ATBC study, supplementation with 50 mg/day alpha-tocopherol was not associated with the end-of-trial prevalence of nuclear, cortical, or posterior subcapsular cataract when adjusted for possible confounders. The authors concluded that supplementation with alpha-tocopherol or beta-carotene for five to eight years does not influence cataract prevalence among middle-aged, male smokers (42).

Vitamin E and Diabetes

- In a double-blind, placebo-controlled, crossover study, 36 type 1 diabetic and 9 nondiabetic subjects received in random order 1,800 IU vitamin E or placebo daily for four months each. Retinal blood flow was measured using video fluorescein angiography and renal function was assessed by normalized creatinine clearance from timed urine collections. After vitamin E treatment, all subjects experienced a significant elevation in serum vitamin E levels. Hemoglobin A_{1c} was not affected by vitamin E. Diabetic patient baseline retinal blood flow was significantly lower than nondiabetic subjects. After vitamin E supplementation, diabetic retinal blood flow significantly increased and was like that of nondiabetic subjects. Vitamin E also resulted in significantly normalized elevated baseline creatine clearance in diabetic patients. The authors suggested that vitamin E supplements might reduce the risk of developing retinopathy or nephropathy in diabetes (43).

- In a double-blind, placebo-controlled study, 21 type 2 patients having diabetes with mild to moderate peripheral neuropathy were randomized to receive 900 mg vitamin E or a placebo daily for six months. There were no significant changes in glycemic indices (fasting plasma glucose, hemoglobin A_{1c}, postprandial plasma glucose) between groups. There was a significant improvement in 2 of 12 studied electrophysiological parameters assessing nerve conduction. Nerve conduction velocity improved significantly in the median motor nerve fibers and tibial motor nerve distal latency after six months with treatment (44).

- In a double-blind, placebo-controlled, crossover study, 20 elderly, nonobese subjects with normal glucose tolerance were randomized to receive 900 mg vitamin E or a placebo daily for four months each. After each study period, subjects underwent a euglycemic hyperinsulinemic glucose clamp. All subjects were eating a weight-maintaining diet providing $\geq$ 250 g carbohydrate/day and 13.8 mg ($\pm$ 0.6 mg) vitamin E/day. (The authors did not provide on diet administration or compliance). In each subject, the pattern of daily vitamin E intake (assessed by dietary records) was accounted for in the statistical analysis. Vitamin E supplementation was related to a significant improvement in whole-body glucose disposal compared to the placebo. Net changes in plasma vitamin E were significantly correlated with net changes in insulin-stimulated glucose disposal. Plasma triglycerides and free fatty acids were significantly reduced with vitamin E supplementation. The authors concluded that vitamin E sup-

V

plements may be useful in improving insulin action in the elderly, however, "further studies will need to clarify the safety and the exact pharmacological mechanisms by which such results may be achieved" (45).

- In a double-blind, placebo-controlled, crossover study, 25 elderly patients with type 2 diabetes were randomly given 900 mg vitamin E or a placebo daily for three months each, separated by a 30-day washout period. Oral hypoglycemic agents were not permitted in this study. Vitamin E supplementation resulted in a significant reduction in plasma glucose, hemoglogin A_{1c}, triglycerides, free fatty acids, total and LDL cholesterol, and apoprotein B levels. There was no effect on beta-cell response to glucose. The authors concluded: "Daily vitamin E supplements seem to produce a minimal but significant improvement in metabolic control in type 2 diabetic patients. More studies are necessary before conclusions can be drawn about the safety of vitamin E during long-term administration" (46).

Vitamin E and Exercise Performance

- In a double-blind, placebo-controlled study, 9 young (aged 22 y to 29 y) and 12 older (aged 55 y to 74 y) male sedentary subjects were randomized to receive 800 IU (≈ 528 mg) alpha-tocopherol or a placebo daily for 48 days. After 48 days, there was a significant increase in vitamin E concentrations in plasma and skeletal muscle (assessed by biopsy). Subjects then performed a bout of eccentric exercise (muscle contraction that involves lengthening of muscle) at 75 percent of their maximum heart rate by running down an inclined treadmill for 45 minutes. All vitamin E-treated subjects excreted significantly less urinary thiobarbituric acid adducts (marker of oxidative damage) after exercise than did placebo subjects at 12 days postexercise (35 percent and 18 percent above baseline in young and old subjects, respectively). Subjects receiving the placebo had a significant decrease in major fatty acids of muscle biopsy taken immediately after exercise. Although not significant, muscle lipid conjugated dienes (an indicator of oxidative damage) tended to increase in placebo subjects compared to the treatment group. The authors concluded: "The alterations in fatty acid composition, vitamin E, and lipid conjugated dienes in muscle and urinary lipid peroxides in controls after eccentric exercise are consistent with the concept that vitamin E provides protection against exercise-induced oxidative injury" (47).

- In a double-blind, placebo-controlled study, 13 mountaineers were given 400 mg vitamin E (divided into two doses) or a placebo for four weeks at the start of an expedition in Nepal. For four weeks prior to the climb, all subjects were given a vitamin/mineral supplement without vitamin E. Erythrocyte filterability, blood viscosity, and three blood coagulation factors were investigated at the baseline (1,500 m) and twice at high altitude (4,300 m) after supplementation. Both groups experienced a marked rise in hematocrit levels during the ascent because of an increase in erythrocytes and leukocytes. The erythrocyte filterability did not change in the vitamin E group but showed a significant impairment in the control group. The placebo group had a significantly higher blood viscosity compared to the vitamin E subjects. The placebo group, but not the vitamin E group, also had a significant fall in the protein C activity (a vitamin K-dependent coagulation factor). The authors concluded: "All the parameters investigated indicate that an extended stay at high altitude in combination with physical exertion can impair the flow characteristics of blood. Supplementation with vitamin E appears to be a suitable prophylactic measure" (48).

- In a placebo-controlled trial, 12 high-altitude mountain climbers were given 400 mg alpha-tocopherol or a placebo during a 10-week expedition. Anaerobic threshold (exercise until exhaustion on a cycle ergometer while assessing serum lactic acid) was determined at 2,500 m and three times in base camp at 5,000 m at 14-day intervals. After two weeks, the anaerobic threshold was higher in both groups. During the experiment, the anaerobic threshold in the vitamin E group showed a significant increase, whereas the placebo group showed a significant decrease. Pentane exhalation (measure of lipid peroxidation) showed no change after four weeks in vitamin E subjects, whereas the exhaled pentane of the placebo group was 100 percent higher than the baseline levels, reaching statistical significance (49).

SAFETY

- The Tolerable Upper Intake Level (UL) for adults is 1,000 mg/day (1,500 IU natural source or 1,100 IU synthetic vitamin E) of any form of alpha-tocopherol from supplements based on the adverse effect of increased tendency to hemorrhage demonstrated in the ATBC study (3).

- In the ATBC Cancer Prevention Study, vitamin E supplements were associated with an increase in the number of deaths from hemorrhagic stroke in male smokers, although risk of ischemic stroke was lower and risk of total stroke death was unaffected by vitamin E (50). Although, the method of determining hemorrhagic stroke in this study has been questioned because incidence of stroke was not reported. In addition, one reviewer pointed out that on average, the participants were heavy smokers who had smoked more than 35 years, a factor that has been associated with increased risk of stroke (1).

- Daily doses of 100 IU to 3,200 IU (66 mg to 2,112 mg) vitamin E for up to five years did not result in any short- or long-term toxicity in healthy volunteers, smokers, and in patients with angina pectoris, diabetes, epilepsy, Parkinson's disease, tardive dyskinesia, and vascular disease (51).

- Use of high-dose vitamin E may be contraindicated in subjects with vitamin K-associated blood coagulation disorders or vitamin K deficiency (3, 52). However, in one study, 800 IU to 1,200 IU (528 mg to 792 mg) doses of vitamin E did not influence prothrombin times in patients on warfarin therapy (53). Another small study reported that 900 IU (594 mg) daily for 12 weeks resulted in no changes in coagulation activity or laboratory values for kidney, liver, or thyroid function (54).

- In a double-blind, placebo-controlled trial supplementing 800 mg alpha-tocopherol for 30 days to elderly subjects (> 65 y) showed no adverse effects. There was no change in body weight, plasma total protein, albumin, glucose, total cholesterol and triglycerides, conjugated and unconjugated bilirubin, alkaline phosphatase, indicators of

V

hepatic and renal function, hematologic status, thyroid hormones, or serum and urinary creatinine levels and creatinine clearance. Supplements caused a significant increase in serum vitamin E and a small significant increase in plasma zinc (55).

- There is some concern about the potential pro-oxidant effects of vitamin E that have been reported *in vitro*. To date, however, there is no evidence of pro-oxidant activity with vitamin E supplements *in vivo* (2).

REFERENCES

1. Weber P, Bendich A, Machlin LJ. Vitamin E and human health: rationale for determining recommended intake levels. *Nutrition.* 1997;13:450–460.
2. Traber MG. Vitamin E. In: Shils ME, Olson JA, Shike M, Ross AC, eds. *Modern Nutrition in Health and Disease.* 9th ed. Baltimore, Md: Williams & Wilkins; 1999:347–362.
3. Food and Nutrition Board, Institute of Medicine. *Dietary Reference Intakes: Vitamin C, Vitamin E, Selenium, and Carotenoids.* Washington, DC: National Academy Press; 2000.
4. Pennington JAT. *Bowes & Church's Food Values of Portions Commonly Used.* 17th ed. Philadelphia, Pa: Lippincott; 1998.
5. Kiyose C, Muramatsu R, Kameyama Y, et al. Biodiscrimination of alpha-tocopherol stereoisomers in humans after oral administration. *Am J Clin Nutr.* 1997;65:785–789.
6. Tribble DL. AHA Science Advisory. Antioxidant consumption and risk of coronary heart disease: emphasis on vitamin C, vitamin E, and beta-carotene: A statement for healthcare professionals from the American Heart Association. *Circulation.* 1999;99:591–595.
7. Ferslew KE, Acuff RV, Daigneault EA, et al. Pharmacokinetics and bioavailability of the RRR and all racemic stereoisomers of alpha-tocopherol in humans after single oral administration. *J Clin Pharmacol.* 1993;33:84–88.
8. National Research Council, Subcommittee on the 10th Edition of the RDAs, Food and Nutrition Board, Commission on Life Sciences. *Recommended Dietary Allowances.* 10th ed. Washington, DC: National Academy Press; 1989.
9. Rexrode KM, Manson JE. Antioxidant and coronary heart disease: observational studies. *J Cardiovasc Risk.* 1996;3:363–367.
10. Kushi LH, Folsom AR, Prineas RJ, et al. Dietary antioxidant vitamins and death from coronary heart disease in postmenopausal women. *N Engl J Med.* 1996;334:1156–1162.
11. Stampfer MJ, Rimm EB. Epidemiologic evidence for vitamin E in prevention of cardiovascular disease. *Am J Clin Nutr.* 1995;62(6 suppl):1365S–1369S.
12. Stampfer MJ, Hennekens CH, Manson JE, et al. Vitamin E consumption and the risk of coronary disease in women. *N Engl J Med.* 1993;328:1444–1449.
13. Losonczy KG, Harris TB, Havlik RJ. Vitamin E and vitamin C supplement use and risk of all-cause and coronary heart disease mortality in older persons: the Established Populations for Epidemiologic Studies of the Elderly. *Am J Clin Nutr.* 1996;64:190–196.
14. Dagenais GR, Marchioli R, Yusuf S, et al. Beta-carotene, vitamin C, and vitamin E and cardiovascular diseases. *Curr Cardiol Rep.* 2000;2:293–299.
15. HOPE study investigators. Vitamin E supplementation and cardiovascular events in high risk patients. *N Engl J Med.* 2000;342:154–160.

16. Gruppo Italiano per lo Studio della Sopravvievenza nell'Infarto Miocardio (GISSI) Prevenzione Investigators. Dietary supplementation with n-3 polyunsaturated fatty acids and vitamin E after myocardial infarction: results of the GISSI-Prevenzione Trial. *Lancet.* 1999;354:447–455.

17. Virtamo J, Rapola JM, Ripatti S, et al. Effect of vitamin E and beta carotene on the incidence of primary nonfatal myocardial infarction and fatal coronary heart disease. *Arch Intern Med.* 1998;158:668–675.

18. Rapola JM, Virtamo J, Ripatti S, et al. Randomized trial of alpha tocopherol and beta-carotene supplements on incidence of major coronary events in men with previous myocardial infarction. *Lancet.* 1997;349:1715–1720.

19. Rapola JM, Virtamo J, Ripatti S, et al. Effects of alpha tocopherol and beta carotene supplements on symptoms, progression, and prognosis of angina pectoris. *Heart.* 1998;79:454–458.

20. Stephens NG, Parsons A, Schofield PM, et al. Randomized controlled trial of vitamin E in patients with coronary disease: Cambridge Heart Antioxidant Study. *Lancet.* 1996;347:781–786.

21. Mensink RP, van Houwelingen AC, Kromhout D, et al. A vitamin E concentrate rich in tocotrienols had no effect on serum lipids, lipoproteins, or platelet function in men with mildly elevated serum lipid concentrations. *Am J Clin Nutr.* 1999;69:213–219.

22. Jacobs EJ, Connell CJ, Patel AV, et al. Vitamin C and vitamin E supplement use and colorectal cancer mortality in a large American Cancer Society cohort. *Cancer Epidemiol Biomarkers Prev.* 2001;10:17–23.

23. Albanes D, Malila N, Taylor PR, et al. Effects of supplemental alpha-tocopherol and beta-carotene on colorectal cancer: results from a controlled trial (Finland). *Cancer Causes Control.* 2000;11:197–205.

24. Albanes D, Heinonen OP, Huttenen JK, et al. Effects of alpha-tocopherol and beta-carotene supplements on cancer incidence in the Alpha-tocopherol Beta-Carotene Cancer Prevention Study. *Am J Clin Nutr.* 1995;62(6 suppl):1427S—1430S.

25. Hartman TJ, Albanes D, Pietinen P, et al. The association between baseline vitamin E, selenium, and prostate cancer in the alpha-tocopherol, beta-carotene cancer prevention study. *Cancer Epidemiol Biomarkers Prev.* 1998;7:335–340.

26. Varis K, Taylor PR, Sipponen P, et al. Gastric cancer and premalignant lesions in atrophic gastritis: a controlled trial on the effect of supplementation with alpha-tocopherol and beta-carotene. The Helsinki Gastritis Study Group. *Scand J Gastroenterol.* 1998;33:294–300.

27. Liede K, Hietanen J, Saxen L, et al. Long-term supplementation with alpha-tocopherol and beta-carotene and prevalence of oral mucosal lesions in smokers. *Oral Dis.* 1998;4:78–83.

28. Pallast EG, Schouten EG, de Waart, et al. Effect of 50- and 100-mg vitamin E supplements on cellular immune function in noninstitutionalized elderly persons. *Am J Clin Nutr.* 1999;69:1273–1281.

29. Meydani SN, Meydani M, Blumberg JB, et al. Vitamin E supplementation and in vivo immune response in healthy elderly subjects. A randomized controlled trial. *JAMA.* 1997;277:1380–1386.

V

30. de Waart FG, Portengen L, Doekes G, et al. Effects of three months of vitamin E supplementation on indices of the cellular and humoral immune response in elderly subjects. *Br J Nutr.* 1997;78:761–774.

31. Sano M, Ernesto C, Thomas RG, et al. A controlled trial of selegiline, alpha-tocopherol, or both as treatment for Alzheimer's disease. The Alzheimer's Disease Cooperative Study. *N Engl J Med.* 1997;336:1216–1222.

32. Lohr JB, Caligiuri MP. A double-blind, placebo-controlled study of vitamin E treatment of tardive dyskinesia. *J Clin Psychiatry.* 1996;57:167–173.

33. Adler LA, Edson R, Lavori P, et al. Long-term treatment effects of vitamin E for tardive dyskinesia. *Biol Psychiatry.* 1998;43:868–872.

34. Dow L, Tracey M, Villar A, et al. Does dietary intake of vitamins C and E influence lung function in older people? *Am J Respir Crit Care Med.* 1996;154:1401–1404.

35. Grievink L, Zijlstra AG, Ke X, et al. Double-blind intervention trial on modulation of ozone effects on pulmonary function by antioxidant supplements. *Am J Epidemiol.* 1999;149:306–314.

36. Rautalahti M, Virtamo J, Haukka J, et al. The effect of alpha-tocopherol and beta-carotene supplementation on COPD symptoms. *Am J Respir Crit Care Med.* 1997;156:1447–1452.

37. Albanes D, Heinonen OP, Taylor PR, et al. Alpha-Tocopherol and beta-carotene supplements and lung cancer incidence in the alpha-tocopherol, beta-carotene cancer prevention study: effects of base-line characteristics and study compliance. *J Natl Cancer Inst.* 1996;88:1560–1570.

38. Jacques PF, Chylack LT, Hankinson SE, et al. Long-term nutrient intake and early age-related nuclear opacities. *Arch Ophthalmol.* 2001;119:1009–1019.

39. Lyle BJ, Mares-Perlman JA, Klein BE, et al. Antioxidant intake and risk of incident age-related nuclear cataracts in the Beaver Dam Eye Study. *Am J Epidemiol.* 1999;149:801–809.

40. Lyle BJ, Mares-Perlman JA, Klein BE, et al. Serum carotenoids and tocopherols and incidence of age-related nuclear cataract. *Am J Clin Nutr.* 1999;69:272–277.

41. Leske MC, Chylack LT, He Q, et al. Antioxidant vitamins and nuclear opacities: the longitudinal study of cataract. *Ophthalmology.* 1998;105:831–836.

42. Teikari JM, Virtamo J, Rautalahti M, et al. Long-term supplementation with alpha-tocopherol and beta-carotene and age-related cataract. *Acta Ophthalmol Scand.* 1997;75:634–640.

43. Bursell SE, Clermont AC, Aiello LP, et al. High-dose vitamin E supplementation normalizes retinal blood flow and creatinine clearance in patients with type 1 diabetes. *Diabetes Care.* 1999;22:1242–1244.

44. Tutuncu NB, Bayraktar M, Varli K. Reversal of defective nerve conduction with vitamin E supplementation in type 2 diabetes: a preliminary study. *Diabetes Care.* 1998;21:1915–1918.

45. Paolisso G, Di Maro G, Galzerano D, et al. Pharmacological doses of vitamin E and insulin action in elderly subjects. *Am J Clin Nutr.* 1994;59:1291–1296.

46. Paolisso G, D'Amore A, Galzerano D, et al. Daily vitamin E supplements improve metabolic control but not insulin secretion in elderly type II diabetic patients. *Diabetes Care.* 1993;16:1433–1437.

47. Meydani M, Evans WJ, Handelman G, et al. Protective effect of vitamin E on exercise-induced oxidative damage in young and older adults. *Am J Physiol.* 1993;264(5 pt 2):R992—R998.

48. Simon-Schnass I, Korniszewski L. The influence of vitamin E on rheological parameters in high altitude mountaineers. *Int J Vitam Nutr Res.* 1990;60:26–34.

49. Simon-Schnass I, Pabst H. Influence of vitamin E on physical performance. *Int J Vitam Nutr Res.* 1988;58:49–54.

50. The effect of vitamin E and beta-carotene on the incidence of lung cancer and other cancers in male smokers. Alpha-Tocopherol, Beta Carotene Cancer Prevention Study Group. *N Engl J Med.* 1994;330:1029–1035.

51. Bendich A. Safety issues regarding the use of vitamin supplements. *Ann N Y Acad Sci.* 1992;669:300–310.

52. Diplock AT. Safety of antioxidant vitamins and beta-carotene. *Am J Clin Nutr.* 1995;62(6 suppl):1510S—1516S.

53. Kim JM, White RH. Effect of vitamin E on the anticoagulant response to warfarin. *Am J Cardiol.* 1996;77:545–546.

54. Kitagawa M, Mino M. Effects of elevated d-alpha (RRR)-tocopherol dosage in man. *J Nutr Sci Vitaminol (Tokyo).* 1989;35:133–142.

55. Meydani SN, Meydani M, Rall LC, et al. Assessment of the safety of high-dose, short-term supplementation with vitamin E in healthy older adults. *Am J Clin Nutr.* 1994;60:704–709.

Wheat Grass and Barley Grass

Wheat and barley are grains that have been farmed for centuries for use in breads and cereals. Wheat grass (also known as intermediate wheat grass or sprouted wheat) is a relative of wheat that is grown for hay or planted on pastures grazed by cattle, sheep, or horses. More recently, the freshly sprouted young leaves of wheat or barley grasses have been crushed to make a "health food" drink or dried into tablets and powders. The dried extract of young barley leaves is widely used in Japan as a supplement. Both of these grasses, like other leafy vegetables, contain vitamins, minerals, and other phytochemicals important in human health (1–3).

Note: Wheat grass and barley grass are not related, and also should not be confused with wheat germ.

Media and Marketing Claims	Efficacy
Antioxidant protection	NR (*in vivo*)
Stimulates immune system	NR (*in vitro*)
A concentrated source of nutrition	↓
Lowers cholesterol level	NR

Advisory

No reported serious adverse effects

Drug/Supplement Interactions

Theoretically, vitamin K content of wheat grass or barley grass may interfere with blood-thinning medications (coumadin, warfarin)

KEY POINTS

- Extracts from wheat and barley grasses have demonstrated antioxidant and antimutagenic properties *in vitro*. This effect may be due to the chlorophyll as well as beta-carotene and alpha-tocopherol contents. Chlorophyll is also present in similar amounts in many green vegetables (leafy lettuce, spinach, broccoli, etc) that also have been shown to possess antimutagenic activity *in vitro*. Animal and human studies are needed to determine whether the *in vitro* antioxidant activity of wheat or barley grasses also occurs *in vivo* (9).

- One laboratory study reported that wheat and barley grasses and the green algae *Chlorella* were potent stimulators of macrophages *in vitro*. Controlled clinical trials are lacking and are necessary to determine the effects of wheat or barley grass extracts on immune function and oxidative DNA damage in humans.

- The liquid or dried extracts of wheat or barley grasses, like any dried extract of a plant, provide a concentrated source of certain nutrients in a small volume (2 tsp to 4 tsp). However, the contribution of these grasses to the overall vitamin and mineral content of the diet is relatively small (*see* Dosage Information/Bioavailability). In addition, pills and powders do not provide the fiber found in whole vegetables. It is also not known whether processing the extracts alters the content or bioavailability of phytochemicals in wheat and barley grasses. Therefore, wheat grass or barley grass pills/powders should not take the place of the Food Guide Pyramid and the National Cancer Institute's recommendation to consume a minimum of five fruit and vegetable servings per day.

- There is currently no evidence from well-controlled, clinical trials demonstrating a lipid-lowering effect of wheat or barley grasses.

FOOD SOURCES

Fresh squeezed wheat grass or barley grass juice (available at health food stores/juice bars)

DOSAGE INFORMATION/BIOAVAILABILITY

Fresh wheat or barley grass juices are available at many health food stores or juice bars. The extract is dried to form tablets or powders usually in doses equivalent to 2 g to 9 grams (usually 2 to 3 tsp of powder). Several supplements combine different ingredients such as wheat and barley grass, algae (*Spirulina, Chlorella*), kelp, brown rice extract, bee pollen, probiotics, and other herbs.

Sprouted wheat grass is approximately 83 percent carbohydrate, 14 percent protein, and 5 percent fat. Nutritional analysis of 10 g (dry weight) of wheat grass indicates that it provides 39 calories, 1.5 g protein, 8.5 g carbohydrates, < 1 g fat, < 1 g fiber, 1.2 RE beta-carotene, 0.04 mg thiamin, 0.02 mg riboflavin, 0.61 mg niacin, 0 µg vitamin B_{12}, 0.01 mg vitamin E, 7.6 µg folate, 0.4 mg iron, 16 mg magnesium, 6 mg calcium, 33 mg potassium, 8.5 µg selenium, and 0.33 mg zinc. (The 10 g sizes were calculated from values from the USDA home page, www.nal.usda/gov/fnic/foodcomp.)

Nutrient analysis provided by one manufacturer's combination of dried wheat and barley grasses (10 g) reportedly contains 1.6 g protein, 7.4 g carbohydrates, 0.08 g fat, 180 RE beta-carotene, 0.08 mg thiamin, 0.12 mg riboflavin, 2.0 µg vitamin B_{12}, 100 mg calcium, 1.6 mg iron.

RELEVANT RESEARCH

- Wheat and Barley Grasses and Immunity and *In Vitro* Antioxidant Activity

- In an *in vitro* study, a flavonoid isolated from freeze-dried young barley leaves (2"-*O*-glycosylisovitexin or 2"-*O*-GIV) demonstrated antioxidant activity almost equivalent to that of alpha-tocopherol. In other *in vitro* studies, 2"-*O*-GIV demonstrated antioxidant activity against glyoxal (potent mutagenic compound) formation from the oxidation of three fatty acid ethyl esters and against malonaldehyde and acetaldehyde formation in lipid peroxidation systems (3–5).

- In an *in vitro* study, green barley enhanced macrophage activity. When a commercial combination of dried plant extracts (young barley, wheat grass, *Chlorella* (a green algae), and *Laminaria*/kelp) was tested, there was a greater effect on macrophage activity. An *in vitro* mutagenicity assay demonstrated that the combination of dried plant extracts inhibited bacterial mutation induced by a chemical procarcinogen alflatoxin B_1 and the binding of this carcinogen to calf thymus DNA (6).

- In an *in vitro* study, extracts from the roots and leaves of wheat sprouts inhibited the mutagenic effect of carcinogens requiring metabolic activation as demonstrated by the Ames *Salmonella*/mammalian-microsome test. Inhibition was directly related to chlorophyll content, with vitamin E and beta-carotene contributing marginally to the overall inhibitory activities. Chlorophyllin, a water-soluble derivative of chlorophyll, demonstrated similar antimutagenic properties (7). In another study by the same authors, the inhibitory effect in the mutagenic assay was apparent with wheat sprouts, mung bean sprouts, and lentil sprouts. Extracts from wheat soaked overnight and unsprouted did not have any effect (8).

SAFETY

- There are no studies testing the safety of supplementing the diet with liquid or dried juices of wheat or barley grasses.

REFERENCES

1. Becker R, Wagoner P, Hanners GD, et al. Compositional, nutritional, and function evaluation of intermediate wheatgrass (*Thinopyrum intermedium*). *J Food Processing and Preservation*. 1991;15:63–77.
2. Osawa T, Katsuzaki H, Hagiwara Y, et al. A novel antioxidant isolated from young green barley leaves. *J Agric Food Chem*. 1992;40:1135–1138.
3. Nishiyama T, Hagiwara Y, Hagiwara H, et al. Inhibitory effect of 2"-0-glycosyl isovitexin on alpha-tocopherol on genotoxic glycoxal formation in lipid peroxidation system. *Food Chem Toxicol*. 1994;32:1047–1051.
4. Miyake T, Shibamoto T. Inhibition of malondehyde and acetaldehyde formation from blood plasma oxidation by naturally occurring antioxidants. *J Agric Food Chem*. 1998;46:3694–3697.
5. Kitta K, Hagiwara Y, Shibamoto T. Antioxidant activity of an isoflavonoid, 2"-O-glycosylisovitexin isolated from green barley leaves. *J Agric Food Chem*. 1992;40:1843–1845.
6. Lau BHS, Lau EW. Edible plant extracts modulate macrophage activity and bacterial mutagenesis. *Int Clin Nutr Rev*. 1992;12:147–155.
7. Lai CN. Chlorophyll: the active factor in wheat sprout extract inhibiting the metabolic activation of carcinogens in vitro. *Nutr Cancer*. 1979;1:19–21.
8. Lai CN, Dabney DJ, Shaw CR. Inhibition of in vitro metabolic activation of carcinogens by wheat sprout extracts. *Nutr Cancer*. 1979;1:27–30.
9. Lai CN, Butler MA, Matney TS. Antimutagenic activities of common vegetables and their chlorophyll content. *Mutat Res*. 1980;77:245–250.

Whey Protein

Whey protein is a generic term that refers to various types of whey, including whey protein concentrates and isolates. Whey protein, a natural by-product of cheese and casein production, is the yellow-green liquid that separates from the curd. Whey contains nearly 100 percent of the milk carbohydrate (lactose) and 20 percent of the total milk protein. β-lactoglobulin and a-lactalbumin make up about 70 to 80 percent of the protein in whey. Other constituents in the protein include rennet whey, bovine serum albumin, lactoferrin, immunoglobulins, cysteine, phospholipoproteins and several enzymes (1).

Media and Marketing Claims	Efficacy
Builds muscle	NR
Improves exercise performance	NR
Improves immune function in HIV+ patients	NR
Anticancer agent	NR

Advisory

• No reported serious adverse effects

- Excess protein could compromise renal function in patients with kidney disease
- Should be avoided if individual is allergic to cow's milk

Drug/Supplement Interactions

No reported adverse interactions

KEY POINTS

- Although whey protein increased weight gain and improved nitrogen retention in injured or starving animals when compared to a diet of free amino acids, these effects need to be examined more closely in humans. More evidence is needed to determine the effect of whey protein supplementation on muscle mass. Currently, there is little evidence to suggest that whey protein is superior to other dietary proteins in healthy individuals.
- Preliminary trials suggest that whey protein supplementation may increase muscular strength in *some* laboratory measures of strength, but *not* all. These results need to be examined further in controlled trials with larger numbers of subjects.
- Whey protein appears to raise the glutathione levels of immune cells in animal studies, which may be beneficial to HIV infected patients and cancer patients. However, controlled trials in large numbers of subjects are needed to determine if supplementation with whey protein improves the clinical outcomes in patients with HIV or cancer.
- Whey protein is equivalent in protein quality to other dietary protein sources including nonfat, low-fat dairy, and lean meats.

FOOD SOURCES

Cow's milk (milk proteins are 20 percent whey and 80 percent casein)

DOSAGE INFORMATION/BIOAVAILABILITY

Whey protein is sold as a powder. Whey protein products are sold in the pure form, hydrolyzed form, or with additional supplements such as creatine, glutamine, branched-chain amino acids (BCAAs), and flavor enhancers. Some products recommend taking 25 g to 50 g whey protein immediately after workouts with a source of high-glycemic carbohydrate, and an additional 25 g between meals and prior to bedtime (total protein intake = 100 g to 125 g). The biological value of whey protein depends on the processing technique. Heat and mechanical processing may lower the biological value of proteins (1).

RELEVANT RESEARCH

Whey Protein and Weight Gain

- Thermally injured guinea pigs (n = 45) fed diets containing whey protein (via gastrostomy feeding tube) maintained body weight and nitrogen retention better than the same diet containing corresponding free amino acids as the nitrogen source (2).

W

- In a rat study (n = 48), whey protein peptide hydrolysate was more effective than purified whole whey protein or free amino acids in increasing weight gain and nitrogen retention (protein anabolism) in starved rats (3).

Whey Protein and Exercise Performance

- In a double-blind, placebo-controlled study, 20 healthy young subjects were randomized to receive whey protein concentrate (Immunocal, 10 g dose, twice daily) or an equivalent amount of casein placebo for three months. Muscular performance was assessed at baseline and at the end of the study by whole leg isokinetic cycle testing (peak power and work capacity during a 30-second cycling sprint). Lymphocyte glutathione was used as a marker of tissue glutathione. (Glutathione is considered a major intracellular antioxidant, the synthesis of which is dependent on cysteine availability. Whey protein is a cysteine donor.) There were no significant differences between subjects at baseline (eg, body composition, height, weight, glutathione levels, performance on muscular tests). Peak power and 30-second work capacity increased significantly in the whey protein group, but did not change in the placebo group. Additionally, lymphocyte glutathione increased in the whey protein group, but not in the placebo group. Body weight did not change significantly in either group, but the whey group had a decrease in percent body fat (4).

- In a double-blind, placebo-controlled study, 36 male subjects were randomized to receive one of three treatments during six weeks of resistance training: (1) whey protein (1.2 g/kg/day), (2) whey protein and creatine monohydrate (0.1 g/kg/day), or a placebo (1.2 g/kg/day maltodextrin). Measures included lean tissue mass by dual energy x-ray absorptiometry, bench press and squat strength (one-repetition maximum), and knee extension/flexion peak torque. Lean tissue mass increased to a greater extent with training in the whey-creatine group compared to the other groups, and in the whey group compared to the placebo group. Bench press strength significantly increased more for the whey-creatine group compared to the whey and placebo groups. Knee extension peak torque increased significantly with training for the whey-creatine and whey groups, but not for the placebo group. All other measures increased to a similar extent across groups. Continued training without supplementation for an additional six weeks resulted in maintenance of strength and lean tissue mass in all groups. However, not all strength measures were improved with supplementation, because subjects who supplemented with creatine and/or whey protein had similar increases in squat strength and knee flexion peak torque compared to subjects who received the placebo (5).

Whey Protein for HIV and Immunity

- In a preliminary study of three HIV-positive patients, a progressive daily dose of whey protein (8 g to 39 g) during three months raised levels of the antioxidant glutathione in mononuclear cells. Subjects also experienced an increase in body weight. The whey protein in this study replaced other protein sources in the diet keeping the total protein intake constant (6).

- A diet enriched with whey protein enhanced the liver and heart glutathione concentration in aging mice and increased their lifespan during a six-month study compared to casein diet-fed and Purina-fed mice (7).

Whey Protein and Cancer

- In an animal study, rats were fed whey, casein, meat, or soy protein-based diets and then injected with dimethylhydrazine to induce colon cancer. Whey and casein diets were more protective against the development and incidence of intestinal tumors than meat or soy protein diets. Intracellular glutathione concentrations in the liver were greatest in whey and casein-fed rats. The authors speculated: "Whey is a source of precursors (cysteine-rich proteins) for glutathione synthesis and may be important in providing protection to the host by stimulating glutathione synthesis" (8).

- A review article discussed animal studies that demonstrated whey protein diets increase tissue glutathione concentrations. It explained the preceding article and suggested that whey may have a chemoprotective effect by enhancing glutathione concentration (9). A follow-up review article presented animal data showing that whey protein concentrates have anticancer activity. The author of this article suggested that "this non-toxic intervention, which is not based on the principles of current cancer chemotherapy, will hopefully attract the attention of laboratory and clinical oncologists" (10).

SAFETY

- There are no long-term studies of whey protein supplementation in humans.
- Many products recommend consuming whey protein in amounts two to three times the recommended dietary allowance for protein (0.8 g/kg). Individuals with hepatic and renal diseases should be cautioned against ingesting excess protein from protein supplements.
- Whey protein should be avoided by those diagnosed with allergies or severe sensitivities to milk or milk proteins.

REFERENCES

1. Smithers GW, Ballard FJ, Copeland AD, et al. New opportunities from the isolation and utilization of whey proteins. *J Dairy Sci.* 1996;79:1454–1459.
2. Trocki O, Mochizuki H, Dominioni L, et al. Intact protein versus free amino acids in the nutrition support of thermally injured animals. *JPEN.* 1986;10:139–145.
3. Poullain MG, Cezard JP, Roger L, et al. Effect of whey proteins, their oligopeptide hydrolysates and free amino acid mixtures on growth and nitrogen retention in fed and starved rats. *JPEN.* 1989;13:382–386.
4. Lands LC, Grey VL, Smountas AA. Effect of supplementation with a cysteine donor on muscular performance. *J Appl Physiol.* 1999;87:1381–1385.

5. Burke DG, Chilibeck PD, Davidson KS, et al. The effect of whey protein supplementation with and without creatine monohydrate combined with resistance training on lean tissue mass and muscle strength.

6. Bounous G, Baruchel S, Falutz J, et al. Whey proteins as a food supplement in HIV-seropositive individuals. *Clin Invest Med.* 1993;16:204–209.

7. Bounous G, Gervais F, Amer V, et al. The influence of dietary whey protein on tissue glutathione and the diseases of aging. *Clin Invest Med.* 1989;12:343–349.

8. McIntosh GH, Regester GO, Le Leu RK, et al. Dairy proteins protect against dimethylhydrazine-induced intestinal cancers in rats. *J Nutr.* 1995;125:809–816.

9. Bounous G, Batist G, Gold P. Whey proteins in cancer prevention. *Cancer Lett.* 1991;57:91–94.

10. Bounous G. Whey protein concentrate (WPC) and glutathione modulation in cancer treatment. *Anticancer Res.* 2000;20:4785–4792.

Yohimbine/Yohimbe

Yohimbine is the major alkaloid present in the bark of the yohimbe (*Pausinystalia yohimbe*) tree indigenous to West Africa. The bark is made up of 6 percent alkaloids, 10 percent to 15 percent of which are yohimbine. Yohimbine is an alpha 2-adrenergic antagonist that stimulates norepinephrine (NE) release. The bark is traditionally used as an aphrodisiac in Africa. Yohimbine, as a prescription drug, has been studied for its potential role in the treatment of sexual disorders and weight control (1).

Media and Marketing Claims	Efficacy
Increases sex drive	↓
Aids in weight loss	NR
Builds muscle	NR

Advisory

- Case reports of nervousness, insomnia, anxiety, urinary frequency, dizziness, tremors, headache, tachycardia, hypotension, hypertension, nausea and vomiting, bronchospasm, and lupus-like syndrome with doses of 4 mg to 20 mg
- Contraindicated in individuals with high or low blood pressure, bipolar disorder, existing liver and kidney disease
- Herb not approved for use in Germany

Drug/Supplement Interactions

Potential for toxic effects when combined with phenothiazines (for mental disorders), monoamine oxidase (MAO) inhibitors, naloxone, antihypertensive drugs, sympathomimetic drugs, tricyclic antidepressants, and antidiabetes drugs

KEY POINTS

- There is a lack of clinical evidence supporting use of yohimbine/yohimbe as an aphrodisiac. A meta-analysis concluded that prescription yohimbine does appear to have a therapeutic benefit over placebo for erectile dysfunction. In the only study of women with hypoactive sexual desire, yohimbine had no benefit.

- There is insufficient evidence on the efficacy and safety of yohimbine/yohimbe to support its use in weight loss.

- Although yohimbine (in the form of the herbal supplement yohimbe bark) is marketed to body builders and athletes, there is currently a lack of research to support its use to enhance sport performance and muscle-building.

DOSAGE INFORMATION/BIOAVAILABILITY

Yohimbine or yohimbine hydrochloride is available in tablet, capsule, and tincture form with labels recommending 10 mg to 20 mg/day divided into four doses. It is also available as a prescription drug. One study by FDA scientists found commercial products contained yohimbine, but contained undeclared diluents and were devoid of other alkaloids normally found in the tree bark (2). In one study of young males, 10 mg yohimbine hydrochloride raised peak plasma levels of yohimbine within 10 minutes to 45 minutes after oral intake (3). Bioavailability ranged from 7 percent to 87 percent with a mean value of 33 percent.

RELEVANT RESEARCH

Yohimbine and Sexual Function

- In a meta-analysis of seven controlled trials examining yohimbine therapy for erectile dysfunction, yohimbine was found to be superior to a placebo. The methodological quality of the studies was rated to be satisfactory. Despite other case reports of adverse effects in the literature, there were few serious adverse reactions reported in these seven trials (4).

- In a placebo-controlled, crossover design study, nine women with clinically diagnosed hypoactive sexual desire were assigned in random order to two treatment phases starting at the beginning of menses and continuing for one month each: (1) a placebo, or (2) 5.4 mg yohimbine three times daily. Daily logs of mood and sexual activity, and trimonthly blood drawings were obtained during an initial baseline month, followed by the two treatment cycles. When compared to healthy controls, subjects with hypoactive sexual desire had an insignificant trend toward lower plasma levels of 3-methyl-4-hydroxyphenylglycol (MHPG), the major metabolite of norepinephrine, at the baseline. Yohimbine treatment caused a sustained rise in plasma MHPG similar to previously reported levels in men. However, in this study, it had no therapeutic effect on improving sexual desire (5).

- In a double-blind, placebo-controlled trial, 86 male patients with erectile dysfunction without clearly detectable organic or psychologic causes were given 30 mg yohimbine

Y

hydrochloride divided into three doses a day or a placebo for eight weeks. Efficacy was determined by subjective criteria (self-evaluation of sexual desire, sexual satisfaction, frequency of intercourse, and quality of erection) and by objective criteria (improvement in penile rigidity). There were no statistical differences on subjective or objective measures alone. However, when objective responders and subjective responders were combined, yohimbine was significantly more effective than the placebo (71 percent vs 45 percent). Seven percent of the patients rated tolerability of yohimbine as fair or poor (the authors did not describe the adverse effects subjects experienced during treatment) (6).

- In a double-blind, placebo-controlled, crossover study, 29 male patients with impotence of mixed etiology (organic or psychogenic) were given two 25-day treatments in random order: (1) 36 mg yohimbine hydrochloride/day, or (2) a placebo. Treatments were separated with a 14-day washout period. Erectile function, ejaculation, interest in sex, physical examination findings, blood pressure, pulse rate, weight, and an audiovisual sexual stimulation test were evaluated before and after treatment. Yohimbine was no more effective than the placebo in treating mixed-type impotence (7).

- In a double-blind, placebo-controlled, partial crossover study, 63 male patients with clinically diagnosed psychogenic impotence were randomly assigned to receive 15 mg yohimbine daily in conjunction with the antidepressant trazodone or a placebo for eight weeks each. Erectile function, ejaculation, interest in sex, and sexual thoughts were investigated at the end of drug treatment and at three- and six-month follow-ups. Fifty-five patients (87 percent) completed the whole trial. Significantly improved clinical results were obtained in 71 percent of the patients who took the combination of yohimbine and trazodone compared to the placebo. However, the experimental design makes it impossible to attribute the effects to yohimbine, trazodone, or a combination of both (8).

- According to one review article, a study of intravenous yohimbine (0.30 mg/kg) administration to young, healthy volunteers reported no beneficial effects on penile circumference or sexual drive (1).

- According to the same review article, several studies in rats have shown yohimbine to enhance different aspects of sexual behavior (frequency of erection, mounting, and ejaculation) (1).

Yohimbine and Weight Loss

- In a double-blind, placebo-controlled, randomized study, 20 obese female outpatients were put on a low-energy diet (1,000 kcal/day) for three weeks (day 1 to 21). After this period, subjects continued on the diet for three more weeks (day 22 to 42) while taking 20 mg yohimbine/day divided into four doses or a placebo. Weight reduction did not differ between groups in the first three weeks of diet alone. During the second three weeks (day 22 to 42) of diet plus yohimbine, the patients displayed a significant increase in mean weight loss compared to the placebo (3.55 kg vs 2.21 kg). Yohimbine had no effect on lipolysis as estimated by plasma glycerol levels measured at baseline and at the end of each three-week period. At day 42, exercise energy expenditure (EEE) and resting energy expenditure (REE) were significantly lower in the placebo group than on day 0 and day 21. In yohimbine-supplemented subjects, REE, but not EEE, was significantly lower at day 42 compared to day 21. The authors speculated that the effect on EEE may account for the weight loss associated with yohimbine. In another group of subjects, the effect of 15 mg yohimbine or placebo on gastric emptying of a radio-labeled solid meal was studied in 15 obese patients in a double-blind manner. There were no differences in gastric emptying time between groups (9).

- In a placebo-controlled, crossover study, 14 healthy, normal weight males were given an acute dose of 0.2 mg/kg of oral yohimbine (average dose for 70-kg subject = 14 mg) after an overnight fast or one hour after a standard 400-kcal breakfast. Blood samples were taken 45, 60, 75, 90, and 105 minutes after yohimbine ingestion. There was a one-week washout period between treatments. Yohimbine increased fat mobilization as measured by plasma glycerol levels and plasma nonesterified fatty acids concentrations in fasting subjects, while the effect was not apparent one hour after a meal. Yohimbine had no significant effects on heart rate or blood pressure. In a second controlled experiment of eight fasting male subjects, the lipid mobilizing action of yohimbine was reinforced during and after 30 minutes of aerobic exercise on a cycle ergometer. Plasma norepinephrine concentrations increased 40 percent to 50 percent after yohimbine intake but were not associated with autonomic symptoms (10).

SAFETY

- There are no long-term studies evaluating the safety of yohimbine/yohimbe.
- Case reports have associated yohimbine ingestion (4 mg to 20 mg) with side-effects including nervousness, insomnia, anxiety, urinary frequency, dizziness, tremors, headache, tachycardia, hypotension, hypertension, nausea and vomiting, bronchospasm, and lupus-like syndrome (1, 11–14).
- Yohimbine/yohimbe is contraindicated in individuals with high or low blood pressure, bipolar disorder, and kidney disease, or patients on tricyclic antidepressants (11, 15).
- Toxicity of yohimbine/yohimbe can be enhanced by other drugs such as phenothiazines (drug used to treat mental disorders), monoamine oxidase (MAO) inhibitors, naloxone, antihypertensive drugs, sympathomimetic drugs, tricyclic antidepressants, and antidiabetic drugs (11, 16).
- Yohimbe bark is not approved for use in Germany, a country that regulates herbal preparations, because of insufficient proof of efficacy and the "unforeseeable correlation between risk and benefit" (15).

REFERENCES

1 Riley AJ. Yohimbine in the treatment of erectile disorder. *Br J Clin Pract.* 1994; 48:133–136.

2 Betz JM, White DK, der Marderosian AH. Gas chromatographic determination of yohimbine in commercial yohimbe products. *J AOAC Int.* 1995;78:1189–1194.

3 Guthrie SK, Hariharan M, Grunhaus LJ. Yohimbine bioavailability in humans. *Eur J Clin Pharmacol.* 1990;39:409–411.

4 Ernst E, Pittler MH. Yohimbine for erectile dysfunction: a systematic review and meta-analysis of randomized clinical trials. *J Urol.* 1998;159:433–436.

5 Piletz JE, Segraves KB, Feng YZ, et al. Plasma MHPG response to yohimbine treatment in women with hypoactive sexual desire. *J Sex Marital Ther.* 1998;24:43–54.

6 Vogt HJ, Brandl P, Kockott G, et al. Double-blind, placebo-controlled safety and efficacy trial with yohimbine hydrochloride in the treatment of nonorganic erectile dysfunction. *Int J Impot Res.* 1997;9:155–161.

7 Kunelius P, Hakkinen J, Lukkarinen O. Is high-dose yohimbine hydrochloride effective in the treatment of mixed-type impotence? A prospective, randomized, controlled double-blind crossover study. *Urology.* 1997;49:441–444.

8 Montorsi F, Strambi LF, Guazzoni G, et al. Effect of yohimbine-trazodone on psychogenic impotence: a randomized, double-blind, placebo-controlled study. *Urology.* 1994;44:732–736.

9 Kucio C, Jonderko K, Piskorska D. Does yohimbine act as a slimming drug? *Isr J Med Sci.* 1991;27:550–556.

10 Galitzky J, Taouis M, Berlan M, et al. Alpha 2-antagonist compounds and lipid mobilization: evidence for a lipid mobilizing effect of oral yohimbine in healthy male volunteers. *Eur J Clin Invest.* 1988;18:587–594.

11 De Smet PA, Smeets OS. Potential risks of health food products containing yohimbe extracts. *BMJ.* 1994;309:958.

12 Sandler B, Aronson P. Yohimbine-induced cutaneous drug eruption, progressive renal failure, and lupus-like syndrome. *Urology.* 1993;41:343–345.

13 Landis E, Shore E. Yohimbine-induced bronchospasm. *Chest.* 1989;96:1424.

14 Price LH, Charney DS, Heninger GR. Three cases of maniac symptoms following yohimbine ingestion. *Am J Psychiatry.* 1984;141:1267–1268.

15 Blumenthal M, ed. *The Complete German Commission E Monographs Therapeutic Guide to Herbal Medicines.* Boston, Mass: Integrative Medicine Communications; 1998.

16 *The Natural Medicines Comprehensive Database.* 3rd ed. Stockton, Calif: Therapeutic Research Faculty; 2001.

Zinc

Zinc, a trace mineral, is part of more than 200 enzymes involved in carbohydrate metabolism, protein synthesis and catabolism, carbon dioxide transport, and the synthesis of nucleic acid and heme, and gene expression. The highest concentrations are located in bone, muscle, integumental tissue (skin, hair, nails), retina, pancreas, and male reproductive organs. Needed for the antioxidant enzyme superoxide dismutase, zinc is thought to play a protective role against damaging superoxide anions (1).

Though overt deficiency is rare, symptoms of zinc depletion are diverse due to zinc's numerous roles in metabolic processes. Clinical signs of deficiency may include: impaired growth, alopecia, diarrhea, delayed sexual maturity, impotence, eye and skin lesions, and anorexia. Individuals most susceptible to inadequate zinc intake and deficiency include the elderly, HIV-positive patients, alcoholics, pregnant and lactating women, diabetics, patients with malabsorption disorders (Crohn's disease, short-bowel syndrome), trauma patients and female athletes (1, 2).

Media and Marketing Claims	Efficacy
Natural way to treat a cold	↔
Improves age-related macular degeneration	?↑
Improves athletic performance	NR
Treats acne	NR
Enhances fertility	NR
Improves immunity in elderly individuals	NR

Advisory

- The Tolerable Upper Intake Level (UL) is 40 mg zinc/day (2).
- Chronic ingestion of doses above the UL may impair immune function, induce copper deficiency, and negatively affect cholesterol levels
- Acute ingestion of high doses of zinc may cause nausea and vomiting

Drug/Supplement Interactions

- Zinc supplements interfere with copper absorption
- Zinc and iron may interfere with the absorption of one another
- Zinc and penicillin bind, interfering with the absorption of both
- Zinc may reduce the absorption of tetracycline (antibiotic)
- Zinc may bind with warfarin (anticoagulant)
- The following drugs may decrease zinc status: angiotensin-converting enzyme (ACE) inhibitors for hypertension (captopril, enalapril); aspirin; oral contraceptives; thiazide diuretics

KEY POINTS

- Studies are conflicting regarding the potential benefit of zinc lozenges on cold symptoms. Some researchers have suggested that the variability of dosage, formulation, and administration of zinc among studies is responsible for the equivocal results. In addition, zinc studies only measured subjective reports of cold symptoms. Further research will need to test immune function and confirm the existence of rhinovirus using microbiological tests.
- Preliminary research suggests that diets rich in zinc may provide a mild protective effect in macular degeneration. Research from the 2001 Age-Related Eye Disease Study reported that zinc supplements (80 mg) plus antioxidants and copper slowed the pro-

Z

gression of advanced age-related macular degeneration (ARM) in subjects at high risk. Individuals with ARM should discuss zinc supplementation with their physician, because this high dose is above the Tolerable Upper Intake Level.

- There is little research on zinc supplementation in athletes and a lack of substantial evidence to suggest that zinc has an ergogenic effect in exercise performance.

- Preliminary research in the 1970s and 1980s suggested some benefit of taking high doses of zinc to treat acne. No further studies have verified these results. Furthermore, the dosages used are associated with potentially dangerous side-effects.

- Although zinc content in the semen of infertile men appears to be lower than in fertile men and short-term zinc-deficient diets are associated with decreased semen volume, there are currently no well-controlled studies beyond animal data demonstrating that zinc supplementation improves fertility in humans. However, it may be advisable for infertile men to take a multivitamin providing the RDA for zinc if dietary intake is inadequate.

- Although zinc deficiency negatively affects the immune response and the elderly tend to have lower plasma zinc levels (1), more controlled research is required to determine the effect of zinc supplements on immunity in the elderly.

- A supplement providing the RDA for zinc may be necessary when dietary intake is not adequate. However, individuals using zinc supplements should not consume amounts above the UL (40 mg) to avoid potential problems including copper deficiency, elevated cholesterol, and impaired immune function.

FOOD SOURCES

Meats, eggs, seafood, whole grains, nuts, and legumes are good sources of zinc. The median daily intake of zinc in the United States is approximately 9 mg for women to 13 mg for men (2). Phytic acid in plants binds with zinc, lowering the intestinal absorption of zinc from these foods. Protein digestibility also influences zinc absorption. In general, zinc uptake is higher from a diet rich in animal protein than a diet rich in plant proteins such as soy (2). Processing whole grains results in the loss of nearly 80 percent of the total zinc (1).

Food	Zinc (mg)
Beef, ground, broiled (3.5 oz)	5.36
Wheat germ, toasted (2 tbsp)	3.22
Beans, garbanzo (1 c)	2.51
Seeds, sunflower (1 oz)	1.50
Chicken, light meat (3.5 oz)	1.23
Rice, brown (1 c)	1.23
Milk, nonfat (1 c)	0.98
Egg (1)	0.53
Codfish (3 oz)	0.49

Source: Data from Pennington JAT (3)

DOSAGE INFORMATION/BIOAVAILABILITY

Zinc is sold in lozenges and tablets bound to gluconate, citrate, sulfate, glycerate, acetate, or picolinate. Several studies have used zinc sulfate or gluconate doses above the RDA ranging from 50 mg to 100 mg elemental zinc/day. Bioavailability of zinc supplements is variable. One study found that excipients in some lozenges such as citrate, mannitol, and sorbitol inhibited the ionization of zinc to free Zn^{2+}, whereas glycine did not interfere with ionization to free zinc (4).

The National Academy of Sciences (NAS) released Dietary Reference Intakes (DRIs) for zinc in 2001. The new adult RDA for zinc is 8 mg for women, 11 mg for men, 11 mg to 13 mg during pregnancy, and 12 mg to 14 mg during lactation (2). Although no vegetarian RDA was specified, the requirement for dietary zinc may be as much as 50 percent greater for vegetarians, especially for strict vegetarians who consume mainly grains and legumes (dietary phytate:zinc molar ratio > 15:1). For people with alcoholism, the daily zinc requirement exceeds the RDA, but an exact amount was not specified in the NAS report (2).

RELEVANT RESEARCH

Zinc and the Common Cold

- A meta-analysis of six randomized, placebo-controlled, double-blind, clinical trials reported no statistical benefit of using zinc lozenges to reduce rhinovirus duration. The studies included in the analysis used zinc gluconate or acetate ranging from 4.3 mg to 23.7 mg taken every two hours while subjects were awake. However, when a study with a low dose of zinc (4.3 mg) was excluded, the analysis did suggest a benefit with zinc treatment. The authors criticized many of the studies for poor blinding because many subjects correctly identified the active treatment, which may have resulted in a false treatment effect. They concluded: "The evidence for effectiveness of zinc salt lozenges in reducing the duration of common colds is still lacking" (5).

- Two additional analyses of randomized, controlled trials of zinc for the common cold reported that evidence that zinc treats cold symptoms is inconclusive (6, 7).

- In a double-blind, placebo-controlled trial, 50 subjects recruited within 24 hours of developing symptoms for the common cold were randomized to receive 12.8 mg zinc (as zinc acetate) or a placebo every two to three hours awake as long as symptoms remained. Subjective symptom scores (sore throat, nasal discharge, congestion, sneezing, cough, scratchy throat, hoarseness, muscle ache, fever, and headache) were recorded daily for 12 days. Plasma zinc and proinflammatory cytokines were measured on day 1 and after subjects were well. Compared with the placebo, the zinc group had shorter mean overall duration of symptoms (4.5 days vs 8.1 days) and significantly decreased severity scores for all symptoms. There were no significant differences between groups on cytokine levels (8).

- In a double-blind, placebo-controlled trial, 249 students (grades 1 to 12) were randomly assigned to take zinc gluconate glycine (ZGG) lozenges (10 mg elemental zinc,

Z

five or six times a day) or a placebo within the first 24 hours of developing a cold. There was no difference in time to resolution of cold symptoms between groups. Compared to the placebo group, the zinc group experienced significantly more adverse effects including bad taste, nausea, diarrhea, and mouth discomfort. The authors concluded: "ZGG lozenges were not effective in treating cold symptoms in children and adolescents" (9).

- In a double-blind, placebo-controlled trial, 100 patients who developed symptoms of the common cold were randomized to receive 13.3 mg zinc as zinc gluconate lozenges (one lozenge every two hours awake) or a placebo for as long as symptoms lasted. Time to complete resolution of symptoms was significantly shorter with zinc than the placebo (4.4 days vs 7.6 days). The zinc-supplemented group had fewer days of coughing, headache, hoarseness, nasal congestion and drainage, and sore throat. There were no differences between groups in fever, muscle ache, scratchy throat, or sneezing. The zinc group had significantly more side effects (nausea, bad taste). Because of the lack of dramatic clinical benefit, the authors concluded that patients must decide whether the possible benefits of zinc gluconate on cold symptoms outweigh the adverse effects (10).

- An article reviewing eight controlled trials with zinc lozenges found four were effective, whereas four were not. The authors suggested the discrepancies may be caused by inadequate placebo control, and differences in lozenge formulation and dosage. They noted that zinc gluconate lozenges appeared to be effective when taken immediately after the onset of symptoms (11).

- One proposed explanation for the mechanism of action behind zinc is that the mineral may bind with proteins of critical nerve endings in the respiratory tract and surface proteins of the human rhinovirus, thereby interrupting virus infection (12).

Zinc and Age-Related Macular Degeneration (AMD)

- In a double-blind, placebo-controlled, multicenter study (Age-Related Eye Disease Study), 3,640 subjects aged 55 y to 80 y with age-related macular degeneration (with at least one eye with the best-corrected vision of 20/32 or better) were randomized to receive one of four treatments: (1) antioxidants (500 mg vitamin C, 400 IU vitamin E, 15 mg beta-carotene); (2) 80 mg zinc (as zinc oxide) and 2 mg copper (added to correct for copper deficiency associated with high dose zinc); (3) antioxidants plus zinc and copper; or (4) a placebo. Subjects were followed for an average of 6.3 years. Nearly two-thirds of the subjects chose to take a multivitamin/mineral supplement in addition to their treatment. Compared to those using the placebo, subjects taking antioxidants plus zinc had a significant odds reduction (28 percent) for the development of advanced AMD. The reduction in risk for subjects taking zinc alone was 25 percent and 20 percent for antioxidants alone. Reduction in risk increased for all three treatments when 1,063 subjects with a low risk of developing advanced ARM were excluded. There was a significant reduction in moderate visual acuity loss only in subjects assigned to antioxidants plus zinc. None of the supplements had any effect on the progression of cataract. There were no significant adverse effects associated with any of the treatments (13).

- In a two-year, double-blind, placebo-controlled study, 112 patients with age-related macular degeneration and exudative lesions in one eye and a 20/40 or better visual acuity and macular degeneration without lesion in the second eye were studied. Subjects were randomized to receive 200 mg zinc sulfate (80 mg elemental zinc) or a placebo daily. Mean serum zinc increased significantly in the treatment group, whereas there was no effect on serum copper, hemoglobin, and red blood cell count. Zinc had no short-term effect on the course of macular degeneration as measured by visual acuity, contrast sensitivity, color discrimination, and retinal grating acuity (14).

- In a double-blind, placebo-controlled trial, 151 patients with bilateral drusen (hyaline deposits beneath retinal pigment epithelium) or age related macular degeneration were randomized to receive 200 mg zinc sulfate (80 mg elemental zinc) for 24 months. There was a significant lower incidence of visual loss in zinc treated subjects at 12 to 24 months. The authors concluded: "Because of the pilot nature of the study and the possible toxic effects and complications of oral zinc administration, widespread use of zinc in macular degeneration is not now warranted" (15).

- In a retrospective longitudinal cohort study, a random sample of Beaver Dam Eye Study participants were examined to determine the relationship of diet to early and late age-related maculopathy (ARM). Subjects in the highest quintiles for zinc intake from foods had lower risk for early but not late ARM. This relationship was stronger for some types of early ARM, such as increased retinal pigment, than for other types. The authors concluded: "The data are weakly supportive of a protective effect of [dietary] zinc on the development of some forms of early ARM" (16).

Zinc and Exercise Performance

- In a nonrandomized, double-blind, placebo-controlled, crossover study, 16 healthy female subjects received 135 mg zinc (formulation not specified) or a placebo for 14 days each. Muscle strength and endurance was measured with an isokinetic, one-leg exercise test before and after both treatments. Zinc supplements significantly increased dynamic isokinetic strength and isometric endurance (17).

- In a double-blind, crossover study, five runners were randomized to receive 50 mg zinc and 3 mg copper or a placebo for six days. On day 4, one hour after supplementation, subjects ran on a treadmill at 70 percent to 75 percent maximal oxygen uptake until exhaustion. Blood samples were taken before, immediately after, and one and two days after the run. Subjects consuming the zinc and copper supplements had significantly reduced production of superoxide anion production compared to the placebo. The authors concluded: "Whether this antioxidant effect of zinc [and copper] will benefit individuals exposed to chronic physical stress remains to be determined" (18).

Zinc and Acne

- In the 1970s and 1980s, several trials investigated the effects of zinc sulfate on acne vulgaris. One placebo-controlled study of 52 patients found that zinc sulfate offered a small benefit in reducing pustules but not on comedones, papules, infiltrates, or cysts

Z

(19). Another double-blind, parallel group study compared zinc sulfate/citrate complex to tetracycline and found the antibiotic to be significantly more effective than zinc in the treatment of moderate to severe acne (20). In contrast, two double-blind, placebo controlled studies showed significant improvement in acne with 400 mg to 600 mg zinc sulfate (≈ 160 mg to 240 mg elemental zinc) during 12 weeks (21, 22). Reported adverse events associated with these high doses of zinc included nausea, vomiting, and abdominal pain. No further research has been completed since 1989.

Zinc and Male Fertility

- Zinc is necessary for growth, sexual maturation, and reproduction. Infertile men have been reported to have reduced seminal and serum zinc levels compared to fertile men (23–25).

- In a randomized, controlled-feeding, crossover study, 11 male subjects living on a metabolic ward were fed a diet composed of a mixture of semisynthetic formula and conventional foods supplemented with zinc sulfate to supply a total of 1.4, 2.5, 3.4, 4.4, or 10.4 mg zinc/day. After an equilibration period of 28 days (10.4 mg zinc/day), all treatments were presented for 35 days each, the first four in random order and the fifth last. Compared to when they were consuming 10.4 mg zinc, subjects consuming 1.4 mg zinc had decreased semen volumes and serum testosterone concentrations, and no change in seminal zinc concentrations. The authors concluded that these measures are sensitive to short-term zinc depletion in young men (26).

- A study of male rats supplemented with zinc sulfate for 30 to 32 days resulted in an increase in the zinc content of the testis and sperm. The incidence of conception from mating between normal females and zinc-fed males was significantly lower than in control males (27).

Zinc and Immunity in the Elderly

- In a double-blind, placebo-controlled, partial crossover study, 63 elderly subjects were given 15 mg or 100 mg zinc as zinc acetate capsules or a placebo daily for 12 months. All subjects were also given a multivitamin/mineral supplement without zinc. Blood samples and immune functions were assessed at 0, 3, 6, 12 and 16 months. Dietary zinc intake was consistently below recommended intakes during the study. Natural killer cell activity was transiently enhanced by the 100-mg dose after three months. Delayed dermal hypersensitivity and lymphocyte proliferation responses to two mitogens were significantly increased in the placebo group, more than either zinc treatment. The authors concluded: "Zinc had a beneficial effect on one measure of cellular immune function while simultaneously having an adverse effect on another measure" (28).

SAFETY

- The Tolerable Upper Intake Level (UL) is set at 40 mg zinc/day based on the adverse effects of higher amounts on copper status (2).

- Chronic intake of doses ranging 100 mg to 300 mg zinc/day are associated with copper deficiency with symptoms of anemia and neutropenia, impaired immune function, and an adverse effect on the ratio of LDL to HDL cholesterol. Some of these effects are also seen with 15-mg to 100-mg doses (29).

- Sideroblastic anemia, leukopenia, and neutropenia, headache, and fatigue were reported in a 17-year-old male who had been taking 300 mg zinc/day for two years as a remedy for his acne. All symptoms resolved 17 months after discontinuing zinc (30).

- An acute toxic dose of zinc (> 200 mg) may be vomited before absorption can occur. Acute high doses of zinc can cause nausea, vomiting, bad taste, and discomfort in the mouth and throat (1).

- Acute ingestion of 85 tablets of zinc gluconate (570 mg elemental zinc) resulted in severe nausea and vomiting within 30 minutes, but no further toxic effects (31).

- A high-calcium diet and supplement providing approximately 1,200 mg calcium decreased zinc absorption by 2 mg/day in postmenopausal women during a 36-day, controlled study. Zinc as part of a calcium supplement can offset the effects of calcium on zinc absorption (32). In contrast, another study using the same zinc balance methodology reported that calcium had no effect on zinc absorption (33).

REFERENCES

1. King JC, Keen CL. Zinc. In: Shils ME, Olson JA, Shike M, Ross AC, eds. *Modern Nutrition in Health and Disease.* 9th ed. Philadelphia, Pa: Lea & Febiger; 1999:223–239.
2. Institute of Medicine, Food and Nutrition Board. *Dietary Reference Intakes for Vitamin A, Vitamin K, Chromium, Copper, Iodine, Iron, Manganese, Molybedenum, Nickel, Silicon, Vanadium, and Zinc.* Washington, DC: National Academy Press; 2001.
3. Pennington JAT. *Bowes and Church's Food Values of Portions Commonly Used.* 17th ed. Philadelphia, Pa: Lippincott-Raven Publishers; 1998.
4. Zarembo JE, Godfrey JC, Godfrey NJ. Zinc (II) in saliva: determination of concentrations produced by different formulations of zinc gluconate lozenges containing common excipients. *J Pharm Sci.* 1992;81:128–130.
5. Jackson JL, Peterson C, Lesho E. A meta-analysis of zinc salts lozenges and the common cold. *Arch Intern Med.* 1997;157:2373–2376.
6. Jackson JL, Lesho E, Peterson C. Zinc and the common cold: a meta-analysis revisited. *J Nutr.* 2000;130:1512S—1515S.
7. Marshall I. Zinc for the common cold. *Cochrane Database Syst Rev.* 2000;2:CD001364.
8. Prasad AS, Fitzgerald JT, Bao B, et al. Duration of symptoms and plasma cytokine levels in patients with the common cold treated with zinc acetate. A randomized, double-blind, placebo-controlled trial. *Ann Intern Med.* 2000;133:245–252.
9. Macknin ML, Piedmonte M, Calendine C, et al. Zinc gluconate lozenges for treating the common cold in children: a randomized controlled trial. *JAMA.* 1998;279:1962–1967.
10. Mossad SB, Macknin ML, Medendorp SV, et al. Zinc gluconate lozenges for treating the common cold. A randomized, double-blind, placebo-controlled study. *Ann Intern Med.* 1996;125:81–88.

Z

11. Garland ML, Hagmeyer KO. The role of zinc lozenges in the treatment of the common cold. *Ann Pharmacother.* 1998;32:63–69.
12. Novick SG, Godfrey JC, Pollack RL, et al. Zinc-induced suppression of inflammation in the respiratory tract, caused by infection with human rhinovirus and other irritants. *Med Hypotheses.* 1997;49:347–357.
13. Age-Related Eye Disease Study Research Group. A randomized, placebo-controlled, clinical trial of high-dose supplementation with vitamins C and E, beta-carotene, and zinc for age-related macular degeneration and vision loss: AREDS report no. 8. *Arch Opthalmol.* 2001;119:1417–1436.
14. Stur M, Tittl M, Reitner A, et al. Oral zinc and the second eye in age-related macular degeneration. *Invest Ophthalmol Vis Sci.* 1996;37:1225–1235.
15. Newsome DA, Swartz M, Leone NC, et al. Oral zinc in macular degeneration. *Arch Ophthalmol.* 1988;106:192–198.
16. Mares-Perlman JA, Klein R, Klein BE, et al. *Arch Ophthalmol.* 1996;114:991–997.
17. Krotkiewski M, Gudmundson M, Backsrtrom P, et al. Zinc and muscle strength and endurance. *Acta Physiol Scand.* 1982;116:309–311.
18. Singh A, Failla ML, Deuster PA. Exercise-induced changes in immune function: effects of zinc supplementation. *J Appl Physiol.* 1994;76: 2290–2303.
19. Weimar VM, Puhl SC, Smith WH, et al. Zinc sulfate in acne vulgaris. *Arch Dermatol.* 1978;114:1776–1778.
20. Cunliffe WJ, Burke B, Dodman B, et al. A double-blind trial of a zinc sulfate/citrate complex and tetracycline in the treatment of acne vulgaris. *Br J Dermatol.* 1979;101:321–325.
21. Verma KC, Saini AS, Dhamija SK. Oral zinc sulfate therapy in acne vulgaris: a double-blind trial. *Acta Derm Venereol.* 1980;60:337–340.
22. Hillstrom L, Pettersson L, Hellbe L, et al. Comparison of oral treatment with zinc sulfate and placebo in acne vulgaris. *Br J Dermatol.* 1977;97:679–684.
23. Mohan H, Verma J, Singh I. Inter-relationship of zinc levels in serum and semen in oligospermic infertile patients and fertile males. *Indian J Pathol Microbiol.* 1997;40:451–455.
24. Kvist U, Bjornadahl L, Kjellberg S. Sperm nuclear zinc, chromatin stability, and male fertility. *Scanning Microsc.* 1987;1:1241–1247.
25. Chia SE, Ong CN, Chua LH, et al. Comparison of zinc concentrations in blood and seminal plasma and the various sperm parameters between fertile and infertile men. *J Androl.* 2000;21:53–57.
26. Hunt CD, Johnson PE, Herbel J, et al. Effects of dietary zinc depletion on seminal volume and zinc loss, serum testosterone concentrations, and sperm morphology in young men. *Am J Clin Nutr.* 1992;56:148–157.
27. Samanta K, Pal B. Zinc feeding and fertility of male rats. *Int J Vitam Nutr Res.* 1986;56:105–108.
28. Bodgen JD, Oleske JM, Lavenhar MA, et al. Effects of one year of supplementation with zinc and other micronutrients on cellular immunity in the elderly. *J Am Coll Nutr.* 1990;9:214–225.
29. Fosmire GJ. Zinc toxicity. *Am J Clin Nutr.* 1990;51:225–227.

Z

30. Porea TJ, Belmont JW, Mahoney DH. Zinc-induced anemia and neutropenia in an adolescent. *J Pediatr.* 2000;136:688–690.

31. Lewis MR, Kokan L. Zinc gluconate: acute ingestion. *J Toxicol Clin Toxicol.* 1998;36:99–101.

32. Wood RJ, Zheng JJ. High dietary calcium intakes reduce zinc absorption and balance in humans. *Am J Clin Nutr.* 1997;65:1803–1809.

33. McKenna AA, Ilich JZ, Andon MB. Zinc balance in adolescent females consuming a low- or high-calcium diet. *Am J Clin Nutr.* 1997;65:1460–1464.

Z

Part Two
APPENDIXES

Government Regulation of Dietary Supplements

This appendix recounts the development of government legislation and bodies that regulate the dietary supplements industry, then discusses quality control and the issues that health professionals face in recommending use of supplements.

HISTORY OF DIETARY SUPPLEMENT REGULATION

Dietary supplements were first regulated as foods "for special dietary use" under the Federal Food Drug and Cosmetic Act of 1938 (FDAC) (1). In 1941, the US Food and Drug Administration (FDA) defined foods for special dietary uses to include supplementing the diet with vitamins, minerals, or other dietary substances. Thirty years later, the agency sought to regulate the dosage and quantity of vitamins and minerals in dietary supplements. However, a 1974 court decision and the Rogers-Proxmire Vitamin Amendments passed in 1976 prevented implementation of these regulations (2).

In 1993, FDA published the work of its Dietary Supplements Task Force as an Advance Notice of Proposed Rulemaking (ANPR), which again suggested limiting the dosage of vitamins and minerals permitted in supplements and declared that some supplements were unapproved food additives or drugs. This ANPR led to a great deal of public debate concerning the importance of dietary supplements in promoting health and the need for consumers to have access to current and accurate information about supplements. The controversy over FDA's consideration of a stricter regulatory approach coupled with a grassroots campaign primarily organized by the supplement industry contributed to the passage of the Dietary Supplement Health Education Act of 1994 (DSHEA) (3).

DSHEA OF 1994

When The Dietary Supplement Health and Education Act was signed into law in October 1994, it provided for the first time that "dietary supplements" had their own set of legal requirements (3). Under this law, supplements would be regulated by FDA similarly to the approach used for food products while prohibiting their regulation as drugs or food additives. DSHEA made significant changes that affected the supplement industry, consumers, and health professionals by providing:

1. A definition of dietary supplement
2. A new framework for addressing safety

3. Guidelines for third-party literature (pamphlets, books, handouts) provided at the point of sale

4. Appropriate use of statements of nutritional support

5. Ingredient and nutrition information labeling standards

6. Granted the FDA authority to establish Good Manufacturing Practices (GMPs)

7. The formation of the Presidential Commission on Dietary Supplements Labels (CDSL) to review and make recommendations on supplement labeling

8. The formation of the Office of Dietary Supplements under the National Institutes of Health (NIH) to facilitate and conduct research exploring the role of dietary supplements in health and disease

Each of these provisions is discussed in this section.

DEFINITION OF DIETARY SUPPLEMENT IN DSHEA

For the first time, DSHEA defined a *dietary supplement* as a product intended to supplement the diet that contains at least one of the following: vitamin, mineral, herb or other botanical, amino acid; or a dietary substance for use to supplement the diet by increasing the total dietary intake; or concentrate, metabolite, constituent, extract, or combination of any of the previously described ingredients. Dietary supplements may be in the form of a tablet, capsule, powder, softgel, gelcap, or liquid; must be labeled as a dietary supplement; and cannot be represented for use as a conventional food or sole item of a meal or diet.

PRODUCT SAFETY

Under DSHEA, dietary supplement manufacturers have the responsibility of providing safe and properly labeled products. However, the FDA bears the burden of showing that a supplement is unsafe or mislabeled before it can restrict or ban a product. Although supplements are legally required to be safe, the FDA lacks the resources to oversee that the numerous supplement companies comply with regulations. Dietary supplements, like conventional foods, are not subject to premarket approval by FDA and are exempt from food additive regulations. Unlike supplements, food additives and drugs must undergo clinical studies to determine their safety, effectiveness, and possible interactions before being approved and allowed on the market.

When a supplement poses a safety issue, the FDA rarely takes formal legal action, but instead chooses other options, such as requesting a recall or issuing a public warning. For example, in 1997, the discovery that a plantain product was contaminated with digitalis resulted in a prompt recall. The same year, after investigating more than 800 adverse events, the agency issued a warning on consuming ephedra and proposed new rules limiting the amount of ephedra alkaloids permitted in products and requiring warning labels. (*See* the Introduction for information about reporting adverse effects related to supplements to FDA MedWatch.)

Because DSHEA specifically excluded "dietary supplements" from the definition of "food additive," ingredients that were on the market before October 1994 are recognized as safe and do not require any formal approval. However, if a new dietary supplement ingredient is introduced that was not marketed before October 1994, manufacturers are required to provide the FDA with evidence that the ingredient is "reasonably expected to be safe" at the level recommended at least 75 days before marketing. The FDA does not formally approve such ingredients but has the opportunity to reject them.

DSHEA REQUIREMENTS FOR LITERATURE

Prior to DSHEA, FDA considered all books, reprints of articles, or other materials displayed next to a product in a store or shipped with a product as "labeling." DSHEA allows "third-party" literature such as reprints, scientific abstracts and articles, book chapters, and other publications used in connection with a sale to be exempt from labeling regulations if they meet all of the following requirements:

- Are not false or misleading
- Do not promote a supplement brand
- Are reprinted in their entirety without any added information
- Present a balanced view of available scientific information
- Are displayed with other similar materials separate from supplement products
- Are not attached to any other product promotional materials

In practice, however, the agency does not have adequate resources to fully monitor and enforce these regulations.

STATEMENTS OF NUTRITIONAL SUPPORT AND HEALTH CLAIMS

Under DSHEA, supplement labels may carry "statements of nutritional support." Nutrition support statements describe the link between a nutrient and a deficiency or the effect of an ingredient on the body's structure or function, or its effect on well-being. Examples of permissible structure function statements include: "Helps maintain healthy intestinal flora," "Helps maintain cardiovascular health," "Promotes relaxation," "Builds strong bones." To make these claims, supplement labels must carry the disclaimer: "*This statement has not been evaluated by the Food and Drug Administration. This product is not intended to diagnose, treat, cure, or prevent any disease.*"

In addition, manufacturers must be able to substantiate that the structure function statements are truthful and not misleading, but are not required to provide this substantiation to the agency. Manufacturers must notify the FDA of statements within 30 days after marketing a product with this type of statement. Although the agency does not approve statements of nutritional support, it can object to them.

The Nutrition Labeling and Education Act of 1990 gave FDA the authority to authorize health claims in food and supplement labeling. Health claims describe a link between specific nutrients or substances in food and a particular a disease or condition and are based on significant scientific agreement. Currently, there are six health claims that are specifically applicable for use on dietary supplement labels provided the product contains sufficient amounts of the nutrient:

- Calcium can reduce the risk of osteoporosis.
- Folic acid protects against neural tube defects.
- Soluble fiber from psyllium seed husks may reduce the risk of coronary heart disease.
- Soluble fiber from oat bran may reduce the risk of coronary heart disease.
- Soy protein may reduce the risk of coronary heart disease in conjunction with a diet low in saturated fat and cholesterol.
- Plant sterol/stanol esters may reduce the risk of coronary heart disease.

Health claims are authorized by the agency after a comprehensive review of scientific evidence. The FDA Modernization Act of 1997 (FDAMA) provided an additional mechanism for manufacturers to use health claims based on authoritative statements by certain scientific bodies.

The underlying legal framework for the health claims system has been challenged, and the courts have ruled that it is a violation of the first amendment for FDA to ban certain statements that may truthfully describe the current evidence, even if "significant scientific agreement" on the subject had not been reached (4). The courts have required FDA to consider whether some "qualified claims" should be permitted. As a result, FDA has determined that the following statements are permissible for dietary supplements:

Omega-3 supplements labels can state that the evidence that omega-3 fatty acid reduces coronary heart disease is "suggestive, but not conclusive" and that it is not known if diets or Omega-3 fatty acids in fish reduce risk of CHD in the general population.

B vitamins supplements containing vitamins B_6, B_{12}, and folic acid may make the statement: "It is known that diets low in saturated fat and cholesterol may reduce the risk of heart disease. The scientific evidence about whether folic acid, vitamin B_6 and vitamin B_{12} may also reduce the risk of heart disease and other vascular diseases is suggestive, but not conclusive. Studies in the general population have generally found that these vitamins lower homcysteine, an amino acid found in the blood. It is not known whether elevated levels of homocysteine may cause vascular disease or whether high homocysteine levels are caused by other factors. Studies that will directly evaluate whether reducing homocysteine may also reduce the risk of vascular disease are not yet complete."

Because the distinction between structure function statements and health claims is often not clear, and the potential for consumer confusion exists, the FDA proposed regulations outlining permissible and prohibited claims on supplement labels in April 1998. In 1999, FDA held several hearings related to the controversies concerning the definition of disease, substantiation, and structure-function claims. These final regulations were published in January 2000 (5). The primary objective of the rule is to provide a consistent standard for distinguishing claims that may be made in labeling without prior FDA review from those that require prior authorizations such as health claims or drug claims. This rule highlights a number of complex issues surrounding the scientific basis of various claims and consumer perceptions and will help to reduce the number of inappropriate disease claims on supplement labels.

LABELING STANDARDS

Under DSHEA, all supplement labels must carry the name of each ingredient, the total quantity of all dietary ingredients (excluding inert ingredients), and the words *dietary supplement* as part of the product name. Alternatively, the term *dietary* can be replaced by a descriptive phrase such as *multivitamin and mineral supplement.* For botanical products, the part of the plant from which the ingredient is derived must be identified. A product is considered "misbranded" if the quality, purity, strength, and identity are misrepresented or if any other statements on the label are false and misleading.

FDA Rules for Supplement Labels

In September 1997, the FDA published final rules for supplement labels that took effect March 1999 (6). The rules require all supplements to carry a "Supplement Facts" panel listing the following information:

- An appropriate serving size is listed.
- Information given includes quantity and percent Daily Values (DV) for 14 nutrients and any other added vitamins or minerals when present at significant levels.
- For products with no established Reference Daily Intakes (RDI), the amount per serving must be stated (eg, 300 mg omega-3 fatty acids).
- If a product contains a proprietary blend, the total amount of the blend must be stated, although the individual amounts of each ingredient do not have to be labeled.
- Below the Supplement Facts panel, ingredients must be listed by common name in descending order by weight. "Other ingredients" such as fillers, excipients, artificial colors or flavors, sweeteners, or binders (eg, gelatin, water, lactose, starch, cellulose) must also be listed.

In addition, labels must print directions for use and the name and place of business of the manufacturer, packager, or distributor. The final rules also mandate that *high potency* can only be used on products that contain 100 percent or more of the established RDI for that vitamin or mineral. *Antioxidant* can only be used with descriptors such as "good source" and "high" if scientific evidence has demonstrated the nutrient inactivates free radicals or prevents free radical-initiated reactions in the body such as has been shown for vitamin C or E (7).

Role of the Federal Trade Commission

Although DSHEA does not directly address the advertising of dietary supplements, the Federal Trade Commission (FTC) is responsible for monitoring claims in advertising including print and broadcast ads, infomercials, and catalogs, as well as direct marketing materials. In November 1998, the FTC issued a guide for the supplement industry to clarify long-

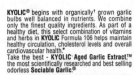

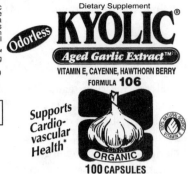

Example of a supplement label by Wakunaga of America Co., Ltd. Used with permission.

standing FTC policies and enforcement practices for dietary supplement advertising. (A copy of the guide can be accessed at http://www.ftc.gov/bcp/conline/pubs/buspubs/dietsupp.htm.)

ESTABLISHMENT OF GOOD MANUFACTURING PRACTICES

DSHEA authorized the FDA to establish Good Manufacturing Practices (GMPs) specifically for dietary supplements, modeled after GMPs for conventional foods. Enforced by the FDA, GMPs are a set of standard procedures for a number of manufacturing components such as production and processing controls, equipment, plant conditions, sanitation, recordkeeping, and employee qualifications. Currently, supplement manufacturers must follow food GMPs, which do not address the unique aspects of supplement manufacturing.

In 1995, in response to DSHEA, the supplement industry submitted a draft of GMPs specifically for dietary supplements to FDA. The proposed GMPs are stricter than food GMPs but not as rigorous as drug GMPs. The stated goals of the proposed draft are to ensure that supplements (1) are safe, not adulterated or misbranded; (2) contain the identity and provide the quantity of dietary ingredients stated in the label; and (3) meet quality specifications that the supplement is represented to meet.

In 1997, the FDA published the dietary supplement GMPs submitted by the supplement industry as an advance notice of proposed rule making, along with a set of questions about appropriate GMPs (8). The FDA expects to issue a formal proposed rule for further comment, then issue a final rule. It commonly takes a year or more for the FDA to evaluate comments received on a proposal, and all proposed and final rules must undergo review by the Office of Management and Budget, which oversees new regulations from all government agencies. Thus, even if the proposed rule is published in 2002, the final rule and implementation may not occur until two or three years later. When final supplement GMPs are adopted, this rule would offer more assurance that all supplement manufacturers are using quality control procedures and are providing reliable products. Some supplement manufacturers have already begun using dietary supplement GMPs, although this practice is not yet legally required.

PRESIDENTIAL COMMISSION ON DIETARY SUPPLEMENT LABELS

In 1995, in accord with DSHEA, a seven-member Presidential Commission on Dietary Supplement Labels (CDSL) was appointed to evaluate and make recommendations about how to provide consumers with truthful, scientifically valid, and not misleading information on supplement labels. In November 1997, the Commission issued its final report (9), in which it:

- Called for improvements in surveillance of supplement safety and in reporting of adverse reactions to supplements

- Made recommendations on the scope and substantiation of nutrition support claims

- Agreed that health claims for dietary supplements should undergo the same authorization procedures as claims for foods

- Urged health professionals to increase their knowledge of dietary supplements to aid consumers in making decisions

- Recommended that the FDA investigate the feasibility of approving botanical remedies for over-the-counter uses when sufficient evidence is available

- Suggested that the supplement industry appoint an expert advisory committee to provide guidance on the safety and efficacy of supplements

- Recommended that Congress fully fund the Office of Dietary Supplements as intended under DSHEA

The FDA published a response to the CDSL report in April 1998 (10). The agency has since begun reevaluating its adverse reaction reporting system (MedWatch) by appointing a working group and dedicating additional funds to improve the system. In response to CDSL recommendation to approve botanical supplements for over-the-counter uses, the FDA noted that the agency lacked the resources to investigate this option. Since the publication of the final report, funding for the Office of Dietary Supplements has been gradually increased by Congress. There continues to be ongoing Congressional interest in fully implementing DSHEA and providing the FDA and the Office of Dietary Supplements (ODS) with additional resources that are needed.

FORMATION OF OFFICE OF DIETARY SUPPLEMENTS

DSHEA mandated the formation of the Office of Dietary Supplements (ODS) under the National Institutes of Health (NIH) to explore the role of dietary supplements in improving health care in the United States. The office is responsible for coordinating research on supplements at the NIH, organizing symposia, and compiling research on supplements into two databases. The International Bibliographic Information on Dietary Supplements (IBIDS) is a database of published, international, scientific literature about dietary supplements, including vitamins, minerals, and botanicals. IBIDS was developed to assist the public, health professionals, and researchers in locating credible, scientific literature on dietary supplements. (IBIDS can be accessed at http://odp.od.nih.gov/ods/databases/ibids.html.) ODS also developed a second database, Computer Access to Research on Dietary Supplements (CARDS), which provides information about current research on dietary supplements and individual nutrients supported by the federal government.

To date, the ODS has coordinated 20 studies, including the effect of chromium on insulin action, L-arginine supplements on cancer, antioxidant supplements on cataracts, and the role of zinc and copper in the nervous system. The office has also awarded grants ($1.5 million yearly for five years) to four research centers to investigate botanical supplements. Additionally, the ODS is developing information fact sheets on supplements that will soon be available to the public. Updates on the activities of ODS can be accessed on its website (http://dietary-supplements.info.nih.gov).

QUALITY CONTROL

Industry Self-Regulation

Because the current food GMPs do not address the specific concerns of supplement manufacturing, many companies set their own standards to ensure quality products. For instance, some pharmaceutical companies also sell dietary supplements, and therefore already follow drug GMPs. Drug GMPs have much stricter regulations for quality control than do food GMPs under which supplements currently are regulated. In addition, some manufacturers hire independent auditors to conduct spot checks and provide feedback about manufacturing processes.

A number of third party voluntary quality assurance programs have been developed to help build consumer confidence in the quality of dietary supplements. Some of these programs include:

- United States Pharmacopoeia (USP) Dietary Supplement Verification Program (see below or http://www.usp.org)

- ConsumerLab.com (*http://www.consumerlab.com*)

- NSF International's Dietary Supplement Certification Program (http://www.nsf.org/dietary/)

United States Pharmacopoeia (USP)

Established in 1820, the US Pharmacopoeia (USP) is a nongovernmental, not-for-profit, voluntary organization that sets standards assuring the integrity and uniform quality of drugs and health care technologies. Officially recognized by federal law in 1906, the standards set by the USP on product strength, quality, and purity of drugs are legally enforceable by FDA. In 1990, USP published the first standards for multi-ingredient vitamin and mineral products including beta-carotene, several calcium salts, vitamin D_2, ferrous fumarate, ferrous gluconate, ferrous sulfate, folic acid, magnesium gluconate, magnesium oxide, and vitamins A, C, E, and K. A supplement containing the "USP" notation indicates that the product has met USP standards for disintegration, dissolution, purity, strength, packaging, labeling, and weight variation. In addition, any supplement labeled with USP is required to display a lot number and expiration date. These standards are voluntary, allowing supplement manufacturers the option of choosing to adopt and implement them.

To assist health professionals and ensure the quality of herbal supplements to consumers, the USP is currently developing public standards for a number of top-selling herbs as well as information for consumers on the safe use of herbal products. Published yearly, the National Formulary (NF) is a reference publication for standards of strength, quality, purity, identity, packaging, labeling, and storage of drugs, dietary supplements, and other healthcare products. The USP is also developing standards for these botanical extracts and their dosage forms that will appear in the NF. Herbal supplement manufacturers may voluntarily apply the "NF" notation to product labels, which indicates that the product complies with the standards in the National Formulary.

USP has developed a voluntary national certification program to assure the quality of dietary supplement ingredients in the marketplace. In November 2001, USP launched the USP Dietary Supplement Verification program, which focuses on conformity testing for ingredient and product specifications and performance standards for good manufacturing practices (according to the proposed dietary supplement GMPs). To ensure that USP-verified products meet their label declarations, USP will test samples at random from the marketplace. The USP-certified verification mark on a label does not address whether a particular supplement is effective, only that USP has provided oversight for the manufacturing of a quality product.

CHOOSING QUALITY DIETARY SUPPLEMENTS

Although the law requires products to have the proper identity and potency, an unscrupulous supplement manufacturer could irresponsibly purchase and use supplement ingredients without adequately testing for purity or identity before packaging. Fortunately, it seems that many quality assurance programs are springing up in an effort to help consumers and health professionals make informed choices about choosing a particular brand. Although there are no set rules or guarantees for selecting supplements, the following tips may be useful.

TIPS FOR SELECTING A REPUTABLE SUPPLEMENT PRODUCT

- Check the manufacturer name—nationally known food and supplement companies often have strict quality control procedures in place, and may be more likely to provide reliable products.
- Look for certifications marks by USP, NSF, or ConsumerLab.com where applicable. A company that is willing to undergo certification through one of these quality assurance programs is more likely to provide a quality product.

- Contact the company—ask to speak to a technical expert to inquire how products are made and quality control procedures and GMPs. Companies should be willing to provide answers to the following questions:
  - Has the particular product been used in any clinical studies published in peer-reviewed journals? Can the company share the scientific studies upon which the structure/function statements or health claims are based? (Obtain citations and ask the representative to send copies of the published articles.)
  - Do you complete an analysis on your final product (not just ingredients) to guarantee the contents in the bottle match those stated on the label?
  - Is the product tested for content uniformity?
  - Does the product meet any existing standards for disintegration and dissolution or other tests of bioavailability?
- Review the label—the label should contain accurate and appropriate information. If statements are unclear or the label makes outrageous claims, the manufacturers are not following DSHEA. If they are not abiding by DSHEA in this regard, it is possible that the company is lax in quality control procedures.

SUMMARY

DSHEA marked a major change in the regulation of the supplement industry. Under this act, dietary supplements are regulated similarly to food even though they may have drug-like actions. Although supplements are legally required to be safe and unadulterated, the 1994 law puts the burden of proof on the FDA to demonstrate a product is unsafe or mis-branded. Unfortunately, the agency lacks the resources to fully monitor and enforce industry compliance with the safety and labeling regulations. Although most products are relatively safe, given the limitations of DSHEA, health professionals must be informed and educated about regulations, efficacy, and potential safety concerns.

REFERENCES

1 Food, Drug, and Cosmetic Act of 1938, Pub L No. 75–717, 52 Stat 1040 (1938).
2 Rogers & Proxmire Vitamins Amendments, Pub L No. 94–278 90 Stat 410 (1976).
3 Dietary Supplement Health and Education Act of 1994 (DSHEA), Pub L No. 103–417 108 Stat (1994).
4 Food Labeling: Health Claims and label statements for dietary supplements; strategy for implementation of Pearson court decision. *Federal Register.* December 1, 1999;64:67289–67291.
5 FDA Final Rule. Regulations on statements made for dietary supplements concerning the effect of the product on the structure or function of the body. *Federal Register.* January 6, 2000;65:999–1050.
6 FDA Final Rule. Food labeling; statement of identity, nutrition labeling and ingredient labeling of dietary supplements; compliance policy guide, revocation; final rules. *Federal Register.* September 23, 1997;62:49826–49858.

7   FDA Final Rule. Food labeling; nutrient content claims: definition for "high potency" and definition of "antioxidant" for use in nutrient content claims for dietary supplements and conventional foods. *Federal Register.* September 23, 1997;62:49868–49881.

8   FDA Advance Notice of Proposed Rulemaking. Current good manufacturing practice in manufacturing, packing, or holding dietary supplements. *Federal Register.* February 6, 1997;62:5700–5709.

9   Commission on Dietary Supplement Labels. *Commission on Dietary Supplement Labels Report to the President, the Congress, and the Secretary of Health and Human Services.* Final Report, November 24, 1997. Available at http://web.health.gov/dietsupp/cover.htm.

10 FDA Notice. Dietary supplements: comments on report of the Commission on Dietary Supplement Labels. *Federal Register.* April 29, 1998;63:23633–23637.

Note: All FDA documents can be viewed in full online at http://www.cfsan.fda.gov/~dms/ds-ind.html.

Appendix B

Ethical Issues and Dietary Supplements

Lisa K. Fieber, MS, RD, and Samuel L. Fieber, JD

As dietary supplements become more popular, health professionals must face some interesting dilemmas, including a maze of ethical and legal considerations. How dietitians manage such problems may well determine their future in this area of practice.

To avoid breaching ethical standards, dietetics practitioners must recognize and address these potential conflicts within their practice. This appendix discusses legal considerations; standards of practice; and challenges for the dietetics professional in complementary care. Further questions about ethical considerations should be directed to the ADA HOD Governance Team at 800/877–1600 ext. 4896 or ethics@eatright.org.

DEFINING ETHICAL STANDARDS

The ADA/CDR Code of Ethics is the primary source of ethical guidance for dietetics professionals (1). However, other resources such as state licensure laws must be consulted in conjunction with a code of ethics to determine the professional's obligation. Ethics are based on standards. Therefore, ethics change as standards change. This subsection discusses the law, positions and standards of professional practice. Together, these resources can help dietetics professionals determine their ethical duty.

Law

The law must remain a primary resource in determining the dietetics professional's ethical duty. Primarily, professionals must understand that simply complying with ethical guidelines may not ensure compliance with the law.

Laws generally come from a state's licensing, certification, or registration agency. Currently 43 states, the District of Columbia, and Puerto Rico have enacted laws regulating dietetics professionals. (*See* the CDR website for the most current information with links to state licensure agencies, http://www.cdrnet.org/certifications/licensure/index.htm.) All practitioners need to be aware of how the laws affect health practitioners both in states with and without licensure.

Association Positions

The ADA publishes positions on current topics of interest to its members. For example, an excerpt of ADA's current position on "Food Fortification and Dietary Supplements" states: [I]t is the position of the American Dietetic Association that the best nutritional strategy for promoting optimal health and reducing the risk of chronic disease is to wisely choose a wide variety of foods. Additional vitamins and minerals from fortified foods and/or supplements can help some people meet their nutritional needs as specified by science-based nutrition standards such as the Dietary Reference Intakes (DRI) (2).

The complete text of this position can be accessed at the ADA Web site (www.eatright.com/positions.html).

STANDARDS OF PROFESSIONAL PRACTICE

The ADA has helped dietetics professionals provide quality services through the development of uniform standards that dietetics professionals may follow in their practice settings (3). Standards of Professional Practice refer to the performance of individual dietetics professionals, regardless of the setting, project, case, or situation. They are defined statements of a dietetics professional's responsibility for providing services in all areas of practice and describe the minimum level of performance expected (3).

The Standards of Professional Practice align with the ADA Code of Ethics and the Professional Development Portfolio (PDP) to achieve a common goal of improving the quality of dietetics practice and promoting professional competence. The PDP offers a framework to develop specific goals, identify learning needs, and pursue continuing professional education to achieve these needs and goals (3).

CHALLENGES: THE DIETETICS PROFESSIONAL AND COMPLEMENTARY CARE

A thorough nutritional assessment may provide the dietetics professional with the information needed to recommend supplementation. Two broad factors related to ethical and legal considerations will determine the recommendation: 1) the practitioner's level of expertise and 2) state regulations in the location of the practitioner's practice.

Practitioner's Level of Expertise

As to the first issue, the ADA Code of Ethics states: "[The] dietetics practitioner assumes responsibility and accountability for personal competence in practice, continually striving to increase professional knowledge and skills and to apply them in practice" (1). The fallacy here is that, depending on the state in which the practice is located, a dietetics professional may not be allowed to make recommendations to the patient. Instead, the practitioner makes recommendations to a physician, who will decide whether to follow the recommendations.

State Laws

Differing state laws regarding recommendation of supplements may present difficulties. The problem is that laws generally define and license the practice of medicine in terms that ingrain the medical profession and that exclude all other forms of healing as the unauthorized practice of medicine (4). The risk of prosecution for practicing medicine unlawfully is a felony in many states. Each state has its own version of the law. All states define the practice of medicine, in part by using such words as *diagnosis, treatment, prevention, cure, advise,* and *prescribe* (5). For example, Michigan, Arkansas, Hawaii, Louisiana, Indiana, and Utah all have state statutes that speak to what constitutes "practice of medicine" (6–8). Dietetics professionals typically "advise" patients. If working in these states, they must walk a fine line to prevent accusations of the illegal practice of medicine.

Debate continues among dietetics professionals regarding the sale of vitamin and mineral supplements, herbs, and botanicals. Practitioners must be alert to situations that might cause a conflict of interest or have the appearance of a conflict and provide "full disclosure when a real or potential conflict of interest arises" (1). In this context, the professional must be extraordinarily cautious, constantly striving to ensure that he or she practices dietetics based on scientific principles and current information (1). The Code of Ethics reminds practitioners to always "promote or endorse products in a manner that is neither false nor misleading" (1).

CONCLUSION

Dietetics professionals need to understand a few basic concepts: 1) Learn the state laws as they pertain to both your practice and the practice of other allied health professionals. 2) Understand and abide by the scope of practice, standards of practice, and code of ethics. 3) Know the underlying science and research that pertains to the specific supplements including strengths and weaknesses of the data.

The trend of increased use of supplements poses a predicament for healthcare professionals: how to responsibly advise patients who use or seek alternative therapies in the face of inconclusive evidence about the safety and effectiveness of these therapies (9).

REFERENCES

1. Code of Ethics for the Profession of Dietetics. The American Dietetic Association. *J Am Diet Assoc.* 1999;99(1):109–113.
2. Position of the American Dietetic Association: Food fortification and dietary supplements. Available at: http://www.eatright.org/images/journal/0101/adap0101.pdf. Published Jan. 2001.
3. Commission on Dietetic Registration. Professional Development Portfolio. Commission on Dietetic Registration; 2001.
4. Buckman R, Lewith G. What does homeopathy do—and how? *BMJ.* 1994;309:103–106.

5. Cohen MH. A fixed star in health care reform; the emerging paradigm of holistic healing. *Ariz St Law J.* 1995;27(1):79.

6. Hawaii Rev Stat S 453–2 (1985 and Supp 1992).

7. La Rev Stat Ann S 37:1262 (West 1988) (same).

8. Utah Code Ann S 58–12-28 (1990).

9 Eisenberg DM. Advising patients who seek alternative medical therapies. *Ann Intern Med.* 1997;127:61–69.

Supplements Sorted by Purported Use

ACNE

Acidophilus
Gamma-linolenic acid (evening
    primrose, black currant, borage seed
    oils)
Vitamin A
Zinc

AGING

Coenzyme Q_{10}
DHEA
Lipoic acid
Melatonin
Royal jelly

ASTHMA/LUNG FUNCTION

Ma huang/ephedra
MSM
Vitamin B_6 (pyridoxine)
Vitamin C
Vitamin E

AUTISM

Vitamin B_6 (pyridoxine)

BIRTH DEFECTS (NEURAL TUBE DEFECTS)

Folic acid/folate

BODY COMPOSITION—ANABOLIC
(see also Exercise Performance)

Androstenedione/androstenediol
Arginine (ornithine and citrulline)
Branched-chain amino acids (BCAAs)
Boron
Chromium
Conjugated linolenic acid (CLA)
Colostrum
Creatine
Gamma-oryzanol
HMB (β-hydroxy β-methylbutyrate)
Vanadium (vanadyl sulfate)
Whey protein
Yohimbine

CANCER PREVENTION/TREATMENT

Acidophilus
Beta-carotene
Bromelain
Calcium (colon cancer)
Coenzyme Q_{10} (breast cancer)
Conjugated linolenic acid (CLA)
DHEA
Flaxseed (breast and colon cancer)
Folic acid/folate (colon and cervical
    cancer)
Fructooligosaccharides (FOS) (colon
    cancer)
Garlic
Green tea extract

Melatonin
Noni juice
Selenium
Shark cartilage
Soy protein and isoflavones
Spirulina/blue-green algae
Vitamin C
Vitamin D (colon and breast cancer)
Vitamin E
Whey protein

CARDIOVASCULAR DISEASE *(see also Circulation, Hypertension, and Hyperlipidemia)*

Arginine
Beta-carotene
Bromelain
Carnitine
Coenzyme Q_{10}
Conjugated linolenic acid (CLA)
Creatine
DHEA
Flaxseed
Folic acid/folate
Garlic
Gamma-linolenic acid (evening primrose, black currant, borage seed oils)
Ginseng
Green tea extract
Lysine
Magnesium
Royal jelly
Selenium
Vitamin B_3 (niacin)
Vitamin B_6 (pyridoxine)
Vitamin B_{12} (cobalamin)
Vitamin C
Vitamin E

CARPAL TUNNEL SYNDROME

Vitamin B_6 (pyridoxine)

CATARACTS/AGE-RELATED MACULOPATHY

Beta-carotene
Vitamin C
Vitamin E
Zinc

CIRCULATION/INTERMITTENT CLAUDICATION

Garlic
Ginkgo biloba

DEMENTIA/ALZHEIMER'S DISEASE *(see also Memory/Neurological Function)*

Carnitine
Ginkgo biloba
Lecithin/choline
Phosphatidylserine
Vitamin B_1 (thiamin)
Vitamin B_{12} (cobalamin)
Vitamin E

DEPRESSION

Folic acid/folate
5-Hydroxy-Tryptophan (5-HTP)
Royal jelly
St. John's wort
SAM-e

DIABETES/GLUCOSE TOLERANCE

Alanine
Chromium
Conjugated linolenic acid (CLA)
Fructooligosaccharides (FOS)
Gamma-linolenic acid (evening primrose, black currant, borage seed oils)
Lipoic acid
Magnesium
Vanadium (vanadyl sulfate)
Vitamin B_3 (niacin)
Vitamin B_{12} (cobalamin)
Vitamin E

DIARRHEA

Bromelain
Colostrum
Goldenseal

DIGESTION

Acidophilus
Bromelain
Colostrum
Fructooligosaccharides (FOS)
MSM
Noni juice
Pancreatin
Spirulina/blue-green algae

EXERCISE PERFORMANCE *(see also Body Composition)*

Androstenedione/androstenediol
Alanine
Bee pollen
Branched-chain amino acids (BCAAs)
Carnitine
Coenzyme Q_{10}
Creatine
Ginseng
Glutamine
Glycerol
HMB (β-Hydroxy β-methylbutyrate)
Lecithin/choline
Lipoic acid
Magnesium
Pantothenic acid
Phosphatidylserine
Pyruvate
Royal jelly
Selenium
Sodium bicarbonate
Vanadium (vanadyl sulfate)
Vitamin C
Vitamin E
Zinc

FATIGUE

Bee pollen
Carnitine
Ginseng
Royal jelly
Vitamin B_1 (thiamin)
Vitamin B_2 (riboflavin)
Vitamin B_{12} (cobalamin)

FERTILITY

Zinc

HAIR LOSS

Gamma-linolenic acid (evening primrose, black currant, borage seed oils)

HERPES VIRUS

Lysine

HIV/AIDS

Arginine
Carnitine
Coenzyme Q_{10}
Colostrum
DHEA
Lipoic acid
N-acetylcysteine
Vitamin B_{12} (cobalamin)
Whey protein

HYPERLIPIDEMIA

Acidophilus
Chitosan
Chromium
Fish oil
Flaxseed
Fructooligosaccharides (FOS)
Gamma-oryzanol
Garlic
Noni juice
Pantothenic acid

Pyruvate
Soy protein and isoflavones
Spirulina/blue-green algae
Vitamin B_3 (niacin)
Wheat grass

HYPERTENSION

Calcium
Fish oil
Garlic
Magnesium
Potassium

IMMUNE FUNCTION

Arginine (ornithine and citrulline)
Beta-carotene
Colostrum
DHEA
Echinacea
Glutamine
Goldenseal
Noni juice
Pancreatin
Selenium
Spirulina/blue-green algae
Vitamin C
Vitamin E
Wheat grass
Zinc

INSOMNIA/SLEEP DISORDERS

Kava
Melatonin
Noni juice
Valerian
Vitamin B_{12} (cobalamin)

JET LAG

Melatonin

LIBIDO/SEX DRIVE

Androstenedione/androstendiol
Boron
DHEA
Ginseng
Melatonin
Yohimbine

LIVER FUNCTION

Alanine
Lecithin/choline
Lipoic acid
SAM-e

LUPUS

DHEA
Flaxseed

MEMORY/NEUROLOGICAL FUNCTION (*see also Dementia/Alzheimer's Disease*)

Bee pollen
Boron
Carnitine
Coenzyme Q_{10}
DHEA
Ginkgo biloba
Lecithin/choline
Phosphatidylserine

MENOPAUSE

Black cohosh
Boron
Dong quai
Soy protein and isoflavones

MIGRAINE HEADACHES

Magnesium
Vitamin B_1 (thiamin)

OSTEOARTHRITIS

Boron
Chondroitin sulfate
Glucosamine
MSM
Noni juice
SAM-e
Vitamin B_3 (niacin)

OSTEOPOROSIS

Boron
Calcium
Soy protein and isoflavones
Vitamin C

PREMENSTRUAL SYNDROME

Black cohosh
Calcium
Dong quai
Gamma-linolenic acid (evening
    primrose, black currant, borage seed
    oils)
Magnesium
Vitamin B_6 (pyridoxine)

PROSTATE FUNCTION

Saw palmetto

RESPIRATORY INFECTION (RHINOVIRUS/INFLUENZA VIRUS)

Bee pollen
Bromelain
Echinacea
Goldenseal
Ma huang/ephedra
N-acetylcysteine (NAC)
Vitamin C
Zinc

RHEUMATOID ARTHRITIS

Fish oil
Flaxseed
Gamma-linolenic acid (evening primrose,
    black currant, borage seed oils)
Pantothenic acid

SKIN DISORDERS (PSORIASIS, ECZEMA, DERMATITIS)

Fish oil
Flaxseed
Gamma-linolenic acid (evening primrose,
    black currant, borage seed oils)

STRESS/ANXIETY

Kava
Valerian
Vitamin B (thiamin, riboflavin,
    pantothenic acid)
5-Hydroxy-tryptophan (5-HTP)

ULCERATIVE COLITIS

Fish oil

WEIGHT REDUCTION

Carnitine
Chitosan
Chromium
DHEA
Hydroxy citrate (*Garcinia cambogia*)
5-Hydroxy-tryptophan (5-HTP)
Ma huang/ephedra
Pyruvate
Yohimbine

VAGINAL YEAST INFECTIONS

Acidophilus

URINARY TRACT INFECTIONS

Cranberry

Appendix D

Dietary Intake Tables

Table D-1: Dietary Reference Intakes (DRIs): Recommended Intakes for Individuals, Vitamins

Food and Nutrition Board, Institute of Medicine, The National Academies

Life Stage Group	Vitamin A (μg/d)[a]	Vitamin C (mg/d)	Vitamin D (μg/d)[b,c]	Vitamin E (mg/d)[d]	Vitamin K (μg/d)	Thiamin (mg/d)	Riboflavin (mg/d)	Niacin (mg/d)[e]	Vitamin B$_6$ (mg/d)	Folate (μg/d)[f]	Vitamin B$_{12}$ (μg/d)	Pantothenic Acid (mg/d)	Biotin (μg/d)	Choline (mg/d)[g]
Infants														
0–6 mo	400*	40*	5*	4*	2.0*	0.2*	0.3*	2*	0.1*	65*	0.4*	1.7*	5*	125*
7–12 mo	500*	50*	5*	5*	2.5*	0.3*	0.4*	4*	0.3*	80*	0.5*	1.8*	6*	150*
Children														
1–3 y	300	15	5*	6	30*	0.5	0.5	6	0.5	150	0.9	2*	8*	200*
4–8 y	400	25	5*	7	55*	0.6	0.6	8	0.6	200	1.2	3*	12*	250*
Males														
9–13 y	600	45	5*	11	60*	0.9	0.9	12	1.0	300	1.8	4*	20*	375*
14–18 y	900	75	5*	15	75*	1.2	1.3	16	1.3	400	2.4	5*	25*	550*
19–30 y	900	90	5*	15	120*	1.2	1.3	16	1.3	400	2.4	5*	30*	550*
31–50 y	900	90	5*	15	120*	1.2	1.3	16	1.3	400	2.4	5*	30*	550*
51–70 y	900	90	10*	15	120*	1.2	1.3	16	1.7	400	2.4[h]	5*	30*	550*
>70 y	900	90	15*	15	120*	1.2	1.3	16	1.7	400	2.4[h]	5*	30*	550*
Females														
9–13 y	600	45	5*	11	60*	0.9	0.9	12	1.0	300	1.8	4*	20*	375*
14–18 y	700	65	5*	15	75*	1.0	1.0	14	1.2	400[i]	2.4	5*	25*	400*
19–30 y	700	75	5*	15	90*	1.1	1.1	14	1.3	400[i]	2.4	5*	30*	425*
31–50 y	700	75	5*	15	90*	1.1	1.1	14	1.3	400[i]	2.4	5*	30*	425*
51–70 y	700	75	10*	15	90*	1.1	1.1	14	1.5	400	2.4[h]	5*	30*	425*
>70 y	700	75	15*	15	90*	1.1	1.1	14	1.5	400	2.4[h]	5*	30*	425*
Pregnancy														
≤18 y	750	80	5*	15	75*	1.4	1.4	18	1.9	600[j]	2.6	6*	30*	450*
19–30 y	770	85	5*	15	90*	1.4	1.4	18	1.9	600[j]	2.6	6*	30*	450*
31–50 y	770	85	5*	15	90*	1.4	1.4	18	1.9	600[j]	2.6	6*	30*	450*
Lactation														
≤18 y	1,200	115	5*	19	75*	1.4	1.6	17	2.0	500	2.8	7*	35*	550*
19–30 y	1,300	120	5*	19	90*	1.4	1.6	17	2.0	500	2.8	7*	35*	550*
31–50 y	1,300	120	5*	19	90*	1.4	1.6	17	2.0	500	2.8	7*	35*	550*

NOTE: This table (taken from the DRI reports, see www.nap.edu) presents Recommended Dietary Allowances (RDAs) in **bold type** and Adequate Intakes (AIs) in ordinary type followed by an asterisk (*). RDAs and AIs may both be used as goals for individual intake. RDAs are set to meet the needs of almost all (97 to 98 percent) individuals in a group. For healthy breastfed infants, the AI is the mean intake. The AI for other life stage and gender groups is believed to cover needs of all individuals in the group, but lack of data or uncertainty in the data prevent stating with confidence the percentage of individuals covered by this intake.

[a] As retinol activity equivalents (RAEs). 1 RAE = 1 mg retinol, 12 mg b-carotene, 24 mg a-carotene, or 24 mg b-cryptoxanthin. To calculate RAEs from REs of provitamin A carotenoids in foods, divide the REs by 2. For preformed vitamin A in foods or supplements and for provitamin A carotenoids in supplements, 1 RE = 1 RAE.

[b] calciferol. 1 µg calciferol = 40 IU vitamin D.

[c] In the absence of adequate exposure to sunlight.

[d] As a-tocopherol. a-Tocopherol includes *RRR*-a-tocopherol, the only form of a-tocopherol that occurs naturally in foods, and the *2R*-stereoisomeric forms of a-tocopherol (*RRR*-, *RSR*-, *RSR*-, *RRS*-, and *RSS*-a-tocopherol) that occur in fortified foods and supplements. It does not include the *2S*-stereoisomeric forms of a-tocopherol (*SRR*-, *SSR*-, *SRS*-, and *SSS*-a-tocopherol), also found in fortified foods and supplements.

[e] As niacin equivalents (NE). 1 mg of niacin = 60 mg of tryptophan; 0–6 months = preformed niacin (not NE).

[f] As dietary folate equivalents (DFE). 1 DFE = 1 µg food folate = 0.6 µg of folic acid from fortified food or as a supplement consumed with food = 0.5 µg of a supplement taken on an empty stomach.

[g] Although AIs have been set for choline, there are few data to assess whether a dietary supply of choline is needed at all stages of the life cycle, and it may be that the choline requirement can be met by endogenous synthesis at some of these stages.

[h] Because 10 to 30 percent of older people may malabsorb food-bound B_{12}, it is advisable for those older than 50 years to meet their RDA mainly by consuming foods fortified with B_{12} or a supplement containing B_{12}.

[i] In view of evidence linking folate intake with neural tube defects in the fetus, it is recommended that all women capable of becoming pregnant consume 400 µg from supplements or fortified foods in addition to intake of food folate from a varied diet.

[j] It is assumed that women will continue consuming 400 µg from supplements or fortified food until their pregnancy is confirmed and they enter prenatal care, which ordinarily occurs after the end of the periconceptional period—the critical time for formation of the neural tube.

Reprinted with permission. Copyright 2001 by the National Academy of Sciences. Courtesy of the National Academy Press, Washington, DC.

Table D-2: Dietary Reference Intakes (DRIs): Recommended Intakes for Individuals, Elements

Food and Nutrition Board, Institute of Medicine, National Academies

Life Stage Group	Calcium (mg/d)	Chromium (µg/d)	Copper (µg/d)	Fluoride (mg/d)	Iodine (µg/d)	Iron (mg/d)	Magnesium (mg/d)	Manganese (mg/d)	Molybdenum (µg/d)	Phosphorus (mg/d)	Selenium (µg/d)	Zinc (mg/d)
Infants												
0–6 mo	210*	0.2*	200*	0.01*	110*	0.27*	30*	0.003*	2*	100*	15*	2*
7–12 mo	270*	5.5*	220*	0.5*	130*	11	75*	0.6*	3*	275*	20*	3
Children												
1–3 y	500*	11*	340	0.7*	90	7	80	1.2*	17	460	20	3
4–8 y	800*	15*	440	1*	90	10	130	1.5*	22	500	30	5
Males												
9–13 y	1,300*	25*	700	2*	120	8	240	1.9*	34	1,250	40	8
14–18 y	1,300*	35*	890	3*	150	11	410	2.2*	43	1,250	55	11
19–30 y	1,000*	35*	900	4*	150	8	400	2.3*	45	700	55	11
31–50 y	1,000*	35*	900	4*	150	8	420	2.3*	45	700	55	11
51–70 y	1,200*	30*	900	4*	150	8	420	2.3*	45	700	55	11
> 70 y	1,200*	30*	900	4*	150	8	420	2.3*	45	700	55	11
Females												
9–13 y	1,300*	21*	700	2*	120	8	240	1.6*	34	1,250	40	8
14–18 y	1,300*	24*	890	3*	150	15	360	1.6*	43	1,250	55	9
19–30 y	1,000*	25*	900	3*	150	18	310	1.8*	45	700	55	8
31–50 y	1,000*	25*	900	3*	150	18	320	1.8*	45	700	55	8
51–70 y	1,200*	20*	900	3*	150	8	320	1.8*	45	700	55	8
> 70 y	1,200*	20*	900	3*	150	8	320	1.8*	45	700	55	8
Pregnancy												
≤ 18 y	1,300*	29*	1,000	3*	220	27	400	2.0*	50	1,250	60	12
19–30 y	1,000*	30*	1,000	3*	220	27	350	2.0*	50	700	60	11
31–50 y	1,000*	30*	1,000	3*	220	27	360	2.0*	50	700	60	11

Lactation											
≤ 18 y	1,300*	44*	1,300	3*	290	10	360	2.6*	50	1,250	70	13
19–30 y	1,000*	45*	1,300	3*	290	9	310	2.6*	50	700	70	12
31–50 y	1,000*	45*	1,300	3*	290	9	320	2.6*	50	700	70	12

NOTE: This table presents Recommended Dietary Allowances (RDAs) in **bold type** and Adequate Intakes (AIs) in ordinary type followed by an asterisk (*). RDAs and AIs may both be used as goals for individual intake. RDAs are set to meet the needs of almost all (97 to 98 percent) individuals in a group. For healthy breastfed infants, the AI is the mean intake. The AI for other life stage and gender groups is believed to cover needs of all individuals in the group, but lack of data or uncertainty in the data prevent stating with confidence the percentage of individuals covered by this intake.

Reprinted with permission from *Dietary Reference Intakes for Calcium, Phosphorous, Magnesium, Vitamin D, and Fluoride* (1997); *Dietary Reference Intakes for Thiamin, Riboflavin, Niacin, Vitamin B_6, Folate, Vitamin B_{12}, Pantothenic Acid, Biotin, and Choline* (1998); *Dietary Reference Intakes for Vitamin C, Vitamine E, Selenium, and Carotenoids* (2000); and *Dietary Reference Intakes for Vitamin A, Vitamin K, Arsenic, Boron, Chromium, Copper, Iodine, Iron, Manganese, Molybdenum, Nickel, Silicon, Vanadium, and Zinc* (2001). Copyright 2001 by the National Academy of Sciences. Courtesy of the National Academy Press, Washington, DC.

Table D-3: Dietary Reference Intakes (DRIs): Tolerable Upper Intake Levels (UL[a]), Vitamins

Food and Nutrition Board, Institute of Medicine, National Academies

Life Stage Group	Vitamin A (µg/d)[b]	Vitamin C (mg/d)	Vitamin D (µg/d)	Vitamin E (mg/d)[c,d]	Vitamin K	Thiamin	Riboflavin	Niacin (mg/d)[d]	Vitamin B$_6$ (mg/d)[d]	Folate (µg/d)[d]	Vitamin B$_{12}$	Pantothenic Acid	Biotin	Choline (g/d)	Carotenoids[e]
Infants															
0–6 mo	600	ND[f]	25	ND	ND	ND	ND	ND	ND	ND	ND	ND	ND	ND	ND
7–12 mo	600	ND	25	ND	ND	ND	ND	ND	ND	ND	ND	ND	ND	ND	ND
Children															
1–3 y	600	400	50	200	ND	ND	ND	10	30	300	ND	ND	ND	1.0	ND
4–8 y	900	650	50	300	ND	ND	ND	15	40	400	ND	ND	ND	1.0	ND
Males, Females															
9–13 y	1,700	1,200	50	600	ND	ND	ND	20	60	600	ND	ND	ND	2.0	ND
14–18 y	2,800	1,800	50	800	ND	ND	ND	30	80	800	ND	ND	ND	3.0	ND
19–70 y	3,000	2,000	50	1,000	ND	ND	ND	35	100	1,000	ND	ND	ND	3.5	ND
>70 y	3,000	2,000	50	1,000	ND	ND	ND	35	100	1,000	ND	ND	ND	3.5	ND
Pregnancy															
≤18 y	2,800	1,800	50	800	ND	ND	ND	30	80	800	ND	ND	ND	3.0	ND
19–50 y	3,000	2,000	50	1,000	ND	ND	ND	35	100	1,000	ND	ND	ND	3.5	ND
Lactation															
≤18 y	2,800	1,800	50	800	ND	ND	ND	30	80	800	ND	ND	ND	3.0	ND
19–50 y	3,000	2,000	50	1,000	ND	ND	ND	35	100	1,000	ND	ND	ND	3.5	ND

[a]UL = The maximum level of daily nutrient intake that is likely to pose no risk of adverse effects. Unless otherwise specified, the UL represents total intake from food, water, and supplements. Due to lack of suitable data, ULs could not be established for vitamin K, thiamin, riboflavin, vitamin B$_{12}$, pantothenic acid, biotin, or carotenoids. In the absence of ULs, extra caution may be warranted in consuming levels above recommended intakes.

[b]As preformed vitamin A only.

[c]As α-tocopherol; applies to any form of supplemental α-tocopherol.

[d]The ULs for vitamin E, niacin, and folate apply to synthetic forms obtained from supplements, fortified foods, or a combination of the two.

[e]β-Carotene supplements are advised only to serve as a provitamin A source for individuals at risk of vitamin A deficiency.

[f]ND = Not determinable due to lack of data of adverse effects in this age group and concern with regard to lack of ability to handle excess amounts. Source of intake should be from food only to prevent high levels of intake.

Reprinted with permission from *Dietary Reference Intakes for Calcium, Phosphorous, Magnesium, Vitamin D, and Fluoride* (1997); *Dietary Reference Intakes for Thiamin, Riboflavin, Niacin, Vitamin B$_6$, Folate, Vitamin B$_{12}$, Pantothenic Acid, Biotin, and Choline* (1998); *Dietary Reference Intakes for Vitamin C, Vitamin E, Selenium, and Carotenoids* (2000); and *Dietary Reference Intakes for Vitamin A, Vitamin K, Arsenic, Boron, Chromium, Copper, Iodine, Iron, Manganese, Molybdenum, Nickel, Silicon, Vanadium, and Zinc* (2001). Copyright 2001 by the National Academy of Sciences. Courtesy of the National Academy Press, Washington, DC.

Table D-4: Dietary Reference Intakes (DRIs): Tolerable Upper Intake Levels (UL[a]), Elements

Food and Nutrition Board, Institute of Medicine, National Academies

Life Stage Group	Arsenic[b]	Boron (mg/d)	Calcium (g/d)	Chromium	Copper (µg/d)	Fluoride (mg/d)	Iodine (µg/d)	Iron (mg/d)	Magnesium (mg/d)[c]	Manganese (mg/d)	Molybdenum (µg/d)	Nickel (mg/d)	Phosphorus (g/d)	Selenium (µg/d)	Silicon[d]	Vanadium (mg/d)[e]	Zinc (mg/d)
Infants																	
0–6 mo	ND[f]	ND	ND	ND	ND	0.7	ND	40	ND	ND	ND	ND	ND	45	ND	ND	4
7–12 mo	ND	ND	ND	ND	ND	0.9	ND	40	ND	ND	ND	ND	ND	60	ND	ND	5
Children																	
1–3 y	ND	3	2.5	ND	1,000	1.3	200	40	65	2	300	0.2	3	90	ND	ND	7
4–8 y	ND	6	2.5	ND	3,000	2.2	300	40	110	3	600	0.3	3	150	ND	ND	12
Males, Females																	
9–13 y	ND	11	2.5	ND	5,000	10	600	40	350	6	1,100	0.6	4	280	ND	ND	23
14–18 y	ND	17	2.5	ND	8,000	10	900	45	350	9	1,700	1.0	4	400	ND	ND	34
19–70 y	ND	20	2.5	ND	10,000	10	1,100	45	350	11	2,000	1.0	4	400	ND	1.8	40
>70 y	ND	20	2.5	ND	10,000	10	1,100	45	350	11	2,000	1.0	3	400	ND	1.8	40
Pregnancy																	
≤18 y	ND	17	2.5	ND	8,000	10	900	45	350	9	1,700	1.0	3.5	400	ND	ND	34
19–50 y	ND	20	2.5	ND	10,000	10	1,100	45	350	11	2,000	1.0	3.5	400	ND	ND	40
Lactation																	
≤18 y	ND	17	2.5	ND	8,000	10	900	45	350	9	1,700	1.0	4	400	ND	ND	34
19–50 y	ND	20	2.5	ND	10,000	10	1,100	45	350	11	2,000	1.0	4	400	ND	ND	40

[a]UL = The maximum level of daily nutrient intake that is likely to pose no risk of adverse effects. Unless otherwise specified, the UL represents total intake from food, water, and supplements. Due to lack of suitable data, ULs could not be established for arsenic, chromium, and silicon. In the absence of ULs, extra caution may be warranted in consuming levels above recommended intakes.

[b]Although the UL was not determined for arsenic, there is no justification for adding arsenic to food or supplements.

[c]The ULs for magnesium represent intake from a pharmacological agent only and do not include intake from food and water.

[d]Although silicon has not been shown to cause adverse effects in humans, there is no justification for adding silicon to supplements.

[e]Although vanadium in food has not been shown to cause adverse effects in humans, this data could be used to set a UL for adults but not children and adolescents. The UL is based on adverse effects in laboratory animals and this data could be used with caution. Source of intake should be from food and vanadium supplements should be used with caution.

[f]ND = Not determinable due to lack of data of adverse effects in this age group and concern with regard to lack of ability to handle excess amounts. Source of intake should be from food only to prevent high levels of intake.

Reprinted with permission from *Dietary Reference Intakes for Calcium, Phosphorous, Magnesium, Vitamin D, and Fluoride* (1997); *Dietary Reference Intakes for Thiamin, Riboflavin, Niacin, Vitamin B₆, Folate, Vitamin B₁₂, Pantothenic Acid, Biotin, and Choline* (1998); *Dietary Reference Intakes for Vitamin C, Vitamin E, Selenium, and Carotenoids* (2000); and *Dietary Reference Intakes for Vitamin A, Vitamin K, Arsenic, Boron, Chromium, Copper, Iodine, Iron, Manganese, Molybdenum, Nickel, Silicon, Vanadium, and Zinc* (2001). Copyright 2001 by the National Academy of Sciences. Courtesy of the National Academy Press, Washington, DC.

Table D-5: Estimated Sodium, Chloride, and Potassium Minimum Requirements of Healthy Persons[a]

Age	Weight (kg)[a]	Sodium (mg)[a,b]	Chloride (mg)[a,b]	Potassium (mg)[c]
Months				
0–5	4.5	120	180	500
6–11	8.9	200	300	700
Years				
1	11.0	225	350	1,000
2–5	16.0	300	500	1,400
6–9	25.0	400	600	1,600
10–18	50.0	500	750	2,000
>18[d]	70.0	500	750	2,000

[a]No allowance has been included for large, prolonged losses from the skin through sweat.
[b]There is no evidence that higher intakes confer any health benefit.
[c]Desirable intakes of potassium may considerably exceed these values (~3,500 mg for adults).
[d]No allowance included for growth. Values for those below 18 years assume a growth rate at the 50th percentile reported by the National Center for Health Statistics and averaged for males and females.

Adapted with permission from Recommended Dietary Allowances, 10th edition, © 1989 by the National Academy of Science. Published by National Academy Press, Washington, DC.

Appendix E

ADDITIONAL RESOURCES

ORGANIZATIONS

American Dietetic Association
216 W. Jackson Blvd.
Chicago, IL 60606-6995
Phone: 800/877-1600
http://www.eatright.org

American Botanical Council
PO Box 201660
Austin TX 78720
Phone: 800/373-7105 (to place orders)
(512) 926-4900
http://www.herbalgram.org

Center for Science in the Public Interest
1875 Connecticut Ave NW
Suite 300
Washington, DC 20009
Phone: 202/332-9110
http://www.cspinet.org

Council for Responsible Nutrition
(trade organization for supplement
   industry)
1875 Eye Street, NW
Suite 400
Washington, DC 20006-5409
Phone: 202/872-1488
http://www.crnusa.org

Food and Drug Administration Center for Food Safety and Applied Nutrition
200 C Street SW
Washington, DC 20204 USA
Phone: 888/INFO-FDA (888/463-6332)
http://www.cfsan.fda.gov

Food and Nutrition Board
Institute of Medicine
2101 Constitution Avenue, NW
Washington, D.C. 20418
http://www.nationalacademies.org/

Herb Research Foundation
1007 Pearl Street
Suite 200
Boulder, CO 80302
Phone: 303/449-2265
http://www.herbs.org

International Food Information Council
1100 Connecticut Ave NW
Suite 430
Washington, DC 20036
Phone: 202/296-6540
http://www.ific.org

National Center for Complementary and Alternative Medicine
NCCAM Clearinghouse
PO Box 7923
Gaithersburg, MD 20898
Phone: 888/644-6226
http://nccam.nih.gov

Office of Dietary Supplements
National Institutes of Health
Building 31, Room 1B25
31 Center Drive, MSC 2086
Bethesda, MD 20892-2086
Phone: 301/435-2920
http://dietary-supplements.info.nih.gov
Website for International Bibliographic
    Information on Dietary Supplements
    (IBIDS): http://dietary-
    supplements.info.nih.gov/databases/
    ibids.html

ORGANIZATIONS PROVIDING INDEPENDENT CERTIFICATION FOR DIETARY SUPPLEMENT PRODUCTS

United States Pharmacopoeia
12601 Twinbrook Parkway
Rockville, MD 20852
Phone: 800/822-8772
http://www.usp.org

NSF International
789 Dixboro Road
Ann Arbor, MI 48105
Phone: 800/NSF—MARK (673-6275)
http://www.nsf.org

ConsumerLab.com
333 Mamaroneck Avenue
White Plains, NY 10605
http://www.consumerlab.com
Phone: 914/722-9149
Email: *info@consumerlab.com*

JOURNALS

Alternative Medicine Review: A Journal of
    Clinical Therapeutics, **bimonthly**
Thorne Research, Inc.
Phone: 208/263-1337
e-mail: altmedrev@thorne.com
$95/year for individuals

Alternative Therapies in Health and
    Medicine, **bimonthly**
InnoVision Communications
Phone: 866/828-2962
$64/year for individuals.

Journal of Nutraceuticals, Functional &
Medical Foods, **quarterly**
The Haworth Press, Inc
http://www.haworthpressinc.com
Phone: 800/429-6784
$50/year

Journal of the American Dietetic
Association, **monthly**
http://www.eatright.org
Phone: 800/877-1600
$150/year individual subscription

Journal of the American Medical
Association, **48 issues/year**
Phone: 800/262-2350
$165/year individual subscription and
    online access

Nutrition Reviews, **monthly**
Phone: 800/627-0629
$122.50/year individual subscription

The Scientific Review of Alternative
Medicine, **quarterly**
http://www.hcrc.org/sram
Phone: 800/421-0351
$50/year for individuals

PUBLICATIONS

HerbalGram, **quarterly**
Joint effort of the American Botanical
    Council and the Herb Research
    Foundation
Phone: 800/373-7105
http://www.herbalgram.org
$35/year

Nutrition Action Healthletter,
monthly (10 issues)
Center for Science in the Public Interest
Phone: 202/332-9110
http://cspinet.org
$24/year

Nutrition Business Journal, monthly
Nutrition Business International
Phone: 619/295-7685
http://www.nutritionbusiness.com
$995/year

**Nutrition in Complementary Care, A
Dietetic Practice Group of the American
Dietetic Association, quarterly newsletter**
$20/year for ADA members
Subscription: Contact the American
    Dietetic Association: 800/877-1600
http://www.complementarynutrition.org

**SCAN's Pulse, Sports, Cardiovascular, and
Wellness Nutritionists (SCAN)**
A Dietetic Practice Group of the American
    Dietetic Association, quarterly
    newsletter
$34.95/year for non–ADA members,
    $29.95 for ADA members
Subscription: Contact the American
    Dietetic Association 800/877-1600 or
    SCAN office: 719/395-9271
http://www.nutrifit.org

**Tufts University Health and Nutrition
Letter, monthly**
Phone: 800/274-7581
$28/year
University of California Berkeley Wellness
    letter, monthly
Phone: 386/447-6328
$28/year

WEB SITES

Web Sites: Scientific Research

**http://ods.od.nih.gov/databases/
    ibids.html**
International Bibliographic Information
    on Dietary Supplements (IBIDS)
This database was created to assist
    researchers, health professionals, and
    the general public in locating scientific
    literature on dietary supplements.

http://www.ncbi.nlm.nih.gov/pubmed
MEDLINE is the National Library of
    Medicine's (NLM) premier
    bibliographic database covering the
    fields of medicine, nursing, dentistry,
    veterinary medicine, the health care
    system, and the preclinical sciences. The
    MEDLINE file contains bibliographic
    citations and author abstracts from
    approximately 3,900 current biomedical
    journals published in the United States
    and 70 foreign countries.

http://www.ag.uiuc.edu/~ffh/napra.htm
NAPALERT—Natural Products Alert
    Database
Program for Collaborative Research/
    Pharmaceutical Sciences College of
    Pharmacy
University of Illinois, Chicago, Ill.

**http://www.ars-grin.gov/duke/
    index.html**
Dr. James Duke's Phytochemical and
    Ethnobotanical Databases

Government Web Sites Related to
    Dietary Supplements

www.fda.gov
Food and Drug Administration: general
    information on dietary supplements

http://www.cfsan.fda.gov/

Food and Drug Administration: Center for
Food Safety and Applied Nutrition:
links to information on dietary
supplement regulations, access to
Federal Register

**http://www.cfsan.fda.gov/~dms/ds-warn.
html**

Food and Drug Administration: warnings
regarding certain dietary supplements

http://nccam.nih.gov

National Center for Complementary and
Alternative Medicine (NIH)

http://dietary-supplements.info.nih.gov

Office of Dietary Supplements (NIH)

Health Fraud Web Sites

http://www.ncahf.org

National Council Against Health Fraud
Nonprofit voluntary health organization
works against health fraud, seeing it as a
public health concern.

http://www.quackwatch.com

Nonprofit organization that aims to
combat health-related frauds, myths,
fads, and fallacies

REPORTING ADVERSE EFFECTS OF DIETARY SUPPLEMENTS

Healthcare Professionals can report to:
800/FDA-1088 (332-1088)

http://www.fda.gov/medwatch/

Consumers can report to:
800/FDA-1088 (332-1088)

http://www.fda.gov/medwatch/

BOOKS

Blumenthal M, Brinckmann J, Dinda K, et
al. *The American Botanical Council's
ABC Clinical Guide to Herbs.* Austin,
Tex: American Botanical Council; 2002.

Blumenthal M, Busse WR, Goldberg A, et
al. (eds.) *The Complete German
Commission E Monographs: Therapeutic
Guide to Herbal Medicines.* Austin, Tex:
American Botanical Council; 1998.

Brinker F. *Herb Contraindications and Drug
Interactions,* 2nd ed. Sandy, Ore: Eclectic
Medical Publications; 1998

Coughlin CM, DeBusk RM. *Integrative
Medicine: Your Quick Reference Guide.*
Boston, Mass: Integrative Medicine
Communications; 1998.
Phone: 505/892-1562.

Duke JA. *The Green Pharmacy: New
Discoveries in Herbal Remedies for
Common Diseases and Conditions from
the World's Foremost Authority on
Healing Herbs.* Emmaus, Pa: Rodale
Press; 1997.

Eskinazi D, ed. *Botanical Medicine: Efficacy,
Quality Assurance and Regulation.*
Larchmont, NY: Mary Ann Liebert Inc;
1999.

Foster S, Tyler VE. *Tyler's Honest Herbal: A
Sensible Guide to the Use of Herbal and
Related Remedies.* 4th ed. New York, NY:
Haworth Herbal Press Inc; 1999.

Jellin JM, Gregory P, Batz F, et al.
*Pharmacist's Letter/Prescriber's Letter
Natural Medicines Comprehensive
Database,* 3rd edition. Stockton, Calif:
Therapeutic Research Faculty; 2000.

Karch SB. *The Consumer's Guide to Herbal
Medicine.* Hauppauge, NY: Advanced
Research Inc; 1999.

Lininger SW, Jr, ed. *A-Z Guide to Drug-
Herb-Vitamin Interactions.* Rocklin,
Calif: Healthnotes; 1999.

Miller LG, Murray WJ, eds. *Herbal Medicinals: A Clinician's Guide.* New York, NY: Pharmaceutical Products Press; 1998.

Peirce A. *The American Pharmaceutical Association Practical Guide to Natural Medicines.* New York, NY: William Morrow & Co; 1999.

Robbers JE, Tyler VE. *Tyler's Herbs of Choice: The Therapeutic Use of Phytomedicinals.* New York, NY; Haworth Herbal Press; 1999.

Schulz V, Hansel R, Tyler VE. *Rational Phytotherapy: A Physician's Guide to Herbal Medicine.* 3rd ed. New York, NY: Springer; 1998.

DIETARY SUPPLEMENT INTAKE ASSESSMENT:
Questions to Ask Patients/Clients

As part of any nutrition assessment, it is important to ask clients or patients questions about dietary supplement intake. The following questions are designed to gather information in order to help your patients/clients make informed decisions about supplement use. (It may be easier to ask your patients/clients to bring in supplement bottles to an appointment to aid with these questions).

- What supplements do you use (vitamin/mineral, herbal, amino acid/protein, fiber, fatty acid, other, etc.)?

- What are your main reasons for taking this supplement(s) (to prevent a disease, to help treat a disease or condition, general health, energy, weight loss, pregnancy, mood, muscle-building, etc.)?

- How long have you used this supplement(s), and how long do you plan on using it?

- How often do you take this supplement(s) (daily, weekly, once in a while)?

- What brand and form of supplement(s) do you take (ie, vitamin E, Brand X, natural *d*-alpha-tocopherol form with mixed tocopherols)?

- What dosage do you take? Do you ever take above the dose specified on the label?

- How much money do you spend on supplements per month? Does this cost make it difficult to buy groceries and/or meals?

- Have you noticed any change in your health or medical condition since you started taking the supplement(s)?

- Have you had any negative reactions since you started using this supplement (skin rash, indigestion, irritability, nervousness)?

- Do you have allergic reactions to any foods, insects, plants/flowers? Are any of your supplements derived from a substance that you may be allergic to (ie, if a patient has an allergy to bee stings or honey, he or she may be have a reaction to bee pollen supplements)?

- What other prescription or over-the-counter medications are you currently taking?

- Do you ever combine alcohol or caffeine-containing beverages while taking this supplement?